Endocrinology

Endocrinology

Pathophysiology to Therapy

Akuffo Quarde MD

Clinical Instructor, University of Minnesota Medical School
Endocrinology, Diabetes and Metabolism Clinic
Sanford Health
Bemidji, Minnesota, USA

WILEY Blackwell

Registered Offices

John Wiley & Sons, Inc., 111 River Street, Hoboken, NJ 07030, USA

John Wiley & Sons Ltd, The Atrium, Southern Gate, Chichester, West Sussex, PO19 8SQ, UK

For details of our global editorial offices, customer services, and more information about Wiley products visit us at www.wiley.com.

Library of Congress Cataloging-in-Publication Data

Names: Quarde, Akuffo, author.

Title: Endocrinology: pathophysiology to therapy / Akuffo Quarde.

Description: Hoboken, NJ: Wiley-Blackwell, 2024. | Includes
   bibliographical references and index.

Identifiers: LCCN 2023046411 (print) | LCCN 2023046412 (ebook) | ISBN
   9781119863533 (paperback) | ISBN 9781119863540 (adobe pdf) | ISBN
   9781119863557 (epub)

Subjects: MESH: Endocrine System Diseases–physiopathology | Endocrine
   Glands–physiopathology | Endocrine System Diseases–therapy

Classification: LCC RC649 (print) | LCC RC649 (ebook) | NLM WK 140 | DDC
   616.4–dc23/eng/20231101

LC record available at https://lccn.loc.gov/2023046411

LC ebook record available at https://lccn.loc.gov/2023046412

Cover Design: Wiley

Cover Image: © SEBASTIAN KAULITZKI/SCIENCE PHOTO LIBRARY/Getty Images

Set in 10.5/13pt STIXTwoText by Straive, Pondicherry, India

SKY10062535_121423

Dedication

To the memory of Dr. Joseph Quartson.

Contents

Preface

This book encourages an integrated understanding of endocrine physiology by examining the mechanisms of action of medical therapies. Relevant endocrine physiology is presented, followed by a review of the detailed mechanism of action of selected medical interventions.

Where applicable, emphasis is placed on clinical pharmacology pearls, such as side effects and therapeutic monitoring guidelines. Supplementary chapters address additional topics, including immune checkpoint inhibitor-related endocrinopathies, anabolic steroid abuse, pseudo-endocrine conditions, and dynamic tests in clinical endocrinology.

As endocrinology is a rapidly evolving subdiscipline of internal medicine, this book avoids focusing on guideline-defined treatment protocols, instead highlighting the pathophysiological basis of endocrine therapies. While not exhaustive in its coverage of endocrine pathophysiology, I hope the discussion of the rationale for using various therapies will enable readers to appreciate complex concepts in a clinically relevant manner.

Endocrinology fellows and practicing physicians should be familiar with landmark clinical trials in the field, so an effort has been made to highlight some practice-changing trials where relevant. This should enrich the training of endocrinology fellows and internal medicine residents, medical students, and other allied health professionals such as pharmacists, nurse practitioners, and physician assistants. Infographics of landmark trials mentioned in this book can be found on this website https://myendo-consult.com/learn/clinical-trials/

I welcome readers' feedback regarding this first edition's limitations and look forward to incorporating valuable suggestions in future editions.

Acknowledgments

I would like to express my heartfelt gratitude to Professor Andrea Manni from Penn State College of Medicine and Professor Alan Sacerdote for their invaluable mentorship and support throughout the development and creation of this book.

I want to acknowledge that the illustrations in this book were created using Adobe InDesign and BioRender, a free online software designed for crafting biomedical diagrams.

CHAPTER 1

Pituitary Gland Therapies

1.1 CUSHING'S DISEASE

1.1.1 Pasireotide

1.1.1.1 Physiology

The Hypothalamic–Pituitary–Adrenal Axis

The hypothalamic–pituitary–adrenal (HPA) axis influences cortisol regulation through a complex balancing act between stimulatory and inhibitory factors. *Corticotrophin-releasing hormone* (CRH), produced in the paraventricular nucleus of the hypothalamus, is transmitted by the hypophyseal portal venous system to corticotroph cells in the anterior pituitary gland [1]. CRH subsequently binds to corticotrophin-releasing hormone type 1 receptor (CRH-R1) on the surface of corticotrophs. As a result, ACTH is released from secretory vesicles in corticotrophs. It should be noted that *Arginine vasopressin* (AVP) further potentiates the anterior pituitary effects of CRH by acting on its cognate Vasopressin subtype 1b receptor (V1b-R) present on corticotrophs. Additionally, CRH promotes the expression of the pro-opiomelanocortin (POMC) gene in the anterior pituitary gland, a process that also increases adrenocorticotropin hormone (ACTH) production as well [2] (see Section 3.1.1).

Subsequently, ACTH binds to the melanocortin-2 receptor (MCR-2) on cells present in the zona fasciculata of the adrenal cortex, leading to increased cortisol synthesis [3]. Adrenal-derived cortisol inhibits the secretion of POMC and ACTH by anterior pituitary corticotrophs through a negative feedback loop [4]. Additional negative feedback inhibition of CRH and AVP synthesis by cortisol occurs at the level of the hypothalamic paraventricular nucleus [5] (see Figure 1.1).

Normal and adenomatous corticotrophs express two subclasses of somatostatin receptors (SSR), namely somatostatin receptor subtype 2 (SSR_2) and somatostatin receptor subtype 5 (SSR_5). Somatostatin, a hypothalamic peptide, inhibits ACTH production through an inhibitory pathway regulated by circulating cortisol. Indeed, SSR_2 receptors are easily downregulated by cortisol, compared to SSR_5 (more resistant to negative feedback by cortisol). As a consequence, SSR_2 receptor modulators (e.g. octreotide) are less effective in Cushing's disease compared to SSR_5 modulators (e.g. pasireotide) [6].

Hypothalamic and pituitary processes: CRH is released under trophic stimulation by various factors, including catecholamines, angiotensin II, serotonin, stress, and cytokines [7]. On the contrary, GABA inhibits CRH release and ultimately ACTH production [8]. CRH from the hypothalamus stimulates anterior pituitary corticotrophs to release their preformed ACTH from secretory vesicles (fast response). Furthermore, CRH increases POMC gene expression by anterior pituitary corticotrophs (slow response).

Endocrinology: Pathophysiology to Therapy, First Edition. Akuffo Quarde.
© 2024 John Wiley & Sons Ltd. Published 2024 by John Wiley & Sons Ltd.

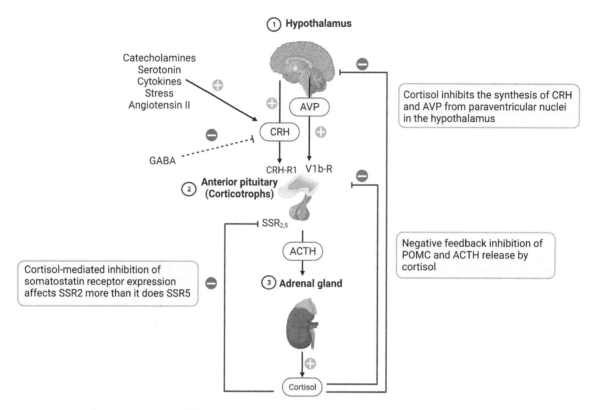

FIGURE 1.1   Schematic representation of the HPA axis, highlighting critical stimulatory and inhibitory feedback loops.

Furthermore, AVP binds to V1b receptors on corticotrophs which further enhances the action of CRH at the level of the anterior pituitary gland [2]. Activation of dopamine D2 receptors (D2Rs) present on corticotroph cells by hypothalamic-derived dopamine inhibits ACTH synthesis and release *(not shown)* [9]. *Adrenal cortex processes:* The binding of ACTH to the MCR-2 receptors present on cells in the zona fasciculata promotes the synthesis of cortisol from cholesterol [3]. *Feedback Loops* Negative feedback inhibition of POMC and ACTH release is mediated by adrenal-derived cortisol [4]. Furthermore, cortisol inhibits the synthesis of CRH and AVP from paraventricular nuclei in the hypothalamus [5]. Cortisol-mediated inhibition of somatostatin receptor expression on corticotrophs affects SSR2 more than it does SSR5 [6]. + = shows stimulatory factors and feedback loops, and − = shows inhibitory factors and feedback loops.

1.1.1.2   Mechanism of Action

Pasireotide is a *near pan-somatostatin* receptor analog because it binds to four of the five isoforms of the somatostatin receptor family, namely (SSR$_1$, SSR$_2$, SSR$_3$, and SSR$_5$). Indeed, pasireotide binds to the SSR$_5$ receptor subtype more avidly than the other SSR, thus

its demonstrable efficacy in Cushing's disease. Corticotroph tumors in the anterior pituitary gland express more SSR$_5$ receptors than other somatostatin receptor subtypes. Furthermore, cortisol's negative feedback inhibition of somatostatin receptor expression by corticotrophs tends to impact SSR$_2$ receptors more than the SSR$_5$ receptor subtype. Due to its affinity for SSR$_5$ receptors, pasireotide is an ideal therapeutic option for Cushing's disease [10]. Also, see Figure 1.1.

1.1.1.3   Practice Guide

Pasireotide *(Signifor)* causes *hyperglycemia, gastrointestinal discomfort,* and *cholelithiasis.* The reported prevalence of hyperglycemia in clinical trials involving patients with Cushing's disease who received pasireotide ranged from 68.4% to 73% [11]. Therefore, it is reasonable to screen for diabetes before and during treatment with pasireotide [12]. Incretin mimetics, metformin, or insulin are preferred for treating pasireotide-mediated hyperglycemia [13]. The proposed mechanisms of pasireotide-mediated hyperglycemia are shown in Table 1.1.

Somatostatin inhibits both hepatic biliary secretions and contraction of the wall of the gallbladder in normal physiology. As a result, patients exposed to

TABLE 1.1 Pathophysiological basis of pasireotide-mediated hyperglycemia.

Hormone	Effects of pasireotide
Insulin	The binding of pasireotide to SSR_5 receptors present on beta cells inhibits pancreatic insulin release [11].
Glucagon	The activation of SSR_2 receptors present on pancreatic alpha cells leads to the inhibition of pancreatic glucagon release. In essence, the reduced affinity of pasireotide for the SSR_2 receptor subtype promotes glucagon-mediated hyperglycemia [11].
Incretins	Pasireotide, through intestinal somatostatin receptors, inhibits the release of the glucagon-like peptide 1(GLP-1) and the glucose-dependent insulinotropic peptide (GIP) from K and L cells, respectively [14, 15]. See Section 4.1.7 for the role of incretins in insulin secretion.

Source: Adapted from refs. [11, 14, 15].

somatostatin analogs (SSAs) are predisposed to forming gallstones [16].

The typical dose range for immediate-release pasireotide is 0.3–0.9 mg (300–900 mcg) as a subcutaneous injection (thigh, upper arm, or abdomen) twice daily. A long-acting release (LAR) formulation is administered once a month (10–30 mg) intramuscularly as a depot injection by a health worker [13]. In practice, the LAR formulation is introduced after patients have demonstrated a response to immediate-release pasireotide.

Clinical Trial Evidence

SSR_5 receptors are abundant in corticotroph tumors, as has been previously mentioned. The *Pasireotide B2305 Study group* trial investigated the efficacy of pasireotide, a SSA with a profound affinity for the SSR_5 receptor, in reducing corticotroph tumor growth [17].

Key Message

Pasireotide led to a halving of median urinary-free cortisol levels in a cohort of patients with confirmed Cushing's disease (persistent, recurrent, or newly diagnosed).

The B2305 pasireotide study group evaluated the efficacy of pasireotide in Cushing's disease. In this pivotal phase 3 trial, 162 subjects with persistent, recurrent, or newly diagnosed Cushing's disease (not considered suitable candidates for transsphenoidal surgery) with urinary-free cortisol (UFC) levels 1.5 times the upper limit of the normal reference range were randomized to subcutaneous pasireotide 600 mcg ($n = 82$) or 900 mcg ($n = 80$), twice daily. The primary outcome was UFC levels below or at the upper limit of the normal reference range. There was approximately a 50% reduction in median UFC levels in the second month of the study, and UFC levels stabilized through to the end of the study for all participants [17].

1.1.2 Retinoic Acid

1.1.2.1 Physiology

Regulation of Corticotroph Physiology by Retinoic Acid

The normal corticotroph cell has a POMC promoter gene, which is critical in POMC synthesis and eventual ACTH secretion. In normal physiology, there are retinoid-sensitive mediators (transcription factors) required for the activation of the POMC promoter gene, namely, *activator protein 1* (AP-1) and *nuclear receptor 77* (Nur77). Retinoic acid (RA), by binding to its nuclear RA receptors inhibits AP-1 and Nur77 expression, thus preventing the activation of the POMC promoter gene [18, 19]. It should be noted that *chicken ovoalbumin upstream promoter transcription factor 1* (COUP-TF1) protects AP-1 and Nur77 from direct inactivation by RA [20]. See Figure 1.2.

The reduced expression of the *"protective transcription factor,"* COUP-TF1 by some corticotroph tumor cells makes RA a reasonable therapeutic option in Cushing's disease [18, 20].

1.1.2.2 Mechanism of Action

RA reduces cortisol synthesis in subjects with Cushings disease through various observed mechanistic pathways.

1. RA reduces the synthesis of ACTH and POMC in corticotroph tumors [20]. This was reviewed earlier.
2. In addition, RA has direct tumoricidal effects on corticotroph tumors [20].

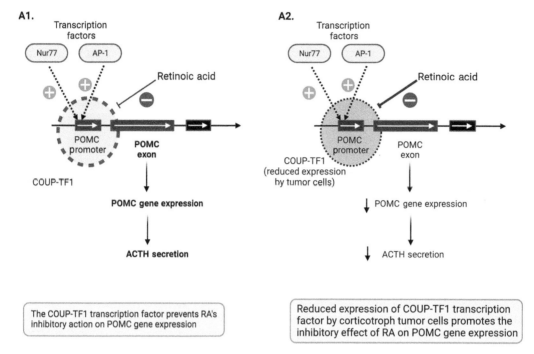

FIGURE 1.2   The role of retinoic acid in anterior corticotroph pathophysiology. AP-1 and Nur77 are critical transcription factors required for activation of the POMC promoter gene in a corticotroph cell. The COUP-TF1 transcription factor prevents RA's inhibitory action on both AP-1 and Nur77, allowing POMC transcription and ACTH secretion to proceed in normal physiology *(image A1)* [18, p. 11]. On the contrary, corticotroph tumors have a reduced expression of COUP-TF1, which allows RA to inhibit AP-1 and Nur77 (critical mediators of POMC promoter gene activation) *(image A2)* [20]. *The thickness of the dashed circle = degree of expression of COUP-TF1. Adapted and modified from Pecori GF et al.* [20].

3. RA reduces adrenal cortisol production through its antiproliferative effects on hyperplastic adrenocortical cells [20].

4. RA also downregulates the expression of the MCR-2 by adrenal cells (see Figure 1.1, [21]).

1.1.2.3   Practice Guide

- RA is teratogenic and should be used with extra caution in women of reproductive age group. Other reported side effects of RA include photosensitivity and mucositis [22].
- RA receptor activation increases the cortisol suppressive effects of dopaminergic agonists (DAs). Combining RA and DA is a suggested therapeutic option in patients with Cushing's disease [23].

Clinical Trial Evidence

The first proof-of-concept study of RA in humans with Cushing's disease was carried out in 7 subjects, with a variable decrease in UFC levels ranging from 22 to 73% [20]. A recent open-label prospective trial evaluated the safety and efficacy of isotretinoin (13-cis RA isomer) in patients with persistent or recurrent Cushing's disease [24].

Key Message

Retinoic acid (a new treatment approach) was associated with a greater than 50% reduction in urinary-free cortisol levels compared to baseline in this small study. Retinoic acid is a potential therapeutic option in patients with persistent or recurrent Cushings disease.

In this single-arm open-label prospective study over a 12-month period, 16 patients with persistent or recurrent Cushings disease after transsphenoidal surgery were treated with isotretinoin monotherapy. All subjects received 20 mg of oral isotretinoin once daily. This was increased by 20 mg every 4 weeks to a maximum dose of 80 mg once daily. The primary outcome was defined as normalization of UFC or > 50% reduction in UFC. At the end of the study, four patients

(25%) had sustained normalization of UFC [24]. The expression of COUP-TF1 (determinant of response to RA) by pituitary corticotrophs was not assessed in this study. This may explain the low response rate observed in the study (see Figure 1.2).

1.1.3 Dopaminergic Agonists

1.1.3.1 Physiology

The Hypothalamic–Pituitary–Adrenal Axis

Refer to Figure 1.1 to review the effects of hypothalamic-derived dopamine on ACTH-producing corticotrophs.

1.1.3.2 Mechanism of Action

Although approximately 80% of corticotroph adenomas express D2 receptors, they have relatively low D2 receptor density, making DAs a less favorable therapeutic option [25]. Bromocriptine and cabergoline reduce cortisol production by binding to D2 receptors present on corticotrophs; however, they are not as effective as SSAs [9].

1.1.3.3 Practice Guide

- Patients taking DAs exhibit an *"escape phenomenon,"* which is characterized by up to a third of patients who previously responded experiencing rebound hypercortisolemia [25].
- Cabergoline is associated with valvular heart disease, especially in patients exposed to doses close to the upper limit of the acceptable dose range [26]. Therefore, serial echocardiograms are reasonable in patients who are taking high doses of cabergoline [26] or are exposed to a cumulatively high lifetime dose [27].
- Common side effects of DAs include postural dizziness, nausea, and headaches [28].
- In contrast to the lower dose range of 0.5–2.0 mg/week of cabergoline used in prolactinomas [29], a much higher dose range between 2.5 and 5 mg/week is required to treat CD [30, 31]. See Section 1.3.1

Clinical Trial Evidence

In this study, the long-term effects of cabergoline therapy in patients with Cushing's disease were explored [32].

Key Message

A third of patients with Cushing's disease treated with cabergoline achieved either normalization or a significant reduction in urinary-free cortisol levels.

This single-arm, retrospective study assessed the efficacy of cabergoline in Cushing's disease. A total of 30 patients received oral cabergoline 0.5–1.0 mg/week, uptitrated weekly. The primary outcome was defined as normalization of UFC levels or > 50% reduction in UFC (this occurred in 36.6% of subjects) [32].

1.1.4 Steroidogenesis Inhibitors

1.1.4.1 Physiology

Adrenal Steroidogenesis

Review of adrenal steroidogenesis (see Section 3.1.1). The role of various adrenal steroidogenic inhibitors, such as ketoconazole, metyrapone, and mitotane in Cushing's syndrome, is shown in Figure 1.3 [37].

1.1.4.2 Mechanism of Action

See Figure 1.3 for a summary of various enzymatic targets of steroidogenic inhibitor therapies. The mechanism of action of metyrapone, mitotane, ketoconazole, and the recently approved steroidogenesis inhibitor, osilodrostat, will be reviewed next.

Metyrapone: Metyrapone has a pyridine moiety, which allows it to alter the activity of 11beta-hydroxylase (critical in the final step of cortisol synthesis). Other metyrapone-inhibited steroidogenic enzymes include the 17 alpha-hydroxylase(17α-OH) and 18-hydroxylase enzymes (less potent inhibition) [36].

Mitotane: Mitotane has both *"adrenolytic"* (adrenal cell death) and *"adrenostatic"* (enzymatic inhibition) properties. Mitotane is a chemotherapeutic agent with a diphenylmethane moiety that causes mitochondrial dysfunction, lysis, and necrosis. Mitotane, as stated earlier, exerts its "adrenostatic" function by inhibiting the side-chain cleavage enzyme, 11beta hydroxylase, and 3βHSD [36].

Ketoconazole: Ketoconazole has an imidazole group (confers its antifungal properties) with demonstrable inhibitory effects on various steroidogenesis enzymes (in particular, the side

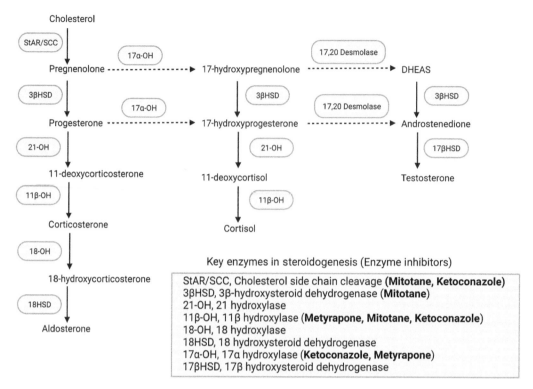

FIGURE 1.3   Schematic representation of adrenal steroidogenesis pathways and the site of action of various enzyme inhibitors. *Metyrapone* primarily inhibits 11 beta-hydroxylase activity (11β-OH), which results in reduced cortisol production of cortisol [33]. Consequently, there is an accumulation of intermediate mineralocorticoid precursors (11-DOC) [34] and a shunting of progesterone and pregnenolone to androgen production [35]. *Mitotane* inhibits various adrenal steroidogenic enzymes, including the side chain cleavage enzyme complex(StAR/SCC), 11beta hydroxylase(11β-OH), and 3βHSD [36]. *Ketoconazole* similarly inhibits various steroidogenic enzymes, including the side chain cleavage enzyme complex, 17alpha hydroxylase (17α-OH), and 11β-OH enzymes [36]. *Source*: Adapted from ref. [37].

chain cleavage complex, 17 alpha-hydroxylase and 11 beta-hydroxylase) in the adrenal cortex and gonads [36].

Osilodrostat: Osilodrostat, like metyrapone, inhibits 11-beta hydroxylase activity in the adrenal cortex. However, unlike metyrapone, osilodrostat has a relatively higher potency and a shorter plasma half-life; thus, it can be administered less frequently (two times daily instead of four times daily) [38].

1.1.4.3   Practice Guide

In practice, these agents are slowly titrated to achieve normal serum cortisol, which can be monitored using late-night salivary cortisol or 24-hour UFC. Overt hypoadrenalism is an inadvertent complication that should be anticipated in patients taking steroidogenesis inhibitors [13].

Metyrapone: Hypokalemia is a known complication of metyrapone treatment due to the accumulation of intermediate steroids with intrinsic mineralocorticoid activity (for example, 11-DOC). Therefore, close monitoring of serum potassium is therefore required [35]. Furthermore, hirsutism (shunting of proximal steroids into androgenic precursors), hypertension, and edema (mineralocorticoid effects of 11-deoxycorticosterone) can occur in patients on metyrapone. Unlike ketoconazole, metyrapone is comparatively safer in pregnancy [39].

Mitotane: Mitotane is lipophilic and, as a result, is stored in a large repository of adipose tissue. This increases the drug's half-life, leading to a delay in its onset of action. Most importantly, the dose of mitotane required to treat Cushing's disease is much lower than the large tumoricidal dose used to treat adrenocortical carcinomas [40]. Mitotane has teratogenic effects and due to its large volume of distribution (stored in adipose tissue), it should be discontinued for at least five years before potential conception [41].

Ketoconazole: Ketoconazole is the recommended first-line medical therapy for nonpregnant adults with confirmed endogenous hypercortisolemia. It is an FDA category C drug and may interfere with androgen-dependent development of the sex organs of an unborn male baby. Despite these apparent antiandrogenic effects, it has been inadvertently used in expectant mothers without overt deleterious fetal effects [39, 41]. Side effects encountered in routine practice include *gynecomastia*, hepatic injury, *male hypogonadism*, and gastrointestinal discomfort. *Electrolyte imbalance* is usually due to either uncontrolled hypercortisolemia (mineralocorticoid receptor activation by cortisol) or hypoadrenalism [42].

Osilodrostat (isturisa): The most common adverse drug events include nausea, headaches, and the clinical effects of either the accumulation of precursor adrenal hormones or overt hypocortisolemia (adrenal insufficiency). Osilodrostat has clinical utility in persistent and recurrent Cushing's disease [43].

Clinical Trial Evidence

This was a retrospective study to evaluate the efficacy of mitotane in Cushing's disease. Seventy-six consecutive patients with proven Cushing's disease reporting to a single facility were followed for a median period of 6.7 months (95% CI of 5.2–8.2 months). The patients received mitotane at a total daily dose of 4 g in three divided doses. Gradual de-escalation to a minimally tolerable dose needed to maintain remission was allowed during the study. There was no placebo or active comparator arm. The primary outcome was defined as Cushing's disease (normalization of 24 hours of UFC). This occurred in 72% of patients [40].

Key Message

Mitotane leads to biochemical amelioration of Cushing's disease (normalization of 24-hour urinary-free cortisol) in more than 70% of patients at doses much lower than required for the treatment of adrenal carcinoma.

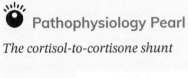

Pathophysiology Pearl

The cortisol-to-cortisone shunt

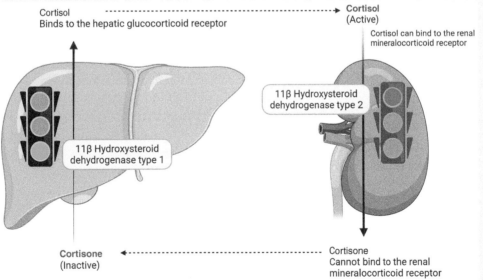

FIGURE 1.4   The cortisol-to-cortisone shunt and the role of two isoforms of 11 beta-hydroxysteroid dehydrogenase (11β-HSD) enzymes. Cortisol and aldosterone bind to the nonselective renal mineralocorticoid receptor under normal physiologic conditions [44]. The 11-beta hydroxysteroid dehydrogenase type 2 (11β-HSD2) isoform converts cortisol to cortisone, thus protecting the renal MCR from direct activation by cortisol. The 11 beta-hydroxysteroid dehydrogenase type 1 (11β-HSD1) isoform converts inactive cortisone to cortisol [45].

Clinical Pearl

Ketoconazole-induced apparent mineralocorticoid excess

There is a reported case of *apparent mineralocorticoid excess* (AME) in a patient treated with ketoconazole. The patient developed hypokalemia and hypertension in a manner that simulated a *"non-glucocorticoid-mediated"* AME. Unlike *metyrapone*, which mainly inhibits 11-beta hydroxylase (not to be confused with 11β-HSD), *ketoconazole* inhibits 11-beta hydroxylase and proximal side-chain cleavage enzymes (see Figure 1.3). This conventionally results in a *relatively lower* concentration of 11-Deoxycorticosterone (a potent mineralocorticoid) in patients treated with ketoconazole compared to metyrapone. Therefore, hypertension and hypokalemia may be inadvertently attributed to refractory hypercortisolemia (effects of excess cortisol overwhelming 11β-HSD2 and activating the renal MCR) rather than accumulation of DOC (see Figure 1.4). In this scenario, an increase in the dose of ketoconazole due to the presumed uncontrolled hypercortisolemia would exacerbate hypertension and hypokalemia (mineralocorticoid effects of DOC). Although DOC-mediated hypertension is more common in patients treated with metyrapone, this rare case report highlights the possibility of ketoconazole-mediated **hypertension** due to DOC accumulation of DOC in Cushing's syndrome [42].

1.1.5   Mifepristone

1.1.5.1   Physiology

Glucocorticoid Receptor Physiology

There are two isoforms of the glucocorticoid receptor (GR), namely, the GRα and GRβ glucocorticoid receptor. The GRα isoform is the proverbial "classic glucocorticoid receptor" in the cytosol, while the GRβ isoform resides in the nucleus. The GRβ receptor exerts a mainly modulatory role by inhibiting the function of GRα [46]. Figure 1.5 shows the mechanism of action of cortisol in normal physiology.

1.1.5.2   Mechanism of Action

Mifepristone, also known as *RU486* (Roussel-Uclaf 38 486), has antiglucocorticoid and anti-progesterone effects. RU486 binds to the *ligand-binding domain* (LBD) of the cytosolic glucocorticoid receptor without directly promoting its downstream effects, such as activation of hormone response elements and transcription factors involved in glucocorticoid-mediated gene function [49].

1.1.5.3   Practice Guide

- Patients taking mifepristone *(Korlym)* may develop significant hypercortisolemia (with elevated ACTH levels), which can increase their risk of *hypokalemia and hypertension (cortisol activating renal MCR)* [50]. Antiprogestin effects predispose female patients to *endometrial hyperplasia (unopposed estrogen action)*.
- Monitor patients for symptoms and signs of adrenal insufficiency. It is worth noting that cortisol levels are unreliable in patients on mifepristone. Indeed, patients may be "adrenally insufficient" despite high cortisol levels (blockade of the GR) [51].
- Mifepristone is approved by the FDA of the United States (Food and Drug Administration) to manage endogenous hypercortisolemia associated with hyperglycemia [52]. Glycemic control improves in up to 60% of patients treated with mifepristone. Thus, doses of antihyperglycemic agents may need to be adjusted [53].
- It is also an abortifacient due to its antiprogesterone effects. Table 1.2 shows the therapeutic sites of action of medical-directed therapies of Cushing's disease.

Clinical Trial Evidence

The Study of the Efficacy and Safety of Mifepristone in the Treatment of Endogenous Cushing's Syndrome (SEISMIC) and its extension sub-study assessed the effects of long-term mifepristone on neuroimaging findings in patients with Cushing's disease [55].

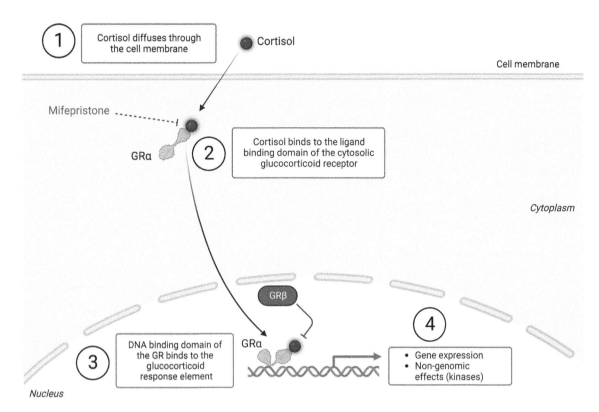

FIGURE 1.5   Glucocorticoid receptor physiology. Cortisol (glucocorticoid), a steroid hormone, diffuses through the plasma membrane to bind to the ligand-binding domain (LBD) of the cytosolic glucocorticoid receptor *(Step 1)*. The hormone–receptor complex undergoes a conformational change and is then translocated from the cytosol into the nucleus to exert its genomic effects *(step 2)*. The glucocorticoid receptor's DNA binding domain (DBD) binds to its assigned hormone response sequence, the Glucocorticoid Response Element (GRE), to exert its intranuclear effects. This leads to the activation of transcription factors, which can activate or inactivate gene expression [46, 47]. Glucocorticoids may also exert nongenomic effects through various kinases *(step 3)*. This typically occurs minutes after ligand–receptor interaction in the cytosol [46]. The nongenomic effects of glucocorticoids include inflammatory and noninflammatory processes (calcium mobilization and muscle function) [48]. GRβ inhibits the intranuclear effects of GRα [46]. *Source*: Adapted from ref. [46].

Key Message

Although mifepristone causes an increase in ACTH among patients with Cushing's disease, it does not significantly increase the size of the pituitary tumor.

The SEISMIC trial was an open-label, multicenter prospective study that evaluated the effects of mifepristone on tumor size and ACTH levels in Cushing's disease over a 24-week period. Subjects received a starting dose of oral mifepristone (300 mg) once daily, steadily increasing to a maximum daily dose of 1200 mg. The primary outcome was defined as a change in ACTH (compared to baseline) and MRI changes (volumetric changes in tumor size). 72% of the subjects had a twofold increase in ACTH compared

TABLE 1.2   Summary of therapeutic targets in Cushing's disease.

Therapy	The primary site of action
Pasireotide	Anterior pituitary gland (SSR$_1$, SSR$_2$, SSR$_3$, and SSR$_5$ receptors)
Retinoic acid	Anterior pituitary gland (Retinoic acid receptors)
Cabergoline	Anterior pituitary gland (Dopaminergic receptors)
Ketoconazole	Adrenal steroidogenesis inhibitor
Metyrapone	Adrenal steroidogenesis inhibitor
Mitotane	Adrenal steroidogenesis inhibitor
Mifepristone	Glucocorticoid receptor antagonist

Source: Adapted from Hinojosa-Amaya et al. [54].

to baseline. ACTH returned to baseline after discontinuing RU486. Tumor progression and regression occurred in two and three subjects, respectively. This was not statistically significant. In fact, there was no evidence that mifepristone predisposes patients to accelerated pituitary tumor growth [55].

In conclusion, there are novel therapies for Cushing's disease which are currently in development. These include cyclin-dependent kinase 2 (CDK2) modulators (*Roscovitine*), epidermal growth factor receptor (EGFR) inhibitors (Gefitinib), and GR antagonists (*Relacorilant*), to mention a few [54].

 Concepts to Ponder Over

Will octreotide, an SSR2 agonist, be a suitable therapeutic option in patients with Nelson syndrome?

Nelson syndrome (NS) may occur after bilateral adrenalectomy in patients with Cushing's disease. NS is characterized by corticotroph tumor expansion and elevated levels of ACTH. However, the underlying pathophysiology of this condition remains unclear at this time [56]. The loss of negative feedback inhibition of cortisol on tumorous corticotroph cells inadvertently leads to their proliferation. Patients may develop hyperpigmentation involving the skin and mucous membranes due to elevated levels of ACTH [57].

It should be noted that cortisol inhibits SSR on corticotroph cells. SSR_2 receptors are preferentially inhibited to a higher degree than SSR_5 receptors [6]. In NS, the lack of cortisol-mediated downregulation of SSR_2 receptors makes SSAs, which bind to this receptor subtype, a reasonable therapeutic option. Although octreotide is less effective in treating Cushing's disease, it has a role in Nelson's syndrome [56, 58].

How does cabergoline (a dopaminergic agonist) cause cardiac valvulopathy?

Compared to bromocriptine, cabergoline is associated with a higher risk of cardiac valvulopathy. The reported cardiac effects of cabergoline include the thickening of the *chordae tendineae* and cardiac valves [59]. The binding of cabergoline to $5HT_{2B}$ *receptors* in the endocardium leads to valvulopathy. The predilection of cabergoline-induced valvulopathy for the tricuspid valve may be due to the disproportionately high amount of this receptor subtype in the right side of the heart [27].

1.2   ACROMEGALY

1.2.1   Somatostatin Analogs

1.2.1.1   Physiology

The role of somatostatin in the regulation of growth hormone.

Growth hormone-releasing hormone (GHRH) is a peptide hormone composed of 44 amino acids synthesized in the arcuate nucleus of the hypothalamus. GHRH is secreted in a pulsatile fashion and is carried from the hypothalamus to the anterior pituitary gland through the hypothalamo-hypophyseal vessels. By binding to receptors on the surface of anterior pituitary somatotrophs, GHRH stimulates gene transcription, translation, and the eventual release of *growth hormone* (GH) from their secretory vesicles. *Somatostatin* (also known as somatostatin receptor inhibitory factor, SRIF), on the other hand, blocks the release of GH by somatotrophs by acting on somatostatin receptors (primarily SSR_2 receptors) [60]. *Ghrelin* (derived from gastric oxyntic cells) is a GH secretagogue that exhibits its effects by acting on hypothalamic GHRH cells in the median eminence [61]. GH and insulin-like growth factor 1 (IGF-1) provide additional negative feedback inhibition of GH secretion (see Figure 1.6). Refer to Table 1.3 for a summary of the various physiological factors which regulate growth hormone secretion.

GH binds to the extracellular component of the hepatic GH receptor (GH-R) and induces a series of intracellular processes required for the transcription and translation of specific genes that encode IGF-1, *IGF-binding protein 3* (IGFBP3), and an *acid-labile subunit* (ALS) [68–70]. These products of GH action at the level of the liver form a ternary complex in circulation that influences the ability of IGF-1 to bind its peripheral insulin-like growth factor 1 receptor (IGF-1R). Indeed, post-translational modification of IGFBP3 (e.g. glycosylation, phosphorylation) is an essential determinant of IGF-1's ability

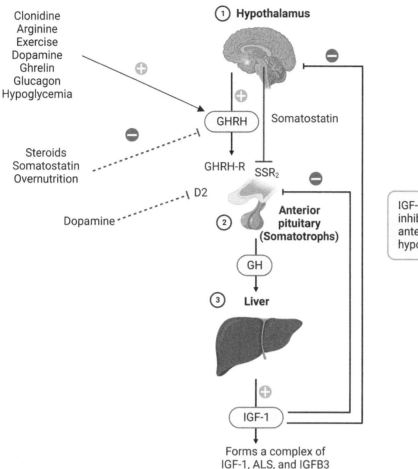

Clonidine
Arginine
Exercise
Dopamine
Ghrelin
Glucagon
Hypoglycemia

Steroids
Somatostatin
Overnutrition

Dopamine

① **Hypothalamus**

Somatostatin

GHRH

GHRH-R   SSR₂

D2

② **Anterior pituitary (Somatotrophs)**

GH

③ **Liver**

IGF-1

Forms a complex of
IGF-1, ALS, and IGFB3

IGF-1 exerts negative feedback inhibition of GH and GHRH at the anterior pituitary and hypothalamus, respectively

FIGURE 1.6 The growth hormone and insulin-like growth factor 1 axis. Hypothalamic-derived GHRH binds to GHRH-R on anterior pituitary somatotrophs and consequently mediates their secretion of GH. Binding of GH to GH-R in the liver promotes the synthesis of IGF-1, ALS, and IGFB3 – a complex that determines the circulating half-life and, therefore, peripheral effects of IGF-1. IGF-1 exerts negative feedback inhibition of GH and GHRH in the anterior pituitary and hypothalamus, respectively. GH exerts negative feedback inhibitory effects on its production at the level of the anterior pituitary gland. Somatostatin inhibits the release of growth hormone by somatotrophs. Important co-inhibitory and co-stimulatory factors influencing net GH secretion are shown *(negative and positive signs)*. *Source*: Adapted from ref. [62].

TABLE 1.3   Regulators of GH.

Promotes GH secretion	Inhibits GH secretion
Arginine [63]	Overnutrition [64]
Clonidine [63]	Glucocorticoids (high doses) [65]
Estrogenᵃ [66]	Somatostatin [60]
Hypoglycemia, Glucagon [67]	
L-dopa [63]	
Exercise [63]	

ᵃ This effect is route-dependent, with the oral route causing an increase in GH and a paradoxically low IGF-1. Transdermal estrogen does not produce this effect [66].
Source: Adapted from refs. [60, 63–67].

to bind to IGF-1R. For example, *glycosylation* of IGFBP3 increases the ability of IGF-1 to bind to IGF-1R. *Deglycosylation*, on the other hand, impairs ligand-to-receptor binding [62]. The consequences of GH action are widely accepted as pivotal for macronutrient metabolism (carbohydrate, lipid, and protein) and cellular growth [71].

1.2.1.2   Mechanism of Action

SSAs activate SSR on somatotroph tumor cells and thus inhibit their production of GH and, consequently, hepatic IGF-1. There is evidence that SSAs also lead to a reduction in the size of GH-secreting tumors [72, 73].

1.2.1.3 Practice Guide

SSAs approved in the United States for the treatment of acromegaly include octreotide (short release), octreotide long-acting release (Sandostatin LAR), and lanreotide (Somatuline). A few practice pearls were shared earlier in Section 1.1.1 (use of pasireotide in Cushing's disease).

- A hallmark side effect of pasireotide is *hyperglycemia*. The risk of hyperglycemia is disproportionately higher among patients with diabetes or prediabetes; it is reasonable to screen for hyperglycemia before and during treatment [74].
- First-generation SSAs (for example, lanreotide and octreotide) have a higher affinity for SSR2 than the SSR5 isoform of the somatostatin receptor [75]. Pasireotide, on the other hand, has a greater affinity for the SSR5 receptor subtype. Tumor response is influenced by the density of specific histological SSR subtypes (e.g. sparsely vs. densely granulated growth hormone-secreting tumors) [76]. This is clinically relevant since it can influence the effectiveness of selected therapies. For example, sparsely granulated somatotroph tumors tend to express SSR5 receptors (pasireotide). Densely granulated somatotrophs, on the other hand, express the SSR2 subtype (octreotide) predominantly [76–78].
- SSAs are associated with an increased risk of cholelithiasis and diarrhea [79].
- Monitoring response to therapy – IGF-1 should normalize to the age and sex-specific reference range for IGF-1. Furthermore, GH should be suppressed to a nadir of <1 ng/mL or <0.4 ng/mL (for newer and more sensitive GH assays) after an oral glucose load with 75 g of anhydrous glucose (Oral glucose tolerance test).

Clinical Trial Evidence

Pasireotide, a second-generation multireceptor SSA, causes a more significant biochemical improvement of acromegaly in contrast to first-generation SSAs (*octreotide* and *lanreotide*) [80, 81].

Key Message

In patients with uncontrolled acromegaly with octreotide or lanreotide, pasireotide produces a treatment response in 15–20% of patients.

The PAOLA study (*Pasireotide versus continued treatment with octreotide or lanreotide in patients with inadequately controlled acromegaly*) was a randomized, prospective, parallel-group study evaluating the safety and efficacy of pasireotide. 198 patients with uncontrolled acromegaly (GH >2.5 mcg/L and IGF > 1.3 times the age- and gender-adjusted upper limit of normal) on octreotide or lanreotide for a minimum of 6 months. Patients were randomized to pasireotide (40 or 60 mg) administered intramuscularly once every 28 days or active comparators (octreotide or lanreotide). The authors defined the primary outcome as a GH level <2.5 mcg/L and normalization of IGF-1. The primary outcome occurred in 15% (40 mg), 20% (60 mg), and 0% (octreotide/lanreotide) [80].

1.2.2 Growth Hormone Receptor Antagonists

1.2.2.1 Physiology

Growth Hormone and IGF-1 Pathway

The growth hormone receptor (GH-R) belongs to the cytokine receptor family [82] and is composed of *extracellular* (binds to its cognate ligand, that is, GH), *transmembrane,* and *cytosolic* domains [83]. See Figure 1.7 and Table 1.4.

1.2.2.2 Mechanism of Action

Pegvisomant has structural homology with endogenous GH except for the substitution of nine amino acids. *Pegylation* (the process of attaching polyethylene glycol to the protein) of GH changes its pharmacokinetic properties, making it hypoallergenic [87].

Due to its similarity to GH, Pegvisomant can occupy the GH receptor pocket, depriving the receptor of direct activation by GH. More importantly, it does not activate GHR (antagonistic action) because it induces defective dimerization of the receptor, thus preventing subsequent signal transduction pathways (JAK–STAT signaling) and eventual production of IGF-1 [88].

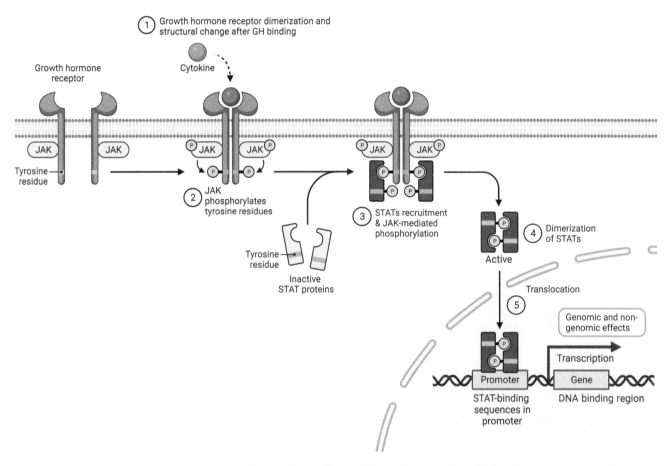

FIGURE 1.7   Growth hormone receptor and intracellular effects of GH to GHR binding. GH binds to the GH-R, leading to dimerization and consequent structural change in the receptor. This critical step initiates the *Janus-Kinase* (JAK) signal *transducer and activator of transcription* (STAT) intracellular signaling pathway. The phosphorylation of tyrosine residues in both the GHR transmembrane domain and STAT molecules is mediated by activated JAK2 tyrosine kinase [84]. There are various STAT molecules involved in specific intracellular processes. STAT5 (transcription factor), for example, is translocated from the cytoplasm to the nucleus and binds to DNA in specific DNA binding regions(DBRs) [85], which encode protein sequences [86]. Mitogen-activated protein kinase (MAPK) activation by JAK2 ultimately exerts genomic (gene expression) and non-genomic effects. GH mediates the production of IGF-1 in various tissues other than the liver, including growth plate chondrocytes, adipose tissue, and skeletal muscle [86]. *Source*: Adapted from ref. [85].

TABLE 1.4   Gene sequences encoding IGF-1 production in specific organs.

Organ	Gene sequence(s)
Liver	Socs2
Skeletal muscle	Igf1
Fat (Adipose tissue)	Fos, Jun, and Igf1
Bone (Chondrocyte)	Igf1

Socs2, suppressor of cytokine signaling 2; Igf1, insulin-like growth factor 1; Jun, proto-oncogene; Fos, proto-oncogene. Source: Adapted from Chia [86].

1.2.2.3   Practice Guide

- Pegvisomant can cause an increase in the size of GH-secreting tumors; it is thus recommended to monitor tumor size with serial pituitary MRIs [89]. Coadministration of SSAs and pegvisomant can reduce the risk of tumor re-expansion compared to pegvisomant monotherapy [90].
- Pegvisomant, a GH-R antagonist, causes an increase in GH levels, thus limiting the utility of GH assessments during monotherapy with this agent. As a result, the evaluation of treatment

response requires serial monitoring of serum IGF-1 levels [89].

- Hepatic enzyme elevation occurs during treatment and resolves after cessation of therapy. Liver function tests (LFT) should therefore be routinely monitored during treatment. Consequently, patients with unexplained elevations in LFT should not start pegvisomant [91].

Clinical Trial Evidence

The pivotal study that led to the approval of pegvisomant was published in 2000. It was a phase III study that compared various doses of pegvisomant with placebo [88]. Additional long-term safety data are available from the ACROSTUDY database. The ACROSTUDY registry is a prospective, Phase IV (post-marketing surveillance) study of patients with acromegaly treated with pegvisomant [92, 93].

Key Message

There is a low but clinically significant risk of tumor re-expansion for patients receiving *pegvisomant* monotherapy, although this should not preclude its use (ACROSTUDY).

A randomized, double-blind, placebo-controlled study comparing various doses of pegvisomant with placebo in patients with acromegaly over a 12-week study period. A total of 112 subjects with confirmed acromegaly, status-post pituitary surgery, radiation therapy, drug therapy, or treatment-naïve. Study participants were randomized to various doses of subcutaneous pegvisomant administered daily (10 mg, 15 mg, or 20 mg) or a comparable placebo. The primary outcome was defined as a mean change in IGF-1 compared to the baseline level. There was a mean decrease in IGF-1 of 4%, 26.7%, 50.1%, and 62.5% in the placebo, 10 mg, 15 mg, and 20 mg, respectively. Various doses of pegvisomant compared to placebo resulted in a clinically significant decrease in IGF-1 and improved clinical features of acromegaly [88].

1.2.3   Dopaminergic Agonists

1.2.3.1   Physiology

Growth Hormone Physiology and the Role of Central Dopaminergic Pathways

The binding of dopamine to D2 receptors in either pituitary somatotrophs or lactotrophs impairs the release of GH and prolactin, respectively [94]. Additionally, dopamine impairs hypothalamic somatostatin release, increasing *GHRH secretion* [95] (See Figure 1.6).

The differential effects of dopamine on GH secretion should be appreciated in normal physiology. The effects of Dopaminergic agonists (DA) at the level of the anterior pituitary gland are more profound than its effects in the hypothalamus. The net effect is a reduction in GH secretion.

1.2.3.2   Mechanism of Action

Growth hormone-secreting tumors express D2R receptors to varying degrees, determining their response to DAs [96]. Indeed, the responsiveness of D2Rs on somatotroph tumors depends on their sensitivity and the concentration of circulating GH [97].

1.2.3.3   Practice Guide

- Cabergoline is more effective than bromocriptine and reduces tumor size in approximately 30% of patients [98]. Also, see Section 1.1.3.

Clinical Trial Evidence

There is a paucity of evidence from randomized, placebo-controlled clinical trials among patients with acromegaly treated with cabergoline [99].

Key Message

Normalization of IGF-1 occurs in a third of acromegalic patients treated with cabergoline monotherapy. There is limited information about the effects of cabergoline on tumor size. Tumor shrinkage was demonstrated in patients with high baseline levels of prolactin (PRL) and IGF-1. It is a reasonable treatment option in *somatomammotrophic tumors* (GH-PRL co-secreting tumors).

This was a meta-analysis of prospective, nonrandomized studies in patients with cabergoline-treated acromegaly. A total of 227 subjects in 15 studies with significant heterogeneity were evaluated. There was no placebo group in this study. The patients were exposed to cabergoline monotherapy at variable doses ranging from 0.3–7 mg/week. The authors defined the primary outcome as the normalization of IGF-1. The primary outcome was achieved in 34% of patients [99].

 Concepts to Ponder Over

What is the effect of estrogen replacement therapy on the GH–IGF-1 axis?

There is a paradoxical effect of estrogen replacement on both GH and IGF-1; this depends on the route of administration of estrogen (oral or transdermal). The oral route leads to an increase in hepatic synthesis of growth hormone binding proteins (*first-pass effect*), which in turn bind GH avidly and somewhat attenuates its peripheral effects at the level of the liver (i.e. GH-induced IGF-1 production). This effect occurs despite an estrogen-mediated increase in pituitary GH production. It has been postulated that oral estrogen is not a GH secretagogue and that GH levels increase due to the loss of negative feedback inhibition of IGF-1 on somatotrophs [66](see Figure 1.6. To further support this hypothesis, women on transdermal estrogen replacement therapy were shown to have GH requirements much lower than those on oral estrogens. Transdermal estrogen escapes the *"hepatic first-pass effect"* and, as such, does not lead to clinically significant changes in GH-binding proteins [100]. It should be noted that women on chronic GH replacement therapy who inadvertently start oral estrogen replacement experience a decline in IGF-1 levels (*GH antagonizing effects of estrogen*), which will require an up-titration in GH doses [101, 102].

What effect does pegvisomant have on glycemic control?

GHR antagonists *improve insulin sensitivity* at the level of the liver, skeletal muscle, and adipose tissue [103]. In a GH excess state like acromegaly, *GH promotes increased lipolysis* in adipose tissue, which liberates free fatty acids (FFAs) (mediators of peripheral insulin resistance). See Figure 1.10 for the effects of GH on fat metabolism. There is a significant reduction in endogenous glucose output among patients with active acromegaly after a 4-week course of pegvisomant. Suppression of GH-induced lipolysis by pegvisomant reduces FFAs, and consequently improves peripheral insulin resistance [104].

1.3 PROLACTINOMA

1.3.1 Dopaminergic Agonists

1.3.1.1 Physiology

Regulation of Prolactin Release

Anterior pituitary lactotrophs release prolactin (a peptide hormone) under trophic stimulation by a hypothalamic-derived *prolactin-releasing factor (a putative hormone), vasoactive intestinal peptide*, or *thyrotropin-releasing hormone (TRH)* [105].

Hypothalamic dopamine (tuberoinfundibular dopaminergic neuronal cells) inhibits the release of prolactin by binding to D2 receptors on anterior pituitary lactotrophs. Prolactin increases hypothalamic dopamine release by upregulating tyrosine hydroxylase activity (dopamine synthesis pathway) in tuberoinfundibular neurons, thus promoting its inhibition by dopamine [106] (Figure 1.8). A summary of the various physiological regulators of prolactin secretion is shown in Table 1.5.

Although classically associated with the function of the mammary glands, prolactin has several extra-mammary effects due to the presence of prolactin receptors in various tissues. There are PRL receptors (PRL-R) in pancreatic beta cells (glucose-mediated insulin release), adipose tissue (thermoregulation), and hematopoietic cells (T-cell activation), to name a few [107, 108].

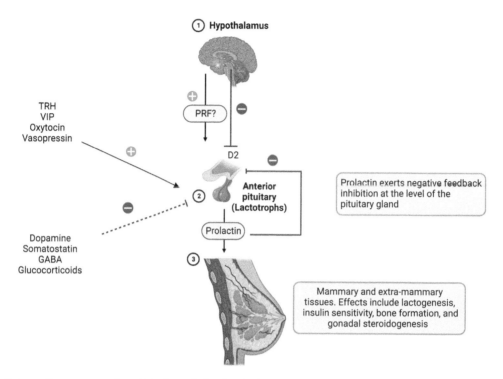

FIGURE 1.8   Schematic representation of the hypothalamic–pituitary-mammary axis. PRF is a putative (unconfirmed) hormone involved in the stimulation of PRL release by lactotrophs in the anterior pituitary gland. Hypothalamic dopamine affects prolactin release by binding and activating D2 receptors present on lactotrophs. Stimulatory and inhibitory factors involved in the regulation of PRL release are represented by + and – signs. Extramammary tissues include gonadal steroidogenesis, skeletal growth, and glucose metabolism, to mention a few.

TABLE 1.5   Regulators of prolactin secretion.

Inhibition of prolactin secretion	Stimulation of prolactin secretion
Dopamine	TRH
Somatostatin	VIP
GABA	Oxytocin
Glucocorticoids	Vasopressin

VIP, vasoactive intestinal peptide; GABA, gamma-aminobutyric acid.
Source: Adapted from Saleem et al. [106].

1.3.1.2   Mechanism of Action

DAs (cabergoline and bromocriptine), synthetic derivatives of ergots, bind to D2 receptors on the surface of pituitary lactotroph tumors and induce dopamine-mediated inhibition of prolactin synthesis and secretion. DAs also exhibit "tumoricidal properties" by promoting programmed cell death of lactotroph tumors through complex intracellular pathways that involve estrogen and neuronal dopamine transporters [109].

1.3.1.3   Practice Guide

- Patients who do not experience a *normalization of serum PRL* or a *50% reduction in tumor size* are classified as dopaminergic agonist resistant. However, no conventionally accepted dose or duration of exposure to DA is required to diagnose a patient as resistant to DA [110, 111].

- Predictors of an inadequate response to DAs include *male gender*, *macroprolactinoma*, *tumor characteristics* (cystic or hemorrhagic), *prolonged latency to euprolactinemia*, and *high PRL at baseline* [112].

- For women in the reproductive age group planning a pregnancy, the use of bromocriptine is a safer therapeutic option compared to cabergoline. This is due to the availability of more safety data for the former compared to the latter [113].

- Side effects of DA include nausea, vomiting, headaches, postural hypotension, psychotropic side effects (hallucinations, psychosis), and nasal congestion [114, 115]. The dictum "start low and go slow" helps mitigate the side effects of DA.

Cabergoline has a longer half-life, a higher affinity for D2R, and a relatively tolerable side-effect profile compared to bromocriptine [116].

- It is reasonable to screen for psychiatric disorders before initiating DAs. Compulsive gambling has been associated with cabergoline use; it is therefore important to alert patients of this potential side effect [117].

 Clinical Pearl

It has been speculated that Mary Tudor, Queen Mary I of England, may have had an undiagnosed prolactinoma based on historical accounts. She experienced a myriad of symptoms, including amenorrhea (from 19 years), headaches, impaired vision, phantom pregnancy, and galactorrhea for most of her adult life [105].

Prolactin-secreting tumors are the most common hormone-secreting tumors in the pituitary gland [106], with a reported prevalence of 50 per 100,000 [107]. Medical therapy using primarily dopaminergic agonists is the mainstay of treatment. Surgery is reserved for patients with medication resistance or intolerance [108].

Clinical Trial Evidence

There was a paradigm shift from surgery to DAs for the treatment of prolactinomas in the 1970s due to the superior efficacy and safety of medical therapy compared to surgery. DAs are now widely recommended as a first-line treatment option for patients with prolactinomas. Due to advancements in transsphenoidal endoscopic procedures, surgery may be a viable option for patients. This was explored in a systematic review investigating surgery as a viable alternative first-line treatment for prolactinoma [118].

Key Message

Dopaminergic agonists remain the first-line therapeutic option in most patients with prolactinomas. However, surgery is more likely to lead to long-term remission in patients regardless of tumor size (macroprolactinoma or microprolactinoma), based on the results of this large meta-analysis.

In this meta-analysis, evaluating long-term remission rates after a dopaminergic holiday or transsphenoidal surgery, patients were grouped into medical ($n = 3564$) and surgical ($n = 1836$) arms. The primary outcome was defined as long-term (≥ 1 year) remission (in other words, maintenance of normal serum prolactin) after either the withdrawal of medical therapy or post-transsphenoidal surgery. The primary outcome after the dopaminergic holiday was 34% (95% CI, 26–46) and 67% (CI, 60–74) after transsphenoidal surgery [118].

1.3.2 Temozolomide

1.3.2.1 Physiology

Cellular Protective Mechanisms Against Mutagens

Endogenous and exogenous factors can promote DNA damage and inadvertently trigger a cascade of events that lead to the formation of tumors. Cells in normal physiology maintain their integrity through a variety of protective pathways such as mismatch repair, nucleotide excision repair, and methylguanine-DNA methyltransferase (MGMT) enzymatic processes [119].

1.3.2.2 Mechanism of Action

Temozolomide (TMZ) is an alkylating chemotherapeutic agent that promotes the methylation of specific residues of guanine (position O-6) and purine (positions N3 and N7) in DNA. This introduces breaks in the DNA of rapidly growing cells, such as lactotrophic tumors, leading to their apoptosis (programmed cell death) [120]. A schematic representation of the mechanism of action of temozolomide is shown in Figure 1.9.

1.3.2.3 Practice Guide

- An evaluation of *MGMT promoter methylation status* is a useful *predictive biomarker* [121] in patients with aggressive prolactinomas or carcinomas [122]. There is an inverse relationship between tumor levels of MGMT and the degree of responsiveness to TMZ [122]. However, MGMT as a biomarker is a novel approach to predict TMZ response in patients with prolactinomas. Therapeutic response after a minimum of 3 cycles of treatment performed better than tumor levels of MGMT in a large cohort of patients with pituitary tumors (including prolactinomas) [123].

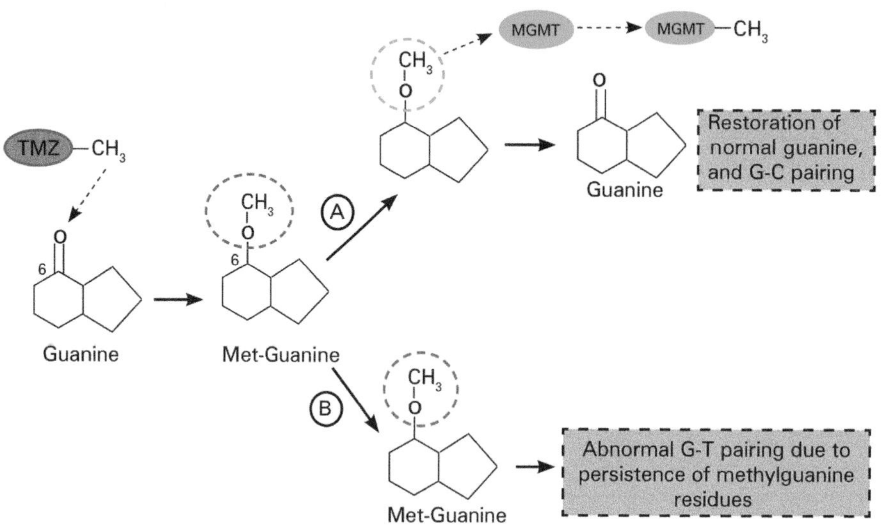

FIGURE 1.9   Schematic representation of the mechanism of action of temozolomide. TMZ promotes the methylation of guanine(G) at the number 6 carbon position, a step that leads to the formation of methylguanine residues in DNA. There is a "suicide enzyme" called methylguanine-DNA methyltransferase (MGMT), whose primary function is to remove these abnormal methyl groups, thus restoring the integrity of guanine residues in DNA *(Step A)*. This defective methylated guanine pairs with thymine (T) instead of cytosine (C) (by convention) during replication. Mismatch repair enzymes excise these **mispaired guanine-thymine** residues, although this is ultimately a futile exercise. Continuous cycles of erroneous G and T pairing and T excisions lead to irreparable DNA breaks that promote cell death *(Step B)* [120]. *Source*: Adapted from ref. [120].

- TMZ, a chemotherapeutic agent, is associated with expected short-term toxicity concerns, such as nausea, emesis, and fatigue [124]. Cytopenias (hematologic toxicity), which require a dose reduction or discontinuation of therapy, are infrequent [123, 124]. Safety data after 5–8 years of exposure to TMZ are very reassuring, making it a valuable long-term salvage therapeutic option [125].

Clinical Trial Evidence

There are no published randomized trials evaluating the safety and efficacy of TMZ compared to placebo. A recent systematic review of all published case reports and case series provided valuable information on the response of dopaminergic agonist-resistant prolactinomas to TMZ [124].

Key Message

Temozolomide has a favorable side-effect profile and is a reasonable rescue therapeutic option in patients who have exhibited a suboptimal response to DAs, radiation therapy, or surgery. Approximately 75% of patients with treatment-resistant prolactinomas achieved a reduction in tumor volume and serum prolactin levels after a temozolomide trial.

This was a meta-analysis of case series and reports that evaluated the tumor response to TMZ in 42 subjects with prolactin-secreting adenoma or carcinoma. Patients with resistance to dopaminergic agonist therapy received oral TMZ dose as 150–200 mg/m^2 in 1–24 therapeutic cycles. The primary outcome was defined as a change in tumor size and hyperprolactinemia improvement. Compared to baseline, a significant reduction in tumor size and prolactin levels occurred in 76.5% and 75% of patients, respectively [124].

 Concepts to Ponder Over

How does primary hypothyroidism contribute to hyperprolactinemia?

Undiagnosed primary hypothyroidism can present with significant hyperprolactinemia and pituitary gland enlargement [126, 127]. Patients with primary hypothyroidism have an upregulation of both TRH and TSH synthesis in the hypothalamus and pituitary gland, respectively [128]. TRH, a prolactin secretagogue, promotes hyperprolactinemia [105](see Figure 1.8). Anterior pituitary thyrotrope hyperplasia under the influence of TRH leads to the formation of a thyrotrope pseudotumor (diffuse enlargement of the pituitary gland).

An inadvertent "stalk effect" due to impingement of the sellar mass on the pituitary stalk disrupts the dopaminergic tracts, leading to impaired tonic inhibition of lactotrophs by dopamine.

Is there a role for SSAs in the treatment of prolactinomas?

Dopaminergic agonist-resistant prolactinomas are usually treated with surgical debulking, radiation therapy, or temozolomide [129]. As you may recall, somatostatin inhibits prolactin release (see Figure 1.8 [106]. Prolactinomas co-express SSR1 and SSR5 predominantly. The low expression of SSR_2 receptors by prolactinomas is responsible for their suboptimal response to octreotide. Pasireotide, being a multireceptor SSA, has an affinity for both SSR_1 and SSR_5 receptors, making it a viable option in the management of prolactinomas (see Section 1.1.1) [130]. There are reports of prolactinomas that have responded to pasireotide [129, 131, 132].

1.4 ADULT GROWTH HORMONE INSUFFICIENCY

1.4.1 Growth Hormone

1.4.1.1 Physiology

Anabolic Effects of Growth Hormone

Basic growth hormone physiology was reviewed earlier in Section 1.2.1. GH exerts its anabolic effects in skeletal tissue, muscle, and adipose tissues [133]. The anabolic effects of growth hormone in various tissues are shown in Table 1.6.

TABLE 1.6 Anabolic effects of growth hormone.

Tissue	Effects
Skeletal tissue	1. Synthesis of type 1 collagen 2. IGF-1-mediated linear growth (stimulation of chondroblasts)
Adipose tissue	1. Promotes lipolysis by potentiating the effects on hormone-sensitive lipase (see Figure 1.10) 2. Glucose uptake
Skeletal muscle	Protein synthesis and muscle growth

Source: Adapted from Root and Root [133].

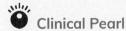

Clinical Pearl

Harvey Cushing was able to associate skeletal undergrowth with a putative growth factor from the anterior pituitary gland. His observations were recorded in his paper, The pituitary body and its disorders, in 1912. *"Doubtless as many cases of infantilism are due to a primary hypophyseal as to a primary thyroid insufficiency ... this is particularly true for cretinoid states – may actually be due to defective hypophyseal activity"* [133]. It was not until the 1950s that growth hormone or somatotrophin was eventually extracted from the anterior pituitary gland. Purified growth hormone was initially utilized in treating short stature in pediatric patients [134]. Although the use of growth hormone in adults took several decades, its utility in a hypopituitary adult was first demonstrated by Raben in 1962 [135]. Adult growth hormone deficiency may present with isolated growth hormone deficiency or coexist with other pituitary hormone insufficiencies [102, 136].

Adipocyte and Growth Hormone Physiology

There are four variants of adipocytes: brown, white, pink, and beige. This classification system is based on their location and physiological role. In this section, we review the physiology of white adipocytes and the importance of growth hormone in fat storage and mobilization. A detailed description of the physiology is covered in Chapter 7.

White adipose tissue (WAT) is primarily involved in the storage and mobilization of fatty acids. Two enzyme systems, lipoprotein lipase (LPL) and hormone-sensitive lipase (HSL), play essential roles in these energy-status-dependent tasks (Figure 1.10).

The Growth Plate and Growth Hormone Physiology

The growth plate (physis) is an anatomically distinct region composed of cartilage with three critical physiological zones in longitudinal bone growth (hypertrophic, proliferative, and resting zones) [138]. Growth hormone promotes the proliferation of chondrocytes in the resting zone. IGF-1, produced by local chondrocytes under trophic stimulation from GH *(see* Table 1.4*)*, promotes the expansion of chondrocytes in all three zones of the growth plate (Figure 1.11) [138, 139].

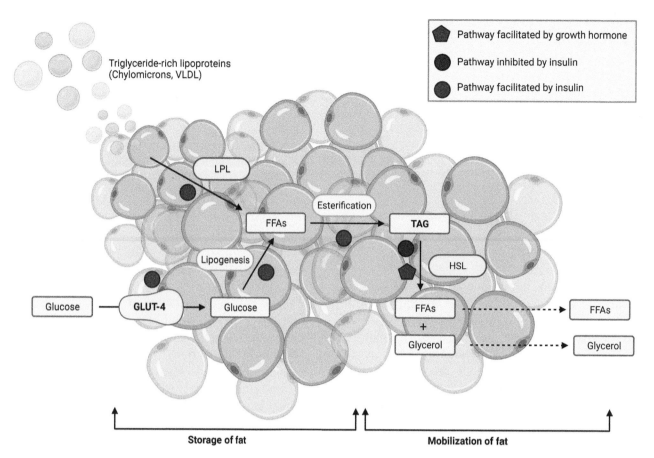

FIGURE 1.10 The regulation of fat storage and mobilization by growth hormone. Fat storage occurs in the prandial period, a process that involves the hydrolysis of triglycerides (TAG) in triglyceride-laden lipoproteins into free fatty acids (FFAs). LPL-induced storage of FFA is facilitated by insulin [134] and inhibited by growth hormone [135]. Also, glucose transporter 4 (GLUT4) transfers glucose from circulation to WAT after a meal. The conversion of glucose to FFA is also facilitated by insulin [136]. Ultimately, FFAs are esterified into TAGs. During periods of energy deficit, hormone-sensitive lipase (HSL) mediates the conversion of TAG repositories to FFA and glycerol. These, in turn, become substrates for gluconeogenesis. Growth hormone facilitates HSL-induced lipolysis of TAG into FFAs and glycerol [137]. On the contrary, insulin inhibits this fat mobilization step. + = shows stimulatory factors, − = shows inhibitory factors. *Source*: Adapted from ref. [134].

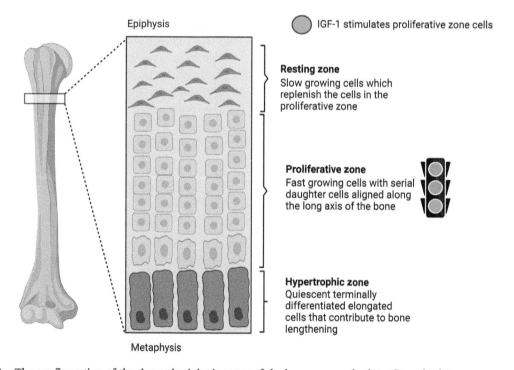

FIGURE 1.11 The configuration of the three physiologic zones of the human growth plate. Growth plates are present at the ends of tubular bones. There is a sequential arrangement of the hypertrophic, proliferative, and resting zones from the epiphyseal to the metaphyseal ends of the bone [138]. *Source*: Adapted from ref. [138].

1.4.1.2   Mechanism of Action

Recombinant human GH (rhGH) with an amino acid sequence similar to endogenous 22-kDa (KDa) growth hormone [140, 141] binds to the GH receptor and promotes the downstream effects of endogenous GH [142].

1.4.1.3   Practice Guide

- Common side effects of GH replacement in adults include *myalgia*, *arthralgia*, *peripheral edema*, and *carpal tunnel syndrome*. The de-escalation of the dose of GH improves and, in some cases, leads to the amelioration of these symptoms [143]. In children on GH therapy, prepubertal breast development, slipped capital femoral epiphysis, and benign intracranial hypertension can occur [144].
- The beneficial effects of growth hormone therapy in patients with AGHD include improving lipid profiles, diastolic blood pressure, insulin sensitivity, and lean body mass to fat body mass ratio [145].

Clinical Trial Evidence

Few large, high-quality, placebo-controlled randomized clinical trials (RCTs) evaluate the safety and efficacy of growth hormone replacement therapy [146].

Key Message

Although GH replacement improves objective cardiovascular risk factors, clinical trials have yet to demonstrate a clinically significant reduction in cardiovascular events [146].

In this randomized controlled trial, 43 hypopituitary subjects with AGHD were randomized to either placebo or rhGH. The primary outcome included various surrogate cardiovascular endpoints, including visceral adiposity, insulin resistance, C-reactive protein (CRP), total cholesterol, and high-density lipoprotein. There was a reduction in high-sensitivity CRP of 38.2 vs. 18.2 (p-value = 0.03), comparing GH with placebo. There was a statistically significant increase in IGF-1 when comparing GH with placebo. Other demonstrable benefits of GH replacement included a decrease in total cholesterol and an increase in high-density lipoprotein [147].

Concepts to Ponder Over

Does GH replacement increase the risk of cancer?

A large cohort of nearly 24,000 patients treated with recombinant human GH during their pediatric years was followed up for an average of 14.8 years per patient. For patients with pediatric growth failure and no known malignancy at baseline, there was no apparent increased risk of most malignancies except for bone and bladder cancers. The incidence rates for bone and bladder cancers were 2.8 (95% confidence intervals 1.1–7.5) and 16.3 (95% confidence intervals 5.2–50.4), respectively. The risk of these new-onset malignancies was not dependent on the cumulative doses of rhGH. However, an increased signal for recurrent primary cancers was observed in patients who received GH therapy in the setting of previously treated malignancies [148].

What are the effects of growth hormone on glycemic control?

GH, a counterregulatory hormone, is expected to cause hyperglycemia in normal physiology [149]. In a long-term observational study, including more than 5000 patients deficient in growth hormone on GH replacement, the incidence of diabetes was 2.6 per 100 patient-years. The risk was significantly higher among older subjects with a high body mass index, triglyceride levels, waist circumference, or blood pressure [150]. Refer to Table 1.7 for a summary of the effects of growth hormone on glucose metabolism.

TABLE 1.7   Glycemic effects of growth hormone.

Mechanism	Glycemic effects
Inhibition of GLUT4 expression by adipose tissue	Reduced peripheral uptake of glucose by adipose tissue
Growth hormone-mediated upregulation of hormone-sensitive lipase activity in adipose tissue.[a]	Liberation of free fatty acids leads to insulin resistance (impairs post-receptor insulin signaling)

(continued)

TABLE 1.7   (Continued)

Mechanism	Glycemic effects
Promotion of gluconeogenesis in the liver and kidneys	Hyperglycemia in the fasting state
Growth hormone-mediated upregulation of lipoprotein lipase in skeletal muscle promotes the accumulation of FFAs in skeletal muscle.‡	Insulin resistance
GH leads to the formation of IGF-1. IGF-1 can bind peripheral insulin receptors and simulate the effects of endogenous insulin-to-insulin receptor interaction	Hypoglycemia

ᵃ Also see Figure 1.11 for the effects of GH on fat storage and mobilization.
Esterification of FFAs into triacylglycerides leads to the formation of intermediate products such as diacylglycerol (impairs post-receptor insulin signaling).
Source: Adapted from Kim and Park [149].

1.5   CENTRAL DIABETES INSIPIDUS

1.5.1   Desmopressin

1.5.1.1   Physiology

Antidiuretic Hormone and Regulation of Serum Osmolarity

AVP is synthesized in the nuclei of paired *hypothal-amohypophyseal* neurons originating from supraoptic and paraventricular nuclei of the hypothalamus and terminating in the posterior pituitary gland [151]. Neurosecretory granules containing AVP are transported along axons that terminate in fenestrated capillaries in the neurohypophysis (posterior pituitary) [152]. The osmolarity sensing center (osmostat), located in the hypothalamus, regulates the release of AVP through relay neurons that project into the cell bodies of the supraoptic and paraventricular nuclei [153].

There is a linear relationship between plasma osmolarity and plasma AVP levels such that significant increases in plasma osmolarity cause a corresponding increase in plasma AVP [154]. In the context of dehydration, AVP, also known as antidiuretic hormone (ADH), increases water conservation at the level of the collecting duct, a process that increases urine osmolarity and leads to the restoration of normal plasma osmolarity [155] (see Figure 1.12).

1.5.1.2   Mechanism of Action

Desmopressin (1-deamino-8-D-arginine vasopressin, DDAVP) is an analog of AVP [158] with a prolonged plasma half-life of approximately 55 minutes (compared to endogenous AVP which has a half-life of 5–10 minutes) [159].

It is worth noting that substituting D-arginine for L-arginine at position 8 of the AVP amino acid chain eliminates the vasopressor effects of this synthetic analog of AVP [160]. Desmopressin promotes water conservation by binding to V2 receptors in the renal collecting ducts [158]. (See Figure 1.12). During periods of significant dehydration, the central thirst mechanism allows free water consumption, which results in the restoration of intravascular volume and osmolarity [155, 163].

 Clinical Pearl

Diabetes insipidus, "tasteless urine," was distinguished from diabetes mellitus in 1674 by Thomas Willis, an English physician. Edward Schafer, a renowned physiologist, discovered the effects of a posterior pituitary extract on urine output in 1901. Paradoxically, the posterior pituitary extract increased urine output according to Schafer's experiments, although this challenged observations of the antidiuretic effects of the posterior pituitary extract on urine output in patients with diabetes insipidus.

Ernest Verney and Ernest H. Starling, in the 1920s, were finally able to demonstrate that pituitrin (posterior pituitary extract) had an antidiuretic effect (and not a diuretic effect as previously reported by Schafer) on the kidneys independent of its effects on blood pressure.

1.5.1.3   Practice Guide

- Desmopressin can be administered safely through various routes (including intravenous, subcutaneous, oral, intranasal, and intramuscular). A simple rule of thumb is to use a conversion factor of 1:10 when converting between administration routes of administration [158].

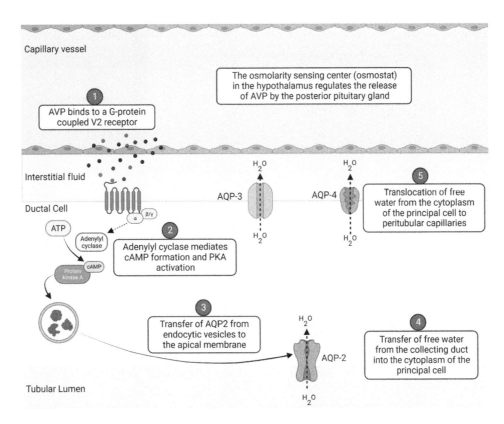

FIGURE 1.12   Schematic representation of AVP-mediated water conservation in the principal cell of the renal collecting duct. AVP binds to G-protein coupled V2 receptors on the principal cell's basolateral membrane (BM) [156]. This initiates a cascade of intracellular processes that involve adenylyl cyclase-mediated cyclic adenosine monophosphate (cAMP) production and subsequent protein kinase A (PKA) activation. Afterward, PKA will promote the release of aquaporins from endocytic vesicles. Aquaporin-2 (AQP2) released from vesicles inserts into the collecting duct apical membrane (AM). This promotes the translocation of free water from the collecting duct into the cytoplasm of the principal cell [157]. Aquaporin-3 (AQP3) and aquaporin-4 (AQP4) water channels, which are integral components (i.e. they are not released from endocytic vesicles) of the BM, facilitate the final transfer of water from the cytoplasm to the peritubular capillaries [155].

> ### Desmopressin Conversion Via the Route of Administration
>
> Intravenous/Subcutaneous: Intranasal: Oral = 1 mcg: 10 mcg: 100 mcg

- Coadministration of NSAIDs and desmopressin can lead to life-threatening hyponatremia [164]. In normal physiology, prostaglandin E2 (PgE_2) impairs the liberation of AQP2 from their endocytic vesicles after AVP to V2 receptor interaction. Cyclooxygenase inhibitors impair the synthesis of PgE_2, thus increasing the availability of AQP2 (water intoxication) [165].
- Consider an intermittent "DDAVP holiday" to reduce the likely risk of hyponatremia. Patients can be advised to delay the administration of a scheduled dose of DDAVP once a week until 2 or 3 successive episodes of breakthrough polyuria [166].

- Gastrointestinal peptidases denature oral desmopressin; as such, patients should be advised of the importance of taking this medication on an empty stomach or at least 90 minutes after a meal [167].
- *Pituitary adenomas* rarely present with central diabetes insipidus (CDI). Therefore, CDI in the setting of a sellar mass is more suggestive of an alternative differential diagnosis, such as craniopharyngiomas or a granulomatous process [166].

> ### Clinical Trial Evidence
>
> In this retrospective study, the incidence of hyponatremia in patients with CDI was evaluated between the intranasal and oral desmopressin routes of administration. Thirty-two subjects who had previously been well-controlled with stable doses of intranasal DDAVP were switched to an oral route of administration for a maximum duration of 18 months [168].

Key Message

Based on the results of this study, the frequency of significant hyponatremia (<130 mmol/L) was 4.2% when subjects were on intranasal desmopressin, compared to 1.3% when on oral desmopressin. This was statistically significant. Normal water and sodium balance are better achieved with oral DDAVP compared to intranasally administered DDAVP [168].

 Pathophysiology Pearl

Conditions masquerading as diabetes insipidus

- Gestational diabetes insipidus occurs in pregnant women due to the degradation of endogenous AVP by a placenta-derived enzyme called vasopressinase. The clinical and biochemical characteristics are similar to those of CDI [169].
- Primary polydipsia (chronic) results in decreased renal concentrating ability due to excessive fluid ingestion. In effect, an abundance of free water promotes the downregulation of aquaporins ("wash-out effect") [170].

1.5.2   Water

1.5.2.1   Physiology

Osmotic Center and the Regulation of Sodium Balance

The previously described osmotic center (also known as the osmostat, see Section 1.5.1) is composed of two discrete structures known as the *organum vasculosum of the lamina terminalis* (OVLT) and the *subfornical organ* (SFO). These structures have projecting from them neurons that supply parts of the forebrain involved in the executive response to thirst, the hypothalamus (SON and PVN), and the sympathetic nervous system [171]. OVLT and SFO are activated by elevated serum osmolarity and angiotensin II levels. The response to the activation of OVLT and SFO includes increased thirst sensation, AVP release, and a sympathoadrenergic increase in blood pressure [172, 173].

1.5.2.2   Mechanism of Action

The role of free water in maintaining hydration status has been discussed. See Figure 1.12.

1.5.2.3   Practice Guide

- Access to free water is essential in the management of CDI. Indeed, in mild diabetes insipidus, optimal water ingestion (as monotherapy) could be enough to maintain sodium and water balance [174].
- Patients with adipsic CDI have all the features of CDI but are unable to sense thirst. It is a complex disease to manage due to marked variability in serum sodium and apparent challenges in maintaining oral hydration [175]

Clinical Trial Evidence

In a long-term retrospective study of 137 CDI-positive subjects at maintenance doses of DDAVP, the risk of sodium imbalance was compared between those with adipsia (impaired thirst sensation) and those with an intact thirst sensation. The risk of hypernatremia between the adipsic and non-adipic groups was 20% and 1.4%, respectively (*P*-value = 0.02). The risk of hyponatremia between the adipsic and non-adipic groups was 50% and 11.1%, respectively (*p*-value = 0.02%) [176].

Key Message

Adipsia increases the risk of a significant sodium imbalance in patients with CDI. Since these patients do not have the ability to respond to increased serum osmolarity, they are prone to profound dehydration in the setting of polyuria [176].

1.5.3   Natriuretic Agents

1.5.3.1   Physiology

Physiology of Diuresis in the Distal Convoluted Tubule (DCT)

The sodium-chloride symporter (secondary active transport system) and the electrochemical gradient created by the sodium-potassium adenosine triphosphatase (Na-K ATPase) (primary active transport system) are both essential for sodium reabsorption in the DCT. However, the DCT is impermeable to water, making urine in this segment hypotonic [177].

1.5.3.2   Mechanism of Action

Thiazide diuretics exert their natriuretic effects by inhibiting thiazide-sensitive Na^+-Cl^- symporters in the distal convoluted tubules of the nephron. The net effect will be the wasting of both sodium and water at the distal nephron (see Figure 1.13). Mechanistically this seems counterintuitive since patients with CDI are polyuric at baseline [178, 180]. See Figure 1.14 for a proposed mechanistic pathway that explains the role of natriuretic agents in the management of CDI.

1.5.3.3   Practice Guide

- Thiazide diuretics, either as monotherapy or dual therapy with amiloride (potassium-sparing diuretic) or indomethacin, are reasonable therapeutic approaches in diabetes insipidus [181].
- A low-salt diet potentiates the paradoxical "antidiuretic effect" of thiazide diuretics [167].

Clinical Pearl

Gitelman syndrome is an inherited form of hypokalemic alkalosis that occurs as a result of a mutation in the gene encoding the sodium chloride symporter. This syndrome simulates exposure to a thiazide diuretic agent [182].

Clinical Trial Evidence

There are no published RCTs on the use of thiazide diuretics in CDI. Some pediatric case reports and retrospective studies exploring the use of thiazide diuretics in CDI gave promising results in terms of treatment efficacy (achievement of eunatremia and control of polyuria) [178, 183, 184]. Most importantly, the use of diuretics is not recommended in the management of CDI. However, diuretic therapy is indicated in treating nephrogenic diabetes insipidus.

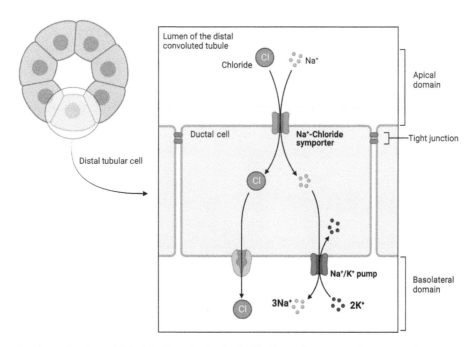

FIGURE 1.13   Mechanism of action of thiazide diuretics in the DCT. The sodium-potassium pump (Na-K ATPase) present on the basolateral membrane of the DCT creates an electrochemical gradient that facilitates the transport of sodium and chloride ions (Cl^-) by the sodium-chloride symporter (luminal or apical membrane) [161]. Chloride ions move from the lumen into the ductal cell against an electrochemical gradient. Cl^- is then ferried from the ductal cell into the peritubular capillaries by chloride channels in the basolateral membrane. Potassium ions (K^+) are also transported from the ductal cell to peritubular capillaries via dedicated K^+ channels. Aldosterone, produced as a consequence of activation of the renin-angiotensin-aldosterone system (RAAS), increases the transcription and translation of the sodium-chloride symporter [162]. *Source*: Adapted from ref. [161].

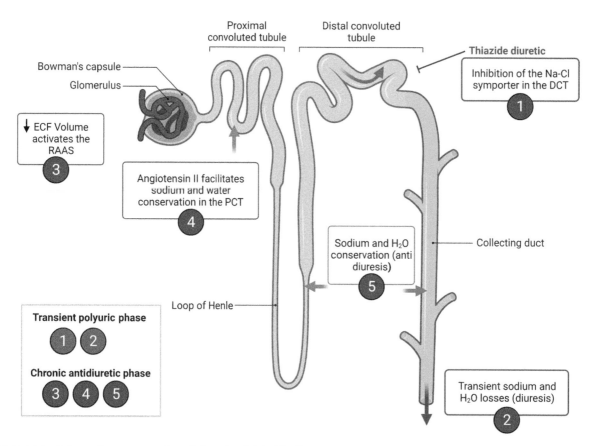

FIGURE 1.14 Schematic representation of the role of thiazide diuretics in central diabetes insipidus. Thiazide diuretics promote sodium wasting in the distal renal tubule. The high sodium load in the renal tubular fluid also increases water loss (osmotic effect). A reduction in extracellular fluid volume causes a decrease in the estimated glomerular filtration rate, ultimately activating the RAAS. Increased levels of Angiotensin II promote a compensatory increase in sodium and water conservation at the proximal tubule (see Section 3.1.2). Consequently, less sodium and water are delivered to collecting tubules, leading to less renal water loss [178, 179].

1.5.4 Clofibrate, Chlorpropamide, and Carbamazepine

1.5.4.1 Physiology

The physiology of central ADH regulation and its peripheral effects is reviewed in Section 1.5.1.

1.5.4.2 Mechanism of Action

Clofibrate: Clofibrate, an antilipidemic agent, has antidiuretic properties. It exerts its antidiuretic effects by increasing ADH release from the neurohypophysis [185]. This drug was withdrawn from the market in 2002 and is mentioned here due to its historical significance [167].

Chlorpropamide: Chlorpropamide, a first-generation sulfonylurea, increases release of ADH and also promotes the antidiuretic effects of ADH at the renal collecting duct [185]. Alternative mechanisms of action include an increase in the

circulating half-life of AVP and a lower osmotic threshold for the release of endogenous AVP [186].

Carbamazepine: Carbamazepine, an antiepileptic agent, potentiates ADH effects at the renal collecting duct [187].

1.5.4.3 Practice Guide

None of these agents are recommended as an alternative to DDAVP in the management of CDI.

Clinical Trial Evidence
There are no RCTs comparing any of these agents with guideline-recommended DDAVP. In a recent case report of a patient with CDI, oxcarbazepine (structurally homologous to carbamazepine) was proposed as an alternative to DDAVP [186].

Concepts to Ponder Over

What is the triphasic response of diabetes insipidus?

The triphasic response of central diabetes insipidus represents a unique state of sodium imbalance characterized by rapid changes in serum sodium and, consequently, intravascular volume among patients with pituitary stalk injury [188]. Disruption of the stalk occurs commonly in the setting of neurosurgery [189] but has also been described in traumatic brain injury [190].

An initial phase of overt CDI occurs due to axonal shock, and it presents with an impaired neuronal transfer of AVP from the hypothalamus to the posterior pituitary gland. The second phase is characterized by axonal death and the release of preformed AVP from their neuronal stores. This is similar to the syndrome of inappropriate ADH (SIADH) secretion. After an 80–90% depletion of AVP stores, the final phase of permanent CDI occurs (see Figure 1.15) [191].

What are the causes of adipsic central diabetes insipidus?

Adipsic CDI manifests itself as an inability to perceive thirst in the setting of AVP deficiency that results in hypotonic polyuria and hypernatremia [192]. It occurs due to the disruption of vascular supply to the osmostat center (OVLT or SFO), infiltrative tumors(craniopharyngioma), autoimmune disease, or congenital malformations of the corpus callosum [193].

Phase I: neuronal shock, which leads to transient diabetes insipidus [191]. This phase lasts for about 72 hours. The timely use of DDAVP or hypotonic fluids is reasonable [189].

Phase II: Neuronal death (distal to the site of stalk transection) and release of preformed AVP (from the neurohypophysis) leads to an SIADH-like picture [191]. This phase may last up to 2 weeks. Careful fluid restriction is key [189].

Phase III: The depletion of neuronal stores of AVP in the paraventricular nucleus (PVN) and supraoptic nucleus (SON) leads to a recurrence of diabetes insipidus. This tends to be permanent, especially in the setting of complete pituitary stalk transection [191].

Source: Adapted from Redrawn and modified from Hoorn and Zietse [189].

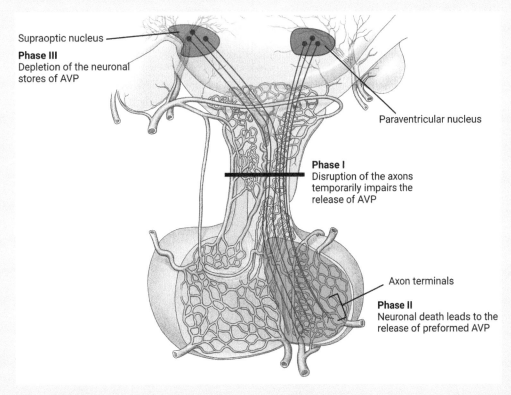

Supraoptic nucleus

Phase III
Depletion of the neuronal stores of AVP

Paraventricular nucleus

Phase I
Disruption of the axons temporarily impairs the release of AVP

Axon terminals

Phase II
Neuronal death leads to the release of preformed AVP

FIGURE 1.15   The triphasic response of central diabetes insipidus. *Source*: Adapter from [181].

1.6 SYNDROME OF INAPPROPRIATE ADH SECRETION

1.6.1 Vaptans

1.6.1.1 Physiology

The *hypothalamic–pituitary-renal* axis with regards to the role of AVP in the conservation of renal water was reviewed in Section 1.5.1. AVP has various effects in different tissues, depending on the AVP receptor subtype expressed in the target tissue (Table 1.8) [194, 195].

 Clinical Pearl

The syndrome of inappropriate antidiuretic hormone (SIADH) secretion is the leading cause of hyponatremia in outpatient and inpatient settings. It is particularly relevant due to morbidity and mortality associated with untreated or poorly managed hyponatremia [194]. Although eponyms are increasingly being replaced by labels that clarify the pathophysiological basis of diseases, the contributions of pioneering physicians should be appreciated. SIADH was previously called the Schwartz–Bartter syndrome. Bartter syndrome, a rare condition of electrolyte imbalance, is also named after Frederic Bartter [196].

TABLE 1.8 Subtypes of AVP receptors and their physiologic effects.

AVP receptor	Tissue	Effect(s)
V1a	Vascular smooth muscle Myocardium	Vasoconstriction and platelet function Cardiac inotropic function
V1b	Pituitary	Pituitary ACTH secretion (see Figure 1.1)
V2	Renal collecting duct Vascular endothelium	Water conservation (see Figure 1.13) Release of vWF and factor VIII

vWF, von Willebrand factor.
Source: Adapted from Verbalis et al. [194].

1.6.1.2 Mechanism of Action

Vaptans are V2 receptor antagonists that impair the binding of endogenous AVP to its cognate V2 receptors. It is essential to appreciate that vaptans cause an *"aquaresis"* (i.e. loss of free water with the conservation of electrolytes) as opposed to the effects of diuretics, which promote both fluid and electrolyte losses. In SIADH, there is an excessive amount of free water (relative to sodium) conservation due to the effects of ADH in the renal collecting tubule. This makes vaptans a more reasonable therapeutic option in SIADH, than monotherapy with conventional diuretic agents [194].

1.6.1.3 Practice Guide

Patients taking vaptans are at risk of dehydration due to polyuria and polydipsia [196].

Although this class of medications has an acceptable safety profile, they should be started in the inpatient setting to avoid significant increases in serum sodium and the risk of osmotic demyelination syndrome [197].

Clinical Trial Evidence
Clinical trials evaluating the safety and efficacy of vaptans in the treatment of euvolemic hyponatremia (SIADH) include SALT-1, SALT-2, and SALTWATER. In the *Study of Ascending Levels of Tolvaptan in Hyponatremia* (SALT-1 and SALT-2), serum sodium increased significantly in the tolvaptan group compared to the placebo group (*p*-value of < 0.001) across a heterogeneous population of hyponatremic patients (euvolemic or hypervolemic hyponatremia) [198]. The *Safety and sodium assessment of Long-term Tolvaptan With hyponatremia: A year-long, open-label Trial to gain Experience under Real-world conditions* (SALTWATER), an extension study of SALT-1 and SALT-2 demonstrated the long-term safety and efficacy of tolvaptan in hyponatremia [196].

1.6.2 Fluid Restriction

1.6.2.1 Physiology

The role of free water in the determination of serum osmolarity was discussed earlier (see Figure 1.13).

1.6.2.2   Mechanism of Action

The mechanistic pathways for the sensation of thirst (see Section 1.5.2) and AVP-mediated regulation of serum osmolarity (see Section 1.5.1) have been discussed.

1.6.2.3   Practice Guide

- Fluid restriction performs abysmally in routine clinical practice, most likely due to the poor selection of patients for this therapeutic option among patients with SIADH [199].

Poor Predictors of Response to Fluid Restriction

Urine osmolarity >500 mOsm/kg/H_2O
Urine output of less than 1500 mL per 24 hours
An estimated "Fürst equation" ratio of >1

Fürst equation

([Urine sodium] + [Urine Potassium]) / [Serum sodium]
[] = concentration.

There are various adjunctive therapies utilized in the management of diabetes insipidus. Their mechanisms of action are shown in Table 1.9.

TABLE 1.9   Mechanism of action of adjunctive therapies in SIADH.

Therapy	Mechanism of action
Loop diuretics[a]	Diuresis (free water and electrolyte losses). Sodium chloride supplementation is mandatory [200, 201]
Sodium chloride[a]	Sodium chloride is best administered with fluid restriction or a diuretic agent ("aquaretic effect") [201]
Lithium	Anti-natriuresis (renal sodium conservation) [202] and limitation of AQP-2 expression in the renal collecting ducts (nephrogenic diabetes insipidus-like presentation) [203].
Demeclocycline	Nephrogenic diabetes insipidus [204]
Urea	Osmotic diuresis and compensatory passive sodium conservation at the level of the ascending limb of the loop of Henle [205].

[a] In the EFFUSE-FLUID clinical trial, a combination of loop diuretics and sodium chloride with fluid restriction did not fare any better than fluid restriction alone.
Source: Adapted from refs. [200–205].

Clinical Trial Evidence

In this retrospective study of 29 patients with SIADH, the efficacy of fluid restriction (1.5–2 L), with or without adjunctive urea supplementation, in the management of SIADH was explored. Changes in serum sodium and urine osmolarity were compared at one year with baseline. The mean serum sodium concentration and urine osmolarity were 129 mEq/L and 274 mOsm/kgH_2O, respectively, at baseline. At the end of 12 months of fluid restriction, serum sodium concentration and urine osmolarity improved to 138.5 mEq/L and 505 mOsm/kgH_2O, respectively. This occurred in 30% of subjects. For patients who had a suboptimal response to fluid restriction alone, most attained eunatremia after the institution of urea supplementation (15–30 g daily) [206].

Key Message

Moderate fluid restriction (1.5–2 L) per day led to eunatremia in 30% of patients with chronic SIADH, according to the results of this retrospective study.

There are other therapies reported for the management of SIADH. These include loop diuretics, urea, hypertonic saline, lithium, demeclocycline, and hemodialysis [207].

 Concepts to Ponder On

What are the diagnostic criteria for SIADH?

The diagnosis of SIADH is based on the criteria proposed by Bartter and Schwartz in 1967 [208].
The classic Bartter and Schwartz criteria

1. Plasma osmolarity <275 mOsm/kg of H_2O
2. Inappropriately concentrated urine >100 mOsm/kg
3. Euvolemia
4. Urine sodium >20 mEq/L
5. Normal thyroid function, normal adrenal function, and no recent exposure to diuretic agents (effects on urine sodium).

Patients who meet ALL of the above criteria are more likely to have SIADH [194].

What conditions can mask the presence of partial central diabetes insipidus?

The coexistence of a paraneoplastic condition manifesting as SIADH may mask the presence of central diabetes insipidus [209].

Partial central diabetes insipidus can also be masked in the presence of glucocorticoid deficiency. It should be noted that glucocorticoids inhibit V2R-mediated water conservation in the collecting duct by impairing the translocation of V2R to the apical membrane of the collecting duct cell. Glucocorticoid deficiency, in part, promotes water reabsorption, thus masking the presence of *partial central diabetes insipidus*. Primary glucocorticoid deficiency leads to increased CRH production (AVP secretagogue) due to loss of negative feedback inhibition of hypothalamic centers by cortisol [209].

PRACTICE-BASED QUESTIONS

1. A 50-year-old woman with a six-month history of easy bruisability, hyperglycemia, and resistant hypertension is admitted to the medicine service. The endocrinologist on call recommends initiating pasireotide. Which of the following receptors is the primary target of Pasireotide in Cushing's disease?

   a. Somatostatin receptor subtype 2 (SSR2)
   b. Somatostatin receptor subtype 5 (SSR5)
   c. Melanocortin-2 receptor (MCR-2)
   d. Dopamine D2 receptor (D2R)

   Correct answer: b) Somatostatin receptor subtype 5 (SSR5). Pasireotide is a "near pan-somatostatin" receptor analog that binds to four of the five somatostatin receptor isoforms (SSR1, SSR2, SSR3, and SSR5). Due to its affinity for SSR5 receptors, pasireotide is an ideal therapeutic option in Cushing's disease. Corticotroph tumors in the anterior pituitary gland express more SSR5 receptors than the other somatostatin receptor subtypes making pasireotide an ideal agent for this tumor.

2. Which of the following transcription factors is inhibited by Retinoic Acid (RA)?

   a. Activator protein 1 (AP-1)
   b. Nuclear receptor 77 (Nur77)
   c. Chicken ovoalbumin upstream promoter transcription factor 1 (COUP-TF1)
   d. Both a and b

Correct answer: d) Both a and b. In normal physiology, there are retinoid-sensitive intermediary mediators (transcription factors) of POMC promoter gene activation, namely, AP-1 and Nur77. Retinoic acid (RA), by binding to its nuclear retinoic acid receptors inhibits AP-1, and Nur77 expression, thus preventing POMC promoter gene activation.

3. What percentage of corticotroph adenomas express D2 receptors?

   a. 10%
   b. 40%
   c. 60%
   d. 80%

   Correct answer: d) 80%. Approximately 80% of corticotroph adenomas express D2 receptors, but they have a relatively low D2 receptor density making, dopaminergic agonists (DAs) a less favorable therapeutic option in Cushings disease, compared to other medical therapies.

4. Which of the following hormones is inhibited by Pasireotide through yet-to-be-characterized intestinal somatostatin receptors?

   a. Insulin
   b. Glucagon-like peptide 1
   c. Glucose-dependent insulinotropic peptide (GIP)
   d. Both b and c

   Correct answer: d) Both b and c. Pasireotide through yet-to-be-characterized intestinal somatostatin receptors inhibits the release of glucagon-like peptide 1(GLP-1) and glucose-dependent insulinotropic peptide (GIP) from K and L cells, respectively. Pasireotide causes hyperglycemia, gastrointestinal discomfort, and cholelithiasis.

5. A 50-year-old man with newly diagnosed Cushing's syndrome is started on medical therapy. What is the typical dose range for Pasireotide immediate-release as a subcutaneous injection?

   a. 0.1 to 0.5 mg
   b. 0.3 to 0.9 mg
   c. 1 to 3 mg
   d. 5–10 mg

   Correct answer: b) 0.3–0.9 mg. The typical dose range for pasireotide immediate-release is 0.3–0.9 mg (300–900 mcg) as a subcutaneous injection (thigh, upper arm, or abdomen) twice a day. A long-acting release (LAR) formulation is administered once a month (10–30 mg) intramuscularly as a depot injection.

6. Which of the following steroidogenesis inhibitors has been recently approved for persistent and recurrent Cushing's disease?

a. Metyrapone
b. Mitotane
c. Ketoconazole
d. Osilodrostat

Correct Answer: d) Osilodrostat. Osilodrostat inhibits 11-beta hydroxylase activity in the adrenal cortex, and it has been recently approved for persistent and recurrent Cushing's disease.

7. Which of the following steroidogenesis inhibitors used in the treatment of Cushings syndrome has been suggested to have both adrenolytic and adrenostatic properties?

a. Metyrapone
b. Mitotane
c. Ketoconazole
d. Osilodrostat

Correct answer: b) Mitotane. Mitotane is suggested to have both adrenolytic and adrenostatic properties. Mitotane is a chemotherapeutic agent with a diphenylmethane moiety that causes mitochondrial dysfunction, lysis, and necrosis.

8. A 28-year-old woman presents with oligomenorrhea and is diagnosed with Cushing's syndrome. Her urine pregnancy test returned negative. Which of the following steroidogenesis inhibitors is the recommended first-line medical therapy for nonpregnant adults with confirmed endogenous hypercortisolemia?

a. Metyrapone
b. Mitotane
c. Ketoconazole
d. Osilodrostat

Correct answer: c) Ketoconazole. Ketoconazole is the recommended first-line medical therapy for nonpregnant adults with confirmed endogenous hypercortisolemia.

9. You are considering various treatment options for Cushing's syndrome in a newly diagnosed patient. You are concerned about the risk of medical therapy on a fetus. Which of the following agents has both anti-glucocorticoid and anti-progesterone effects?

a. Metyrapone
b. Mitotane
c. Ketoconazole
d. Mifepristone

Correct answer: d) Mifepristone. Mifepristone has both anti-glucocorticoid and anti-progesterone effects. It actually exerts its effects by binding to the ligand-binding domain of the cytosolic glucocorticoid receptor without directly promoting its downstream effects.

10. An endocrinologist on call evaluates a newly diagnosed patient with a small 4 mm pituitary adenoma. He makes a diagnosis of Cushing's disease. What is the recommended first-line treatment for Cushing's disease?

a. Ketoconazole
b. Metyrapone
c. Mitotane
d. Transsphenoidal surgery

Correct answer: d) Transsphenoidal surgery. Transsphenoidal surgery is the recommended first-line treatment for Cushing's disease. However, a high recurrence rate of about 20% makes medical therapies an essential adjunctive approach.

11. A 54-year-old man with poor libido, excessive diaphoresis, and wide spaced teeth is noted to have elevated growth hormone levels after an oral glucose tolerance test. His IGF-1 level remains elevated on two occasions. You are considering the use of somatostatin analogs in his treatment. What is the role of somatostatin in growth hormone regulation?

a. Promotes the release of growth hormone from somatotrophs
b. Blocks the release of growth hormone from somatotrophs
c. Enhances the sensitivity of the liver to growth hormone
d. Enhances the synthesis of insulin-like growth factor 1 in the liver

Correct answer: b. Blocks the release of growth hormone from somatotrophs. Somatostatin inhibits the release of GH by somatotrophs by acting on somatostatin receptors (primarily the SSR2 receptor subtype).

12. Which of the following organs does not produce insulin-like growth factor 1 (IGF-1)?

    a. Liver
    b. Skeletal muscle
    c. Adipose tissue
    d. Brain

    Correct answer: d. Brain. IGF-1 is produced in various tissues, including the liver, skeletal muscle, and adipose tissue, but not by the brain.

13. A 63-year-old woman is diagnosed with acromegaly. What is the mechanism of action of pegvisomant?

    a. It activates the growth hormone receptor and induces IGF-1 production
    b. It inhibits the growth hormone receptor and blocks IGF-1 production
    c. It activates the somatostatin receptor and inhibits growth hormone production
    d. It inhibits the somatostatin receptor and enhances growth hormone production

    Correct answer: b. It inhibits the growth hormone receptor and blocks IGF-1 production. Pegvisomant occupies the GH receptor pocket, depriving the receptor of direct activation by GH. This subsequently induces defective dimerization of the receptor, thus preventing key signal transduction pathways (JAK–STAT signaling) and the eventual production of IGF-1.

14. A 38-year-old obese patient is diagnosed with a pituitary adenoma. You are considering the use of pasireotide. What is the hallmark side effect of pasireotide?

    a. Hypoglycemia
    b. Hyperglycemia
    c. Diarrhea
    d. Cholelithiasis

    Correct answer: b. Hyperglycemia. Pasireotide is associated with a disproportionate risk of hyperglycemia, particularly in patients with diabetes or prediabetes, and should be screened for before and during treatment.

15. You are considering the use of dopaminergic modulators in the management of acromegaly. What is the differential effect of dopamine on growth hormone secretion in normal physiology?

    a. It increases growth hormone secretion at the level of the anterior pituitary gland
    b. It increases growth hormone secretion at the level of the hypothalamus
    c. Growth hormone decreases growth hormone secretion at the level of the anterior pituitary gland
    d. Growth hormone decreases growth hormone secretion at the level of the hypothalamus

    Correct answer: c. It decreases growth hormone secretion at the level of the anterior pituitary gland. The effects of dopamine on GH secretion are more profound at the level of the anterior pituitary gland than at the level of the hypothalamus. The net effect is a reduction in GH secretion.

16. A 56-year-old woman presents with polyuria. You have scheduled a formal water deprivation test. What is the relationship between plasma osmolarity and plasma AVP levels?

    a. Plasma AVP levels are independent of plasma osmolarity
    b. Significant decreases in plasma osmolarity cause a corresponding increase in plasma AVP levels
    c. Significant increases in plasma osmolarity cause a corresponding decrease in plasma AVP levels
    d. Plasma AVP levels are not affected by changes in plasma osmolarity

    Correct answer: b. Significant increases in plasma osmolarity cause a corresponding increase in plasma AVP levels. This linear relationship between plasma osmolarity and plasma AVP levels ensures the proper regulation of water balance in the body, allowing for the conservation of water when necessary.

17. A patient with central diabetes insipidus reports a significant improvement in polyuria after starting desmopressin therapy. Which receptors are involved in the water-conserving properties of desmopressin?

    a. V1 receptors
    b. V2 receptors
    c. Beta-1 receptors
    d. Alpha-2 receptors

Correct answer: b. Desmopressin binds to V2 receptors on the basolateral membrane of the principal cell in the renal collecting duct. This initiates a cascade of intracellular processes that ultimately lead to the promotion of water conservation at the level of the collecting duct, resulting in the restoration of normal plasma osmolarity.

18. What is adipsic CDI?

    a. A form of CDI in which patients are unable to sense thirst
    b. A form of CDI in which the kidneys are unresponsive to vasopressin
    c. A form of CDI caused by a pituitary adenoma
    d. A form of CDI caused by a genetic mutation

Correct answer: a. Adipsic CDI is a condition in which patients with CDI are unable to sense thirst. This makes management of the condition challenging, as patients may have difficulty maintaining oral hydration, leading to significant sodium imbalances.

19. What is the recommended timing of administration for oral desmopressin?

    a. With food
    b. On an empty stomach
    c. With a high-fat meal
    d. With a glass of water

Correct answer: b. Gastrointestinal peptidases denature oral Desmopressin, which can lead to reduced efficacy of the medication. Patients should be advised to take this medication either on an empty stomach or at least 90 minutes after a meal to ensure optimal absorption.

20. A 26-year-old woman presents with seizures after starting an antidepressant medication. What is the likely explanation for her presentations

    a. Hypernatremia
    b. Polyuria
    c. Hyperkalemia
    d. Hyponatremia

Correct answer: d. Syndrome of inappropriate antidiuretic hormone secretion (SIADH) is characterized by excessive release of ADH, which results in increased water reabsorption in the kidneys. A state of dilutional hyponatremia therefore results, a condition where there is a low concentration of sodium in the blood due to an excessive amount of water. The other options, hypernatremia, polyuria, and hyperkalemia, are not typically associated with SIADH.

REFERENCES

1. Martin-Grace, J., Dineen, R., Sherlock, M., and Thompson, C.J. (2020). Adrenal insufficiency: Physiology, clinical presentation and diagnostic challenges. *Clin. Chim. Acta Int. J. Clin. Chem.* 505: 78–91.

2 Rotondo, F., Butz, H., Syro, L.V. et al. (2016). Arginine vasopressin (AVP): a review of its historical perspectives, current research and multifunctional role in the hypothalamo-hypophysial system. *Pituitary* 19 (4): 345–355.

3. Spencer, R.L. and Deak, T. (2017). A users guide to HPA axis research. *Physiol. Behav.* 178: 43–65.

4. Osterlund, C.D., Rodriguez-Santiago, M., Woodruff, E.R. et al. (2016). Glucocorticoid fast feedback inhibition of stress-induced ACTH secretion in the male rat: rate independence and stress-state resistance. *Endocrinology* 157 (7): 2785–2798.

5. Myers, B., McKlveen, J.M., and Herman, J.P. (2012). Neural regulation of the stress response: The many faces of feedback. *Cell. Mol. Neurobiol.* 32 (5): 683–694.

6. Hofland, L.J., Lamberts, S.W.J., and Feelders, R.A. (2010). Role of somatostatin receptors in normal and tumoral pituitary corticotropic cells. *Neuroendocrinology* 92 (Suppl 1): 11–16.

7. Herman, J.P., McKlveen, J.M., Ghosal, S. et al. (2016). Regulation of the hypothalamic-pituitary-adrenocortical stress response. *Compr. Physiol.* 6 (2): 603–621.

8. Giordano, R., Pellegrino, M., Picu, A. et al. (2006). Neuroregulation of the hypothalamus-pituitary-adrenal (HPA) axis in humans: effects of GABA-, mineralocorticoid-, and GH-Secretagogue-receptor modulation. *Sci. World J.* 6: 1–11.

9. Tateno, T., Kato, M., Tani, Y. et al. (2009). Differential expression of somatostatin and dopamine receptor subtype genes in adrenocorticotropin (ACTH)-secreting pituitary tumors and silent corticotroph adenomas. *Endocr. J.* 56 (4): 579–584.

10. Lacroix, A., Gu, F., Schopohl, J. et al. (2020). Pasireotide treatment significantly reduces tumor volume in patients with Cushing's disease: results from a Phase 3 study. *Pituitary* 23 (3): 203–211.

11. Silverstein, J.M. (2016). Hyperglycemia induced by pasireotide in patients with Cushing's disease or acromegaly. *Pituitary* 19 (5): 536–543.

12. Novartis Pharmaceuticals. (2016). A randomized, double-blind study to assess the safety and efficacy of different dose levels of pasireotide (SOM230) subcutaneous (sc) over a 6 month treatment period in patients with de Novo, persistent or recurrent Cushing's disease.

13. Tritos, N.A. and Biller, B.M.K. (2020). Advances in the medical treatment of Cushing disease. *Endocrinol. Metab. Clin. N. Am.* 49 (3): 401–412.

14. Henry, R.R., Ciaraldi, T.P., Armstrong, D. et al. (2013). Hyperglycemia associated with pasireotide: results from a mechanistic study in healthy volunteers. *J. Clin. Endocrinol. Metab.* 98 (8): 3446–3453.

15. Colao, A., De Block, C., Gaztambide, M.S. et al. (2014). Managing hyperglycemia in patients with Cushing's disease treated with pasireotide: medical expert recommendations. *Pituitary* 17 (2): 180–186.

16. Ahrendt, S.A., McGuire, G.E., Pitt, H.A., and Lillemoe, K.D. (1991). Why does somatostatin cause gallstones? *Am. J. Surg.* 161 (1): 177–182. discussion 182–183.

17. Colao, A., Petersenn, S., Newell-Price, J. et al. (2012). A 12-month phase 3 study of pasireotide in Cushing's disease. *N. Engl. J. Med.* 366 (10): 914–924.

18. Sano, T. (2010). The 11th meeting of the international pituitary pathology society October 16–20, 2009 Awaji Island, Japan. *Endocr. Pathol.* 21 (1): 48–68.

19. Mason, D., Hassan, A., Chacko, S., and Thompson, P. (2002). Acute and chronic regulation of pituitary receptors for vasopressin and corticotropin releasing hormone. *Arch. Physiol. Biochem.* 110 (1–2): 74–89.

20. Pecori Giraldi, F., Ambrogio, A.G., Andrioli, M. et al. (2012). Potential role for retinoic acid in patients with Cushing's disease. *J. Clin. Endocrinol. Metab.* 97 (10): 3577–3583.

21. Sesta, A., Cassarino, M.F., Tapella, L. et al. (2016). Effect of retinoic acid on human adrenal corticosteroid synthesis. *Life Sci.* 151: 277–280.

22. Theodoropoulou, M. and Reincke, M. (2019). Tumor-directed therapeutic targets in Cushing disease. *J. Clin. Endocrinol. Metab.* 104 (3): 925–933.

23. Occhi, G., Regazzo, D., Albiger, N.M. et al. (2014). Activation of the dopamine receptor type-2 (DRD2) promoter by 9-cis retinoic acid in a cellular model of Cushing's disease mediates the inhibition of cell proliferation and ACTH secretion without a complete corticotroph-to-melanotroph transdifferentiation. *Endocrinology* 155 (9): 3538–3549.

24. Vilar, L., Albuquerque, J.L., Lyra, R. et al. (2016). The role of isotretinoin therapy for Cushing's disease: results of a prospective study. *Int. J. Endocrinol.* 2016: 8173182.

25. Cuevas-Ramos, D., Lim, D.S.T., and Fleseriu, M. (2016). Update on medical treatment for Cushing's disease. *Clin. Diabetes Endocrinol.* 2 (1): 16.

26. Auriemma, R.S., Pivonello, R., Ferreri, L. et al. (2015). Cabergoline use for pituitary tumors and valvular disorders. *Endocrinol. Metab. Clin. N. Am.* 44 (1): 89–97.

27. Stiles, C.E., Tetteh-Wayoe, E.T., Bestwick, J.P. et al. (2019). A meta-analysis of the prevalence of cardiac valvulopathy in patients with hyperprolactinemia treated with cabergoline. *J. Clin. Endocrinol. Metab.* 104 (2): 523–538.

28. Verhelst, J., Abs, R., Maiter, D. et al. (1999). Cabergoline in the treatment of hyperprolactinemia: a study in 455 patients. *J. Clin. Endocrinol. Metab.* 84 (7): 2518–2522.

29. Vroonen, L., Jaffrain-Rea, M.-L., Petrossians, P. et al. (2012). Prolactinomas resistant to standard doses of cabergoline: a multicenter study of 92 patients. *Eur. J. Endocrinol.* 167 (5): 651–662.

30. Burman, P., Edén-Engström, B., Ekman, B. et al. (2016). Limited value of cabergoline in Cushing's disease: a prospective study of a 6-week treatment in 20 patients. *Eur. J. Endocrinol.* 174 (1): 17–24.

31. Ferriere, A., Cortet, C., Chanson, P. et al. (2017). Cabergoline for Cushing's disease: a large retrospective multicenter study. *Eur. J. Endocrinol.* 176 (3): 305–314.

32. Godbout, A., Manavela, M., Danilowicz, K. et al. (2010). Cabergoline monotherapy in the long-term treatment of Cushing's disease. *Eur. J. Endocrinol.* 163 (5): 709–716.

33. Liddle, G.W., Estep, H.L., Kendall, J.W. et al. (1959). Clinical application of a new test of pituitary reserve. *J. Clin. Endocrinol. Metab.* 19: 875–894.

34. Kamenický, P., Droumaguet, C., Salenave, S. et al. (2011). Mitotane, metyrapone, and ketoconazole combination therapy as an alternative to rescue adrenalectomy for severe ACTH-dependent Cushing's syndrome. *J. Clin. Endocrinol. Metab.* 96 (9): 2796–2804.

35. Daniel, E., Aylwin, S., Mustafa, O. et al. (2015). Effectiveness of metyrapone in treating Cushing's

syndrome: a retrospective multicenter study in 195 patients. *J. Clin. Endocrinol. Metab.* 100 (11): 4146–4154.

36. Pivonello, R., De Leo, M., Cozzolino, A., and Colao, A. (2015). The treatment of Cushing's disease. *Endocr. Rev.* 36 (4): 385–486.

37. Daniel, E. and Newell-Price, J.D.C. (2015). Therapy of endocrine disease: steroidogenesis enzyme inhibitors in Cushing's syndrome. *Eur. J. Endocrinol.* 172 (6): R263–R280.

38. Fleseriu, M., Pivonello, R., Young, J. et al. (2016). Osilodrostat, a potent oral 11β-hydroxylase inhibitor: 22-week, prospective, Phase II study in Cushing's disease. *Pituitary* 19 (2): 138–148.

39. Bronstein, M., Machado, M., and Fragoso, M. (2015). Management of pregnant patients with Cushing's syndrome. *Eur. J. Endocrinol.* 173 (2): R85–R91.

40. Baudry, C., Coste, J., Khalil, R.B. et al. (2012). Efficiency and tolerance of mitotane in Cushing's disease in 76 patients from a single center. *Eur. J. Endocrinol.* 167 (4): 473–481.

41. Lindsay, J.R., Jonklaas, J., Oldfield, E.H., and Nieman, L.K. (2005). Cushing's syndrome during pregnancy: personal experience and review of the literature. *J. Clin. Endocrinol. Metab.* 90 (5): 3077–3083.

42. Luque-Ramírez, M., Ortiz-Flóres, A.E., Nattero-Chávez, L., and Escobar-Morreale, H.F. (2020). Apparent mineralocorticoid excess as a side effect of ketoconazole therapy in a patient with Cushing's disease. *Clin. Endocrinol.* 92 (1): 80–83.

43. Pivonello, R., Fleseriu, M., Newell-Price, J. et al. (2020). Efficacy and safety of osilodrostat in patients with Cushing's disease (LINC 3): a multicentre phase III study with a double-blind, randomised withdrawal phase. *Lancet Diabetes Endocrinol.* 8 (9): 748–761.

44. Manni, A. and Quarde, A. (2020). *Endocrine Pathophysiology: A Concise Guide to the Physical Exam*. Springer International Publishing.

45. Edwards, C.R. and Stewart, P.M. (1991). The cortisol-cortisone shuttle and the apparent specificity of glucocorticoid and mineralocorticoid receptors. *J. Steroid Biochem. Mol. Biol.* 39 (5B): 859–865.

46. Oakley, R.H. and Cidlowski, J.A. (2013). The biology of the glucocorticoid receptor: new signaling mechanisms in health and disease. *J. Allergy Clin. Immunol.* 132 (5): 1033–1044.

47. Weikum, E.R., Knuesel, M.T., Ortlund, E.A., and Yamamoto, K.R. (2017). Glucocorticoid receptor control of transcription: precision and plasticity via allostery. *Nat. Rev. Mol. Cell Biol.* 18 (3): 159–174.

48. Panettieri, R.A., Schaafsma, D., Amrani, Y. et al. (2019). Non-genomic effects of glucocorticoids: an updated view. *Trends Pharmacol. Sci.* 40 (1): 38–49.

49. Cadepond, F., Ulmann, A., and Baulieu, E.E. (1997). RU486 (mifepristone): mechanisms of action and clinical uses. *Annu. Rev. Med.* 48: 129–156.

50. Cohan, P. (2013). Pasireotide and mifepristone: new options in the medical management of cushing's disease. *Endocr. Pract.* 20 (1): 84–93.

51. Yuen, K.C.J., Moraitis, A., and Nguyen, D. (2017). Evaluation of evidence of adrenal insufficiency in trials of normocortisolemic patients treated with mifepristone. *J. Endocr. Soc.* 1 (4): 237–246.

52. Carmichael, J.D. and Fleseriu, M. (2013). Mifepristone: is there a place in the treatment of Cushing's disease? *Endocrine* 44 (1): 20–32.

53. Fleseriu, M., Biller, B.M.K., Findling, J.W. et al. (2012). Mifepristone, a glucocorticoid receptor antagonist, produces clinical and metabolic benefits in patients with Cushing's syndrome. *J. Clin. Endocrinol. Metab.* 97 (6): 2039–2049.

54. Hinojosa-Amaya, J.M., Cuevas-Ramos, D., and Fleseriu, M. (2019). Medical management of cushing's syndrome: current and emerging treatments. *Drugs* 79 (9): 935–956.

55. Fleseriu, M., Findling, J.W., Koch, C.A. et al. (2014). Changes in plasma ACTH levels and corticotroph tumor size in patients with Cushing's disease during long-term treatment with the glucocorticoid receptor antagonist mifepristone. *J. Clin. Endocrinol. Metab.* 99 (10): 3718–3727.

56. Fountas, A. and Karavitaki, N. (2020). Nelson's syndrome: an update. *Endocrinol. Metab. Clin. N. Am.* 49 (3): 413–432.

57. Shraga-Slutzky, I., Shimon, I., and Weinshtein, R. (2006). Clinical and biochemical stabilization of Nelson's syndrome with long-term low-dose cabergoline treatment. *Pituitary* 9 (2): 151–154.

58. van der Hoek, J., Lamberts, S.W.J., and Hofland, L.J. (2004). The role of somatostatin analogs in Cushing's disease. *Pituitary* 7 (4): 257–264.

59. Budayr, A., Tan, T.C., Lo, J.C. et al. (2020). Cardiac valvular abnormalities associated with use and cumulative exposure of cabergoline for hyperprolactinemia: the CATCH study. *BMC Endocr. Disord.* 20 (1): 25.

60. Blum, W.F., Alherbish, A., Alsagheir, A. et al. (2018). The growth hormone–insulin-like growth factor-I

axis in the diagnosis and treatment of growth disorders. *Endocr. Connect.* 7 (6): R212–R222.

61. Anderson, L.L. and Scanes, C.G. (2012). Nanobiology and physiology of growth hormone secretion. *Exp. Biol. Med.* 237 (2): 126–142.

62. Ranke, M.B. and Wit, J.M. (2018). Growth hormone - past, present and future. *Nat. Rev. Endocrinol.* 14 (5): 285–300.

63. de Fátima Borges, M., Teixeira, F.C.C., Feltrin, A.K. et al. (2016). Clonidine-stimulated growth hormone concentrations (cut-off values) measured by immunochemiluminescent assay (ICMA) in children and adolescents with short stature. *Clinics* 71 (4): 226–231.

64. Fazeli, P.K. and Klibanski, A. (2014). Determinants of growth hormone resistance in malnutrition. *J. Endocrinol.* 220 (3): R57–R65.

65. Mazziotti, G. and Giustina, A. (2013). Glucocorticoids and the regulation of growth hormone secretion. *Nat. Rev. Endocrinol.* 9 (5): 265–276.

66. Leung, K.-C., Johannsson, G., Leong, G.M., and Ho, K.K.Y. (2004). Estrogen regulation of growth hormone action. *Endocr. Rev.* 25 (5): 693–721.

67. Hawkes, C.P., Grimberg, A., Dzata, V.E., and De Leon, D.D. (2016). Adding glucagon-stimulated GH testing to the diagnostic fast increases the detection of GH-sufficient children. *Horm. Res. Paediatr.* 85 (4): 265–272.

68. Donaghy, A.J., Delhanty, P.J.D., Ho, K.K. et al. (2002). Regulation of the growth hormone receptor/binding protein, insulin-like growth factor ternary complex system in human cirrhosis. *J. Hepatol.* 36 (6): 751–758.

69. Domené, H.M., Hwa, V., Jasper, H.G., and Rosenfeld, R.G. (2011). Acid-labile subunit (ALS) deficiency. *Best Pract. Res. Clin. Endocrinol. Metab.* 25 (1): 101–113.

70. Poyrazoğlu, Ş., Hwa, V., Baş, F. et al. (2019). A novel homozygous mutation of the acid-labile subunit (IGFALS) gene in a male adolescent. *J. Clin. Res. Pediatr. Endocrinol.* 11 (4): 432–438.

71. Devesa, J., Almengló, C., and Devesa, P. (2016). Multiple effects of growth hormone in the body: is it really the hormone for growth? *Clin. Med. Insights Endocrinol. Diabetes* 9: 47–71.

72. Carmichael, J.D., Bonert, V.S., Nuño, M. et al. (2014). Acromegaly clinical trial methodology impact on reported biochemical efficacy rates of somatostatin receptor ligand treatments: a meta-analysis. *J. Clin. Endocrinol. Metab.* 99 (5): 1825–1833.

73. Gariani, K., Meyer, P., and Philippe, J. (2013). Implications of Somatostatin Analogues in the Treatment of Acromegaly. *Eur. Endocrinol.* 9 (2): 132–135.

74. McKeage, K. (2015). Pasireotide in acromegaly: a review. *Drugs* 75 (9): 1039–1048.

75. Dineen, R., Stewart, P.M., and Sherlock, M. (2017). Acromegaly. *QJM Int. J. Med.* 110 (7): 411–420.

76. Iacovazzo, D., Carlsen, E., Lugli, F. et al. (2016). Factors predicting pasireotide responsiveness in somatotroph pituitary adenomas resistant to first-generation somatostatin analogues: an immunohistochemical study. *Eur. J. Endocrinol.* 174 (2): 241–250.

77. Mayr, B., Buslei, R., Theodoropoulou, M. et al. (2013). Molecular and functional properties of densely and sparsely granulated GH-producing pituitary adenomas. *Eur. J. Endocrinol.* 169 (4): 391–400.

78. Amarawardena, W.K.M.G., Liyanarachchi, K.D., Newell-Price, J.D.C. et al. (2017). Pasireotide: successful treatment of a sparsely granulated tumour in a resistant case of acromegaly. *Endocrinol. Diabetes Metab. Case Rep.* 2017: 17-0067.

79. Gomes-Porras, M., Cárdenas-Salas, J., and Álvarez-Escolá, C. (2020). Somatostatin analogs in clinical practice: a review. *Int. J. Mol. Sci.* 21 (5): 1682. https://doi.org/10.3390/ijms21051682.

80. Gadelha, M.R., Bronstein, M.D., Brue, T. et al. (2014). Pasireotide versus continued treatment with octreotide or lanreotide in patients with inadequately controlled acromegaly (PAOLA): a randomised, phase 3 trial. *Lancet Diabetes Endocrinol.* 2 (11): 875–884.

81. Gadelha, M., Bex, M., Colao, A. et al. (2020). Evaluation of the efficacy and safety of switching to pasireotide in patients with acromegaly inadequately controlled with first-generation somatostatin analogs. *Front. Endocrinol.* 10: 931.

82. Waters, M.J., Shang, C.A., Behncken, S.N. et al. (1999). Growth hormone as a cytokine. *Clin. Exp. Pharmacol. Physiol.* 26 (10): 760–764.

83. Brooks, A.J., Wooh, J.W., Tunny, K.A., and Waters, M.J. (2008). Growth hormone receptor; mechanism of action. *Int. J. Biochem. Cell Biol.* 40 (10): 1984–1989.

84. Waters, M.J. and Brooks, A.J. (2015). JAK2 activation by growth hormone and other cytokines. *Biochem. J.* 466 (1): 1–11.

85. Dehkhoda, F., Lee, C.M.M., Medina, J., and Brooks, A.J. (2018). The growth hormone receptor: mechanism of receptor activation, cell signaling, and physiological aspects. *Front. Endocrinol.* 9: 35.

86. Chia, D.J. (2014). Minireview: mechanisms of growth hormone-mediated gene regulation. *Mol. Endocrinol.* 28 (7): 1012–1025.

87. Veldhuis, J.D., Bidlingmaier, M., Bailey, J. et al. (2010). A pegylated growth hormone receptor antagonist, pegvisomant, does not enter the brain in humans. *J. Clin. Endocrinol. Metab.* 95 (8): 3844–3847.

88. Trainer, P.J., Drake, W.M., Katznelson, L. et al. (2000). Treatment of acromegaly with the growth hormone-receptor antagonist pegvisomant. *N. Engl. J. Med.* 342 (16): 1171–1177.

89. Tritos, N.A. and Biller, B.M.K. (2017). Pegvisomant: a growth hormone receptor antagonist used in the treatment of acromegaly. *Pituitary* 20 (1): 129–135.

90. Giustina, A., Arnaldi, G., Bogazzi, F. et al. (2017). Pegvisomant in acromegaly: an update. *J. Endocrinol. Investig.* 40 (6): 577–589.

91. Hodish, I. and Barkan, A. (2008). Long-term effects of pegvisomant in patients with acromegaly. *Nat. Clin. Pract. Endocrinol. Metab.* 4 (6): 324–332.

92. Grottoli, S., Maffei, P., Bogazzi, F. et al. (2015). ACROSTUDY: the Italian experience. *Endocrine* 48 (1): 334–341.

93. Tritos, N.A., Mattsson, A.F., Vila, G. et al. (2020). All-cause mortality in patients with acromegaly treated with pegvisomant: an ACROSTUDY analysis. *Eur. J. Endocrinol.* 182 (3): 285–292.

94. Lu, M., Flanagan, J.U., Langley, R.J. et al. (2019). Targeting growth hormone function: strategies and therapeutic applications. *Signal Transduct. Target. Ther.* 4 (1): 3.

95. Vance, M.L., Kaiser, D.L., Frohman, L.A. et al. (1987). Role of dopamine in the regulation of growth hormone secretion: dopamine and bromocriptine augment growth hormone (GH)-releasing hormone-stimulated GH secretion in normal man. *J. Clin. Endocrinol. Metab.* 64 (6): 1136–1141.

96. Cooper, O. and Greenman, Y. (2018). Dopamine agonists for pituitary adenomas. *Front. Endocrinol.* 9: 469.

97. Lawton, N.F., Evans, A.J., and Weller, R.O. (1981). Dopaminergic inhibition of growth hormone and prolactin release during continuous in vitro perifusion of normal and adenomatous human pituitary. *J. Neurol. Sci.* 49 (2): 229–239.

98. Chanson, P. (2016). Medical treatment of acromegaly with dopamine agonists or somatostatin analogs. *Neuroendocrinology* 103 (1): 50–58.

99. Sandret, L., Maison, P., and Chanson, P. (2011). Place of cabergoline in acromegaly: a meta-analysis. *J. Clin. Endocrinol. Metab.* 96 (5): 1327–1335.

100. Cook, D.M., Ludlam, W.H., and Cook, M.B. (1999). Route of estrogen administration helps to determine growth hormone (GH) replacement dose in GH-deficient adults. *J. Clin. Endocrinol. Metab.* 84 (11): 3956–3960.

101. Janssen, Y.J., Helmerhorst, F., Frölich, M., and Roelfsema, F. (2000). A switch from oral (2 mg/day) to transdermal (50 microg/day) 17beta-estradiol therapy increases serum insulin-like growth factor-I levels in recombinant human growth hormone (GH)-substituted women with GH deficiency. *J. Clin. Endocrinol. Metab.* 85 (1): 464–467.

102. Molitch, M.E., Clemmons, D.R., Malozowski, S. et al. (2011). Evaluation and treatment of adult growth hormone deficiency: an endocrine society clinical practice guideline. *J. Clin. Endocrinol. Metab.* 96 (6): 1587–1609.

103. Lindberg-Larsen, R., Møller, N., Schmitz, O. et al. (2007). The impact of pegvisomant treatment on substrate metabolism and insulin sensitivity in patients with acromegaly. *J. Clin. Endocrinol. Metab.* 92 (5): 1724–1728.

104. Higham, C.E., Rowles, S., Russell-Jones, D. et al. (2009). Pegvisomant improves insulin sensitivity and reduces overnight free fatty acid concentrations in patients with acromegaly. *J. Clin. Endocrinol. Metab.* 94 (7): 2459–2463.

105. Freeman, M.E., Kanyicska, B., Lerant, A., and Nagy, G. (2000). Prolactin: structure, function, and regulation of secretion. *Physiol. Rev.* 80 (4): 1523–1631.

106. Saleem, M., Martin, H., and Coates, P. (2018). Prolactin biology and laboratory measurement: an update on physiology and current analytical issues. *Clin. Biochem. Rev.* 39 (1): 3–16.

107. Gorvin, C.M. (2015). The prolactin receptor: diverse and emerging roles in pathophysiology. *J. Clin. Transl. Endocrinol.* 2 (3): 85–91.

108. Brooks, C.L. (2012). Molecular mechanisms of prolactin and its receptor. *Endocr. Rev.* 33 (4): 504–525.

109. Liu, X., Tang, C., Wen, G. et al. (2019). The mechanism and pathways of dopamine and dopamine agonists in prolactinomas. *Front. Endocrinol.* 9: 768–768.

110. Shimazu, S., Shimatsu, A., Yamada, S. et al. (2012). Resistance to dopamine agonists in prolactinoma is

correlated with reduction of dopamine D2 receptor long isoform mRNA levels. *Eur. J. Endocrinol.* 166 (3): 383–390.

111. Molitch, M.E. (2005). Pharmacologic resistance in prolactinoma patients. *Pituitary* 8 (1): 43–52.

112. Vermeulen, E., D'Haens, J., Stadnik, T. et al. (2020). Predictors of dopamine agonist resistance in prolactinoma patients. *BMC Endocr. Disord.* 20 (1): 68.

113. Almalki, M.H., Alzahrani, S., Alshahrani, F. et al. (2015). Managing prolactinomas during pregnancy. *Front. Endocrinol.* 6: 85.

114. Huang, H.Y., Lin, S.J., Zhao, W.G., and Wu, Z.B. (2018). Cabergoline versus bromocriptine for the treatment of giant prolactinomas: A quantitative and systematic review. *Metab. Brain Dis.* 33 (3): 969–976.

115. Sabuncu, T., Arikan, E., Tasan, E., and Hatemi, H. (2001). Comparison of the effects of cabergoline and bromocriptine on prolactin levels in hyperprolactinemic patients. *Intern. Med. Tokyo Jpn.* 40 (9): 857–861.

116. Brichta, C.M., Wurm, M., Krebs, A. et al. (2019). Start low, go slowly – Mental abnormalities in young prolactinoma patients under cabergoline therapy. *J. Pediatr. Endocrinol. Metab.* 32 (9): 969–977.

117. Miura, J., Kikuchi, A., Fujii, A. et al. (2009). Pathological gambling associated with cabergoline in a case of recurrent depression. *Drug Discov. Ther.* 3 (4): 190–192.

118. Zamanipoor Najafabadi, A.H., Zandbergen, I.M., de Vries, F. et al. (2020). Surgery as a viable alternative first-line treatment for prolactinoma patients. a systematic review and meta-analysis. *J. Clin. Endocrinol. Metab.* 105 (3): e32–e41.

119. Sharma, S., Salehi, F., Scheithauer, B.W. et al. (2009). Role of MGMT in tumor development, progression, diagnosis, treatment and prognosis. *Anticancer Res.* 29 (10): 3759–3768.

120. Zhang, J., Stevens, M.F.G., and Bradshaw, T.D. (2012). Temozolomide: mechanisms of action, repair and resistance. *Curr. Mol. Pharmacol.* 5 (1): 102–114.

121. Cankovic, M., Nikiforova, M.N., Snuderl, M. et al. (2013). The role of MGMT testing in clinical practice: a report of the association for molecular pathology. *J. Mol. Diagn.* 15 (5): 539–555.

122. Whitelaw, B.C., Dworakowska, D., Thomas, N.W. et al. (2012). Temozolomide in the management of dopamine agonist–resistant prolactinomas. *Clin. Endocrinol.* 76 (6): 877–886.

123. Raverot, G., Sturm, N., de Fraipont, F. et al. (2010). Temozolomide treatment in aggressive pituitary tumors and pituitary carcinomas: a french multicenter experience. *J. Clin. Endocrinol. Metab.* 95 (10): 4592–4599.

124. Almalki, M.H., Aljoaib, N.N., Alotaibi, M.J. et al. (2017). Temozolomide therapy for resistant prolactin-secreting pituitary adenomas and carcinomas: a systematic review. *Hormones (Athens)* 16 (2): 139–149.

125. Khasraw, M., Bell, D., and Wheeler, H. (2009). Long-term use of temozolomide: Could you use temozolomide safely for life in gliomas? *J. Clin. Neurosci.* 16 (6): 854–855.

126. Kocova, M., Netkov, S., and Sukarova-Angelovska, E. (2001). Pituitary pseudotumor with unusual presentation reversed shortly after the introduction of thyroxine replacement therapy. *J. Pediatr. Endocrinol. Metab. JPEM* 14 (9): 1665–1669.

127. Khawaja, N.M., Taher, B.M., Barham, M.E. et al. (2006). Pituitary enlargement in patients with primary hypothyroidism. *Endocr. Pract. Off. J. Am. Coll. Endocrinol. Am. Assoc. Clin. Endocrinol.* 12 (1): 29–34.

128. Kostoglou-Athanassiou, I. and Ntalles, K. (2010). Hypothyroidism - new aspects of an old disease. *Hippokratia* 14 (2): 82–87.

129. Coopmans, E.C., van Meyel, S.W.F., Pieterman, K.J. et al. (2019). Excellent response to pasireotide therapy in an aggressive and dopamine-resistant prolactinoma. *Eur. J. Endocrinol.* 181 (2): K21–K27.

130. Jaquet, P., Ouafik, L., Saveanu, A. et al. (1999). Quantitative and functional expression of somatostatin receptor subtypes in human prolactinomas. *J. Clin. Endocrinol. Metab.* 84 (9): 3268–3276.

131. Ceccato, F., Lombardi, G., Albiger, N. et al. (2019). Temozolomide cytoreductive treatment in a giant cabergoline-resistant prolactin-secreting pituitary neuroendocrine tumor. *Anti-Cancer Drugs* 30 (5): 533–536.

132. Felker, J., Patterson, B., Wrubel, D., and Janss, A. (2016). Successful treatment of a child with a prolactin secreting macroadenoma with temozolomide. *J. Pediatr. Endocrinol. Metab. JPEM* 29 (12): 1413–1415.

133. Root, A.W. and Root, M.J. (2002). Clinical pharmacology of human growth hormone and its secretagogues. *Curr. Drug Targets Immune Endocr. Metabol. Disord.* 2 (1): 27–52.

134. Frayn, K.N., Coppack, S.W., Fielding, B.A., and Humphreys, S.M. (1995). Coordinated regulation of hormone-sensitive lipase and lipoprotein lipase in human adipose tissue in vivo: Implications for the control of fat storage and fat mobilization. *Adv. Enzym. Regul.* 35: 163–178.

135. Hjelholt, A.J., Søndergaard, E., Pedersen, S.B. et al. (2020). Growth hormone upregulates ANGPTL4 mRNA and suppresses lipoprotein lipase via fatty acids: Randomized experiments in human individuals. *Metabolism* 105: 154188.

136. Song, Z., Xiaoli, A.M., and Yang, F. (2018) Regulation and metabolic significance of de novo lipogenesis in adipose tissues. *Nutrients*, 10 (10): 1383. https://doi.org/10.3390/nu10101383.

137. Kopchick, J.J., Berryman, D.E., Puri, V. et al. (2020). The effects of growth hormone on adipose tissue: old observations, new mechanisms. *Nat. Rev. Endocrinol.* 16 (3): 135–146.

138. Nilsson, O., Marino, R., De Luca, F. et al. (2005). Endocrine regulation of the growth plate. *Horm. Res.* 64 (4): 157–165.

139. Shim, K.S. (2015). Pubertal growth and epiphyseal fusion. *Ann. Pediatr. Endocrinol. Metab.* 20 (1): 8–12.

140. Wallace, J.D., Cuneo, R.C., Bidlingmaier, M. et al. (2001). Changes in non-22-kilodalton (kDa) isoforms of growth hormone (GH) after administration of 22-kDa recombinant human GH in trained adult males. *J. Clin. Endocrinol. Metab.* 86 (4): 1731–1737.

141. Saugy, M., Robinson, N., Saudan, C. et al. (2006). Human growth hormone doping in sport. *Br. J. Sports Med.* 40 (Suppl 1): i35–i39.

142. Rezaei, M. and Zarkesh-Esfahani, S.H. (2012). Optimization of production of recombinant human growth hormone in *Escherichia coli. J. Res. Med. Sci. Off. J. Isfahan Univ. Med. Sci.* 17 (7): 681–685.

143. Díez, J.J., Sangiao-Alvarellos, S., and Cordido, F. (2018). Treatment with growth hormone for adults with growth hormone deficiency syndrome: benefits and risks. *Int. J. Mol. Sci.* 19 (3).

144. Souza, F.M. and Collett-Solberg, P.F. (2011). Adverse effects of growth hormone replacement therapy in children. *Arq. Bras. Endocrinol. Metabol.* 55 (8): 559–565.

145. Maison, P., Griffin, S., Nicoue-Beglah, M. et al. (2004). Impact of growth hormone (GH) treatment on cardiovascular risk factors in GH-deficient adults: a metaanalysis of blinded, randomized, placebo-controlled trials. *J. Clin. Endocrinol. Metab.* 89 (5): 2192–2199.

146. Ramos-Leví, A.M. and Marazuela, M. (2018). Treatment of adult growth hormone deficiency with human recombinant growth hormone: an update on current evidence and critical review of advantages and pitfalls. *Endocrine* 60 (2): 203–218.

147. Beauregard, C., Utz, A.L., Schaub, A.E. et al. (2008). Growth hormone decreases visceral fat and improves cardiovascular risk markers in women with hypopituitarism: a randomized, placebo-controlled study. *J. Clin. Endocrinol. Metab.* 93 (6): 2063–2071.

148. Swerdlow, A.J., Cooke, R., Beckers, D. et al. (2017). Cancer risks in patients treated with growth hormone in childhood: the SAGhE European cohort study. *J. Clin. Endocrinol. Metab.* 102 (5): 1661–1672.

149. Kim, S.-H. and Park, M.-J. (2017). Effects of growth hormone on glucose metabolism and insulin resistance in human. *Ann. Pediatr. Endocrinol. Metab.* 22 (3): 145–152.

150. Luger, A., Mattsson, A.F., KoŁtowska-Häggström, M. et al. (2012). Incidence of diabetes mellitus and evolution of glucose parameters in growth hormone–deficient subjects during growth hormone replacement therapy: a long-term observational study. *Diabetes Care* 35 (1): 57–62.

151. Ishunina, T.A. and Swaab, D.F. (1999). Vasopressin and oxytocin neurons of the human supraoptic and paraventricular nucleus; size changes in relation to age and sex. *J. Clin. Endocrinol. Metab.* 84 (12): 4637–4644.

152. Miyata, S. (2015). New aspects in fenestrated capillary and tissue dynamics in the sensory circumventricular organs of adult brains. *Front. Neurosci.* 9: 390.

153. Verbalis, J.G. (2007). How does the brain sense osmolality? *J. Am. Soc. Nephrol.* 18 (12): 3056–3059.

154. Terwel, D. and Jolles, J. (1994). The relationship between plasma osmolality and plasma vasopressin concentration is altered in old male Lewis rats. *Eur. J. Endocrinol.* 131 (1): 86–90.

155. Kanbay, M., Yilmaz, S., Dincer, N. et al. (2019). Antidiuretic hormone and serum osmolarity physiology and related outcomes: what is old, what is new, and what is unknown? *J. Clin. Endocrinol. Metab.* 104 (11): 5406–5420.

156. Bankir, L., Bichet, D.G., and Morgenthaler, N.G. (2017). Vasopressin: physiology, assessment and osmosensation. *J. Intern. Med.* 282 (4): 284–297.

157. Boone, M. and Deen, P.M.T. (2008). Physiology and pathophysiology of the vasopressin-regulated renal water reabsorption. *Pflugers Arch.* 456 (6): 1005–1024.

158. Elder, C.J. and Dimitri, P.J. (2017). Diabetes insipidus and the use of desmopressin in hospitalised children. *Arch. Dis. Child. Educ. Pract. Ed.* 102 (2): 100–104.

159. Vilhardt, H. (1990). Basic pharmacology of desmopressin. *Drug Investig.* 2 (5): 2–8.

160. Sawyer, W.H., Acosta, M., Balaspiri, L. et al. (1974). Structural changes in the arginine vasopressin molecule that enhance antidiuretic activity and specificity. *Endocrinology* 94 (4): 1106–1115.

161. Subramanya, A.R. and Ellison, D.H. (2014). Distal Convoluted Tubule. *Clin. J. Am. Soc. Nephrol.* 9 (12): 2147–2163.

162. McCormick, J.A. and Ellison, D.H. (2015). The distal convoluted tubule. *Compr. Physiol.* 5 (1): 45–98.

163. Bichet, D.G. (2018). Vasopressin and the regulation of thirst. *Ann. Nutr. Metab.* 72 (Suppl 2): 3–7.

164. García, E.B.G., Ruitenberg, A., Madretsma, G.S., and Hintzen, R.Q. (2003). Hyponatraemic coma induced by desmopressin and ibuprofen in a woman with von Willebrand's disease. *Haemophilia* 9 (2): 232–234.

165. Verrua, E., Mantovani, G., Ferrante, E. et al. (2013). Severe water intoxication secondary to the concomitant intake of non-steroidal anti-inflammatory drugs and desmopressin: a case report and review of the literature. *Hormones (Athens)* 12 (1): 135–141.

166. Garrahy, A., Moran, C., and Thompson, C.J. (2019). Diagnosis and management of central diabetes insipidus in adults. *Clin. Endocrinol.* 90 (1): 23–30.

167. Oiso, Y., Robertson, G.L., Nørgaard, J.P., and Juul, K.V. (2013). Treatment of neurohypophyseal diabetes insipidus. *J. Clin. Endocrinol. Metab.* 98 (10): 3958–3967.

168. Kataoka, Y., Nishida, S., Hirakawa, A. et al. (2015). Comparison of incidence of hyponatremia between intranasal and oral desmopressin in patients with central diabetes insipidus. *Endocr. J.* 62 (2): 195–200.

169. Barron, W.M., Cohen, L.H., Ulland, L.A. et al. (1984). Transient vasopressin-resistant diabetes insipidus of pregnancy. *N. Engl. J. Med.* 310 (7): 442–444.

170. Cadnapaphornchai, M.A., Summer, S.N., Falk, S. et al. (2003). Effect of primary polydipsia on aquaporin and sodium transporter abundance. *Am. J. Physiol.-Ren. Physiol.* 285 (5): F965–F971.

171. Leib, D.E., Zimmerman, C.A., and Knight, Z.A. (2016). Thirst. *Curr. Biol.* 26 (24): R1260–R1265.

172. Zimmerman, C.A., Leib, D.E., and Knight, Z.A. (2017). Neural circuits underlying thirst and fluid homeostasis. *Nat. Rev. Neurosci.* 18 (8): 459–469.

173. Fitzsimons, J.T. (1998). Angiotensin, thirst, and sodium appetite. *Physiol. Rev.* 78 (3): 583–686.

174. Saifan, C., Nasr, R., Mehta, S., Sharma Acharya, P., Perrera, I., Faddoul, G., Nalluri, N., Kesavan, M., Azzi, Y., and El-Sayegh, S. (2013). Diabetes insipidus: a challenging diagnosis with new drug therapies. *ISRN Nephrol.*, 2013:797620. https://doi.org/10.5402/2013/797620.

175. Cuesta, M., Hannon, M.J., and Thompson, C.J. (2017). Adipsic diabetes insipidus in adult patients. *Pituitary* 20 (3): 372–380.

176. Behan, L.A., Sherlock, M., Moyles, P. et al. (2015). Abnormal plasma sodium concentrations in patients treated with desmopressin for cranial diabetes insipidus: results of a long-term retrospective study. *Eur. J. Endocrinol.* 172 (3): 243–250.

177. Mistry, A.C., Wynne, B.M., Yu, L. et al. (2016). The sodium chloride cotransporter (NCC) and epithelial sodium channel (ENaC) associate. *Biochem. J.* 473 (19): 3237–3252.

178. Raisingani, M., Palliyil Gopi, R., and Shah, B. (2017). Use of chlorothiazide in the management of central diabetes insipidus in early infancy. *Case Rep. Pediatr.* 2017: 2407028.

179. Magaldi, A.J. (2000). New insights into the paradoxical effect of thiazides in diabetes insipidus therapy. *Nephrol. Dial. Transplant.* 15 (12): 1903–1905.

180. Loffing, J. (2004). Paradoxical antidiuretic effect of thiazides in diabetes insipidus: another piece in the puzzle. *J. Am. Soc. Nephrol.* 15 (11): 2948–2950.

181. Rivkees, S.A., Dunbar, N., and Wilson, T.A. (2007). The management of central diabetes insipidus in infancy: desmopressin, low renal solute load formula, thiazide diuretics. *J. Pediatr. Endocrinol. Metab. JPEM* 20 (4): 459–469.

182. Graziani, G., Fedeli, C., Moroni, L. et al. (2010). Gitelman syndrome: pathophysiological and clinical aspects. *QJM Mon. J. Assoc. Physicians* 103 (10): 741–748.

183. Al Nofal, A. and Lteif, A. (2015). Thiazide diuretics in the management of young children with central diabetes insipidus. *J. Pediatr.* 167 (3): 658–661.

184. Abraham, M.B., Rao, S., Price, G., and Choong, C.S. (2014). Efficacy of hydrochlorothiazide and low renal solute feed in neonatal central diabetes insipidus with transition to oral desmopressin in early infancy. *Int. J. Pediatr. Endocrinol.* 2014 (1): 11.

185. Moses, A.M., Howanitz, J., Gemert, M.V., and Miller, M. (1973). Clofibrate-induced antidiuresis. *J. Clin. Invest.* 52 (3): 535–542.

186. Abdallah, B., Hodgins, S., Landry, D. et al. (2018). Oxcarbazepine therapy for complete central diabetes insipidus. *Case Rep. Nephrol. Dial.* 8 (1): 20–24.

187. Kamiyama, T., Iseki, K., Kawazoe, N. et al. (1993). Carbamazepine-induced hyponatremia in a patient with partial central diabetes insipidus. *Nephron* 64 (1): 142–145.

188. Goel, A., Farhat, F., Zik, C., and Jeffery, M. (2018). Triphasic response of pituitary stalk injury following TBI: a relevant yet uncommonly recognised endocrine phenomenon. *Case Rep. Dermatol.* 2018: bcr-2018-226725.

189. Hoorn, E.J. and Zietse, R. (2010). Water balance disorders after neurosurgery: the triphasic response revisited. *NDT Plus* 3 (1): 42–44.

190. Capatina, C., Paluzzi, A., Mitchell, R., and Karavitaki, N. (2015). Diabetes insipidus after traumatic brain injury. *J. Clin. Med.* 4 (7): 1448–1462.

191. Loh, J.A. and Verbalis, J.G. (2008). Disorders of water and salt metabolism associated with pituitary disease. *Endocrinol. Metab. Clin. N. Am.* 37 (1): 213–234.

192. Eisenberg, Y. and Frohman, L.A. (2015). Adipsic diabetes insipidus: a review. *Endocr. Pract.* 22 (1): 76–83.

193. Dalan, R., Chin, H., Hoe, J. et al. (2019). Adipsic diabetes insipidus—The challenging combination of polyuria and adipsia: a case report and review of literature. *Front. Endocrinol.* 10: 630.

194. Verbalis, J.G., Goldsmith, S.R., Greenberg, A. et al. (2013). Diagnosis, evaluation, and treatment of hyponatremia: expert panel recommendations. *Am. J. Med.* 126 (10): S1–S42.

195. Izumi, Y., Miura, K., and Iwao, H. (2014). Therapeutic potential of vasopressin-receptor antagonists in heart failure. *J. Pharmacol. Sci.* 124 (1): 1–6.

196. Berl, T., Quittnat-Pelletier, F., Verbalis, J.G. et al. (2010). Oral tolvaptan is safe and effective in chronic hyponatremia. *J. Am. Soc. Nephrol. JASN* 21 (4): 705–712.

197. Peri, A. (2013). The use of vaptans in clinical endocrinology. *J. Clin. Endocrinol. Metab.* 98 (4): 1321–1332.

198. Schrier, R.W., Gross, P., Gheorghiade, M. et al. (2006). Tolvaptan, a selective oral vasopressin V2-receptor antagonist, for hyponatremia. *N. Engl. J. Med.* 355 (20): 2099–2112.

199. Cuesta, M., Ortolá, A., Garrahy, A. et al. (2017). Predictors of failure to respond to fluid restriction in SIAD in clinical practice; time to re-evaluate clinical guidelines? *QJM Int. J. Med.* 110 (8): 489–492.

200. Decaux, G., Waterlot, Y., Genette, F., and Mockel, J. (1981). Treatment of the syndrome of inappropriate secretion of antidiuretic hormone with furosemide. *N. Engl. J. Med.* 304 (6): 329–330.

201. Krisanapan, P., Vongsanim, S., Pin-On, P. et al. (2020). Efficacy of furosemide, oral sodium chloride, and fluid restriction for treatment of syndrome of inappropriate antidiuresis (SIAD): An open-label randomized controlled study (the effuse-fluid trial). *Am. J. Kidney Dis.* 76 (2): 203–212.

202. Finsterer, U., Beyer, A., Jensen, U. et al. (1982). The syndrome of inappropriate secretion of antidiuretic hormone (SIADH) – treatment with lithium. *Intensive Care Med.* 8 (5): 223–229.

203. Kazama, I., Arata, T., Michimata, M. et al. (2007). Lithium effectively complements vasopressin V2 receptor antagonist in the treatment of hyponatraemia of SIADH rats. *Nephrol. Dial. Transplant. Off. Publ. Eur. Dial. Transpl. Assoc. - Eur. Ren. Assoc.* 22 (1): 68–76.

204. Miell, J., Dhanjal, P., and Jamookeeah, C. (2015). Evidence for the use of demeclocycline in the treatment of hyponatraemia secondary to SIADH: a systematic review. *Int. J. Clin. Pract.* 69 (12): 1396–1417.

205. Pierrakos, C., Taccone, F.S., Decaux, G. et al. (2012). Urea for treatment of acute SIADH in patients with subarachnoid hemorrhage: a single-center experience. *Ann. Intensive Care* 2: 13.

206. Decaux, G., Gankam Kengne, F., Couturier, B. et al. (2018). Mild water restriction with or without urea for the longterm treatment of syndrome of inappropriate antidiuretic hormone secretion (SIADH): Can urine osmolality help the choice? *Eur. J. Intern. Med.* 48: 89–93.

207. Gross, P. (2012). Clinical management of SIADH. *Ther. Adv. Endocrinol. Metab.* 3 (2): 61–73.

208. Bartter, F.C. and Schwartz, W.B. (1967). The syndrome of inappropriate secretion of antidiuretic hormone. *Am. J. Med.* 42 (5): 790–806.

209. Chin, H.X., Quek, T.P., and Leow, M.K. (2017). Central diabetes insipidus unmasked by corticosteroid therapy for cerebral metastases: beware the case with pituitary involvement and hypopituitarism. *J. R. Coll. Physicians Edinb.* 47 (3): 247–249.

CHAPTER 2

Thyroid Gland Therapies

2.1 HASHIMOTO'S THYROIDITIS

2.1.1 Levothyroxine

2.1.1.1 Physiology

Types of Thyroid Hormones

Thyroid hormones are important regulators of various physiological processes, such as cellular growth and metabolism. The thyroid gland present in the anterior neck is responsible for the synthesis and secretion of thyroid hormones: thyroxine (T4) and triiodothyronine (T3).

First, T4 is the predominant thyroid hormone secreted by the thyroid gland, accounting for approximately 90% of endogenous total thyroid hormone production [1]. It should be noted that T4 is, in fact, a prohormone with relatively low biological activity compared to T3 [1, 2]. Structurally, T4 comprises four iodine atoms bound to a tyrosine-derived backbone. Most T4 is bound to carrier proteins, such as thyroxine-binding globulin (TBG), transthyretin, and albumin in circulation, with only a tiny fraction (approximately 0.03%) present as free thyroxine (FT4) [3]. Free T4 is the unbound form that can enter target cells and exert various intracellular effects.

On the other hand, T3, the biologically active thyroid hormone, accounts for almost 10% of the total endogenous thyroid hormone production [1]. T3 has approximately three to five times greater potency than T4 and is produced through peripheral deiodination.

T3 circulates bound to carrier proteins (mainly TBG and albumin), with a small fraction (approximately 0.3%) existing as free triiodothyronine (FT3). Free T3 exerts its effects by binding to its cognate intracellular thyroid hormone receptors (TRs) [3].

Reverse T3 (rT3) is an inactive metabolite of T4, generated by the action of type 3 deiodinase [4, 5], which selectively removes an iodine atom from the inner ring of T4 [5]. Although rT3 shares structural similarity with T3, it does not bind to thyroid receptors TRs with high affinity and, therefore, does not exhibit any significant biological activity. rT3 is a by-product of thyroid hormone inactivation and is clinically useful as an important marker of the sick euthyroid syndrome [6].

Transport of Thyroid Hormones in Plasma

As was previously mentioned, thyroid hormones, specifically T4 and T3 are bound to carrier proteins in the general circulation. These carrier proteins ferry thyroid hormones throughout the body, thus regulating their availability to target tissues. Indeed, more than 95% of thyroid hormones in serum are bound to three major carrier proteins, leaving a small, unbound

Endocrinology: Pathophysiology to Therapy, First Edition. Akuffo Quarde.
© 2024 John Wiley & Sons Ltd. Published 2024 by John Wiley & Sons Ltd.

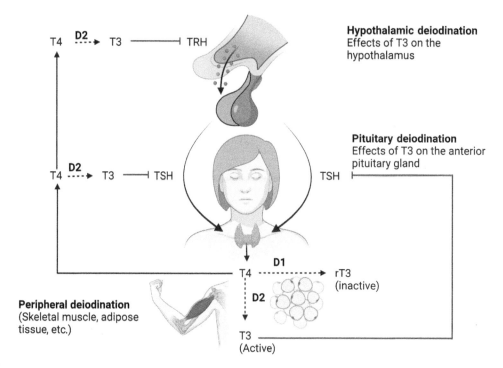

FIGURE 2.1   Role of deiodinases in the regulation of thyroid hormones. The role of various deiodinases (D1, D2, and D3) in regulating the hypothalamic-pituitary-thyroid axis. D2 is required to convert T4–T3 not only in peripheral tissues but also in the hypothalamus and pituitary gland.

fraction [2]. Thyroid-binding globulin (TBG) is the primary and most abundant carrier protein, which binds approximately 70% of T4 and 80% of T3 [7].

Transthyretin, or *thyroxine-binding prealbumin (TBPA)*, binds about 10–15% of T4 and a negligible proportion of T3 [8]. Finally, albumin, the most abundant protein in human serum, has the lowest affinity for thyroid hormone among all carrier proteins. Albumin binds approximately 15–20% of T4 and 5–10% of T3 [9]. Although albumin has a relatively lower affinity for thyroid hormones than TBG and transthyretin, its high concentration in the bloodstream means it plays a significant role in the transport of thyroid hormones.

Only a tiny fraction of T4 (approximately 0.03%) and T3 (approximately 0.3%) remains unbound or "free" in the serum [10]. The free fraction of total thyroid hormones in circulation is readily available for cell uptake, where it exerts its intracellular effects. In contrast, protein-bound thyroid hormones are considered a readily accessible store of thyroid hormones that are biologically inert [11].

Mechanisms of Thyroid Hormone Metabolism

Deiodination is the most significant pathway that metabolizes thyroid hormones and regulates T3

bioavailability in human tissues. The thyroid gland produces only a small amount of T3, while most of T3 (roughly 80%) in peripheral tissues is produced by enzymatic deiodination via outer ring deiodination (ORD) of T4. Similarly, the metabolite rT3 is produced through inner ring deiodination (IRD) of T4 [12, 13]. Hence, the metabolism of thyroid hormones by deiodinase enzymes results in either their activation or inactivation (see Figure 2.1).

2.1.1.2   Mechanism of Action

Levothyroxine (LT4) is a synthetic preparation of endogenous thyroid hormone T4, utilized for the treatment of hypothyroidism, irrespective of the underlying cause [14]. In order to exert its physiological effects, levothyroxine is converted by various deiodinases into the biologically active hormone T3. As a result, T3 interacts with nuclear TRs to ultimately modulate gene transcription [15] (see Figure 2.2).

Levothyroxine is converted to the active hormone T3 by the action of deiodinase enzymes, primarily type 1 (D1) and type 2 (D2) deiodinases [16, 17]. For example, type I deiodinase (D1), which is found predominantly in hepatic and renal tissues, is responsible for the conversion of the prohormone T4 to its

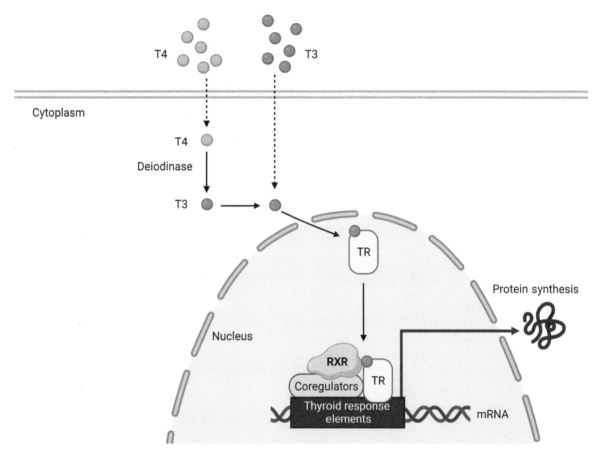

FIGURE 2.2   Intracellular effects of T3. T3 exerts its intracellular effects by binding to a nuclear thyroid hormone receptor. Along with retinoid X receptors and various coregulators, thyroid hormone facilitates the transcription of regulatory proteins required for metabolism.

biologically active form, T3 [10]. Furthermore, D1 converts T4 to rT3, its inactive metabolite [18].

Type 2 deiodinase (D2) is present mainly in the brain, pituitary gland, brown adipose tissue (BAT), skeletal muscle, and other peripheral tissues. D2 primarily converts T4 to T3 for intracellular use, thus playing a critical role in the local concentration of active thyroid hormone [4]. It is worth noting that negative feedback regulation of the hypothalamic-pituitary-thyroid (HPT) axis depends on T3 generated in the pituitary gland itself [19].

Once formed, T3 enters the nucleus of target cells and binds to nuclear TRs, which are members of the nuclear receptor superfamily. TRs form heterodimers with retinoid X receptors (RXR) and bind to specific DNA sequences called thyroid hormone response elements (TREs) located in the promoter regions of target genes [10, 20]. The thyroid hormone receptor that is already bound as a heterodimer with RXR (retinoid X receptors) binds to the specific TH response element

sequences (TRE) found in the promoter regions of T3 target genes in the nucleus and controls the expression of these genes in a ligand-dependent manner. On the contrary, unliganded TRs connect with TREs in T3 target genes and control transcriptional repression. In the absence of T3, corepressor proteins are recruited into the RXR-TR heterodimer and inhibit the expression of the target gene [21, 22]. Different types of mRNAs are produced as a result of transcription; these mRNAs then migrate from the nucleus into the cytosol, where they undergo translation to produce proteins [23] (refer to Figure 2.2).

Transcriptional regulation mediated by T3-bound TRs impacts various physiological processes, including basal metabolic rate (BMR), protein synthesis, carbohydrate and lipid metabolism, bone growth and development, and nervous system maturation [24, 25]. The net effect of levothyroxine treatment is restoring normal thyroid hormone levels and alleviating hypothyroid symptoms (Table 2.1).

Pathophysiology Pearl

TABLE 2.1 Altered thyroid hormone levels: effects on physiological functions.

System	Hypothyroidism	Hyperthyroidism
Basal metabolic rate (BMR) and temperature regulation	Low BMR Decreased body temperature Cold intolerance	High BMR Increased body temperature Heat intolerance
Carbohydrate metabolism	Decreased glucose metabolism	Increased glucose metabolism. Enhanced glycolysis and gluconeogenesis
Cardiac	Bradycardia and hypotension	Tachycardia and hypertension
Gastrointestinal (GI) tract	Decreased GI motility and smooth muscle tone	Increased GI motility
Hematopoietic	Anemia	—
Musculoskeletal	Slow relaxation of contracted muscle	Muscle atrophy

Source: Adapted from ref. [24].

Practice Pearl(s)

The dose of levothyroxine in treating hypothyroidism is highly variable, depending on the patient's comorbidities, body weight, and severity of hypothyroidism (overt or subclinical). In healthy young patients, the recommended full replacement dose of levothyroxine is (1.6 mcg/kg/day). This dose is suggested in athyroidal patients (e.g. postsurgical hypothyroidism) [26].

On the other hand, for elderly patients and subjects with known or suspected cardiovascular disease, "start low and go slow." These patients should start with levothyroxine (25–50 mcg/day). These can increase by 25 mcg/day every 4–6 weeks until TSH reaches the expected goal [27, 28]. Additionally, it is best to start 50–75% of the predicted full replacement dose of levothyroxine for patients with subclinical hypothyroidism [29].

Interpretation of Thyroid Function Tests

Circulating serum TSH levels exhibit a circadian rhythm reaching a nadir in the late afternoon and early evening, between 4 pm and 7 pm [30].

TSH levels are elevated even in very mild primary hypothyroidism and are suppressed to <0.1 µU/mL in mild hyperthyroidism. Consequently, a normal plasma TSH level effectively excludes hyperthyroidism and primary hypothyroidism. Furthermore, changes in plasma TSH tend to lag behind changes in plasma T4. For this reason, TSH levels can be misleading when plasma T4 levels are changing rapidly, as may occur during hyperthyroidism treatment or in the first few weeks after changes in the dose of T4 [31]. A schematic representation of the treatment targets in primary and secondary hypothyroidism is shown in Figure 2.3.

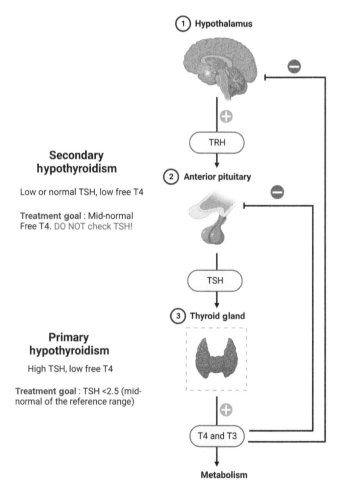

FIGURE 2.3 Comparison of treatment targets in primary and secondary hypothyroidism.

The TSH Goal for the Treatment of Primary Hypothyroidism

The goal of treatment for patients with primary hypothyroidism is the TSH range of 0.5–2.0 mU/L [32]. Historically, the conventional TSH range of 0.5–5 mU/L was based on a cohort of subjects that included those with antithyroid antibodies (occult autoimmune thyroid disease). For this reason, the "normal" range of TSH is thought to be skewed toward higher TSH values. In fact, when normal subjects without thyroid autoimmunity were evaluated, most had TSH values below the mid-normal point, that is, 2.5 mU/L [33].

Refer to Table 2.2 for important clinical pearls in managing primary hypothyroidism.

TABLE 2.2 Summary of treatment recommendations of primary hypothyroidism.

Plan	Recommendations
Initial dose	Low dose (25–50 mcg once daily), especially in the elderly and those with significant heart disease. Standard dose: 1.6 mcg/kg body weight (young, healthy patients). For subclinical hypothyroidism (high TSH, normal free T4) start with 50% of the weight-based estimate.
Dose adjustments	TSH should be checked every 6 weeks until TSH is at the goal. TSH goal <2.5 (not the typical reference range of 0.5–4.5).
Monitoring	After stabilization of thyroid function, check TSH every 6–12 months or if the clinical situation warrants it.
Conditions requiring escalating doses	Malabsorption (celiac disease), medications that alter LT4 absorption (divalent cations such as iron, magnesium, and calcium) are separated at least 4 hours from thyroid pills, medications that increase thyroxine metabolism (phenytoin, carbamazepine, rifampicin), Obesity, low protein states (nephrotic syndrome, severe chronic liver disease).
Conditions requiring lower doses	Recent significant weight loss.

Source: Adapted from [32].

2.1.2 Liothyronine

2.1.2.1 Physiology

Importance of Thyroid Hormone in Protein Synthesis

The primary mode of action involves binding of T3 (active thyroid hormone) to TRs, which function as nuclear transcription factors [35]. Once bound, the hormone receptor complex interacts with specific DNA sequences known as TREs on target genes. This interaction can either stimulate or repress the transcription of genes, ultimately influencing protein synthesis and degradation(see Figure 2.2) [36, 37].

In addition to their genomic effects, thyroid hormones can also have nongenomic actions on target cells. These effects are typically faster and do not involve direct interaction with DNA. An example of a non-genomic action of thyroid hormone is its role in stimulating amino acid transport into target cells. This process may involve the interaction of thyroid hormones with membrane-bound proteins or other components of the cell membrane, which influence the transport and availability of amino acids for protein synthesis [38].

Regulation of Metabolism

T3 crosses the plasma membrane of the targeted cells and binds to mitochondrial receptors, increasing adenosine triphosphate (ATP) production through oxidative phosphorylation. Furthermore, T3 in the nucleus activates genes involved in the transcription of various proteins involved in energy production. This effect of T3 is often called the "calorigenic effect of thyroid hormones" [39].

Furthermore, thyroid hormones play a crucial role in regulating various metabolic processes. Hyperthyroxinemia promotes a hypermetabolic state characterized by increased resting energy expenditure, weight loss, and decreased lipolysis. Conversely, hypothyroxinemia decreases resting energy expenditure, weight gain, and increased lipolysis [40].

Finally, thyroid hormone regulates carbohydrate metabolism through various effects. T3 enhances insulin-dependent glucose uptake into cells, gluconeogenesis, and glycogenolysis, leading to a net increase in plasma glucose [41].

Effects of Thyroid Hormones on Growth and Development

Thyroid hormone (TH) is crucial for healthy endochondral ossification, skeletal development, linear growth, bone mass maintenance, and optimal fracture repair [42]. Also, iodothyronine transporters and TRs are present in osteoblasts and osteoclasts, which are important cells involved in bone formation and remodeling [43].

Dysregulation of thyroid hormone production has differential effects on bone turnover. For example, hypothyroidism is characterized by a decrease in bone turnover and a prolonged remodeling phase of bone formation, leading to increased bone mass [44]. On the other hand, hyperthyroidism is associated with increased bone turnover and accelerated bone resorption. Consequently, hyperthyroxinemia promotes a decrease in bone mass and increases the risk of osteoporosis [45, 46].

Importance of Thyroid Hormones in thermogenesis

Thyroid hormones regulate the basal metabolic rate through their effects on thermogenesis, primarily in brown adipose tissue BAT. BAT, a specialized type of fat tissue, contains many mitochondria, essential in generating energy in the form of ATP (via oxidative phosphorylation). Interestingly, in BAT mitochondria, some of this energy is dissipated as heat [39]. The role of thyroid hormone in thermogenesis is shown in Figure 2.4.

2.1.2.2 Mechanism of Action

Liothyronine (LT3), a synthetic form of the endogenous thyroid hormone T3 is absorbed in the gastrointestinal tract and enters the systemic circulation after oral administration. T3 then enters target cells, primarily through thyroid hormone transporters, such as monocarboxylate transporter 8 (MCT8) and organic anion transport polypeptide 1C1 (OATP1C1) [51].

Once inside target cells, liothyronine, the biologically active form of thyroid hormone, binds directly to nuclear TRs. The intracellular effects of T3 were reviewed earlier (see Section 2.1.1)

Practice Pearl(s)

When Should You Consider Combination T4/T3 Therapy?

For patients who continue to experience subjective hypothyroid symptoms, a brief trial of a combination therapy consisting of levothyroxine and liothyronine may be considered [52, 53]. However, it is crucial to rule out other potential causes of fatigue, a common complaint of hypothyroid patients, prior to initiating a trial of dual LT3 and LT4.

When implementing the combination of levothyroxine (T4) and liothyronine (T3), a reasonable conversion factor is 25–50 mcg of levothyroxine to 5–10 mcg of liothyronine. For instance, the daily dose of levothyroxine can be decreased by 25 mcg when initiating liothyronine at a dose of 5 mcg, which should be administered in the morning [54].

It is important to note that for patients undergoing dual therapy, the TSH nadir, or the lowest point in the TSH levels, occurs approximately 10 hours after the administration of T3 [55]. Therefore, it is recommended to monitor TSH levels early in the morning before administering the liothyronine dose. This approach will provide a more accurate assessment of the patient's thyroid hormone status and allow for any necessary adjustments in the treatment plan.

Clinical Trial Evidence

The study aimed to evaluate the effects of combined levothyroxine and liothyronine (LT4/LT3) therapy in primary hypothyroidism patients. Using a randomized, double-blind, crossover design with 32 adult participants either continued on LT4 treatment or began dual LT4/LT3 therapy (75/15 µg/day) for 8 weeks, after which they switched treatments for an additional 8 weeks.

The study found that the combination therapy led to significantly lower free T4 levels compared to monotherapy, but TSH and T3 levels remained unaffected in both treatment arms. More patients on LT4/LT3 had T3 levels above the upper limit (15% vs. 3%). Additionally, there was an increase in heart rate, but no significant changes were observed in the electrocardiogram, arterial blood pressure, lipid profile, body weight, or quality of life of study participants. The study concluded that combination therapy did not yield significant clinical benefits. Dual levothyroxine and liothyronine are, therefore, not the standard treatment for primary hypothyroidism [56].

2.1.3 Selenium

2.1.3.1 Physiology

Role of Selenium in Thyroid Hormone Metabolism

Selenium is an essential trace element that regulates various physiological processes by acting as a key component of selenoproteins. These critical proteins contain a unique amino acid known as selenocysteine. Selenoproteins are involved in critical metabolic processes such as antioxidant defense, thyroid hormone metabolism, and redox signaling [57]. In regards to thyroid hormone metabolism, selenium is required

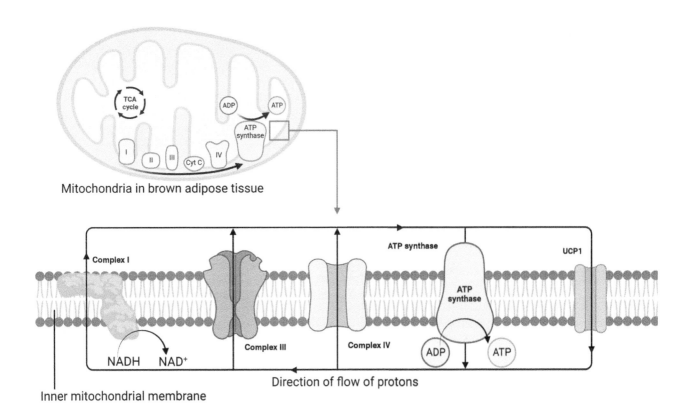

FIGURE 2.4 A simplified chemiosmotic proton circuit in BAT mitochondria. Electrons generated as a result of nutrient metabolism (e.g. fatty acids and glucose) are transferred along the electron transport chain (ETC), creating a proton gradient across the inner mitochondrial membrane. Protons accumulate in the intermembrane space before being transferred to the mitochondrial matrix. Indeed, instead of driving ATP synthesis, protons flow back into the mitochondrial matrix through a shuttle protein known as Uncoupling Protein 1 (UCP1). The energy of the proton flow is dissipated as heat, which contributes to thermogenesis [47]. T3 promotes the expression of UCP1, increasing the availability of uncoupling proteins in BAT mitochondria. This enhances the proton leak, which augments subsequent heat production. Furthermore, T3 stimulates lipolysis (the breakdown of triglycerides into free fatty acids), which serves as substrates for the production of energy and activators of UCP1 [48]. T3 also promotes the generation of new mitochondria in BAT, increasing the capacity of adipose tissue for heat production [49]. Finally, T3 interacts with the sympathetic nervous system, which releases norepinephrine, a hormone that stimulates thermogenesis in BAT [50].

for the optimal function of deiodinase enzymes (D1, D2, and D3), which are responsible for the activation and inactivation of thyroid hormones [58].

Role of Deiodinase Enzymes in Thyroid Hormone Regulation

Type 1 (D1), type 2 (D2), and type 3 (D3) iodothyronine deiodinases are the three known enzymes that catalyze the deiodination of thyroid hormone.

The outer ring deiodinase activity of D1 and D2 converts prohormone T4 into its bioactive form, T3 [59]. In contrast, D3 has inner ring deiodinase activity, which results in the degradation of T4 to rT3 and T3 to 3,3'-T2. Therefore, IRD is an inactivating pathway through which T4 and T3 are transformed to the metabolites rT3 and 3,3'T2, respectively, while ORD is an activating pathway through which the prohormone T4 is converted to active T3 [60].

To exert their catalytic action, all deiodinases require selenium; thus, defects in selenoprotein synthesis can result in abnormal thyroid hormone metabolism [61].

D1 was the first enzyme to be identified and cloned and is the only selenodeiodinase that has both ORD and IRD activities. Although D1 contributes a significant portion of T3 levels in human serum, the catalytic activity of D2 (for 5'-deiodination of T4) has been found to be 700-fold greater than that of D1 [62].

D2 is the main enzyme that causes the rapid rise in intracellular T3 levels in particular tissues [63, 64]. As serum T4 levels fall, T3 is preserved in important thyroid-responsive tissues such as the brain, skeletal muscle, and brown fat since D2 is highly expressed in these tissues. T3 is produced intracellularly by D2, which is then transported to the nucleus to regulate gene transcription [65].

Also, it has been shown that the placenta, the uterus during pregnancy, as well as several fetal tissues have significant D3 activity. The high D3 activity at these locations seems to protect fetal tissues from high T3 concentrations [60].

2.1.3.2 Mechanism of Action

In addition to its effects on the activity of deiodinase enzymes, selenium is a key component of several antioxidant selenoproteins, such as glutathione peroxidases (GPx) and thioredoxin reductases (TrxR) [66–68]. Selenium supplementation may enhance the activity of antioxidant selenoproteins, thus counteracting the oxidative stress generated in the setting of Hashimoto's thyroiditis [69, 70].

Practice Pearl(s)

There is a limited role for the use of selenium in the management of Hashimoto's thyroiditis (a cause of primary hypothyroidism). Historically its use in this condition has been mainly attributed to the importance of selenium in the functioning of deiodinase enzymes and antioxidant defense systems [71].

It is important to emphasize that selenium supplementation may not be beneficial for all patients with Hashimoto's thyroiditis and should be considered on an individual basis, taking into account factors such as baseline selenium status and the presence of comorbidities. Based on a recent Cochrane systematic review, there is no evidence to either support or refute the efficacy of selenium supplementation in Hashimoto's thyroiditis [72]. Further more, excessive selenium intake can be toxic and should be avoided [73].

Clinical Trial Evidence

Meta-analysis of various studies evaluating the clinical utility of selenium in hypothyroidism failed to show a benefit of selenium in the management of primary hypothyroidism, including Hashimoto's thyroiditis [73].

 Concepts to Ponder

Is Liothyronine Supplementation Suitable for Patients with Hypothyroidism?

Due to the increasing popularity of internet blogs, various patients are being exposed to incorrect information about thyroid hormone supplementation. Indeed, these "expert thyroid blogs" advocate for routine monitoring of free T3 levels in patients with primary hypothyroidism. Furthermore, a treat-to-target approach with liothyronine (LT3), which includes progressively escalating doses of thyroid hormone in order to "improve" free T3, is, unfortunately, being recommended by non-endocrinologists, in contrast to clinical practice guidelines.

Nonetheless, there are unique, rare circumstances where T3 supplementation is acceptable. Recent research indicates that individuals with hypothyroidism who possess a unique D2 gene variant (Thr92Ala) show an improvement in symptoms when treated with a combination of LT4 and LT3 therapy, as opposed to using T4 monotherapy. This suggests that the presence of this genetic variation may lead to a dysfunction in the conversion of T4 to T3 in both peripheral tissues and the brain [74].

2.2   GRAVES' DISEASE AND THYROID EYE DISEASE

2.2.1   Thionamides

2.2.1.1   Physiology

Mechanism of Thyroid Hormone Synthesis

Thyroid hormone synthesis is a highly regulated process that occurs in the thyroid gland, specifically within the thyroid follicular cells.

Sodium-iodide symporters (NIS) actively transport iodide ions from the bloodstream into thyroid follicular cells against a sodium electrochemical gradient, which is maintained by the sodium-potassium pump (Na+/K+-ATPase). This results in an elevated intrafollicular iodide concentration compared to the plasma.

Iodide ions are then transported to the apical membrane of the thyroid follicular cells by the action of pendrin, an anion exchanger protein. At the apical membrane of the thyroid follicular cell, the thyroid peroxidase (TPO) enzyme, in the presence of hydrogen peroxide (H_2O_2), catalyzes the oxidation of iodide to form reactive iodine species [75]. Subsequently, thyroglobulin (Tg), a large glycoprotein containing multiple tyrosine residues, is synthesized in the rough endoplasmic reticulum of thyroid follicular cells. After posttranslational modifications in the Golgi apparatus, Tg is secreted into the follicular lumen (colloid) through exocytosis.

Next, reactive iodine species generated at the apical membrane react with the tyrosine residues present on Tg, a process known as organification. This results in the formation of monoiodotyrosine (MIT) and diiodotyrosine (DIT), iodinated tyrosine derivatives [76].

TPO enzyme also catalyzes the coupling of iodotyrosines (MIT and DIT). The coupling of one DIT and one MIT yields T3, while the coupling of two DIT molecules produces tetraiodothyronine (T4, also known as thyroxine).

Colloid-containing iodinated Tg is internalized by the thyroid follicular cells through endocytosis. The colloid-laden endosomes fuse with lysosomes containing proteolytic enzymes, which cleave Tg and release T3 and T4 [77].

T3 and T4 are transported across the basolateral membrane of thyroid follicular cells into the perifollicular capillaries. Most T3 and T4 molecules circulate bound to carrier proteins, such as TBG, transthyretin, and albumin [78] (see Figure 2.5).

2.2.1.2   Mechanism of Action

Thionamides, mainly methimazole (MMI) and propylthiouracil (PTU), are a class of medications used in the treatment of hyperthyroidism. These drugs exert their effects at the level of the thyroid gland by inhibiting various critical steps in thyroid hormone synthesis [79, 80].

Thionamides primarily inhibit TPO, an essential enzyme in thyroid hormone synthesis. In normal physiology, TPO catalyzes the oxidation of iodide (I^-) to iodine (I_2) and the iodination of tyrosine residues on Tg to form MIT and DIT. Both MMI and PTU act as competitive inhibitors of TPO, preventing the enzyme from binding to its substrates and subsequently halting the formation of iodinated tyrosines [81].

Furthermore, TPO is responsible for coupling iodinated tyrosine residues, MIT and DIT, on Tg to form the thyroid hormones, T3 and T4. Thionamides interfere with this coupling process by inhibiting TPO, thereby reducing the synthesis of T3 and T4 within the thyroid gland [82].

PTU also blocks the peripheral conversion of T4 to T3 by type 1 and 2 deiodinase enzymes. By promoting a rapid decline in circulating T3 levels, PTU can be particularly beneficial in the management of severe hyperthyroidism as occurs in the setting of thyroid storm [83].

Finally, there is evidence that thionamide therapies may have immunomodulatory effects that contribute to their efficacy in the treatment of Graves' disease [84, 85]. Thionamides may reduce TSI levels and modulate T-cell function, potentially attenuating the autoimmune response and improving disease outcomes [86].

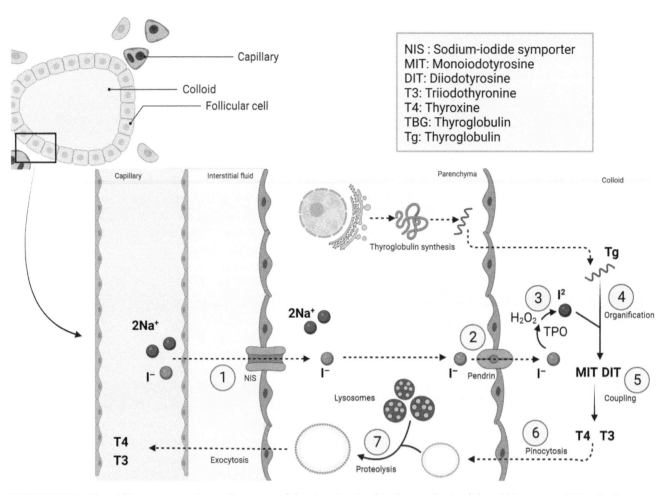

FIGURE 2.5 Thyroid hormone synthesis. Summary of the steps involved in the synthesis of thyroid hormone. NIS = Sodium iodide symporter, T4 = tetraiodothyronine, T3 = triiodothyronine, MIT = monoiodotyrosine (MIT), DIT = diiodotyrosine.

Practice Pearl(s)

A practical approach to treating hyperthyroidism is summarized in Table 2.3.

TABLE 2.3   Thionamide therapy in hyperthyroidism.

Management	Comments
Initial assessment	Evaluate the patient's clinical status, including signs and symptoms of hyperthyroidism. Assess the size of the thyroid gland through physical examination or imaging. Obtain baseline laboratory tests, including free T4, T3, TSH, and thyroid antibodies if applicable [87].
Initiation of methimazole	• The initial dose is based on free T4 levels and gland size, as follows: • Free T4 levels 1–1.5 times the upper limit of normal (ULN): Initiate with 5–10 mg of methimazole once daily. • Free T4 levels >1.5–2 times ULN (or iodine-induced thyrotoxicosis): Initiate with 10–20 mg of methimazole once daily. • Free T4 levels >2 times ULN: Initiate with 20–40 mg of methimazole daily [88].
Monitoring and adjusting therapy	• Monitor thyroid function tests (TFTs), including free T4, T3, and TSH, every 4–6 weeks during the initial phase of therapy. Adjust the methimazole dose based on TFTs and the patient's clinical response.

TABLE 2.3 (Continued)

Management	Comments
	• Once the patient achieves euthyroidism, gradually decrease the methimazole dose to the lowest effective maintenance dose (typically 5–20 mg daily) to minimize the risk of hypothyroidism. • Continue monitoring TFTs every 4–8 weeks during the maintenance phase, adjusting the methimazole dose as needed to maintain euthyroidism. • Regularly assess the patient for signs and symptoms of adverse effects, including hepatotoxicity and agranulocytosis.
Duration of therapy	• The duration of therapy depends on the underlying cause of hyperthyroidism, the patient's clinical response, and the development of adverse effects. • In patients with Graves' disease, methimazole therapy typically lasts 12–18 months, followed by a gradual tapering of the dose to assess for disease remission. • If hyperthyroidism relapses or is refractory to treatment, consider alternative therapeutic options, such as radioactive iodine ablation or thyroidectomy [89].

Source: Based on [87–89].

Clinical Trial Evidence

In this multicenter study carried out in 18 thyroid centers in Europe, the authors compared the safety and efficacy of two fixed doses of methimazole in the treatment of Graves' disease. 509 patients with Graves' disease were randomized to either 10 or 40 mg of methimazole along with levothyroxine supplementation. Although patients on the 40 mg dose of methimazole achieved euthyroidism faster compared to the 10 mg dose, relapse rates were equal between both groups. As expected, adverse drug reactions were notably higher in the 40 mg group compared to the 10 mg group [90].

2.2.2 Lugol's Iodine

2.2.2.1 Physiology

The mechanism of thyroid hormone synthesis was reviewed in Section 2.2.1.

2.2.2.2 Mechanism of Action

Lugol's iodine, also known as potassium iodide solution, is used in the management of Graves' disease and other hyperthyroid conditions as an adjunct therapy or preoperative treatment [91–93]. The mechanism of action of Lugol's iodine in Graves' disease is primarily attributed to the Wolff–Chaikoff effect. The Wolff–Chaikoff effect is a phenomenon where acute exposure to high concentrations of iodide leads to a temporary inhibition of thyroid hormone synthesis, thereby reducing the production of T4 and T3 [94]. Administration of Lugol's iodine therefore results in a rapid increase in plasma iodide concentration [95].

The high iodide levels are taken up by the thyroid gland via the NIS. The increased intrathyroidal iodide concentration inhibits the organification process, which is the incorporation of iodine into Tg, a crucial step in thyroid hormone synthesis. This inhibition occurs through the temporary suppression of the TPO enzyme, which is responsible for both the oxidation of iodide and the iodination of Tg [96].

The inhibition of the organification process leads to a decrease in the synthesis of T4 and T3. This transient suppression of thyroid hormone synthesis results in lower circulating levels of T4 and T3, thus alleviating the symptoms of hyperthyroidism [97].

The Wolff–Chaikoff effect is typically transient, lasting for a few days to a couple of weeks. The thyroid gland eventually escapes from the inhibitory effects of high iodide concentrations by downregulating the NIS, thus reducing the uptake of iodide. As a result, thyroid hormone synthesis resumes, albeit at a lower rate, which helps maintain a euthyroid state [98].

Practice Pearl(s)

The management guidelines for the use of potassium iodide in Graves' disease are outlined in Table 2.4

TABLE 2.4   Dosing suggestions for potassium iodide in Graves' disease.

Management	Comments
Preoperative stabilization	0.05–0.1 mL (1–2 drops, 50 mg/drop) every 8 hours
Acute management of thyroid storm	0.25 mL (5 drops) every 6 hours
Adjunct to radioactive iodine (RAI) therapy	0.15 mL (3 drops) every 12 hours

Source: Adapted from ref. [99].

Clinical Trial Evidence

There is limited clinical trial evidence showing the efficacy of iodine-containing solutions in the treatment of thyroid storm [100] or preoperative preparation for Graves' disease [101]. Nonetheless, potassium iodide has been shown to be efficacious in reducing the severity of hyperthyroidism when utilized as add-on therapy for patients exposed to radioiodine or thionamides.

In a randomized trial of 134 untreated patients with Graves' disease, a low dose of potassium iodide tablets (50 mg) or matching placebo was added to varying regimens of methimazole. The combination of potassium iodide with methimazole (15 or 30 mg) resulted in a normalization of free thyroxine levels in 54% and 59% of the patients respectively. However, only 27% and 29% of patients on monotherapy with methimazole achieved normal thyroxine levels on 15 mg and 30 mg of methimazole, respectively [102].

2.2.3   Iodide Transport Inhibitors

2.2.3.1   Physiology

The mechanism of thyroid hormone synthesis was reviewed in Section 2.2.1.

2.2.3.2   Mechanism of Action

Thiocyanate, an iodide uptake inhibitor, impedes iodide transport into thyroid follicular cells. As a result, thiocyanate reduces the availability of iodide for thyroid hormone synthesis, decreasing the production of thyroid hormones [103].

Thiocyanate and other iodide uptake inhibitors, such as perchlorate and pertechnetate, competitively inhibit the NIS by binding to the iodide binding site on the symporter [104]. These inhibitors share similar chemical properties to iodide, allowing them to compete for NIS binding. By binding to NIS, these inhibitors block the entry of iodide into the thyroid follicular cells, thus reducing the intracellular concentration of iodide available for thyroid hormone synthesis [105].

With reduced intracellular iodide concentrations, the essential steps of thyroid hormone synthesis, including the oxidation, organification, and coupling of iodide, are hindered [106, 107].

Practice Pearl(s)

These agents are not conventionally utilized in the treatment of Graves' disease.

Thiocyanate and other iodide uptake inhibitors can be used as adjunctive therapy in the management of hyperthyroidism, particularly during the preoperative preparation of patients for thyroidectomy or in cases of thyroid storm [108]. However, their use is typically limited to short-term treatment, as prolonged exposure to these inhibitors can lead to an escape phenomenon, in which the thyroid gland adapts to the reduced iodide availability and resumes hormone synthesis.

Clinical Trial Evidence

There are no clinical trials evaluating the effectiveness of these agents in Graves' disease.

2.2.4   Glucocorticoids

2.2.4.1   Physiology

See Section 3.1.1 for a review of glucocorticoid physiology.

2.2.4.2   Mechanism of Action

Firstly, glucocorticoids inhibit the conversion of T4, a prohormone, to its more biologically active form, T3 [95], through its suppressive effects on the activity of type 1 and type 2 deiodinase enzymes [109].

Also, glucocorticoid therapy is useful in the management of autoimmune conditions like Graves' disease complicated by thyroid storm [110]. These immunomodulatory effects can help to attenuate the autoimmune process underlying Graves' disease, potentially reducing the production of thyroid-stimulating immunoglobulins (TSIs), a key driver of hyperthyroidism [111].

Practice Pearl(s)

The typical dose of intravenous hydrocortisone is 100 mg every 6 hours. These can then be rapidly tapered off and discontinued when the patient's clinical condition improves [95].

Clinical Trial Evidence

Researchers conducted a retrospective nationwide cohort study in Japan which included 811 patients admitted for a thyroid storm. Of these, 600 were treated with glucocorticoids, and 211 were treated without glucocorticoids. The results showed no significant improvement in in-hospital mortality or 30-day mortality in the patients treated with glucocorticoids [112].

2.2.5   Selenium

2.2.5.1   Physiology

The role of selenium in thyroid hormone physiology has been previously reviewed.

2.2.5.2   Mechanism of Action

Selenium, an essential component of various antioxidant enzymes, such as GPx and thioredoxin reductase, is important in protecting cellular components from oxidative stress by neutralizing reactive oxygen species (ROS). In the context of thyroid eye disease (TED), excessive ROS production contributes to inflammation and tissue damage in the retroorbital region. Selenium enhances the antioxidant defense system in extrathyroidal tissue, thus reducing oxidative stress, limiting tissue damage, and mitigating the inflammatory response in the orbit [113].

Also, selenium promotes various immunomodulatory processes, such as T-cell proliferation and cytokine production. Indeed, there is evidence that selenium promotes the differentiation of T helper (Th) cells toward an anti-inflammatory Th2 phenotype while suppressing the more pro-inflammatory Th1 responses [114]. In TED, the immunomodulatory effects of selenium may contribute to the attenuation of the autoimmune process, reducing inflammation and potentially slowing disease progression [57].

Furthermore, selenium plays an essential role in thyroid hormone metabolism as a cofactor for deiodinase enzymes, as has been previously discussed. Therefore, by regulating thyroid hormone levels through its effects on deiodinases, selenium may indirectly impact the severity of TED [115, 116].

Finally, in TED, activated orbital fibroblasts contribute to the deposition of glycosaminoglycans (GAGs), leading to increased periorbital tissue volume and inflammation. Selenium has been shown to inhibit both the activation of orbital fibroblasts and the deposition of GAGs in periorbital tissues. This suggests selenium's potential protective effect against the tissue remodeling that occurs in TED [117].

Practice Pearl(s)

The typical dose of selenium used in the treatment of thyroid eye disease is 100mcg twice daily [118].

Clinical Trial Evidence

In this clinical trial, individuals over the age of 18 who were experiencing mild Graves' orbitopathy (GO) were randomized to a placebo or selenium. The active arm of the study received 100 µg selenium tablets twice a day for 6 months, while the comparator arm was placed on placebo. Researchers examined the patients using the clinical activity score (CAS) for GO prior to treatment and again after the first, third, and sixth months of treatment.

After 6 months, the group supplemented with selenium demonstrated meaningful improvements

(continued)

(continued)

in both palpebral fissure and clinical activity scores. In contrast, the placebo group had no significant difference in CAS scores.

Supplements of selenium taken orally have proven effective at stalling progression and reducing clinical activity in those with mild GO, according to this study [119].

2.2.6   Beta-Blockers

2.2.6.1   Physiology

Elevated levels of thyroid hormone (primarily T3) have various cardiac effects.

A summary of the cardiac effects of thyroid hormone includes the following:

1. It prolongs myocardial sodium channel activation, increasing intracellular sodium and stimulating the sodium–calcium antiport system. This raises intramyocardial calcium and promotes contractility [120].

2. T3 upregulates β1 adrenergic receptor expression in the myocardium and kidney juxtaglomerular cells (JGCs). Catecholamine activation of β1 receptors in JGCs releases renin, activating the renin-angiotensin-aldosterone system (RAAS), leading to sodium and fluid retention, which increases cardiac preload and contractility [120].

3. T3 binds to TREs, promoting calcium adenosine triphosphatase (Ca-ATPase) transcription and translation in the myocardial sarcoplasmic reticulum. This increases intramuscular calcium concentration, enhancing T3's inotropic effects [121].

4. T3 exerts a positive inotropic effect on cardiac muscle by directly activating myocardial L-type calcium channels, increasing myocardial calcium uptake [122].

5. T3 upregulates a myocardial gap junction protein important for electrical impulse transmission, which has been linked to hyperthyroidism-induced atrial fibrillation [123].

6. T3's effects include reduced cardiac parasympathetic tone and increased tissue sensitivity to circulating catecholamines [124].

2.2.6.2   Mechanism of Action

It is important to note that beta-blockers, including propranolol, are used as supportive therapy to manage symptoms and are not a definitive treatment for thyroid storm or severe Graves' disease. The primary treatment for these conditions involves addressing the underlying cause, such as antithyroid medications, radioactive iodine therapy, or surgery.

The mechanism of action of beta blockers in hyperthyroidism is shown in Figure 2.6.

Propranolol, when taken in high doses, inhibits type 1 deiodinase, which is the enzyme that converts

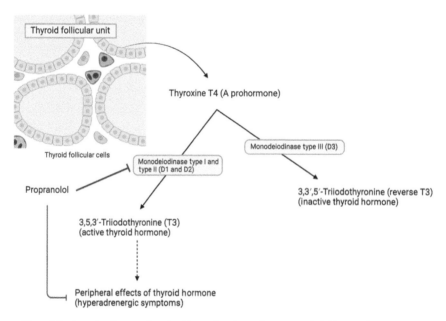

FIGURE 2.6   Effects of beta-blockers in thyrotoxicosis. Sites of action of propranolol (the preferred beta-blocker) in patients with hyperthyroidism.

T4–T3, the active form of T3. This can reduce the level of T3, a key contributor to symptoms in these conditions [126].

Propranolol and other beta-blockers can calm the central nervous system by crossing the blood–brain barrier [127]. This can alleviate symptoms such as anxiety, nervousness, and tremors, which are common among patients with Graves' disease or thyroid storm [128].

Beta-blockers may also reduce peripheral resistance by blocking beta-2 receptors. This can lower blood pressure and increase blood flow for patients with Graves' disease or thyroid storm [120].

Propranolol, a beta-blocker that blocks cardiac beta-1 receptors, reduces heart rate (chronotropy) as well as the force of heart contractions(inotropy). This can relieve symptoms like palpitations and tachycardia that are common with Graves' or thyroid storm [129].

Practice Pearl(s)

In patients with thyroid storm, treatment typically begins with a beta-blocker, such as propranolol, to adequately control heart rate and blood pressure. Beta-blockers are contraindicated in patients with systolic dysfunction. Furthermore, caution is advised when administering beta-blockers to patients with asthma or severe peripheral vascular disease (review the effects of adrenergic receptor activation in Table 2.5) [129].

In patients with reactive airway disease, more cardioselective beta-blockers like metoprolol or atenolol are preferred [130]. Nonetheless, for patients with severe asthma, where beta-blockers are relatively contraindicated, calcium channel blockers can be employed to achieve rate control [131].

Propranolol is administered in doses of 60–80 mg every 4 hours, with the cardiac function closely monitored. Propranolol can also be administered intravenously as a slow, 10-minute bolus, followed by 1–3 mg doses scheduled every 4 hours. This should only be done in a monitored setting [132].

TABLE 2.5   Location of adrenergic receptors and the effects of catecholamines.

Adrenergic receptor (location)	Cardiac-specific effects
α1 adrenergic receptor (smooth muscle of vessels)	• Increases peripheral vasoconstriction. • Positive inotropy.
α2 adrenergic receptor (presynaptic area of sympathetic ganglia and smooth muscles)	• Promotes arterial vasodilation
β1 adrenergic receptors (cardiac muscle)	Positive inotropy Positive chronotropy Promotes the release of renin by juxtaglomerular cells.
β2 adrenergic receptors (sympathetic ganglia and smooth muscles)	Vasodilation Promotes the release of norepinephrine by sympathetic ganglia.
D1 dopaminergic receptor (kidney vasculature)	Promotes vasodilation of renal arteries.
D2 dopaminergic receptor (presynaptic neurons)	Negative inotropy via its effects on sympathetic neurons (inhibits the release of norepinephrine).

Source: Adapted from ref. [125].

Clinical Trial Evidence

The study aimed to determine the effects of beta-blockers on antithyroid drug treatment in patients who have mild Graves' Disease (GD). The authors randomly assigned 28 patients to either receive methimazole with or without beta-blockers (14 patients: 1 woman, 13 men). The groups did not differ in the improvement of thyroid function, but beta-blockers caused a greater decrease in heart rate. Only the beta-blocker group showed significant improvement in "physical functioning," as measured by SF36 questionnaires. The authors concluded beta-blockers can reduce heart rate and alleviate specific symptoms in patients with mild GD. They however did not improve thyroid function tests [133].

2.2.7   Cholestyramine

2.2.7.1   Physiology

See Section 7.1.1.

2.2.7.2   Mechanism of Action

Cholestyramine binds to bile acids in the intestine, forming an insoluble complex that is excreted via the enteric route. This interrupts the enterohepatic circulation of not only bile acids but also thyroid hormone, which is dependent on the biliary system for its enterohepatic cycling [134].

Practice Pearl(s)

Since cholestyramine interferes with the enterohepatic circulation of bile, other oral medications will need to be administered either 2 hours before or after its administration. It is typically administered orally at a dose of 4 g every 6 hours [135].

Clinical Trial Evidence

This study evaluated the effectiveness of combining cholestyramine and propylthiouracil in the treatment of Graves' hyperthyroidism. The authors randomized 30 patients into two groups. Group I received propranolol and cholestyramine, while Group II received propranolol and PTU. After 2 and 4 weeks, the serum total T3 (TT3) levels in Group I were significantly lower than those of Group II. The authors concluded that cholestyramine is an effective and well-tolerated adjunctive treatment of Graves' hyperthyroidism [136].

2.2.8   Lithium

2.2.8.1   Physiology

See Section 2.2.1 to review thyroid hormone synthesis.

2.2.8.2   Mechanism of Action

Hyperthyroidism can be treated with lithium, an agent that is primarily used for treating bipolar disorder.

Lithium competes against iodine for uptake by the NIS present on thyroid follicular cells. This results in a reduced availability of iodine for thyroid hormone synthesis [137]. Furthermore, lithium can inhibit thyroid hormone production by interfering with the coupling reaction between various iodotyrosines, a critical step in the formation of T4 and T3 [138].

Lithium can also suppress TPO activity, an enzyme responsible for the oxidation and organification of iodine [139].

Lastly, lithium can also reduce the peripheral conversion of T4 to the more biologically active thyroid hormone, T3. Lithium exerts this effect by blocking the deiodinase enzyme needed for the deactivation of T3 [139].

Practice Pearl(s)

Lithium, at doses of 600–1000 mg/day, is an effective alternative for hyperthyroidism treatment in patients allergic to iodine or intolerant of thionamides. Its effects on thyroid hormone secretion are similar to iodide [138]. Indeed, lithium prolongs radioiodine retention within the thyroid gland, potentially increasing the effectiveness of radioiodine therapy.

Clinical Trial Evidence

This study examined the clinical effects of lithium carbonate in patients with Graves' disease (GD) in the setting of hepatic injury or leukopenia, for which thionamide therapies are relatively contraindicated. 51 patients received lithium carbonate in combination with hepatoprotective medications or medications that increase the white blood cell count. After 36 weeks, thyroid hormone levels and liver function tests improved. At the 1-year follow-up, 23.5% of patients achieved remission. The study concluded lithium carbonate effectively treated mild-to-moderate hyperthyroidism due to GD, particularly for patients with hepatic injury or leukopenia [140].

2.2.9 Teprotumumab

2.2.9.1 Physiology

Thyroid eye disease, also known as Graves' ophthalmopathy, is an autoimmune inflammatory condition primarily affecting extraocular muscle, periorbital fat, and connective tissues surrounding the orbits. Next, we will briefly review the mechanisms underlying the development of this ocular complication of Graves' disease.

Firstly, in patients with Graves' disease, the production of autoantibodies that target the thyroid-stimulating hormone receptor (TSHR) cross-react with other tissues, for example, orbital fibroblasts which express the TSHR and insulin-like Growth Factor-1 receptor (IGF-1R). These receptors are activated by TSHR antibodies, which trigger an inflammatory cascade that promotes the remodeling of periorbital soft tissues [141].

Furthermore, the activated orbital fibroblasts also produce an extracellular matrix, mainly GAGs and collagen. These components contribute to the remodeling of tissue in the orbital fossa. Indeed, the deposition of collagen leads to soft tissue fibrosis, whereas the accumulation of GAGs results in increased tissue swelling, changes that may cause significant expansion of the extraocular muscle and orbital fat. These extensive changes in the periorbital tissues culminate in the pathognomonic feature of exophthalmos [142].

These changes can cause enlargement of the extraocular muscles and expansion of the orbital fat, leading to proptosis (bulging of the eyes) and other characteristic features of TED [143].

Additionally, the lymphatic drainage system of the orbit may be compromised in TED due to inflammation or fibrosis. This can lead to an increase in interstitial fluid, further exacerbating periorbital swelling [143].

While the exact etiology is yet to be fully characterized, it is postulated that both genetic and environmental factors play a part in the pathogenesis of TED. Most importantly, environmental factors such as smoking have also been shown to exacerbate this disease [144, 145]. These mechanisms contribute collectively to the characteristic TED features, such as proptosis and orbital swelling.

2.2.9.2 Mechanism of Action

Teprotumumab is a human monoclonal antibody that targets the IGF-1R and has shown clinical benefits for patients with TED. Teprotumumab binds to IGF-1R and blocks its activation by TSH receptor antibodies and IGF-1. This treatment offers a novel way to treat this complicated disease [146].

Graves' disease-specific autoantibodies, that is, TSH receptor antibodies, can react with orbital fibroblasts that express thyroid-stimulating hormonal receptors (TSHR) and IGF-1R. TSH autoantibodies or endogenous insulin-like growth factors-1 (IGF-1) activate IGF-1R on orbital fibroblasts, stimulating signaling cascades that promote inflammation, tissue remodeling, and fibrosis [142, 147, 148].

Practice Pearl(s)

An intravenous infusion of teprotumumab (10 mg/kg initially, followed by 20 mg/kg for subsequent doses) is administered every 3 weeks for a total of 8 doses [149].

Clinical Trial Evidence

In this study, authors investigated the effectiveness of IGF-IR inhibitor teprotumumab in patients with active thyroid eye disease in a randomized double-blind placebo-controlled phase 3 multicenter study. Participants received intravenous teprotumumab infusions or placebo every 3 weeks over a 21-week period. The primary outcome at week 24 was a response to proptosis. At week 24, 83% in the teprotumumab-treated group showed a response to proptosis compared with 10% in the placebo-treated group. All secondary outcomes, including overall response, Clinical Activity Score, diplopia response, and Graves' ophthalmopathy-specific quality-of-life GO-QOL overall score, showed significant improvement in the teprotumumab group. Most adverse events were mild to moderate, with only two serious events occurring in the teprotumumab-treated group. The authors concluded that patients with active thyroid eye disease who received teprotumumab had better outcomes than those receiving placebo [150].

Concepts to Ponder

What Is the Pathophysiologic Basis for Upper Eyelid Retraction in Graves' Disease?

Under the sympathetic stimulation caused by excess circulating thyroid hormones, Muller's (superior-tarsal) muscle contracts and contributes toward lid retraction [151].

The levator palpebrae superioris muscle is infiltrated with inflammatory cells due to extensive orbital inflammation. This leads to its fibrosis and contraction [151].

2.3   RIEDEL'S THYROIDITIS

2.3.1   Glucocorticoids

2.3.1.1   Physiology

Read Chapter 3 for the effects of glucocorticoids on metabolism.

2.3.1.2   Mechanism of Action

Riedel's thyroiditis (RT), a rare chronic inflammatory condition, is characterized by dense fibrosis that replaces normal thyroid tissue. The fibrotic process may extend beyond the thyroid gland and causes compression of surrounding structures. RT is not known to have a specific cause. It is however considered a fibrosing form of Hashimoto thyroiditis or an IgG4-related disease [152].

Glucocorticoids, such as prednisone, are often used in the management of RT. Exogenous steroids suppress the production of inflammatory mediators involved in the pathogenesis of this condition [153, 154].

Practice Pearl(s)

Glucocorticoids have been effective in reducing thyroid enlargement in some Riedel's thyroiditis patients, particularly when initiated early in the disease course. Long-term treatment is typically required, as disease recurrence may occur upon dose tapering. Oral prednisone 40 mg daily for 3 months or more [152].

Clinical Trial Evidence

This systematic review and meta-analysis examined RT presentation, management, and outcomes. Data from 212 patients showed common symptoms, including neck swelling, dyspnea, and neck pain. Elevated inflammatory markers were observed in 70–97% of cases, while thyroid antibody positivity was present in less than 50%. Most patients underwent surgical intervention, with total thyroidectomy being the most common. Glucocorticoids were used in 70% of cases, with a median duration of 3 months. The prognosis was generally favorable, with 90% experiencing symptom resolution or improvement. This analysis offers valuable insights for clinicians regarding RT presentation and management [155].

2.3.2   Rituximab

2.3.2.1   Physiology

B cells are essential components of the immune system and play a crucial role in the pathophysiology of autoimmune disorders. In autoimmune diseases, the immune system mistakenly targets and attacks the body's own cells and tissues, leading to inflammation and tissue damage [156].

B cells produce and secrete antibodies, which can recognize specific antigens on foreign pathogens. However, in autoimmune diseases, B cells produce autoantibodies that mistakenly target self-antigens, leading to tissue damage and inflammation [157].

Also, B cells can act as antigen-presenting cells (APCs) by capturing and processing self-antigens and presenting them to T cells. This interaction can lead to the activation of autoreactive T cells, which can contribute to the pathogenesis of autoimmune diseases [158].

Furthermore, B cells can produce and secrete various cytokines, including pro-inflammatory and anti-inflammatory cytokines, that modulate the immune response. In autoimmune disorders, B cells may contribute to the inflammatory environment by secreting pro-inflammatory cytokines, such as interleukin (IL)-6 and tumor necrosis factor (TNF)-α [159].

Indeed, in some autoimmune diseases, B cells can promote the differentiation of autoreactive Th cells, such as Th1, Th2, and Th17 cells, which can exacerbate inflammation and tissue damage [160].

Finally, B cells can form ectopic lymphoid structures within target tissues, leading to a localized immune response and tissue destruction [161].

2.3.2.2 Mechanism of Action

Although rituximab has not been extensively studied for the treatment of RT, the mechanism of its action in other autoimmune or inflammatory conditions may suggest potential benefits for RT patients.

Rituximab binds CD20 on B cell surfaces, causing their depletion by various mechanisms such as cellular cytotoxicity, and apoptosis [126]. Rituximab can reduce the production of autoantibodies by depleting the B cells.

B cells, by interacting with T cells, play a direct role in the activation and differentiation of T cells [127]. Rituximab, by depleting B cells, can indirectly affect T-cell responses, thereby decreasing inflammation and autoimmunity in RT [128].

Finally, B cells secrete and produce pro-inflammatory cytokines, which contribute to inflammation in autoimmune diseases [129]. The cytokines can be reduced by rituximab, which leads to a decrease in inflammation in RT.

Practice Pearl(s)

Intravenous Rituximab (375 mg/m²) was administered monthly over a three-month period [162].

Clinical Trial Evidence

There are no large or well-powered studies evaluating the efficacy of rituximab in Graves' disease. There are, however, a few published cases of off-label utilization of rituximab [162–164].

 Concepts to Ponder

Effects of Smoking on the Clinical Course of Thyroid Eye Disease

The relationship between smoking and thyroid eye disease (TED) has been extensively investigated, with numerous studies highlighting the detrimental effects of smoking on the clinical course and management of TED [144, 165]. Smoking has been shown to exacerbate the severity of TED by promoting orbital inflammation, increasing proptosis, and worsening diplopia [165]. These clinical manifestations can significantly impair patients' quality of life and increase the risk of sight-threatening complications, such as optic neuropathy [144].

The pathophysiological mechanisms underlying the relationship between smoking and TED are complex and multifactorial. One proposed mechanism involves the direct toxic effects of cigarette smoke on orbital fibroblasts, inducing an inflammatory response and the production of cytokines, which can lead to the activation of orbital fibroblasts and the expansion of orbital adipose/connective tissues [142]. Smoking may also increase the risk of Graves' disease by stimulating autoantibodies to the thyrotropin receptor [166].

Considering the significant role of smoking in the pathophysiology and clinical course of TED, it is crucial for physicians to address smoking cessation as a key component of disease management. Smoking cessation interventions such as nicotine replacement therapy and pharmacological agents, like varenicline and bupropion, can improve patient outcomes and reduce the risk for sight-threatening complications [167].

2.4 THYROID HORMONE RESISTANCE

2.4.1 Beta-Blockers

2.4.1.1 Physiology

Overview of Thyroid Hormone Receptor Isoforms

TRs are a group of nuclear receptors involved in the actions of thyroid hormones (THs) in target cells [22]. TRs regulate metabolism, growth, and development in normal physiology [21]. TRs exist in multiple isoforms, encoded by two distinct genes: THRA (encoding TRα) and THRB (encoding TRβ) [168]. The expression and function of these isoforms vary quite widely across different tissues, contributing to the diversity of effects of THs in the body [169].

The THRA gene encodes two major isoforms: TRα1 and TRα2. TRα1 is the predominant isoform and is the functional intracellular receptor for THs, binding to TREs present in target genes [170]. Furthermore, TRα1 is widely expressed in tissues such as the brain, heart, and skeletal muscle [171]. Consequently, TRα1 plays a key role in regulating heart rate, cardiac output, and skeletal muscle function [172].

Unlike TRα1, TRα2 does not bind THs, acting predominantly as a negative regulator of TRα1 function [173]. The tissue expression of TRα2 is more restricted compared to TRα1, with high levels of the former being found primarily in the brain. Nonetheless, the exact physiological roles of TRα2 are yet to be elucidated [10].

The THRB gene encodes two major isoforms, these are TRβ1 and TRβ2. Both isoforms bind THs and regulate target gene transcription [41]. TRβ1 is predominantly expressed in the liver, kidneys, and thyroid gland, playing a key role in the regulation of metabolism, cholesterol homeostasis, and thyroid hormone synthesis [10]. TRβ2 is mainly found in the hypothalamus, pituitary gland, and retina and is involved in the regulation of the HPT axis [174].

Molecular Basis of Thyroid Hormone Resistance

Thyroid hormone resistance (THR) is a rare genetic disorder characterized by reduced tissue responsiveness to thyroid hormones, primarily T3 and T4. This results in elevated serum levels of thyroid hormones with normal or elevated thyrotropin (TSH) levels, leading to an incongruity between the clinical and biochemical manifestations of the condition [175].

The molecular basis of thyroid hormone resistance primarily involves mutations in the thyroid hormone receptor (TR) genes. The two main subtypes of TRs, TRα and TRβ, encoded by the THRA and THRB genes, respectively, are involved in mediating the effects of thyroid hormones on target tissues [22]. Among the two, mutations in the THRB gene are more commonly associated with THR, while THRA gene mutations are rarer [176].

Mutations in the THRB gene causes defects in the ligand-binding domain of the TRβ protein, impairing its ability to bind to thyroid hormones. This leads to reduced sensitivity of target tissues to thyroid hormone signaling, thus requiring higher levels of thyroid hormones to maintain normal physiological function [10].

2.4.1.2   Mechanism of Action

The role of beta-blockers in hyperthyroxinemia was reviewed in Section 2.2.6.

Practice Pearl(s)

In thyroid hormone resistance, the use of beta-blockers can be beneficial in managing symptoms associated with the hyperadrenergic state, which may occur due to elevated thyroid hormone levels [175]. Although tissue resistance to thyroid hormones is the primary issue in THR, specific tissues or organs, such as the cardiovascular system, may still be sensitive to the effects of thyroid hormones [10].

Beta-blockers such as propranolol or atenolol can alleviate symptoms such as palpitations and tremors [177]. They reduce heart rate, blood pressure, and myocardial contraction by blocking catecholamines' effects on beta-adrenergic receptors [178]. Thus, beta-blockers can help to reduce myocardial stress caused by elevated thyroid hormone levels [179].

Although beta-blockers do not address the underlying cause of thyroid hormone resistance, they can be a useful adjunct in the management of symptomatic patients [180]. The primary goal of treating THR is to optimize thyroid hormone levels and suppress TSH levels if necessary, which may involve the use of supraphysiologic doses of levothyroxine [181]. Beta-blockers can be used alongside these treatments to manage the cardiovascular effects of hyperthyroxinemia and improve the quality of life for individuals with THR. Oral Propranolol, 30–60 mg/day, is typically used as adjunctive therapy in patients with persistent cardiovascular effects [182].

Clinical Trial Evidence

There are no well-powered studies evaluating the role of beta-blockers in thyroid hormone resistance syndromes.

2.4.2   Thyroid Hormone Replacement Therapy

2.4.2.1   Physiology

THR is a rare genetic disorder that affects the responsiveness of tissues to thyroid hormones. There are two main subtypes: resistance to thyroid hormone alpha (RTHα) and resistance to thyroid hormone beta (RTHβ), which are caused by mutations in the THRA and THRB genes, respectively [175]. These genes encode TRs, TRα, and TRβ, which are responsible for mediating the effects of thyroid hormones in various tissues [183].

2.4.2.2 Mechanism of Action

RTHα is a rare form of THR characterized by resistance to thyroid hormones in tissues predominantly expressing TRα, such as the heart, bone, and gastrointestinal tract [184]. Patients with RTHα may present with growth retardation, delayed bone maturation, constipation, anemia, and sometimes mild intellectual disabilities. The typical treatment for these patients is to use supraphysiologic levothyroxine doses to overcome RTH [176]. This should only be done with caution since higher doses of the thyroid hormone may have adverse effects on tissues that are usually sensitive to thyroid hormones.

RTHβ is a more common form of THR and affects tissues predominantly expressing TRβ, such as the liver, kidneys, and pituitary gland [185]. Patients with RTHβ may exhibit elevated T4 and T3 levels, normal or slightly elevated TSH levels, and a variable range of clinical symptoms, including goiter, attention deficit hyperactivity disorder (ADHD), and tachycardia. The treatment for RTHβ varies depending on the severity of the symptoms and the degree of hormone resistance [186].

Practice Pearl(s)

Thyroid hormone replacement plays a crucial role in managing thyroid hormone resistance syndromes, particularly in patients with resistance to thyroid hormone alpha (RTHα) and resistance to thyroid hormone beta (RTHβ). The choice of treatment, dose, and duration depends on the subtype of thyroid hormone resistance and the severity of the clinical symptoms [175, 187].

In RTHα patients, thyroid hormone replacement with supraphysiologic doses of levothyroxine may be necessary to overcome the resistance in TRα-expressing tissues like the heart, bone, and gastrointestinal tract [176]. However, caution is required, as higher doses of thyroid hormones might negatively affect other tissues with normal sensitivity to thyroid hormones [184].

For RTHβ patients, the management approach varies depending on the severity of symptoms and the degree of hormone resistance. In many cases, no specific treatment is required, and patients are managed conservatively with regular monitoring of thyroid hormone levels [188]. In some instances,

---

thyroid hormone replacement therapy may be considered for patients with severe symptoms or specific clinical indications [189].

Clinical Trial Evidence

Due to the rarity of thyroid hormone resistance, there are no well-powered studies investigating the efficacy of levothyroxine.

 Concepts to Ponder

What Is the Biochemical Profile of Patients with Thyroid Hormone Resistance?

Thyroid hormone resistance syndrome is a rare genetic disorder characterized by a reduced responsiveness of target tissues to the action of thyroid hormones [190]. An important clinical pearl in the evaluation of thyroid hormone resistance syndrome is the importance of recognizing the biochemical hallmark of the disorder: elevated serum free thyroxine (FT4) and triiodothyronine (T3) levels with non-suppressed or even elevated thyroid-stimulating hormone (TSH) levels [186]. Identifying this unique biochemical profile is crucial for distinguishing thyroid hormone resistance syndrome from other thyroid disorders. The gold standard for diagnosing thyroid hormone resistance syndrome is genetic testing for mutations in the THRB or THRA genes, encoding the thyroid hormone receptor β and α, respectively [186, 191].

What Is the Difference Between Pituitary and Generalized Resistance to Thyroid Hormone?

The lack of consistency in clinical findings among patients with THR is due to the variable expression of thyroid hormone receptors across various tissues [192, 193].

Pituitary or central thyroid hormone resistance is caused by reduced negative feedback inhibition of thyroid hormone on the anterior pituitary, resulting in an increased secretion of both TSH and thyroid hormones. Patients with pituitary or central thyroid hormone resistance are clinically hyperthyroid [194]. Conversely, patients with generalized resistance to thyroid hormones may be either euthyroid or hypothyroid, depending on which tissue-specific subtype of thyroid hormone receptor is affected [176].

2.5   TSH-SECRETING TUMORS

2.5.1   Somatostatin Receptor Ligands

2.5.1.1   Physiology

Somatostatin, also known as somatotropin release-inhibiting factor (SRIF), is a hypothalamic peptide hormone [195] that exerts negative feedback effects on the HPT axis [196].

Somatostatin is synthesized and released by specific neurons in the hypothalamus, where it acts as an inhibitor of TRH release [197]. By inhibiting TRH release, somatostatin contributes to negative feedback regulation of the HPT axis [169].

Furthermore, somatostatin acts directly on the anterior pituitary gland to inhibit TSH secretion. Somatostatin binds to specific somatostatin receptors on the surface of thyrotrope cells in the anterior pituitary, leading to a reduction in intracellular cAMP levels [198]. This ultimately leads to decreased TSH synthesis and secretion [199].

2.5.1.2   Mechanism of Action

Somatostatin analogs, such as octreotide and lanreotide, are synthetic compounds that mimic the action of the naturally occurring hormone somatostatin [200]. Somatostatin analogs bind to specific somatostatin receptor subtypes (SSTRs) present on the surface of pituitary adenoma cells [201]. The most common receptor subtypes involved in the inhibition of TSH secretion are SSTR2 and SSTR5 [202]. By binding to these receptors, somatostatin analogs that bind to SSTRs activate inhibitory G proteins (Gi), inhibiting adenylate cyclase activity. This leads to a decrease in the intracellular levels of cyclic AMP (cAMP), an important second messenger involved in hormone secretion. Reduced cAMP levels result in decreased TSH synthesis and secretion [203].

In addition to their inhibitory effects on hormone secretion, somatostatin analogs have also been shown to exert antiproliferative effects on pituitary adenoma cells. They can induce cell cycle arrest and promote apoptosis, thereby reducing tumor size and alleviating mass effects [200].

Overall, somatostatin analogs act by binding to specific somatostatin receptors on TSH-secreting pituitary adenoma cells, leading to reduced hormone synthesis and secretion through multiple intracellular mechanisms [201, 203]. This results in decreased TSH levels, alleviating the symptoms of hyperthyroidism caused by the adenoma [201].

Practice Pearl(s)

An important differential diagnosis of TSH-secreting pituitary adenomas is thyroid hormone resistance syndrome. Distinguishing between a TSH-secreting pituitary tumor (TSHoma) and thyroid hormone resistance (RTH) can be challenging, as both conditions can present with elevated thyroid hormone levels (free T3 and T4) and either high or inappropriately normal serum TSH [188] (see Table 2.6).

The dose range, side effects, and relevant clinical pearls were discussed in Chapter 1.

TABLE 2.6   Comparison of TSH-secreting pituitary tumors and thyroid hormone resistance.

Clinical feature	TSHoma	Thyroid hormone resistance
T3 suppression test	No effect on TSH suppression	Suppresses TSH
MRI	Positive	Negative
SHBG	High	Normal
Alpha subunit	High	Normal
Family history	Negative history of thyroid dysfunction	Positive
TRH test	No response	Normal or exaggerated response

Clinical Trial Evidence

This study evaluated the effects of a slow-release formulation of the somatostatin analog lanreotide (SR-L) on hormone secretion, tumor size, and tolerance in 18 patients with TSH-secreting pituitary adenomas over 6 months. Clinical signs of hyperthyroidism improved within 1 month for 16 patients. Plasma TSH, free alpha-subunit, and thyroid hormone levels significantly decreased during treatment, with normalization observed in 13 out of 16 cases.

No significant change in adenoma size was observed after 6 months, and side effects were mild and transient. No gallstones occurred during the study. The findings suggest that SR-L is a safe and effective treatment for thyrotropinomas, maintaining its effect throughout treatment [204].

2.5.2 Dopaminergic Agonists

2.5.2.1 Physiology

Dopamine, a neurotransmitter, exerts negative feedback inhibition on the HPT axis [196]. This is because dopamine has an inhibitory effect on both thyrotropin-releasing hormone (TRH) and thyroid-stimulating hormone (TSH) secretion [205]. The effects of dopamine on the HPT axis were discussed in Chapter 1.

2.5.2.2 Mechanism of Action

Dopaminergic agonists (DAs) are generally used to treat prolactinomas; however, they have also been shown to be efficacious in treating TSH-secreting pituitary tumors (thyrotropinomas) [188]. The mechanism of action of dopaminergic agonists in TSH-producing pituitary tumors is based on the ability of these agents to bind and activate D2 receptors on the surface of thyrotropinoma cells [188]. The activation of these dopamine receptors results in a suppression of TSH secretion and synthesis. Dopaminergic receptor agonists can also have an antiproliferative impact on tumor cells which may inhibit the growth of tumor cells [206].

> **Practice Pearl(s)**
>
> The dose range, side effects, and relevant clinical pearls of dopaminergic agonists were discussed in Chapter 1.

> **Clinical Trial Evidence**
>
> There are various case reports of the use of dopaminergic agonists in TSHomas, with variable degrees of efficacy [207–209].

> **Concepts to Ponder**
>
> **What Is the Primary Treatment Modality for TSH-Secreting Adenomas?**
>
> Transsphenoidal surgery is the first-line treatment for TSH-producing tumors, followed by adjuvant therapy, such as radiation therapy or medical therapy [188].

2.6 THYROID CANCER

2.6.1 Tyrosine Kinase Inhibitors

2.6.1.1 Physiology

Tyrosine kinases are a family of intracellular enzymes that modulate various cellular signaling processes [210]. This family of receptors can be classified into two main categories. These are receptor tyrosine kinases (RTKs) and non-receptor tyrosine kinases [210].

Receptor tyrosine kinases are composed of an extracellular ligand-binding domain, a transmembrane domain (spanning the cell membrane), and an intracellular kinase domain [210]. RTKs include epidermal growth factor receptor (EGFR), vascular endothelial growth factor receptor (VEGFR), and platelet-derived growth factor receptor (PDGFR) (see Figure 2.7). Non-receptor tyrosine kinases, on the other hand, are cytoplasmic proteins that lack a transmembrane domain and are beyond the scope of this text.

The role of tyrosine kinases in cellular signaling and tumor growth, showing the sites of action of various tyrosine kinase inhibitors is shown in Figure 2.7.

The extracellular domain of RTK is bound by a specific ligand, such as growth factors or cytokines [210] which causes receptor dimerization. Tyrosine residues within the kinase region are autophosphorylated. This results in the activation of the receptor kinase [210]. Tyrosine kinases, once activated, promote the phosphorylation of specific tyrosine residues on target protein [211]. The activation of downstream signaling pathways, such as MAPK/ERK and PI3K/AKT or JAK/STAT, is triggered by this. The activation of these downstream pathways leads to multiple cellular processes, including cell growth and survival [212].

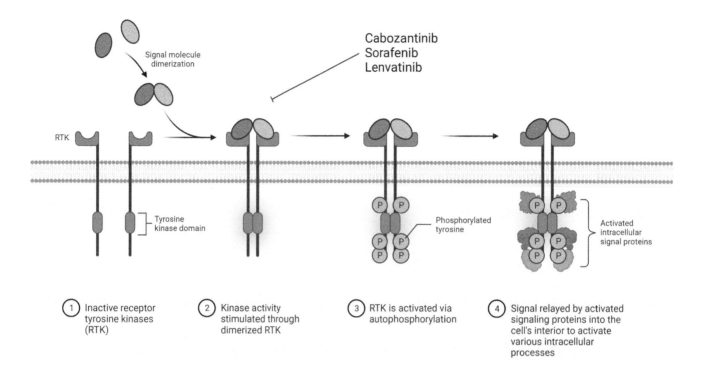

FIGURE 2.7   Sites of action of tyrosine kinase inhibitors.

Genetic alterations in malignancies (e.g. gain of function mutations) can result in the constitutive activation of tyrosine-kinases and their downstream signaling pathway [212]. This process can lead to uncontrolled cell proliferation, resistance against apoptosis, and increased tumor invasion and metastasis [212]. Additionally, aberrant tyrosine-kinase signals can contribute to therapy resistance and tumor recurrence [213].

2.6.1.2   Mechanism of Action

Tyrosine Kinase Inhibitors (TKIs), a group of targeted anticancer agents, are essential in treating thyroid cancers of all types. This is especially true in cases of advanced or metastatic disease [214]. They inhibit the activity of specific enzymes called tyrosine-kinases, which are important components of cell signaling pathways, such as those that control cell growth, differentiation, and survivability [215].

The mechanism of action of TKIs in thyroid cancer involves the following steps:

Several types of thyroid cancer have been found to contain mutations or overexpression of tyrosine kinase receptors such as RET and BRAF. These alterations can lead to constitutive activation of downstream signaling pathways (e.g. MAPK and PI3K/AKT), promoting tumor growth, survival, and angiogenesis [216–218]. TKIs target these aberrantly activated tyrosine kinases, blocking their activity and disrupting the oncogenic signaling cascades [215, 218].

The Vascular Endothelial Growth Factor (VEGF), and its receptors, the VEGFRs, play a key role in the promotion of angiogenesis in thyroid carcinoma [214]. TKIs that target VEGFRs inhibit angiogenesis and deprive the tumor of oxygen and nutrients essential for its growth [219].

TKIs also induce programmed cell death in cancer cells by blocking the activation and downstream signaling pathways of certain tyrosine kinases [215]. This results in a decrease in the size of tumors and, in some instances, tumor regression [220].

Some TKIs also inhibit thyroid cancer cell migration and invasion, reducing their potential to spread to other organs.

The target profiles of different TKIs are distinct, allowing for specific drug selection based on the molecular features of the tumor. TKIs are commonly used in thyroid cancer, including sorafenib and lenvatinib [220].

Practice Pearl(s)

Tyrosine Kinase inhibitors are indicated in patients with significant differentiated thyroid cancer (DTC) tumor burden, symptomatic, rapidly progressive, and imminently threatening disease [221]. The typical doses of selected TKIs are shown in Table 2.7.

TABLE 2.7 Dosing schedule of various TKIs.

TKI	Dosing schedule
Cabozantinib	60 mg once daily administered orally in either locally advanced or metastatic DTC [222].
Lenvatinib	24 mg once daily, administered orally [220].
Sorafenib	400 mg twice daily, administered orally [223].

DTC differentiated thyroid carcinoma.
Derived from references [220, 222, 223].

Clinical Trial Evidence

The DECISION phase 3 trial assessed the efficacy and safety of sorafenib in patients with radioactive iodine-refractory, locally advanced or metastatic differentiated thyroid cancer. The study found that sorafenib significantly improved median progression-free survival (10.8 months) compared to placebo (5.8 months), with a hazard ratio of 0.59 ($p < 0.0001$). The treatment was beneficial across all prespecified clinical and genetic biomarker subgroups. Adverse events were mostly grade 1 or 2, with the most common being hand-foot skin reaction, diarrhea, alopecia, and rash or desquamation. The results suggest sorafenib as an effective treatment for patients with progressive, radioactive iodine-refractory differentiated thyroid cancer.[223]

2.6.2 Radioactive Iodine Ablation

2.6.2.1 Physiology

The role of iodine in thyroid hormone synthesis was reviewed earlier in this chapter. See Section 2.2.1.

2.6.2.2 Mechanism of Action

Radioactive iodine (RAI) (I-131) is an effective treatment for thyroid cancer due to its mechanism of action, which exploits the thyroid gland's natural ability to take up iodine via the NIS [221]. Most differentiated thyroid cancer (DTC) cells, including papillary and follicular thyroid cancers, preserve this physiologic ability to concentrate iodine thus making radioactive iodine a suitable treatment for DTCs.

RAI is typically administered orally in the form of a capsule, either as the I-123 or I-131 capsule. Once ingested, it enters the general circulatory system. Both healthy thyroid cells and DTC cells with functional NIS actively take up iodine to synthesize thyroid hormones. RAI is preferentially absorbed by these cells due to their high affinity for iodine [224].

I-131 is a beta-emitting radionuclide, which means it releases high-energy beta particles as it decays. When absorbed by thyroid cells, the emitted beta particles damage cellular structures, including DNA, leading to cell death [225]. Radioactive iodine is mainly absorbed by thyroid follicular cells mediated by the NIS, selectively destroying both normal thyroid tissue and thyroid cancer cells while sparing most other healthy nonthyroidal tissues in the body [226].

The body excretes any remaining radioactive iodine through urine, feces, sweat, and saliva. The radioactive iodine's half-life is about 8 days, meaning the radiation level reduces by half every 8 days [225].

Practice Pearl(s)

Radioactive iodine (RAI) treatment is an effective therapeutic modality for differentiated thyroid cancer. However, it requires strict adherence to radiation safety precautions to protect patients, healthcare professionals, and the general public [227]. The following are detailed radiation precautions and their rationale for patients receiving RAI therapy.

RAI treatment can cause fetal thyroid ablation and is contraindicated during pregnancy. For this reason, women of childbearing age must undergo pregnancy testing before RAI administration and should use effective contraception during and for up to six months post-treatment [228]. Also, radioactive iodine concentrates in breast milk and poses a risk to nursing infants. Breastfeeding should therefore be discontinued before RAI treatment and not resumed afterward to prevent inadvertent infant exposure to radioactive iodine [229].

Patients receiving RAI may emit radiation for several days, necessitating isolation in a hospital

(continued)

(continued)

setting or at home to minimize exposure to others. The duration of isolation depends on the administered dose, local regulations, and individual patient factors [230].

Radioactive iodine is excreted primarily through urine, and proper hygiene practices can reduce contamination risk. Patients should wash their hands thoroughly after using the bathroom, clean bathroom surfaces regularly, and flush toilets multiple times after use to minimize residual radiation [230].

To reduce contamination risk, patients should use disposable utensils, plates, and cups [230]. Consuming sufficient fluids can promote renal clearance of radioactive iodine, decreasing the duration of radiation exposure.

To prevent cross-contamination, clothing, bed linens, and towels used during the isolation period should be washed separately from those of other household members. Instructions for handling contaminated laundry should follow local radiation safety guidelines [231].

Finally, radioactive iodine can accumulate in salivary glands, causing inflammation (sialoadenitis) and xerostomia. Chewing gum or sucking on hard candy can stimulate saliva production, enhancing radioactive iodine clearance from the glands and reducing potential side effects [232].

Clinical Trial Evidence

This retrospective study assessed the survival of 96 patients with lung metastases from differentiated thyroid carcinoma. Longer survival times were observed in patients under 45 years of age at diagnosis, those with metastases concentrating 131I, and those with fine miliary metastases. Multivariate analysis revealed a 5.4-fold increased risk of death in patients over 45 years old, while 131I treatment could reduce this risk to nearly 1/6. The study concluded that young age at diagnosis and 131I uptake by metastases positively affected survival time, and radioiodine therapy, even with high cumulative 131I activity, could lead to longer survival or complete recovery [233].

2.6.3   mTOR Inhibitors

2.6.3.1   Physiology

The mammalian target of the rapamycin (mTOR) signaling pathway is essential for cellular pathways that are required for cell growth, proliferation, metabolism, and survival [234].

2.6.3.2   Mechanism of Action

mTOR inhibitors in thyroid cancer block the activity of the mTOR protein, thus inhibiting its downstream signaling responses required for tumor proliferation [235].

Practice Pearl(s)

There is limited use of these medications in general endocrinology. Patients requiring mTOR inhibitors should be referred to oncologists.

Clinical Trial Evidence

See the practice pearl above.

 Concepts to Ponder

What Is the Role of Thyroid Hormone Replacement in the Management of Thyroid Cancer?

Thyroid hormone suppression plays a critical role in the management of differentiated thyroid cancer (DTC), which includes papillary and follicular thyroid cancer. The primary goal of thyroid hormone suppression therapy is to reduce the levels of thyroid-stimulating hormone (TSH) in the bloodstream, thereby inhibiting the growth and proliferation of thyroid cancer cells [221].

The rationale for TSH suppression lies in the understanding that TSH promotes the growth of both normal thyroid tissue and thyroid cancer cells. By maintaining low TSH levels through exogenous thyroid hormone administration, the risk of cancer recurrence and progression can be minimized [236].

Levothyroxine (LT4) is the most commonly used medication for TSH suppression therapy. The dosage of LT4 is carefully adjusted to maintain TSH levels below the reference range without causing overt hyperthyroidism [237]. The target TSH level depends on the individual patient's risk of recurrence and the presence of any comorbidities. In high-risk patients, TSH suppression may be more aggressive, whereas in low-risk patients, a more conservative approach may be taken to minimize the potential side effects of LT4 therapy [221].

TSH suppression therapy is generally continued for several years after the initial treatment of DTC, with regular monitoring to assess the patient's response and to adjust the LT4 dosage as needed [238]. The duration of therapy and the degree of TSH suppression is individualized based on the patient's risk factors, response to therapy, and overall clinical situation.

PRACTICE-BASED QUESTIONS

1. Which of the following is the primary carrier protein for thyroid hormones in the bloodstream?

   a. Albumin
   b. Transthyretin
   c. Thyroxine-binding globulin (TBG)
   d. Type 1 deiodinase

   Correct answer: c. Thyroxine-binding globulin (TBG). **Explanation:** Thyroxine-binding globulin (TBG) is the primary and most abundant carrier protein in the bloodstream for thyroid hormones, binding about 70% of T4 and 80% of T3. TBG has a high affinity for thyroid hormones and plays a significant role in maintaining a stable concentration of free thyroid hormones in circulation.

2. What is the main difference between T4 and T3 in terms of biological activity?

   a. T4 has greater biological activity than T3.
   b. T3 has greater biological activity than T4.
   c. T4 and T3 have equal biological activity.
   d. T4 and T3 have no biological activity.

   Correct answer: b. T3 has greater biological activity than T4. **Explanation:** T3 is the biologically

active thyroid hormone and possesses approximately three to five times greater potency than T4. Although T4 is the predominant thyroid hormone secreted by the thyroid gland, it is a prohormone with relatively low biological activity compared to T3.

3. Which of the following enzymes is mainly responsible for converting T4–T3 in peripheral tissues like the liver and kidneys?

   a. Type 1 deiodinase (D1)
   b. Type 2 deiodinase (D2)
   c. Type 3 deiodinase (D3)
   d. Transthyretin

   Correct answer: a. Type 1 deiodinase (D1). **Explanation:** Type 1 deiodinase (D1) is predominantly found in peripheral tissues such as the liver and kidneys and is responsible for converting most of the prohormone thyroxine (T4) to the biologically active hormone triiodothyronine (T3) in circulation.

4. Which form of thyroid hormone is used as a first-line treatment for hypothyroidism?

   a. Dessicated thyroid hormone
   b. Liothyronine
   c. Levothyroxine (L-T4)
   d. Reverse T3 (rT3)

   Correct answer: c. Levothyroxine (L-T4). **Explanation:** Levothyroxine, also known as L-thyroxine or L-T4, is a synthetic form of the endogenous thyroid hormone thyroxine (T4). It is widely used as a first-line treatment for hypothyroidism, a condition characterized by insufficient thyroid hormone production. The mechanism of action of levothyroxine involves its conversion to the biologically active hormone triiodothyronine (T3) and subsequent interaction with nuclear thyroid hormone receptors (TRs) to modulate gene transcription.

5. Which enzyme is primarily responsible for converting T4–T3 in the brain, pituitary gland, brown adipose tissue, skeletal muscle, and other tissues?

   a. Type 1 deiodinase (D1)
   b. Type 2 deiodinase (D2)
   c. Type 3 deiodinase (D3)
   d. Transthyretin

Correct answer: b. Type 2 deiodinase (D2). **Explanation:** Type 2 deiodinase (D2) is mainly present in the brain, pituitary gland, brown adipose tissue, skeletal muscle, and other tissues. D2 primarily converts T4–T3 for intracellular use, providing a localized source of active thyroid hormone.

6. A patient diagnosed with Graves' disease presents with severe hyperthyroidism. Which of the following medications helps to inhibit the peripheral conversion of T4–T3, in addition to inhibiting the thyroid peroxidase enzyme?

   a. Methimazole
   b. Propylthiouracil
   c. Iodide
   d. Selenium

Correct answer: b) Propylthiouracil. **Explanation:** Propylthiouracil (PTU) is a thionamide medication that inhibits the thyroid peroxidase enzyme, thereby inhibiting the synthesis of thyroid hormones. In addition, PTU also inhibits the peripheral conversion of T4–T3 by blocking the activity of type 1 and 2 deiodinase enzymes, which can be particularly beneficial in the management of severe hyperthyroidism or thyroid storm.

7. Which of the following medications used in the management of Graves' disease inhibits iodide transport into the thyroid gland?

   a. Methimazole
   b. Lugol's iodine
   c. Thiocyanate
   d. Glucocorticoids

Correct answer: c) Thiocyanate. **Explanation:** Thiocyanate and other iodide uptake inhibitors, such as perchlorate and pertechnetate, impede iodide transport into the thyroid gland. By blocking the entry of iodide into the thyroid follicular cells, these inhibitors reduce the intracellular concentration of iodide available for thyroid hormone synthesis, ultimately decreasing the production of thyroid hormones.

8. In the management of thyroid eye disease, which essential trace element is known to modulate the immune response and enhance the antioxidant defense system?

   a. Iron
   b. Zinc
   c. Copper
   d. Selenium

Correct answer: d) Selenium. **Explanation:** Selenium is an essential trace element that plays a crucial role in thyroid eye disease management. It is a crucial component of various antioxidant enzymes, such as glutathione peroxidase (GPx) and thioredoxin reductase. These enzymes help protect cellular components from oxidative stress by neutralizing reactive oxygen species (ROS). Selenium also modulates the immune response by regulating various immune cell functions, such as T-cell proliferation and cytokine production.

9. A 35-year-old female presents with symptoms of tachycardia, palpitations, and tremors. Laboratory results show elevated levels of T3 and T4, and normal TSH levels. Which of the following is the most appropriate pharmacological treatment for managing her cardiovascular symptoms?

   a. Propranolol
   b. Levothyroxine
   c. Octreotide
   d. Cabergoline

Correct answer: a) Propranolol. **Explanation:** Propranolol is a beta-blocker that can help alleviate symptoms related to increased sensitivity to catecholamines, such as tachycardia, palpitations, and tremors. It works by blocking the effects of catecholamines on beta-adrenergic receptors, thereby reducing heart rate, blood pressure, and the force of myocardial contraction. This can help to reduce the cardiovascular strain associated with elevated thyroid hormone levels.

10. A 40-year-old male with a history of thyroid hormone resistance presents with elevated T4 and T3 levels and normal TSH levels. He is experiencing severe constipation, anemia, and mild intellectual disabilities. Which of the following treatments should be considered for this patient?

    a. Propranolol
    b. Supraphysiologic doses of levothyroxine
    c. Octreotide
    d. Cabergoline

Correct answer: b) Supraphysiologic doses of levo-thyroxine. **Explanation:** This patient is likely experiencing resistance to thyroid hormone alpha (RTHα), which affects tissues predominantly expressing TRα, such as the gastrointestinal tract. Treatment with supraphysiologic doses of levothyroxine may be necessary to overcome the resistance in TRα-expressing tissues and alleviate symptoms.

11. A 28-year-old female presents with elevated T4 and T3 levels, normal TSH levels, and a pituitary adenoma on MRI. Which of the following treatments is most appropriate for her condition?

    a. Propranolol
    b. Supraphysiologic doses of levothyroxine
    c. Octreotide
    d. Cabergoline

    Correct answer: c) Octreotide. **Explanation:** This patient likely has a TSH-secreting pituitary tumor (TSHoma). Octreotide, a somatostatin analog, is an appropriate treatment for TSHomas as it reduces hormone synthesis and secretion through its inhibitory effects on TSH secretion.

12. A 45-year-old male with a TSH-secreting pituitary adenoma is treated with octreotide. Which of the following is a possible side effect of this treatment?

    a. Hypertension
    b. Hyperglycemia
    c. Hypothyroidism
    d. Weight gain

    Correct answer: b) Hyperglycemia. **Explanation:** Somatostatin analogs, such as octreotide, can cause hyperglycemia as a side effect. This is due to their inhibitory effects on insulin and glucagon secretion, leading to impaired glucose regulation.

13. A patient presents with elevated T4 and T3 levels, inappropriately normal TSH levels, and a negative pituitary MRI. Which test is likely to help differentiate between a TSH-secreting pituitary tumor and thyroid hormone resistance?

    a. T3 suppression test
    b. TRH stimulation test
    c. Alpha subunit measurement
    d. SHBG measurement

    Correct answer: a) T3 suppression test. **Explanation:** The T3 suppression test can help differentiate between a TSH-secreting pituitary tumor (TSHoma) and thyroid hormone resistance (RTH).

14. What is the primary reason propranolol is often used for initial therapy in thyroid storm or severe Graves' disease?

    a. It increases the heart rate and the force of the heart's contractions
    b. It inhibits the conversion of thyroxine (T4) to triiodothyronine (T3)
    c. It blocks the blood–brain barrier
    d. It increases peripheral vascular resistance

    Correct answer: b) It inhibits the conversion of thyroxine (T4) to triiodothyronine (T3). **Explanation:** Propranolol is often used for initial therapy in thyroid storm or severe Graves' disease because, in high doses, it inhibits the conversion of thyroxine (T4) to the more active triiodothyronine (T3) by inhibiting the type 1 deiodinase enzyme. This can help reduce the levels of circulating T3, which is a primary contributor to the symptoms associated with these conditions.

15. How do beta-blockers like propranolol help alleviate symptoms of anxiety, nervousness, and tremors in patients with thyroid storm or severe Graves' disease?

    a. By blocking cardiac beta-1 receptors
    b. By crossing the blood–brain barrier and calming the central nervous system
    c. By blocking the beta-2 receptors in the blood vessels
    d. By inhibiting the conversion of thyroxine (T4) to triiodothyronine (T3)

    Correct answer: b) By crossing the blood–brain barrier and calming the central nervous system. **Explanation:** Beta-blockers, such as propranolol, can cross the blood–brain barrier and calm the central nervous system. This can help alleviate symptoms like anxiety, nervousness, and tremors that are common in patients with thyroid storm or severe Graves' disease.

16. How does cholestyramine impact thyroid hormone metabolism?

    a. By inhibiting thyroid peroxidase
    b. By binding to bile acids and disrupting the normal absorption and reabsorption of thyroid hormones in the intestine
    c. By increasing the peripheral conversion of T4–T3
    d. By competing with iodine for uptake by thyroid cells

    Correct answer: b) By binding to bile acids and disrupting the normal absorption and reabsorption of thyroid hormones in the intestine. **Explanation:** Cholestyramine binds to bile acids in the intestine, forming an insoluble complex that is excreted in the feces. This interrupts the enterohepatic circulation of bile acids and prevents their reabsorption. Since thyroid hormones, such as thyroxine (T4) and triiodothyronine (T3), are partly metabolized in the liver and excreted into the bile, cholestyramine's binding to bile acids indirectly impacts thyroid hormone metabolism.

17. How does lithium affect thyroid hormone synthesis and secretion?

    a. By increasing the activity of thyroid peroxidase
    b. By competing with iodine for uptake by thyroid cells and inhibiting thyroid hormone release
    c. By promoting the conversion of T4–T3
    d. By increasing the availability of iodine for thyroid hormone synthesis

    Correct answer: b) By competing with iodine for uptake by thyroid cells and inhibiting thyroid hormone release. **Explanation:** Lithium is concentrated in the thyroid gland, where it competes with iodine for uptake by the thyroid cells. This competition reduces the availability of iodine for thyroid hormone synthesis. Moreover, lithium can inhibit thyroid hormone release by interfering with the coupling of iodotyrosine residues, which are essential for the formation of thyroxine (T4) and triiodothyronine (T3).

18. A patient with thyroid storm is experiencing severe asthma. Which medication is relatively contraindicated, and what alternative can be used for rate control?

    a. Propranolol, use Metoprolol
    b. Metoprolol, use Propranolol
    c. Propranolol, use Calcium channel blockers
    d. Metoprolol, use Calcium channel blockers

    Correct answer: c) Propranolol, use Calcium channel blockers. **Explanation:** In patients with severe asthma, beta-blockers like propranolol are relatively contraindicated due to their potential to exacerbate respiratory symptoms. Instead, calcium channel blockers can be employed to achieve rate control in such patients.

19. What is the primary purpose of using beta-blockers like propranolol in the treatment of thyroid storm or severe Graves' disease?

    a. To act as a definitive treatment for thyroid storm
    b. To provide symptomatic relief and improve overall condition
    c. To replace antithyroid medications or radioactive iodine therapy
    d. To reverse the underlying cause of the condition

    Correct answer: b) To provide symptomatic relief and improve overall condition. **Explanation:** Beta-blockers, including propranolol, are used as supportive therapy to manage symptoms in thyroid storm or severe Graves' disease. They are not a definitive treatment, and their primary purpose is to provide symptomatic relief and improve the patient's overall condition while other treatments address the underlying cause.

20. Which of the following statements about cholestyramine is true?

    a. Cholestyramine binds to thyroid hormones directly, leading to their excretion.
    b. Cholestyramine interferes with the enterohepatic circulation of bile acids and indirectly affects thyroid hormone metabolism.
    c. Cholestyramine directly inhibits the conversion of T4–T3.
    d. Cholestyramine can be administered alongside other oral medications without any concern for interactions.

Correct answer: b) Cholestyramine interferes with the enterohepatic circulation of bile acids and indirectly affects thyroid hormone metabolism. **Explanation:** Cholestyramine binds to bile acids in the intestine, forming an insoluble complex that is excreted in the feces. This interrupts the enterohepatic circulation of bile acids and prevents their reabsorption. Since thyroid hormones are partly metabolized in the liver and excreted into the bile, cholestyramine's binding to bile acids indirectly impacts thyroid hormone metabolism.

REFERENCES

1. Armstrong, M., Asuka, E., and Fingeret, A. (2023). *Physiology, Thyroid Function.* StatPearls.
2. Stathatos, N. (2012). Thyroid physiology. *Med. Clin. North Am.* 96: 165–173.
3. Dunlap, D.B. (1990). Chapter 142 – Thyroid function tests. In: *Clinical Methods: The History, Physical, and Laboratory Examinations*, 3e (ed. H.K. Walker, W.D. Hall, and J.W. Hurst). Boston: Butterworths https://www.ncbi.nlm.nih.gov/books/NBK249/.
4. Larsen, P.R. and Zavacki, A.M. (2012). The role of the iodothyronine deiodinases in the physiology and pathophysiology of thyroid hormone action. *Eur. Thyroid J.* 1: 232–242.
5. Luongo, C., Trivisano, L., Alfano, F., and Salvatore, D. (2013). Type 3 deiodinase and consumptive hypothyroidism: A common mechanism for a rare disease. *Front. Endocrinol (Lausanne)* 4: 115.
6. Burmeister, L.A. (1995). Reverse T3 does not reliably differentiate hypothyroid sick syndrome from euthyroid sick syndrome. *Thyroid* 5: 435–441.
7. Hennemann, G., Krenning, E.P., and Docter, R. (1986). Thyroid hormone-binding plasma proteins. In: *Frontiers in Thyroidology: Volume 1* (ed. G. Medeiros-Neto and E. Gaitan), 97–101. Boston, MA: Springer US.
8. Purkey, H.E., Dorrell, M.I., and Kelly, J.W. (2001). Evaluating the binding selectivity of transthyretin amyloid fibril inhibitors in blood plasma. *Proc. Natl. Acad. Sci.* 98: 5566–5571.
9. Hoffenberg, R. and Ramsden, D.B. (1983). The Transport of Thyroid Hormones. *Clin. Sci.* 65: 337–342.
10. Yen, P.M. (2001). Physiological and molecular basis of thyroid hormone action. *Physiol. Rev.* 81: 1097–1142.
11. Stepien, B.K. and Huttner, W.B. (2019). Transport, metabolism, and function of thyroid hormones in the developing mammalian brain. *Front. Endocrinol. (Lausanne)* 10: 209. https://doi.org/10.3389/fendo.2019.00209.
12. Visser, T.J., Kaptein, E., Terpstra, O.T., and Krenning, E.P. (1988). Deiodination of thyroid hormone by human liver. *J. Clin. Endocrinol. Metab.* 67: 17–24.
13. Visser, T.J. (1994). Role of sulfation in thyroid hormone metabolism. *Chem. Biol. Interact.* 92: 293–303.
14. Benvenga, S. and Carlé, A. (2019). Levothyroxine formulations: Pharmacological and clinical implications of generic substitution. *Adv. Ther.* 36: 59–71.
15. Zhang, J. and Lazar, M.A. (2000). The mechanism of action of thyroid hormones. *Annu. Rev. Physiol.* 62: 439–466.
16. Dentice, M. and Salvatore, D. (2011). Deiodinases: The balance of thyroid hormone: Local impact of thyroid hormone inactivation. *J. Endocrinol.* 209: 273–282.
17. Chaker, L., Razvi, S., Bensenor, I.M. et al. (2022). Hypothyroidism. *Nat. Rev. Dis. Primers.* 8: 1–17.
18. Sabatino, L., Vassalle, C., Del Seppia, C., and Iervasi, G. (2021). Deiodinases and the three types of thyroid hormone deiodination reactions. *Endocrinol Metab (Seoul)* 36: 952–964.
19. Lechan, R.M. and Fekete, C. (2005). Role of thyroid hormone deiodination in the hypothalamus. *Thyroid* 15: 883–897.
20. Hsu, J.H., Zavacki, A.M., Harney, J.W., and Brent, G.A. (1995). Retinoid-X receptor (RXR) differentially augments thyroid hormone response in cell lines as a function of the response element and endogenous RXR content. *Endocrinology* 136: 421–430.
21. Lazar, M.A. (1993). Thyroid hormone receptors: Multiple forms, multiple possibilities. *Endocr. Rev.* 14: 184–193.
22. Cheng, S.-Y., Leonard, J.L., and Davis, P.J. (2010). Molecular aspects of thyroid hormone actions. *Endocr. Rev.* 31: 139–170.
23. Grøntved, L., Waterfall, J.J., Kim, D.W. et al. (2015). Transcriptional activation by the thyroid hormone receptor through ligand-dependent receptor recruitment and chromatin remodelling. *Nat. Commun.* 6: 7048.
24. Kirsten, D. (2000). The thyroid gland: Physiology and pathophysiology. *Neonatal Netw.* 19: 11–26.
25. Singh, B.K., Sinha, R.A., and Yen, P.M. (2018). Novel transcriptional mechanisms for regulating metabolism by thyroid hormone. *Int. J. Mol. Sci.* 19: 3284.
26. Santini, F., Pinchera, A., Marsili, A. et al. (2005). Lean body mass is a major determinant of levothyroxine dosage in the treatment of thyroid diseases. *J. Clin. Endocrinol. Metab.* 90: 124–127.

27. Bensenor, I.M., Olmos, R.D., and Lotufo, P.A. (2012). Hypothyroidism in the elderly: Diagnosis and management. *Clin. Interv. Aging* 7: 97–111.

28. Biondi, B., Cappola, A.R., and Cooper, D.S. (2019). Subclinical hypothyroidism: A review. *JAMA* 322: 153–160.

29. Fatourechi, V. (2009). Subclinical hypothyroidism: An update for primary care physicians. *Mayo Clin. Proc.* 84: 65–71.

30. Brabant, G., Prank, K., Ranft, U. et al. (1990). Physiological regulation of circadian and pulsatile thyrotropin secretion in normal man and woman*. *J. Clin. Endocrinol. Metabol.* 70: 403–409.

31. Sheehan, M.T. (2016). Biochemical testing of the thyroid: TSH is the best and, oftentimes, only test needed – A review for primary care. *Clin. Med. Res.* 14: 83–92.

32. Laurberg, P., Andersen, S., Bülow Pedersen, I., and Carlé, A. (2005). Hypothyroidism in the elderly: Pathophysiology, diagnosis and treatment. *Drugs Aging* 22: 23–38.

33. Spencer, C.A., Hollowell, J.G., Kazarosyan, M., and Braverman, L.E. (2007). National Health and Nutrition Examination Survey III thyroid-stimulating hormone (TSH)-thyroperoxidase antibody relationships demonstrate that TSH upper reference limits may be skewed by occult thyroid dysfunction. *J. Clin. Endocrinol. Metab.* 92: 4236–4240.

34. Grozinsky-Glasberg, S., Fraser, A., Nahshoni, E. et al. (2006). Thyroxine-triiodothyronine combination therapy versus thyroxine monotherapy for clinical hypothyroidism: Meta-analysis of randomized controlled trials. *J. Clin. Endocrinol. Metab.* 91: 2592–2599.

35. Davis, P.J., Mousa, S.A., and Lin, H.-Y. (2021). Nongenomic actions of thyroid hormone: The integrin component. *Physiol. Rev.* 101: 319–352.

36. De Stefano, M.A., Ambrosio, R., Porcelli, T. et al. (2021). Thyroid hormone action in muscle atrophy. *Metabolites* 11: 730.

37. Riis, A.L.D., Jørgensen, J.O.L., Ivarsen, P. et al. (2008). Increased protein turnover and proteolysis is an early and primary feature of short-term experimental hyperthyroidism in healthy women. *J. Clin. Endocrinol. Metab.* 93: 3999–4005.

38. Bassett, J.H.D. (2011). Thyroid hormone action: genomic and non-genomic effects. Presented at Society for Endocrinology BES 2011, Birmingham, UK. Endocr. Abstr. 25: S6.1.

39. McAninch, E.A. and Bianco, A.C. (2014). Thyroid hormone signaling in energy homeostasis and energy metabolism. *Ann. N. Y. Acad. Sci.* 1311: 77–87.

40. Müller, M.J., Lautz, H.U., Plogmann, B. et al. (1992). Energy expenditure and substrate oxidation in patients with cirrhosis: The impact of cause, clinical staging and nutritional state. *Hepatology* 15: 782–794.

41. Mullur, R., Liu, Y.-Y., and Brent, G.A. (2014). Thyroid hormone regulation of metabolism. *Physiol. Rev.* 94: 355–382.

42. Xing, W., Cheng, S., Wergedal, J., and Mohan, S. (2014). Epiphyseal chondrocyte secondary ossification centers require thyroid hormone activation of Indian hedgehog and osterix signaling. *J. Bone Miner. Res.* 29: 2262–2275.

43. Williams, G.R. (2013). Thyroid hormone actions in cartilage and bone. *Eur Thyroid J* 2: 3–13.

44. Galliford, T.M., Murphy, E., Williams, A.J. et al. (2005). Effects of thyroid status on bone metabolism: A primary role for thyroid stimulating hormone or thyroid hormone? *Minerva Endocrinol.* 30: 237–246.

45. Lademann, F., Tsourdi, E., Hofbauer, L.C., and Rauner, M. (2020). Thyroid hormone actions and bone remodeling – The role of the wnt signaling pathway. *Exp. Clin. Endocrinol. Diabetes* 128: 450–454.

46. Delitala, A.P., Scuteri, A., and Doria, C. (2020). Thyroid hormone diseases and osteoporosis. *J. Clin. Med.* 9: 1034.

47. Nicholls, D.G. (2021). Mitochondrial proton leaks and uncoupling proteins. *Biochim. Biophys. Acta Bioenerg.* 1862: 148428.

48. Katz, L.S., Xu, S., Ge, K. et al. (2017). T3 and glucose coordinately stimulate ChREBP-mediated Ucp1 expression in brown adipocytes from male mice. *Endocrinology* 159: 557–569.

49. Yau, W.W., Singh, B.K., Lesmana, R. et al. (2019). Thyroid hormone (T3) stimulates brown adipose tissue activation via mitochondrial biogenesis and MTOR-mediated mitophagy. *Autophagy* 15: 131–150.

50. Zekri, Y., Guyot, R., Suñer, I.G. et al. (2022). Brown adipocytes local response to thyroid hormone is required for adaptive thermogenesis in adult male mice. *elife* 11: e81996.

51. Groeneweg, S., van Geest, F.S., Peeters, R.P. et al. (2020). Thyroid hormone transporters. *Endocr. Rev.* 41: 146–201.

52. Wiersinga, W.M. (2019). T4 + T3 combination therapy: Any progress? *Endocrine* 66: 70–78.

53. Daniel, E. and Newell-Price, J.D.C. (2015). Therapy of endocrine disease: Steroidogenesis enzyme inhibitors in Cushing's syndrome. *Eur. J. Endocrinol.* 172: R263–R280.

54. Madan, R. and Celi, F.S. (2020). Combination therapy for hypothyroidism: Rationale, therapeutic goals, and design. *Front Endocrinol (Lausanne)* 11: 371.

55. Jonklaas, J., Burman, K.D., Wang, H., and Latham, K.R. (2015). Single dose T3 administration: Kinetics and effects on biochemical and physiologic parameters. *Ther. Drug Monit.* 37: 110–118.

56. Kaminski, J., Miasaki, F.Y., Paz-Filho, G. et al. (2016). Treatment of hypothyroidism with levothyroxine plus liothyronine: A randomized, double-blind, crossover study. *Arch Endocrinol Metab* 60: 562–572.

57. Ventura, M., Melo, M., and Carrilho, F. (2017). Selenium and thyroid disease: From pathophysiology to treatment. *Int. J. Endocrinol.* 2017: 1297658.

58. Arthur, J.R., Nicol, F., and Beckett, G.J. (1992). The role of selenium in thyroid hormone metabolism and effects of selenium deficiency on thyroid hormone and iodine metabolism. *Biol. Trace Elem. Res.* 34: 321–325.

59. Moreno, M., Berry, M.J., Horst, C. et al. (1994). Activation and inactivation of thyroid hormone by type I iodothyronine deiodinase. *FEBS Lett.* 344: 143–146.

60. Russo, S.C., Salas-Lucia, F., and Bianco, A.C. (2021). Deiodinases and the metabolic code for thyroid hormone action. *Endocrinology* 162: bqab059.

61. Darras, V.M., Hume, R., and Visser, T.J. (1999). Regulation of thyroid hormone metabolism during fetal development. *Mol. Cell. Endocrinol.* 151: 37–47.

62. Kuiper, G.G.J.M., Kester, M.H.A., Peeters, R.P., and Visser, T.J. (2005). Biochemical mechanisms of thyroid hormone deiodination. *Thyroid* 15: 787–798.

63. Grozovsky, R., Ribich, S., Rosene, M.L. et al. (2009). Type 2 deiodinase expression is induced by peroxisomal proliferator-activated receptor-γ agonists in skeletal myocytes. *Endocrinology* 150: 1976–1983.

64. Rosene, M.L., Wittmann, G., Arrojo e Drigo, R. et al. (2010). Inhibition of the type 2 iodothyronine deiodinase underlies the elevated plasma TSH associated with amiodarone treatment. *Endocrinology* 151: 5961–5970.

65. Sentis, S.C., Oelkrug, R., and Mittag, J. (2021). Thyroid hormones in the regulation of brown adipose tissue thermogenesis. *Endocr. Connect.* 10: R106–R115.

66. Metere, A., Frezzotti, F., Graves, C.E. et al. (2018). A possible role for selenoprotein glutathione peroxidase (GPx1) and thioredoxin reductases (TrxR1) in thyroid cancer: Our experience in thyroid surgery. *Cancer Cell Int.* 18: 7.

67. Hu, Y., Feng, W., Chen, H. et al. (2021). Effect of selenium on thyroid autoimmunity and regulatory T cells in patients with Hashimoto's thyroiditis: A prospective randomized-controlled trial. *Clin. Transl. Sci.* 14: 1390–1402.

68. Köhrle, J. (2023). Selenium, iodine and iron–essential trace elements for thyroid hormone synthesis and metabolism. *Int. J. Mol. Sci.* 24: 3393.

69. Negro, R. (2008). Selenium and thyroid autoimmunity. *Biologics* 2: 265–273.

70. Leoni, S.G., Kimura, E.T., Santisteban, P., and De la Vieja, A. (2011). Regulation of thyroid oxidative state by thioredoxin reductase has a crucial role in thyroid responses to iodide excess. *Mol. Endocrinol.* 25: 1924–1935.

71. Duntas, L.H. (2010). Selenium and the thyroid: A close-knit connection. *J. Clin. Endocrinol. Metab.* 95: 5180–5188.

72. van Zuuren, E.J., Albusta, A.Y., Fedorowicz, Z. et al. (2014). Selenium supplementation for Hashimoto's thyroiditis: Summary of a cochrane systematic review. *Eur Thyroid J* 3: 25–31.

73. Winther, K.H., Wichman, J.E.M., Bonnema, S.J., and Hegedüs, L. (2017). Insufficient documentation for clinical efficacy of selenium supplementation in chronic autoimmune thyroiditis, based on a systematic review and meta-analysis. *Endocrine* 55: 376–385.

74. Panicker, V., Saravanan, P., Vaidya, B. et al. (2009). Common variation in the DIO2 gene predicts baseline psychological well-being and response to combination thyroxine plus triiodothyronine therapy in hypothyroid patients. *J. Clin. Endocrinol. Metab.* 94: 1623–1629.

75. Carvalho, D.P. and Dupuy, C. (2017). Thyroid hormone biosynthesis and release. *Mol. Cell. Endocrinol.* 458: 6–15.

76. Citterio, C.E., Targovnik, H.M., and Arvan, P. (2019). The role of thyroglobulin in thyroid hormonogenesis. *Nat. Rev. Endocrinol.* 15: 323–338.

77. Van Herle, A.J., Vassart, G., and Dumont, J.E. (1979). Control of thyroglobulin synthesis and secretion. (First of two parts). *N. Engl. J. Med.* 301: 239–249.

78. Bianco, A.C. and Kim, B.W. (2006). Deiodinases: Implications of the local control of thyroid hormone action. *J. Clin. Invest.* 116: 2571–2579.

79. García-Mayor, R.V. and Larrañaga, A. (2010). Treatment of Graves' hyperthyroidism with thionamides-derived drugs: Review. *Med. Chem.* 6: 239–246.

80. Burch, H.B. and Cooper, D.S. (2018). Anniversary review: Antithyroid drug therapy: 70 years later. *Eur. J. Endocrinol.* 179: R261–R274.

81. Abdi, H., Amouzegar, A., and Azizi, F. (2019). Antithyroid Drugs. *Iran J. Pharm Res* 18: 1–12.

82. Yoshihara, A., Luo, Y., Ishido, Y. et al. (2019). Inhibitory effects of methimazole and propylthiouracil on iodotyrosine deiodinase 1 in thyrocytes. *Endocr. J.* 66: 349–357.

83. Manna, D., Roy, G., and Mugesh, G. (2013). Antithyroid drugs and their analogues: Synthesis, structure, and mechanism of action. *Acc. Chem. Res.* 46: 2706–2715.

84. Volpé, R. (2001). The immunomodulatory effects of anti-thyroid drugs are mediated via actions on thyroid cells, affecting thyrocyte-immunocyte signalling: A review. *Curr. Pharm. Des.* 7: 451–460.

85. Rajasoorya, C. (1993). Examining the therapeutic options in hyperthyroidism – A personal perspective. *Ann. Acad. Med. Singap.* 22: 617–623.

86. Rittmaster, R.S., Zwicker, H., Abbott, E.C. et al. (1996). Effect of methimazole with or without exogenous L-thyroxine on serum concentrations of thyrotropin (TSH) receptor antibodies in patients with Graves' disease. *J. Clin. Endocrinol. Metab.* 81: 3283–3288.

87. De Leo, S., Lee, S.Y., and Braverman, L.E. (2016). Hyperthyroidism. *Lancet* 388: 906–918.

88. Pokhrel, B. and Bhusal, K. (2023). *Graves Disease.* StatPearls.

89. Ross, D.S., Burch, H.B., Cooper, D.S. et al. (2016). 2016 American thyroid association guidelines for diagnosis and management of hyperthyroidism and other causes of thyrotoxicosis. *Thyroid* 26: 1343–1421.

90. Reinwein, D., Benker, G., Lazarus, J.H., and Alexander, W.D. (1993). A prospective randomized trial of antithyroid drug dose in Graves' disease therapy. European Multicenter Study Group on Antithyroid Drug Treatment. *J. Clin. Endocrinol. Metab.* 76: 1516–1521.

91. Chai, J., Zhang, R., Zheng, W. et al. (2022). Effect of Lugol's solution on 131I therapy efficacy in Graves' disease. *Clin. Exp. Med.* doi: 10.1007/s10238-022-00859-4.

92. Huang, S.-M., Liao, W.-T., Lin, C.-F. et al. (2016). Effectiveness and mechanism of preoperative lugol solution for reducing thyroid blood flow in patients with Euthyroid Graves' disease. *World J. Surg.* 40: 505–509.

93. Erbil, Y., Ozluk, Y., Giriş, M. et al. (2007). Effect of lugol solution on thyroid gland blood flow and microvessel density in the patients with Graves' disease. *J. Clin. Endocrinol. Metabol.* 92: 2182–2189.

94. Markou, K., Georgopoulos, N., Kyriazopoulou, V., and Vagenakis, A.G. (2001). Iodine-induced hypothyroidism. *Thyroid* 11: 501–510.

95. Carroll, R. and Matfin, G. (2010). Endocrine and metabolic emergencies: Thyroid storm. *Ther. Adv. Endocrinol. Metab.* 1: 139–145.

96. Ahad, F. and Ganie, S.A. (2010). Iodine, iodine metabolism and iodine deficiency disorders revisited. *Indian J Endocrinol Metab* 14: 13–17.

97. Emerson, C.H., Anderson, A.J., Howard, W.J., and Utiger, R.D. (1975). Serum thyroxine and triiodothyronine concentrations during iodide treatment of hyperthyroidism. *J. Clin. Endocrinol. Metab.* 40: 33–36.

98. Wolff, J. and Chaikoff, I.L. (1949). The temporary nature of the inhibitory action of excess iodine on organic iodine synthesis in the normal thyroid. *Endocrinology* 45: 504–513. illust.

99. Ross, D.S., Daniels, G.H., De Stefano, P. et al. (1983). Use of adjunctive potassium iodide after radioactive iodine (131I) treatment of Graves' hyperthyroidism. *J. Clin. Endocrinol. Metab.* 57: 250–253.

100. De Almeida, R., McCalmon, S., and Cabandugama, P.K. (2022). Clinical review and update on the management of thyroid storm. *Mo. Med.* 119 (4): 366–371.

101. Tsai, C.H., Yang, P.S., Lee, J.J. et al. (2019). Effects of preoperative iodine administration on thyroidectomy for hyperthyroidism: a systematic review and meta-analysis. *Otolaryngol. Head Neck Surg.* 160 (6): 993–1002.

102. Takata, K., Amino, N., Kubota, S. et al. (2010). Benefit of short-term iodide supplementation to antithyroid drug treatment of thyrotoxicosis due to Graves' disease. *Clin. Endocrinol. (Oxf).* 72 (6): 845–850.

103. Ajjan, R.A., Findlay, C., Metcalfe, R.A. et al. (1998). The modulation of the human sodium iodide symporter activity by Graves' disease Sera1. *J. Clin. Endocrinol. Metabol.* 83: 1217–1221.

104. Mitchell, M.L. and O'Rourke, M.E. (1960). Response of the thyroid gland to thiocyanate and thyrotropin. *J. Clin. Endocrinol. Metabol.* 20: 47–56.

105. Knight, B.A., Shields, B.M., He, X. et al. (2018). Effect of perchlorate and thiocyanate exposure on

thyroid function of pregnant women from South-West England: A cohort study. *Thyroid. Res.* 11: 9.

106. Felker, P., Bunch, R., and Leung, A.M. (2016). Concentrations of thiocyanate and goitrin in human plasma, their precursor concentrations in brassica vegetables, and associated potential risk for hypothyroidism. *Nutr. Rev.* 74: 248–258.

107. Willemin, M.-E. and Lumen, A. (2017). Thiocyanate: A review and evaluation of the kinetics and the modes of action for thyroid hormone perturbations. *Crit. Rev. Toxicol.* 47: 537–563.

108. Braverman, L.E., He, X., Pino, S. et al. (2005). The effect of perchlorate, thiocyanate, and nitrate on thyroid function in workers exposed to perchlorate long-term. *J. Clin. Endocrinol. Metabol.* 90: 700–706.

109. Martinez-deMena, R., Calvo, R.-M., Garcia, L., and Obregon, M.J. (2016). Effect of glucocorticoids on the activity, expression and proximal promoter of type II deiodinase in rat brown adipocytes. *Mol. Cell. Endocrinol.* 428: 58–67.

110. Hu, Y., Man, Y., Sun, X., and Xue, Y. (2021). Effects of glucocorticoid pulse therapy on thyroid function and thyroid antibodies in children with Graves' disease. *Ital. J. Pediatr.* 47: 46.

111. Siomkajło, M., Mizera, Ł., Szymczak, D. et al. (2021). Effect of systemic steroid therapy in Graves' orbitopathy on regulatory T cells and Th17/Treg ratio. *J. Endocrinol. Investig.* 44: 2475–2484.

112. Senda, A., Endo, A., Tachimori, H. et al. (2020). Early administration of glucocorticoid for thyroid storm: Analysis of a national administrative database. *Crit. Care* 24: 470.

113. Winther, K.H., Rayman, M.P., Bonnema, S.J., and Hegedüs, L. (2020). Selenium in thyroid disorders – Essential knowledge for clinicians. *Nat. Rev. Endocrinol.* 16: 165–176.

114. Ma, C. and Hoffmann, P.R. (2021). Selenoproteins as regulators of T cell proliferation, differentiation, and metabolism. *Semin. Cell Dev. Biol.* 115: 54–61.

115. Lanzolla, G., Marinò, M., and Marcocci, C. (2020). Selenium in the treatment of Graves' hyperthyroidism and eye disease. *Front Endocrinol (Lausanne)* 11: 608428.

116. Wang, F., Li, C., Li, S. et al. (2023). Selenium and thyroid diseases. *Front Endocrinol (Lausanne)* 14: 1133000.

117. Dharmasena, A. (2014). Selenium supplementation in thyroid associated ophthalmopathy: An update. *Int. J. Ophthalmol.* 7: 365–375.

118. Marcocci, C., Kahaly, G.J., Krassas, G.E. et al. (2011). Selenium and the course of mild Graves' orbitopathy. *N. Engl. J. Med.* 364: 1920–1931.

119. Almanza-Monterrubio, M., Garnica-Hayashi, L., Dávila-Camargo, A., and Nava-Castañeda, Á. (2021). Oral selenium improved the disease activity in patients with mild Graves' orbitopathy. *J. Fr. Ophtalmol.* 44: 643–651.

120. Ertek, S. and Cicero, A.F. (2013). Hyperthyroidism and cardiovascular complications: A narrative review on the basis of pathophysiology. *Arch. Med. Sci.* 9: 944–952.

121. Dillmann, W. and h. (2002). Cellular action of thyroid hormone on the heart. *Thyroid* 12: 447–452.

122. Panagoulis, C., Halapas, A., Chariatis, E. et al. (2008). Hyperthyroidism and the heart. *Hell. J. Cardiol.* 49: 169–175.

123. Almeida, N.A.S., Cordeiro, A., Machado, D.S. et al. (2009). Connexin40 messenger ribonucleic acid is positively regulated by thyroid hormone (TH) acting in cardiac atria via the TH receptor. *Endocrinology* 150: 546–554.

124. Cacciatori, V., Bellavere, F., Pezzarossa, A. et al. (1996). Power spectral analysis of heart rate in hyperthyroidism. *J. Clin. Endocrinol. Metab.* 81: 2828–2835.

125. Zuber, S.M., Kantorovich, V., and Pacak, K. (2011). Hypertension in pheochromocytoma: Characteristics and treatment. *Endocrinol. Metab. Clin. N. Am.* 40: 295–311.

126. Abubakar, H., Singh, V., Arora, A., and Alsunaid, S. (2017). Propranolol-induced circulatory collapse in a patient with thyroid crisis and underlying thyrocardiac disease: A word of caution. *J. Investig. Med. High Impact Case Rep.* 5: 2324709617747903.

127. Laurens, C., Abot, A., Delarue, A., and Knauf, C. (2019). Central effects of beta-blockers may be due to nitric oxide and hydrogen peroxide release independently of their ability to cross the blood-brain barrier. *Front. Neurosci.* 13: 33.

128. Henderson, J.M., Portmann, L., Van Melle, G. et al. (1997). Propranolol as an adjunct therapy for hyperthyroid tremor. *Eur. Neurol.* 37: 182–185.

129. Geffner, D.L. and Hershman, J.M. (1992). Beta-adrenergic blockade for the treatment of hyperthyroidism. *Am. J. Med.* 93: 61–68.

130. Huang, K.-Y., Tseng, P.-T., Wu, Y.-C. et al. (2021). Do beta-adrenergic blocking agents increase asthma exacerbation? A network meta-analysis of randomized controlled trials. *Sci. Rep.* 11: 452.

131. Reid, J.R. and Wheeler, S.F. (2005). Hyperthyroidism: Diagnosis and Treatment. *Am. Fam. Physician* 72: 623–630.

132. De Groot, L.J., Bartalena, L. and Feingold, K.R. (2000). Thyroid storm. Endotext.

133. Tagami, T., Yambe, Y., Tanaka, T. et al. (2012). Short-term effects of β-adrenergic antagonists and methimazole in new-onset thyrotoxicosis caused by Graves' disease. *Intern. Med.* 51: 2285–2290.

134. Sebastián-Ochoa, A., Quesada-Charneco, M., Fernández-García, D. et al. (2008). Dramatic response to cholestyramine in a patient with Graves' disease resistant to conventional therapy. *Thyroid* 18: 1115–1117.

135. Alswat, K.A. (2015). Role of cholestyramine in refractory hyperthyroidism: A case report and literature review. *Am J Case Rep* 16: 486–490.

136. Tsai, W.-C., Pei, D., Wang, T.-F. et al. (2005). The effect of combination therapy with propylthiouracil and cholestyramine in the treatment of Graves' hyperthyroidism. *Clin. Endocrinol.* 62: 521–524.

137. Bagchi, N., Brown, T.R., and Mack, R.E. (1978). Studies on the mechanism of inhibition of thyroid function by lithium. *Biochim. Biophys. Acta* 542: 163–169.

138. Prakash, I., Nylen, E.S., and Sen, S. (2015). Lithium as an alternative option in Graves thyrotoxicosis. *Case Rep Endocrinol* 2015: 869343.

139. Sharma, P.P. (2022). Use of lithium in hyperthyroidism secondary to Graves' disease: A case report. *Am J Case Rep.* doi: 10.12659/AJCR.935789.

140. Zheng, R., Liu, K., Chen, K. et al. (2015). Lithium carbonate in the treatment of Graves' disease with ATD-induced hepatic injury or leukopenia. *Int. J. Endocrinol.* 2015: 694023.

141. Gupta, S. and Douglas, R. (2011). The pathophysiology of thyroid eye disease (TED): Implications for immunotherapy. *Curr. Opin. Ophthalmol.* 22: 385–390.

142. Bahn, R.S. (2010). Graves' ophthalmopathy. *N. Engl. J. Med.* 362: 726–738.

143. Bahn, R.S. (2003). Pathophysiology of Graves' ophthalmopathy: The cycle of disease. *J. Clin. Endocrinol. Metabol.* 88: 1939–1946.

144. Thornton, J., Kelly, S.P., Harrison, R.A., and Edwards, R. (2007). Cigarette smoking and thyroid eye disease: A systematic review. *Eye (Lond.)* 21: 1135–1145.

145. O'Dell, J.M., Mussatto, C.C., Chu, R.L. et al. (2023). Effects of smoking on outcomes of thyroid eye disease treated with teprotumumab: A retrospective cohort study. *Kans J Med* 16: 62–64.

146. Girnita, L., Smith, T.J., and Janssen, J.A.M.J.L. (2022). It takes two to tango: IGF-I and TSH receptors in thyroid eye disease. *J. Clin. Endocrinol. Metab.* 107: S1–S12.

147. Smith, T.J. and Hoa, N. (2004). Immunoglobulins from patients with Graves' disease induce hyaluronan synthesis in their orbital fibroblasts through the self-antigen, insulin-like growth factor-I receptor. *J. Clin. Endocrinol. Metab.* 89: 5076–5080.

148. Weightman, D.R., Perros, P., Sherif, I.H., and Kendall-Taylor, P. (1993). Autoantibodies to IGF-1 binding sites in thyroid associated ophthalmopathy. *Autoimmunity* 16: 251–257.

149. Xin, Y., Xu, F., Gao, Y. et al. (2021). Pharmacokinetics and exposure-response relationship of teprotumumab, an insulin-like growth factor-1 receptor-blocking antibody, in thyroid eye disease. *Clin. Pharmacokinet.* 60: 1029–1040.

150. Douglas, R.S., Kahaly, G.J., Patel, A. et al. (2020). Teprotumumab for the treatment of active thyroid eye disease. *N. Engl. J. Med.* 382: 341–352.

151. Khatavi, F., Nasrollahi, K., Zandi, A. et al. (2017). A promising modified procedure for upper eyelid retraction-associated Graves' ophthalmopathy: Transconjunctival lateral levator aponeurectomy. *Med Hypothesis Discov Innov Ophthalmol* 6: 44–48.

152. Falhammar, H., Juhlin, C.C., Barner, C. et al. (2018). Riedel's thyroiditis: Clinical presentation, treatment and outcomes. *Endocrine* 60: 185–192.

153. Barnes, P.J. (1998). Anti-inflammatory actions of glucocorticoids: Molecular mechanisms. *Clin. Sci. (Lond.)* 94: 557–572.

154. Moulik, P.K., Al-Jafari, M.S., and Khaleeli, A.A. (2004). Steroid responsiveness in a case of Riedel's thyroiditis and retroperitoneal fibrosis. *Int. J. Clin. Pract.* 58: 312–315.

155. Zala, A., Berhane, T., Juhlin, C.C. et al. (2020). Riedel thyroiditis. *J. Clin. Endocrinol. Metab.* 105: dgaa468.

156. Davidson, A. and Diamond, B. (2001). Autoimmune diseases. *N. Engl. J. Med.* 345: 340–350.

157. Shlomchik, M.J. (2008). Sites and stages of autoreactive B cell activation and regulation. *Immunity* 28: 18–28.

158. Lund, F.E. (2008). Cytokine-producing B lymphocytes-key regulators of immunity. *Curr. Opin. Immunol.* 20: 332–338.

159. Mauri, C. and Bosma, A. (2012). Immune regulatory function of B cells. *Annu. Rev. Immunol.* 30: 221–241.

160. Fillatreau, S., Sweenie, C.H., McGeachy, M.J. et al. (2002). B cells regulate autoimmunity by provision of IL-10. *Nat. Immunol.* 3: 944–950.

161. Pitzalis, C., Jones, G.W., Bombardieri, M., and Jones, S.A. (2014). Ectopic lymphoid-like structures in infection, cancer and autoimmunity. *Nat. Rev. Immunol.* 14: 447–462.

162. Mammen, S.V. and Gordon, M.B. (2019). Successful use of rituximab in a case of riedel thyroiditis resistant to treatment with prednisone and tamoxifen. *AACE Clinical Case Reports* 5: e218–e221.

163. Soh, S.-B., Pham, A., O'Hehir, R.E. et al. (2013). Novel use of rituximab in a case of riedel's thyroiditis refractory to glucocorticoids and tamoxifen. *J. Clin. Endocrinol. Metabol.* 98: 3543–3549.

164. Shafi, A.A., Saad, N.B., and AlHarthi, B. (2020). Riedel's thyroiditis as a diagnostic dilemma – A case report and review of the literature. *Ann Med Surg (Lond)* 52: 5–9.

165. Bartalena, L., Pinchera, A., and Marcocci, C. (2000). Management of Graves' ophthalmopathy: Reality and perspectives. *Endocr. Rev.* 21: 168–199.

166. McAlinden, C. (2014). An overview of thyroid eye disease. *Eye Vis (Lond).* doi: 10.1186/s40662-014-0009-8.

167. Clinical Practice Guideline Treating Tobacco Use and Dependence 2008 Update Panel, Liaisons, and Staff (2008). A clinical practice guideline for treating tobacco use and dependence: 2008 Update. *Am. J. Prev. Med.* 35: 158–176.

168. Williams, G.R. (2000). Cloning and characterization of two novel thyroid hormone receptor beta isoforms. *Mol. Cell Biol.* 20: 8329–8342.

169. Ortiga-Carvalho, T.M., Sidhaye, A.R., and Wondisford, F.E. (2014). Thyroid hormone receptors and resistance to thyroid hormone disorders. *Nat. Rev. Endocrinol.* 10: 582–591.

170. Tylki-Szymańska, A., Acuna-Hidalgo, R., Krajewska-Walasek, M. et al. (2015). Thyroid hormone resistance syndrome due to mutations in the thyroid hormone receptor α gene (THRA). *J. Med. Genet.* 52: 312–316.

171. Flamant, F. and Gauthier, K. (2013). Thyroid hormone receptors: The challenge of elucidating isotype-specific functions and cell-specific response. *Biochim. Biophys. Acta* 1830: 3900–3907.

172. Davis, P.J., Goglia, F., and Leonard, J.L. (2016). Nongenomic actions of thyroid hormone. *Nat. Rev. Endocrinol.* 12: 111–121.

173. Mitsuhashi, T., Tennyson, G.E., and Nikodem, V.M. (1988). Alternative splicing generates messages encoding rat c-erbA proteins that do not bind thyroid hormone. *Proc. Natl. Acad. Sci. U. S. A.* 85: 5804–5808.

174. Singh, B.K. and Yen, P.M. (2017). A clinician's guide to understanding resistance to thyroid hormone due to receptor mutations in the TRα and TRβ isoforms. *Clin Diabetes Endocrinol.* https://doi.org/10.1186/s40842-017-0046-z.

175. Refetoff, S., Weiss, R.E., and Usala, S.J. (1993). The syndromes of resistance to thyroid hormone. *Endocr. Rev.* 14: 348–399.

176. Moran, C. and Chatterjee, K. (2015). Resistance to thyroid hormone due to defective thyroid receptor alpha. *Best Pract. Res. Clin. Endocrinol. Metab.* 29: 647–657.

177. Kahaly, G.J. and Dillmann, W.H. (2005). Thyroid hormone action in the heart. *Endocr. Rev.* 26: 704–728.

178. Frishman, W.H. (2016). Beta-adrenergic receptor blockers in hypertension: Alive and well. *Prog. Cardiovasc. Dis.* 59: 247–252.

179. Biondi, B. and Cooper, D.S. (2008). The clinical significance of subclinical thyroid dysfunction. *Endocr. Rev.* 29: 76–131.

180. Refetoff, S. and Dumitrescu, A.M. (2007). Syndromes of reduced sensitivity to thyroid hormone: Genetic defects in hormone receptors, cell transporters and deiodination. *Best Pract. Res. Clin. Endocrinol. Metab.* 21: 277–305.

181. Rastogi, M.V. and LaFranchi, S.H. (2010). Congenital hypothyroidism. *Orphanet J. Rare Dis.* 5: 17.

182. Aguilar Diosdado, M., Escobar-Jimenez, L., Fernandez Soto, M.L. et al. (1991). Hyperthyroidism due to familial pituitary resistance to thyroid hormone: Successful control with 3, 5, 3' triiodothyroacetic associated to propranolol. *J. Endocrinol. Investig.* 14: 663–668.

183. Bassett, J.H.D. and Williams, G.R. (2016). Role of thyroid hormones in skeletal development and bone maintenance. *Endocr. Rev.* 37: 135–187.

184. Bochukova, E., Schoenmakers, N., Agostini, M. et al. (2012). A mutation in the thyroid hormone receptor alpha gene. *N. Engl. J. Med.* 366: 243–249.

185. Kowalik, M.A., Perra, A., Pibiri, M. et al. (2010). TRbeta is the critical thyroid hormone receptor isoform in T3-induced proliferation of hepatocytes and pancreatic acinar cells. *J. Hepatol.* 53: 686–692.

186. Pappa, T. and Refetoff, S. (2021). Resistance to thyroid hormone beta: A focused review. *Front Endocrinol (Lausanne)* 12: 656551.

187. Weiss, R.E., Dumitrescu, A., and Refetoff, S. (2010). Approach to the patient with resistance to thyroid hormone and pregnancy. *J. Clin. Endocrinol. Metab.* 95: 3094–3102.

188. Beck-Peccoz, P., Brucker-Davis, F., Persani, L. et al. (1996). Thyrotropin-secreting pituitary tumors. *Endocr. Rev.* 17: 610–638.

189. Dumitrescu, A.M. and Refetoff, S. (2013). The syndromes of reduced sensitivity to thyroid hormone. *Biochim. Biophys. Acta* 1830: 3987–4003.

190. Rivas, A.M. and Lado-Abeal, J. (2016). Thyroid hormone resistance and its management. *Proc. (Baylor Univ. Med. Cent.)* 29: 209–211.

191. Refetoff, S., Bassett, J.H.D., Beck-Peccoz, P. et al. (2014). Classification and proposed nomenclature for inherited defects of thyroid hormone action, cell transport, and metabolism. *European Thyroid Journal* 3: 7–9.

192. Moran, C., Agostini, M., Visser, W.E. et al. (2014). Resistance to thyroid hormone due to a mutation in thyroid hormone receptor α1 and the α2 variant protein. *Lancet Diabetes Endocrinol.* 2: 619–626.

193. Lee, J.H. and Kim, E.Y. (2014). Resistance to thyroid hormone due to a novel mutation of thyroid hormone receptor beta gene. *Ann Pediatr Endocrinol Metab* 19: 229–231.

194. Agrawal, N.K., Goyal, R., Rastogi, A. et al. (2008). Thyroid hormone resistance. *Postgrad. Med. J.* 84: 473–477.

195. Patel, Y.C. (1999). Somatostatin and its receptor family. *Front. Neuroendocrinol.* 20: 157–198.

196. Fliers, E., Kalsbeek, A., and Boelen, A. (2014). Beyond the fixed setpoint of the hypothalamus-pituitary-thyroid axis. *Eur. J. Endocrinol.* 171: R197–R208.

197. Epelbaum, J. (1986). Somatostatin in the central nervous system: Physiology and pathological modifications. *Prog. Neurobiol.* 27: 63–100.

198. Theodoropoulou, M. and Stalla, G.K. (2013). Somatostatin receptors: From signaling to clinical practice. *Front. Neuroendocrinol.* 34: 228–252.

199. Hershman, J.M. (2004). Physiological and pathological aspects of the effect of human chorionic gonadotropin on the thyroid. *Best Pract. Res. Clin. Endocrinol. Metab.* 18: 249–265.

200. Lamberts, S.W., Hofland, L.J., van Koetsveld, P.M. et al. (1990). Parallel in vivo and in vitro detection of functional somatostatin receptors in human endocrine pancreatic tumors: Consequences with regard to diagnosis, localization, and therapy. *J. Clin. Endocrinol. Metab.* 71: 566–574.

201. Colao, A., Filippella, M., Di Somma, C. et al. (2003). Somatostatin analogs in treatment of non-growth hormone-secreting pituitary adenomas. *Endocrine* 20: 279–283.

202. Strowski, M.Z. and Blake, A.D. (2008). Function and expression of somatostatin receptors of the endocrine pancreas. *Mol. Cell. Endocrinol.* 286: 169–179.

203. Appetecchia, M. and Baldelli, R. (2010). Somatostatin analogues in the treatment of gastroenteropancreatic neuroendocrine tumours, current aspects and new perspectives. *Journal of Experimental & Clinical Cancer Research : CR* 29: 19.

204. Kuhn, J.M., Arlot, S., Lefebvre, H. et al. (2000). Evaluation of the treatment of thyrotropin-secreting pituitary adenomas with a slow release formulation of the somatostatin analog lanreotide. *J. Clin. Endocrinol. Metab.* 85: 1487–1491.

205. Lyons, D.J., Horjales-Araujo, E., and Broberger, C. (2010). Synchronized network oscillations in rat tuberoinfundibular dopamine neurons: Switch to tonic discharge by thyrotropin-releasing hormone. *Neuron* 65: 217–229.

206. Melmed, S., Casanueva, F.F., Hoffman, A.R. et al. (2011). Diagnosis and treatment of hyperprolactinemia: An Endocrine Society clinical practice guideline. *J. Clin. Endocrinol. Metab.* 96: 273–288.

207. Kao, Y.-H., Chang, T.-J., and Huang, T.-S. (2013). Thyrotropin-secreting pituitary tumor presenting with congestive heart failure and good response to dopaminergic agonist cabergoline. *J. Formos. Med. Assoc.* 112: 721–724.

208. Yang, C., Wu, H., Wang, J. et al. (2017). Successful management of octreotide-insensitive thyrotropin-secreting pituitary adenoma with bromocriptine and surgery. *Medicine (Baltimore)* 96: e8017.

209. Rimareix, F., Grunenwald, S., Vezzosi, D. et al. (2015). Primary medical treatment of thyrotropin–secreting

pituitary adenomas by first-generation somatostatin analogs: A case study of seven patients. *Thyroid* 25: 877–882.

210. Lemmon, M.A. and Schlessinger, J. (2010). Cell signaling by receptor tyrosine kinases. *Cell* 141: 1117–1134.

211. Hunter, T. (2009). Tyrosine phosphorylation: Thirty years and counting. *Curr. Opin. Cell Biol.* 21: 140–146.

212. Hanahan, D. and Weinberg, R.A. (2011). Hallmarks of cancer: The next generation. *Cell* 144: 646–674.

213. Liu, R. and Xing, M. (2016). TERT promoter mutations in thyroid cancer. *Endocr. Relat. Cancer* 23: R143–R155.

214. Cabanillas, M.E., McFadden, D.G., and Durante, C. (2016). Thyroid cancer. *Lancet* 388: 2783–2795.

215. Roskoski, R. (2020). Properties of FDA-approved small molecule protein kinase inhibitors: A 2020 update. *Pharmacol. Res.* 152: 104609.

216. Pešorda, M., Kusačić Kuna, S., Huić, D. et al. (2020). Kinase inhibitors in the treatment of thyroid cancer: Institutional experience. *Acta Clin. Croat.* 59: 73–80.

217. Cabanillas, M.E., Ryder, M., and Jimenez, C. (2019). Targeted therapy for advanced thyroid cancer: Kinase inhibitors and beyond. *Endocr. Rev.* 40: 1573–1604.

218. Porter A, Wong DJ (2021). Perspectives on the treatment of advanced thyroid cancer: Approved therapies, resistance mechanisms, and future directions *Front. Oncol.* 10: 592202. https://doi.org/10.3389/fonc.2020.592202.

219. Cabanillas, M.E., Hu, M.I., Durand, J.-B., and Busaidy, N.L. (2011). Challenges associated with tyrosine kinase inhibitor therapy for metastatic thyroid cancer. *J. Thyroid. Res.* 2011: e985780.

220. Schlumberger, M., Tahara, M., Wirth, L.J. et al. (2015). Lenvatinib versus placebo in radioiodine-refractory thyroid cancer. *N. Engl. J. Med.* 372: 621–630.

221. Haugen, B.R., Alexander, E.K., Bible, K.C. et al. (2016). 2015 American thyroid association management guidelines for adult patients with thyroid nodules and differentiated thyroid cancer: The American thyroid association guidelines task force on thyroid nodules and differentiated thyroid cancer. *Thyroid* 26: 1–133.

222. Capdevila, J., Klochikhin, A., Leboulleux, S. et al. (2022). A randomized, double-blind noninferiority study to evaluate the efficacy of the Cabozantinib tablet at 60 mg per day compared with the cabozantinib capsule at 140 mg per day in patients with progressive, metastatic medullary thyroid cancer. *Thyroid* 32: 515–524.

223. Brose, M.S., Nutting, C.M., Jarzab, B. et al. (2014). Sorafenib in radioactive iodine-refractory, locally advanced or metastatic differentiated thyroid cancer: A randomised, double-blind, phase 3 trial. *Lancet* 384: 319–328.

224. Maxon, H.R. and Smith, H.S. (1990). Radioiodine-131 in the diagnosis and treatment of metastatic well differentiated thyroid cancer. *Endocrinol. Metab. Clin. N. Am.* 19: 685–718.

225. Szumowski, P., Abdelrazek, S., Iwanicka, D. et al. (2021). Dosimetry during adjuvant 131I therapy in patients with differentiated thyroid cancer-clinical implications. *Sci. Rep.* 11: 13930.

226. Portulano, C., Paroder-Belenitsky, M., and Carrasco, N. (2014). The Na+/I- symporter (NIS): Mechanism and medical impact. *Endocr. Rev.* 35: 106–149.

227. American Thyroid Association Taskforce On Radioiodine Safety, Sisson, J.C., Freitas, J. et al. (2011). Radiation safety in the treatment of patients with thyroid diseases by radioiodine 131I : Practice recommendations of the American thyroid association. *Thyroid* 21: 335–346.

228. Lazarus, J.H. (1998). The effects of lithium therapy on thyroid and thyrotropin-releasing hormone. *Thyroid* 8: 909–913.

229. Van Nostrand, D., Neutze, J., and Atkins, F. (1986). Side effects of "rational dose" iodine-131 therapy for metastatic well-differentiated thyroid carcinoma. *J. Nucl. Med.* 27: 1519–1527.

230. Barrington, S.F., Kettle, A.G., O'Doherty, M.J. et al. (1996). Radiation dose rates from patients receiving iodine-131 therapy for carcinoma of the thyroid. *Eur. J. Nucl. Med.* 23: 123–130.

231. Williamson, M. (2006). Radiological protection for medical exposure to ionizing radiation. *Health Phys.* 90: 597.

232. Mandel, S.J. and Mandel, L. (2003). Radioactive iodine and the salivary glands. *Thyroid* 13: 265–271.

233. Ronga, G., Filesi, M., Montesano, T. et al. (2004). Lung metastases from differentiated thyroid carcinoma. A 40 years' experience. *Q. J. Nucl. Med. Mol. Imaging* 48: 12–19.

234. Laplante, M. and Sabatini, D.M. (2012). mTOR signaling in growth control and disease. *Cell* 149: 274–293.

235. Chappell, W.H., Steelman, L.S., Long, J.M. et al. (2011). Ras/Raf/MEK/ERK and PI3K/PTEN/Akt/mTOR inhibitors: Rationale and importance to inhibiting these pathways in human health. *Oncotarget* 2: 135–164.

236. Jonklaas, J., Bianco, A.C., Bauer, A.J. et al. (2014). Guidelines for the treatment of hypothyroidism: Prepared by the American thyroid association task force on thyroid hormone replacement. *Thyroid* 24: 1670–1751.

237. Biondi, B. and Cooper, D.S. (2010). Benefits of thyrotropin suppression versus the risks of adverse effects in differentiated thyroid cancer. *Thyroid* 20: 135–146.

238. Jonklaas, J., Sarlis, N.J., Litofsky, D. et al. (2006). Outcomes of patients with differentiated thyroid carcinoma following initial therapy. *Thyroid* 16: 1229–1242.

CHAPTER 3

Adrenal Gland Therapies

3.1 PRIMARY ADRENAL INSUFFICIENCY

3.1.1 Glucocorticoids

3.1.1.1 Physiology

Physiological Effects of Cortisol

Cortisol is a glucocorticoid hormone produced exclusively by the zona fasciculata of the adrenal cortex [1].

A summary of the physiological effects of glucocorticoids is summarized next.

1. Cortisol is required for the maintenance of normoglycemia through its modulatory effects on gluconeogenesis and glycogen synthesis in the postabsorptive period [2].
2. It has potent anti-inflammatory and immunosuppressive effects by inhibiting the synthesis of pro-inflammatory cytokines, thus, suppressing the activation and function of various immune cells [3].
3. Cortisol helps regulate the sleep–wake cycle and other circadian processes. Furthermore, superimposed on this diurnal rhythm (circadian rhythm) is an ultradian rhythm of cortisol pulses every hour, which is facilitated by ACTH [4, 5]. The significance of the hypothalamic–pituitary–adrenal (HPA) axis with respect to cortisol regulation was reviewed in Section 1.1.1.
4. Cortisol influences the renal handling of electrolytes, such as sodium and potassium, through its effects on vasopressin secretion and the renal mineralocorticoid receptor (MR) [6].

Glucocorticoid receptor (GR) physiology was reviewed earlier in Section 1.1.5.

3.1.1.2 Mechanism of Action

The mechanism of action of hydrocortisone involves binding to the GR and eliciting subsequent post-receptor effects [7] (See Figure 1.5).

Hydrocortisone, a steroid hormone, diffuses through the cell membrane and binds to the intracellular GR, which is present in the cytoplasm. This binding leads to a conformational change in the receptor, causing the release of heat shock proteins (HSPs) and other chaperone proteins bound to the receptor [7].

The hydrocortisone–GR complex is then translocated to the cell nucleus. Once inside the nucleus, the complex binds to specific DNA sequences known as **glucocorticoid response elements** (GREs) [8].

The binding of the hydrocortisone–GR complex to GRE regulates the transcription of target genes, which involves either the upregulation or downregulation of a target gene, depending on the tissue [9].

Endocrinology: Pathophysiology to Therapy, First Edition. Akuffo Quarde.
© 2024 John Wiley & Sons Ltd. Published 2024 by John Wiley & Sons Ltd.

Pathophysiology Pearl

What is the cortisol to cortisone shunt?

Cortisol can bind to both glucocorticoid and mineralocorticoid receptors, and under physiological conditions, plasma levels of cortisol can be up to 1000-fold higher than those of aldosterone. 11β-hydroxysteroid dehydrogenase type 2 (11β-HSD2) inactivates cortisol to cortisone, thus protecting the mineralocorticoid receptor from direct activation of cortisol [10].

11β-hydroxysteroid dehydrogenase type 1 (11β-HSD1) and 11β-hydroxysteroid dehydrogenase type 2 (11β-HSD2) are involved in the regulation of cortisol levels in circulation [11].

11β-HSD1 is expressed primarily in hepatic and adipose tissues, converting cortisone (inactive) to cortisol (active) [10]. 11β-HSD2, on the other hand, is predominantly found in aldosterone-sensitive tissues, such as the kidneys, colon, and salivary glands, where it converts cortisol to cortisone. In other words, 11β-HSD2 protects the mineralocorticoid receptor (MR) from cortisol by reducing local cortisol concentrations and thus permitting aldosterone to bind to the MR to exert its effects on sodium and water retention [12]. See Figure 1.4.

In states of hypercortisolemia, such as Cushing's syndrome, excessive cortisol production overwhelms 11β-HSD2 activity, an enzyme required for the inactivation of cortisol to cortisone. This ultimately promotes the activation of mineralocorticoid receptors (MRs) by supraphysiological levels of cortisol. It should be noted that cortisol activates the MRs similarly to aldosterone, promoting sodium and water reabsorption and contributing to hypertension [13].

Practice Pearl(s)

In patients with adrenal insufficiency, the recommended starting dose of hydrocortisone is usually 15–25 mg/day, divided into two or three doses [13]. Alternatively, the dose can be calculated based on estimating the body surface area (mg/m²/day). The recommended daily dose of hydrocortisone based on estimates of body surface area ranges from 8–12 mg/m²/day [13]. Generally, these estimates of the total daily dose of hydrocortisone should serve as a guide, as the final selected dose should be tailored to the patient's needs, considering factors such as age, body weight, preexisting comorbidities, and clinical response [14]. See Table 3.1 for a summary of suggested dosing schedules of selected glucocorticoid therapies.

In an acute adrenocortical crisis, hydrocortisone is the preferred glucocorticoid because it has dual glucocorticoid and mineralocorticoid properties, closely similar to endogenous cortisol [16]. In addition, hydrocortisone is rapidly absorbed and has a relatively short half-life, making it suitable for the management of life-threatening adrenocortical crises [17].

For several reasons, dexamethasone, a longer-acting glucocorticoid, is usually not recommended as a first-line treatment for an adrenal crisis. This is because although dexamethasone has potent glucocorticoid effects, it lacks mineralocorticoid activity. This means it will not address the potential mineralocorticoid deficiency that can occur in primary adrenal insufficiency [16]. Additionally, dexamethasone has a much longer half-life, which may complicate the transition to oral medications and maintenance therapy after initial stabilization [13].

Prednisone has optimal glucocorticoid activity but relatively weak mineralocorticoid activity compared to hydrocortisone. Prednisone exists in an oral formulation and is, therefore, more commonly used in the long-term treatment of adrenal insufficiency but is not the first choice for stress dosing during an adrenal crisis [13]. Refer to Table 3.2 for the glucocorticoid and mineralocorticoid potencies of various glucocorticoid preparations.

TABLE 3.1   Dosing schedules for glucocorticoid replacement therapies.

Type of steroid	Equivalent total daily dose (mg)	Doses per day
Hydrocortisone	15–25	2–3
Prednisone	5–7.5	2
Prednisolone	4–6	2
Dexamethasone	0.25–0.5	1
Fludrocortisone	0.05–0.2	1

Source: Based on refs. [13, 15].

TABLE 3.2 Comparison of the potencies of glucocorticoid and mineralocorticoid of various glucocorticoid preparations.

Glucocorticoids	Equivalent dose (mg)	Glucocorticoid potency	Mineralocorticoid potency	Half-life (hrs)	Physiologic dose
Short-acting					
Hydrocortisone	20	1	1	2	6–12 mg/m²/day
Cortisone	25	0.8	0.8	0.5	
Intermediate-acting					
Prednisone	5	4	0.3	2.5	1.5–3 mg/m²/day
Prednisolone	5	5	0.3	2	1.5–3 mg/m²/day
Methylprednisolone	4	5	0	2	1.2–2.4 mg/m²/day
Long-acting					
Dexamethasone	0.75	30	0	4.5	0.2–0.4 mg/m²/day
Betamethasone	0.6	25–40	0	6.5	

Source: Adapted from ref. [17].

Clinical Trial Evidence

This study aimed to assess the suitability of glucocorticoid replacement in hypoadrenal patients and its impact on bone markers. The prospective and cross-sectional study involved 32 patients on replacement glucocorticoid therapy. Measurements included serum and urinary cortisol, osteocalcin, N-telopeptide of type I collagen (NTX), and bone mineral density. The results showed that 88% of the patients required a change in glucocorticoid therapy, with 75% required a dose reduction. After reducing the hydrocortisone dose, the median osteocalcin increased, with no change in the NTX/creatinine ratio. The study concluded that many patients on conventional corticosteroid replacement therapy are overtreated or on inappropriate regimens. An individual assessment should be performed to reduce the long-term risk of osteoporosis [18].

3.1.2   Mineralocorticoids

3.1.2.1   Physiology

The Renin Angiotensin Aldosterone Axis

The renin-angiotensin-aldosterone system (RAAS) is a critical hormonal system involved in regulating blood pressure, fluid balance, and electrolyte homeostasis [19]. The discovery of renin, the initial enzyme in this cascade, dates back to 1898 when the Finnish physiologist Robert Tigerstedt first observed its vasopressor effects. However, this discovery took almost three decades to gain widespread recognition [20].

Renin is a proteolytic enzyme mainly produced by the juxtaglomerular cells (JGCs) in the kidney's juxtaglomerular apparatus (JGA) [19]. It is derived from preprorenin, which is cleaved and processed into prorenin, an inactive molecule [21]. The majority of circulating renin exists in its inactive form, with a prorenin-to-renin ratio of approximately 9 : 1 [21].

Several pathways regulate renin synthesis and secretion, including the baroreceptor pathway, macula densa cells, and the sympathoadrenal system.

1. The baroreceptor pathway, first proposed by Skinner, is based on the principle that changes in the tensile stretch of blood vessels (blood pressure) can inhibit or stimulate renin release [22]. A significant decrease in blood pressure, primarily at the level of preglomerular vessels (afferent arteriole), stimulates renin release by the JGCs [22].

2. The macula densa is a group of specialized cells in the early distal tubule sensitive to sodium load. These cells transmit paracrine signals to nearby JGCs in response to changes in urinary sodium excretion, thus regulating renin secretion [23]. It is worth noting that prostaglandins, nitric oxide, and adenosine can also stimulate the macula densa pathway [24].

3. Catecholamines released from the adrenal medulla or renal sympathetic nerve endings

activate beta 1 adrenergic receptors on JGCs, promoting renin release [25].

The role of renin as the rate-limiting enzyme of the RAAS will be reviewed next. Angiotensinogen, an alpha globulin (plasma protein) synthesized primarily by the liver, serves as the substrate for renin [26]. Renin cleaves angiotensinogen to produce angiotensin I (an inactive decapeptide). It is worth noting that hormones such as cortisol, thyroid hormone, estrogens, and angiotensin II can further enhance the effects of renin on angiotensinogen [26].

Angiotensin Converting Enzyme (ACE) is widely expressed in the vascular endothelium of various tissues, including the brain, skeletal muscle, skin, heart, kidneys, and lungs [27]. It is particularly abundant in the endothelium of the pulmonary vasculature, where it converts inactive angiotensin I into potent vasoconstrictor angiotensin II [27]. Angiotensin II exerts multiple effects on distant tissues, primarily through binding to the receptors of the angiotensin receptor type 1 (AT1) and type 2 (AT2) receptors [28].

In contrast, ACE2 serves as a negative feedback regulator for RAAS. It converts angiotensin I into angiotensin (1–9), which is further cleaved by ACE to form angiotensin (1–7) [28]. This heptapeptide exerts various effects, such as peripheral vasodilation and inhibition of antidiuretic hormone release, by binding to AT2 receptors. Consequently, angiotensin (1–7) counterbalances the fluid-retentive and vasoconstrictive effects of angiotensin II [29]. A summary of RAAS is shown in Figure 3.1.

Angiotensin II acts primarily on two receptor subtypes: AT1 and AT2 receptors. The AT1 receptor, a G protein-coupled receptor, is expressed in various tissues such as blood vessels, the liver, lung, kidneys, adrenal gland, and the integument [30]. Activation of AT1 receptors by angiotensin II leads to various effects:

- Vasoconstriction [31].
- Enhanced inotropic effects on cardiac muscle [32].
- Potentiation of catecholamine release from sympathetic nerve endings [33].
- Stimulation of aldosterone release by the zona glomerulosa of the adrenal cortex [34].
- Cardiac muscle proliferation [35].
- Promotion of atherosclerosis and proliferation of vascular smooth muscle [36].
- Increased activity of NADPH oxidase, which generates reactive oxygen species (ROS) [37].

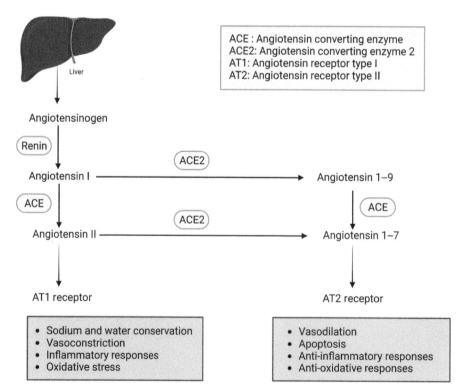

FIGURE 3.1   Schematic representation of the effects of angiotensinogen activation. The effects of AT1 and AT2 receptor activation and the respective peptides required for their activation are shown.

AT2 receptors are widely expressed in organs such as the brain, kidneys, heart, adrenals, and integument [38].

Activation of AT2 receptors counteracts the effects of AT1 receptor stimulation, resulting in various effects. These include the following:

- Inhibition of sympathetic activation [39].
- Suppression of the inflammatory effects of AT1 receptor activation [40].
- Vasodilation and urinary sodium loss [41].
- Antithrombotic and antifibrotic effects [42].

Refer to Figure 3.2 for a summary of the hemodynamic effects of renin-angiotensin-aldosterone system activation.

Aldosterone, a mineralocorticoid produced by the zona glomerulosa of the adrenal cortex, is a key component of the RAAS [43]. Aldosterone exerts a range of effects on fluid and electrolyte balance.

1. Aldosterone promotes sodium and water reabsorption in the renal tubules, particularly in the distal convoluted tubules (DCTs) and collecting ducts (CDs) [44]. In exchange for sodium reabsorption, aldosterone stimulates the excretion of potassium and hydrogen ions, helping to maintain electrolyte homeostasis [45–47].

2. Hypothalamic osmoreceptors are activated in response to increased serum osmolarity due to aldosterone-mediated sodium retention. This triggers the release of vasopressin (antidiuretic hormone) from the posterior pituitary gland, leading to enhanced reabsorption of free water in the CDs. As a result, extracellular volume increases, diluting the sodium pool and reducing plasma osmolarity [48].

3. Vasopressin release in response to aldosterone-mediated sodium retention also exerts vasoconstrictive effects on peripheral tissues, further contributing to blood pressure regulation [48]. Vasopressin in high concentrations, as could occur during periods of significant hypotension, binds to the vasopressin type 1 receptor (V1R) in vascular smooth muscle. V1R activation

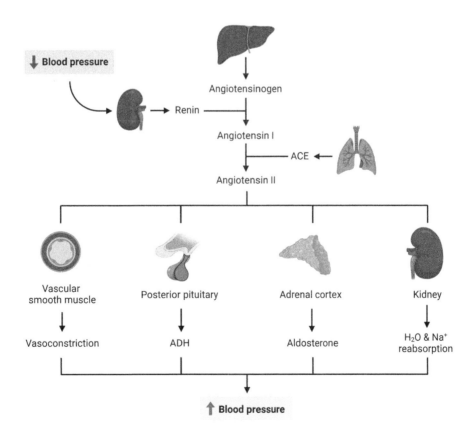

FIGURE 3.2 A schematic diagram of the renin-angiotensin-aldosterone axis. The steps involved in activating the renin-angiotensin-aldosterone axis and its peripheral effects are shown.

causes smooth muscle contraction and maintenance of blood pressure [49].

4. Aldosterone directly enhances vascular tone by increasing the responsiveness of blood vessels to the vasoconstrictive effects of catecholamines such as epinephrine and norepinephrine [50].

5. Aldosterone limits the vasodilatory effects of nitric oxide, a potent endogenous vasodilator, by reducing its bioavailability and activity [51].

Beyond its essential role in fluid and electrolyte balance, aldosterone can exert deleterious effects on the cardiovascular system, particularly in the setting of hyperaldosteronism. These effects are summarized next.

1. Aldosterone stimulates the proliferation of vascular smooth muscle cells, contributing to increased vessel wall thickness [52].

2. Aldosterone also facilitates the release of various pro-inflammatory cytokines that result in vascular dysfunction and the subsequent development of atherosclerosis [53].

3. Aldosterone increases the production of Reactive oxygen species (ROS) and reduces antioxidant defenses required to maintain the integrity of vascular endothelium [52].

How Does Cortisol Influence RAAS?

Cortisol plays a significant role in modulating the RAAS through various mechanisms. First, cortisol stimulates the production of the renin substrate, angiotensinogen, in the liver [54]. Angiotensinogen is then cleaved by renin, an enzyme released by JGCs in the kidneys, to form angiotensin I, marking the beginning of the RAAS cascade.

Secondly, cortisol has been found to upregulate the expression of the angiotensin-converting enzyme (ACE), which is responsible for converting angiotensin I to angiotensin II, a potent vasoconstrictor [55]. By increasing the availability of ACE, cortisol indirectly increases angiotensin II levels.

Finally, cortisol can bind to MRs when 11β-HSD2 activity is insufficient, mimicking the effects of aldosterone on sodium and water reabsorption. This contributes to increased blood volume and hypertension [43]. The cortisol to cortisone shunt was reviewed in Sections 3.1.1 and 1.1.1.

3.1.2.2 Mechanism of Action

Mineralocorticoids are a class of steroid hormones primarily involved in regulating electrolyte balance and blood pressure [56]. The most important and well-known mineralocorticoid is aldosterone, produced by the zona glomerulosa cells of the adrenal cortex [57]s The primary target of aldosterone is the DCT and the CDs in the kidneys [58].

MRs are ligand-dependent transcription factors that belong to the nuclear receptor superfamily [59]. In the absence of aldosterone, MRs are sequestered in the cytoplasm, bound to HSPs [60] (See Figure 3.3).

When aldosterone binds to the MR, it induces a conformational change, leading to the release of HSPs and the exposure of the nuclear localization signal [61]. The aldosterone–MR complex then translocates to the nucleus, where it binds to specific DNA sequences called hormone response elements (HREs) in the promoter regions of target genes [62].

The binding of the aldosterone–MR complex to HREs modulates the transcription of target genes [63]. The primary genes regulated by aldosterone include those that encode the epithelial sodium channel (ENaC) and the Na^+/K^+-ATPase pump-regulated kinase 1 (SGK1) [64].

The transcriptional regulation by aldosterone leads to the synthesis of new proteins that play an essential role in ion transport [65]. ENaC is located on the apical membrane of the principal cells of DCT and CD and is responsible for sodium reabsorption from the renal filtrate [66]. The Na^+/K^+-ATPase pump located on the basolateral membrane of the same cells is responsible for transporting sodium out of the cell into the bloodstream while pumping potassium into the cell [67]. Upregulation of these proteins by aldosterone increases sodium reabsorption and potassium excretion [68].

As sodium is reabsorbed in the DCT and CD, water passively follows along an osmotic gradient. This process increases the overall reabsorption of water, leading to an increase in blood volume and, consequently, blood pressure [69].

Aldosterone also has indirect effects on other ion channels and transporters [70]. For example, increased expression of SGK1 can modulate the function of several ion channels and transporters, such as the renal outer medullary potassium channel (ROMK) and the Na-Cl cotransporter (NCC), further fine-tuning the electrolyte balance and blood pressure regulation [71, 72] (see Figure 3.3).

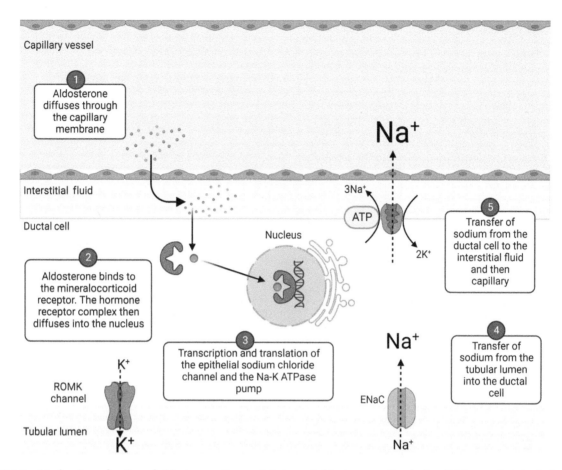

FIGURE 3.3 Mechanism of action of aldosterone. Sequential steps of aldosterone action in the distal convoluted tubule: from hormone binding to enhanced sodium reabsorption and potassium excretion.

Practice Pearl(s)

In practice, the recommended dose of fludrocortisone is 0.05–0.2 mg/day, administered as a single oral dose upon awakening in the morning. The prescribed dose of fludrocortisone should be individualized based on the patient's clinical response and biochemical parameters, such as plasma renin activity (treatment goal is the upper limit of the normal reference range), serum electrolytes, and blood pressure [13].

Clinical Trial Evidence

In a study of 193 patients with primary adrenal insufficiency (PAI), researchers investigated the relationship between fludrocortisone (FC) dose, glucocorticoid therapy, and various clinical and endocrine parameters. They found that FC's mineralocorticoid (MC) activity was dose-dependent and that renin and electrolyte levels can be used to titrate the FC dose. The study concluded that renin and electrolytes should be routinely evaluated in patients with PAI, and the dose of FC may need to be reduced in long-term follow-up of patients [73].

3.1.3 Androgens

3.1.3.1 Physiology

What Are Androgens?

The adrenal glands are responsible for the secretion of various androgens, including dehydroepiandrosterone (DHEA) (4 mg/day), dehydroepiandrosterone sulfate (DHEA-S)(7–15 mg/day), androstenedione (1.5 mg/day), and testosterone (0.05 mg/day) [74].

3.1.3.2 Mechanism of Action

The effects of androgens on normal physiology were reviewed in Section 6.2.1.

Practice Pearl(s)

Androgen supplementation in primary or secondary adrenal insufficiency, although not a critical component of treatment, has been shown to improve mood, libido, and energy levels in patients with these conditions, especially women [75, 76]. It is worth noting that current evidence on the efficacy of DHEA supplementation is limited in this population [77].

The usual starting dose of DHEA is 25 mg a day [76]. Laboratory monitoring includes the measurement of DHEA-S and testosterone concentrations in the morning before oral DHEA. It is also reasonable to monitor for clinical signs of androgen excess, such as acne and hirsutism.

Clinical Trial Evidence

In this meta-analysis, various randomized controlled trials assessing the impact of dehydroepiandrosterone (DHEA) on health-related quality of life (HRQOL) in women with primary or secondary adrenal insufficiency were evaluated. A total of 10 eligible trials were included in the analysis. The results showed a modest improvement in HRQOL and depression scores in women treated with DHEA compared to placebo, with an effect size of 0.21 (95% confidence interval, 0.08–0.33; heterogeneity $[I^2]$ = 32%). Nonetheless, the observed effects on anxiety and sexual well-being were small and not statistically significant. Hence, based on these findings, the authors concluded that the current evidence does not sufficiently support the routine administration of DHEA in women with adrenal insufficiency [78].

 Concepts to Ponder

Are they any unique clinical situations where routine management of adrenal insufficiency would need to be modified?

The timing of glucocorticoid therapy should be tailored to a patient's clinical status. A summary of suggested dosing schedules for various medical comorbidities is outlined in Table 3.3.

TABLE 3.3 Management of steroid replacement in unique clinical situations.

Clinical scenario	Recommendations
Shift workers with dysregulated sleep–wake cycles	Designate the odd time of awakening of the patient as the morning. Hence, the patient should take a larger dose of hydrocortisone upon waking up. The second dose should be administered 6–8 h later. Fludrocortisone should be taken upon waking up [79].
Pregnancy	Estrogen increases cortisol binding globulin, and this can reduce the levels of bioavailable exogenous steroids. Increasing hydrocortisone by 20–40% is recommended in the second to third trimester of pregnancy. Also, an increase in progesterone (anti-mineralocorticoid activity) in the last trimester of pregnancy requires a possible increase in fludrocortisone. Renin increases in pregnancy; as such, it should not be monitored. Sodium and potassium levels can, however, be useful [80].
Dialysis (hemodialysis or peritoneal)	Discontinue fludrocortisone therapy. Also, adjust glucocorticoid replacement since steroid replacement therapy is dialyzable [81].
Hypertension	The dose of fludrocortisone should be reduced. Calcium channel blockers are favored over RAAS modulators (ACE inhibitors or ARBs) [82].

ACE, angiotensin-converting enzymes; ARB's, angiotensin receptor blockers.
Source: Based on refs. [79–81].

Can opioids cause adrenal insufficiency?

There is evidence that long-term exposure to opioids can lead to suppression of the hypothalamic–pituitary–adrenal axis, leading to the development of central adrenal insufficiency. The primary mechanism of opioid-induced adrenal insufficiency (OIAI) is unclear. Nonetheless, discontinuation of opioids can lead to a complete resolution of OIAI [83].

3.2   PRIMARY HYPERALDOSTERONISM

3.2.1   Mineralocorticoid Antagonists

3.2.1.1   Physiology

The physiology of the RAAS was reviewed in Section 3.1.2.

3.2.1.2   Mechanism of Action

The mechanism of action of aldosterone antagonists in primary hyperaldosteronism involves the competitive inhibition of the MRs in the distal tubules and CDs of the nephron. These receptors mediate the effects of aldosterone on sodium and potassium transport, as was mentioned earlier (See Figure 3.3) [84].

When aldosterone antagonists bind to the MRs, they prevent aldosterone from exerting its effects on sodium and water reabsorption and potassium excretion. As a result, aldosterone antagonists promote sodium and water losses while reducing potassium excretion. This leads to decreased blood pressure and the normalization of electrolyte levels, thus alleviating the symptoms associated with primary hyperaldosteronism [84].

Examples of aldosterone antagonists used to treat primary hyperaldosteronism include spironolactone and eplerenone. Spironolactone is a nonselective MR antagonist, while eplerenone is a more selective antagonist with fewer side effects [85].

Practice Pearl(s)

The dosing of spironolactone and eplerenone for the treatment of primary hyperaldosteronism may vary depending on the individual patient's needs, the severity of the condition, and the response to the medication [84].

Below are general dosing guidelines for spironolactone and eplerenone in the treatment of primary hyperaldosteronism:

1. The initial dose of spironolactone is 12.5–25 mg once daily, which can be titrated based on the patient's response and tolerability. The maintenance dose typically ranges from 25 to 100 mg, divided into one or two doses per day. In some cases, doses up to 400 mg/day may be required for optimal control of blood pressure and aldosterone blockade [86].

2. The usual starting dose for eplerenone is 50 mg once daily. Based on the patient's response and tolerability, the dose can be increased to 50 mg twice daily or 100 mg once daily [87].

3. Monitoring blood pressure, serum potassium levels, and renal function during treatment with spironolactone or eplerenone is essential, as these medications can cause significant hyperkalemia [84].

Clinical Trial Evidence

In a multicenter, randomized, double-blind study comparing the efficacy of aldosterone antagonists, the authors evaluated the safety and tolerability of eplerenone and spironolactone in patients with hypertension associated with primary aldosteronism. Spironolactone showed a greater antihypertensive effect than eplerenone. The mean change from baseline in seated diastolic blood pressure (DBP) was −5.6 mmHg for eplerenone and −12.5 mmHg for spironolactone, with a difference of −6.9 mmHg (−10.6, −3.3), P value<0.001. However, spironolactone was associated with a higher incidence of male gynecomastia (21.2 vs. 4.5%) and female mastodynia (21.1 vs. 0.0%). Despite the lower antihypertensive effect of eplerenone, it had fewer antiandrogenic side effects than spironolactone [88].

 Clinical Pearl

How do mineralocorticoid receptor antagonists affect aldosterone-renin ratio (ARR) testing?

Mineralocorticoid receptor antagonists (eplerenone and spironolactone) bind to and block the mineralocorticoid receptor, thereby inhibiting

(continued)

(continued)

aldosterone from binding to its receptor. This leads to sodium excretion and a decrease in extracellular volume [84]. Consequently, plasma renin levels rise due to volume contraction (a feedback mechanism required for maintaining blood pressure and vascular volume) [89]. An increase in plasma renin levels can result in a false-negative aldosterone-renin ratio which may result in some cases of primary hyperaldosteronism being missed in patients on MR antagonists [90].

If patients on mineralocorticoid receptor antagonists continue to exhibit hypokalemia despite treatment, it suggests insufficient blockade of the mineralocorticoid receptors. In this scenario, renin remains suppressed, and the aldosterone-to-renin ratio is interpretable (or valid) [91–93].

What is the appropriate method for evaluating the aldosterone-to-renin ratio in patients receiving mineralocorticoid receptor antagonists?

It is not necessary to discontinue mineralocorticoid receptor antagonists before testing the ARR. If renin is suppressed, case-detection testing, confirmatory testing, and adrenal vein sampling can be conducted without discontinuing mineralocorticoid receptor antagonists [93].

Conversely, if renin is not suppressed (normal or elevated), it is advised to cease these interfering medications for 4–6 weeks before repeating case-detection testing [91].

How do ACE inhibitors (ACEi), Angiotensin Receptor Blockers (ARBs), or direct renin inhibitors affect aldosterone-renin ratio testing?

These agents interfere with renin receptor activation, reflexively increasing plasma renin levels, which may result in a falsely negative aldosterone-renin ratio [94]. Therefore, if plasma renin activity is >1 ng/mL/hr., primary aldosteronism cannot be ruled out without discontinuing these agents [95]. In contrast, if plasma renin activity is <1 ng/mL/hr. while on these agents, it strongly suggests a diagnosis of primary aldosteronism [96].

3.2.2   Amiloride

3.2.2.1   Physiology

The mechanism of action of mineralocorticoids was reviewed in Section 3.1.2.

3.2.2.2   Mechanism of Action

Amiloride and triamterene are potassium-sparing diuretics that act on the DCTs and CDs in the nephron of the kidney [97]. They are used in the management of primary hyperaldosteronism to counteract the effects of excessive plasma aldosterone, such as, hypertension, hypokalemia, and metabolic alkalosis [95].

The mechanism of action of amiloride and triamterene is summarized next:

1. *Inhibition of epithelial sodium channels (ENaC):* Both amiloride and triamterene work by inhibiting ENaC on the apical membrane of principal cells in the DCT and CDs [98]. These channels are responsible for the reabsorption of sodium from the renal filtrate back into the bloodstream. By blocking these channels, amiloride and triamterene prevent excessive sodium reabsorption and thus promoting natriuresis (sodium excretion in urine) [99].

2. *Preservation of potassium:* As a consequence of inhibiting ENaC, the electrochemical gradient across the apical membrane is altered, reducing the driving force for potassium secretion through potassium channels [100]. This results in the preservation of potassium levels in the blood, counteracting the hypokalemia caused by excessive aldosterone in primary hyperaldosteronism [96].

3. *Attenuation of aldosterone-induced effects:* In primary hyperaldosteronism, excessive aldosterone production leads to increased sodium reabsorption and potassium excretion [85].

4. *Mild diuretic effect:* Amiloride and triamterene, by promoting natriuresis, exert a mild diuretic effect, which contributes to the reduction of blood pressure in patients with primary hyperaldosteronism [101].

Pathophysiology Pearl

What is aldosterone Escape

Hyperaldosteronism enhances the reabsorption of sodium and water while facilitating renal potassium and H+ excretion. As a result, hyperaldosteronism induces plasma volume expansion, hypokalemia, and metabolic alkalosis [102]. Plasma volume expansion augments renal blood flow, subsequently reducing renin and angiotensin II production [102]. Elevated peritubular capillary hydrostatic pressure facilitates sodium transport from the interstitium back into the renal tubules (natriuresis) [103]. Stretching of atrial myocytes leads to the release of atrial natriuretic factor (ANF), which, despite hyperaldosteronism, encourages sodium excretion [104]. So what is aldosterone escape?

Under normal physiological conditions, sodium and water are reabsorbed from the renal tubular lumen and transported into the interstitium. Starling's forces subsequently determine the gradient of sodium and water movement from the interstitium into the peritubular capillaries and ultimately into the systemic circulation [102].

It is noteworthy that hydrostatic pressures across the renal tubules, interstitium, and peritubular capillaries are balanced in normal physiology. Consequently, oncotic pressures govern the flow of sodium and water. Due to the higher protein concentration in the peritubular capillary compared to the interstitium, sodium and water are transported from the interstitium into the capillaries (via oncotic forces) [102].

In contrast, hyperaldosteronism-associated plasma volume expansion results in an overwhelming hydrostatic pressure compared to the oncotic pressure in the peritubular capillaries. This pathological alteration in Starling's forces promotes the "backflow" of sodium and water from the interstitium into the renal tubular lumen (pressure natriuresis). This adaptation prevents hypernatremia and fluid retention (edema) in primary hyperaldosteronism [103]. See Figure 3.4.

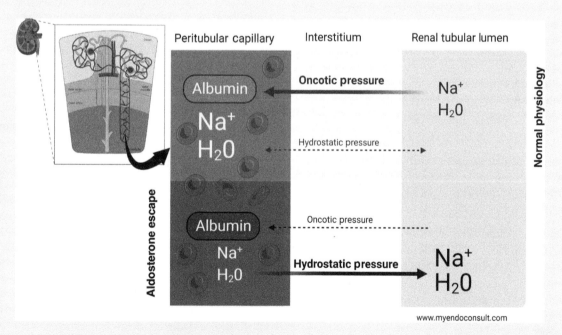

www.myendoconsult.com

FIGURE 3.4 Mechanism of aldosterone escape. Oncotic and hydrostatic pressures determine the direction of the flow of fluid in both normal physiology and pathological states.

Practice Pearl(s)

The optimal treatment of primary hyperaldosteronism involves the use of mineralocorticoid receptor antagonists, such as spironolactone or eplerenone. The initial dose of spironolactone is 12.5–25 mg daily (typical dose range of 100–400 mg/day) [84]. While eplerenone has a starting dose of 25 mg twice daily (maximum dose of 100 mg/day) [105].

Spironolactone has traditionally been the preferred choice due to its longer duration of action compared to eplerenone. Eplerenone, although shorter-acting, has a higher specificity for the aldosterone receptor and is associated with fewer side effects [105].

The goals of therapy for primary hyperaldosteronism include the following:

- Raising serum potassium levels to the high-normal range to prevent complications related to hypokalemia [84].
- Plasma renin activity can be monitored with the aim of achieving a level higher than 1 ng/mL/hour. This approach ensures sufficient mineralocorticoid receptor blockade and excessive aldosterone effects are mitigated [84].
- Normalizing blood pressure to reduce the risk of cardiovascular events [106].
- Reversing the detrimental effects of hyperaldosteronism on the heart and kidneys, such as left ventricular hypertrophy and renal impairment, respectively [106].

Plasma aldosterone-to-renin ratio (ARR) is a useful screening test; however, certain medications (e.g. ACE inhibitors, ARBs, and mineralocorticoid receptor antagonists) can interfere with the results [107]. Confirmatory tests, such as saline infusion, captopril challenge, or fludrocortisone suppression tests, may be required for a definitive diagnosis [107].

Adrenal vein sampling can help differentiate between unilateral (e.g. aldosterone-producing adenoma) and bilateral (idiopathic hyperaldosteronism) causes [108].

In patients with unilateral primary hyperaldosteronism, adrenalectomy is the treatment of choice and can lead to significant improvements in blood pressure control and potassium levels [108]. Medical therapy is recommended for patients with bilateral adrenal hyperplasia [84].

Clinical Trial Evidence

This study aimed to compare the efficacy and safety of eplerenone and spironolactone in treating bilateral idiopathic hyperaldosteronism (IHA). 34 patients with IHA were randomly assigned to receive either spironolactone ($n = 17$) or eplerenone ($n = 17$) for 24 weeks. The primary outcome was the percentage of patients with blood pressure (BP) < 140/90 mmHg at 16 weeks. BP was normalized in 76.5% of spironolactone patients and 82.4% of eplerenone patients, with no significant difference ($p = 1.00$) between both groups. Systolic BP decreased more rapidly with eplerenone. Serum potassium levels normalized in all patients at 4 weeks. Mild hyperkalemia was observed in two patients on 400 mg spironolactone and three patients on 150 mg eplerenone. Two patients experienced painful bilateral gynecomastia at week 16 while on 400 mg spironolactone. Switching to 150 mg, eplerenone resolved gynecomastia and maintained BP control. At the end of the study, 19 patients were on eplerenone, and 15 were on spironolactone. The study concluded that eplerenone was as effective as spironolactone in reducing BP in IHA patients, with a similar risk of mild hyperkalemia [109].

 Pathophysiology Pearl

Pseudohyperaldosteronism refers to endocrine disorders that display certain clinical characteristics similar to primary hyperaldosteronism, such as hypertension and hypokalemia. However, unlike primary hyperaldosteronism, these conditions do not show an expected rise in the plasma aldosterone-to-plasma renin ratio. Instead, patients with pseudohyperaldosteronism exhibit low levels of both aldosterone and renin.

Liddle's syndrome: A gain-of-function mutation of the gene encoding the amiloride-sensitive epithelial sodium chloride transporter [110].

Gordon syndrome: A gain-of-function mutation in the thiazide-responsive sodium-chloride transporter found in the distal nephron differentiates Gordon Syndrome from other pseudohyperaldosteronism causes. Contrary to other conditions, this syndrome is linked with elevated potassium levels rather than reduced potassium levels [111].

Defects in adrenal steroidogenesis: A deficiency in the 11β-hydroxylase enzyme leads to an accumulation of 11-Deoxycorticosterone, a hormone with inherent mineralocorticoid activity [112].

Cushing's syndrome: Elevated cortisol levels can lead to the saturation of the 11β-hydroxysteroid dehydrogenase 2 enzyme, resulting in cortisol binding to the mineralocorticoid receptor (refer to the cortisol-to-cortisone shunt) [113].

Apparent mineralocorticoid excess: A hereditary condition marked by an autosomal recessive inheritance pattern involving a nonfunctional mutation in the 11β-hydroxysteroid dehydrogenase 2 enzyme [114].

Excessive consumption of licorice, grapefruits, or carbenoxolone: Inhibition of 11β-hydroxysteroid dehydrogenase 2 [113].

 Concepts to Ponder

What is Adrenal Vein Sampling?

Adrenal vein sampling (AVS) was initially proposed and demonstrated as a reliable diagnostic method for localizing the origin of hyperaldosteronism in the 1960s by James Melby and his colleagues at the Boston University School of Medicine [115].

The diagnostic accuracy of computed tomography (CT) for identifying the origin of hyperaldosteronism is limited, with a success rate of approximately 50% [116]. Therefore, adrenal vein sampling (AVS) plays a crucial role in localizing the source of hyperaldosteronism for patients who choose surgical intervention [117]. It is important to note that AVS outcomes are operator-dependent,

and the procedure is best performed in high-volume centers with expertise in performing the procedure [117]. In fact, when conducted by experienced professionals, the technical success rate surpasses 90% [118].

Vascular Supply of the adrenal glands

Vascular supply of the adrenal glands is shown in Figure 3.5.

The right adrenal vein directly drains into the inferior vena cava. Cannulation of the right adrenal vein can be challenging due to factors such as its short trajectory, small diameter, and occasional anomalous origin (which may arise alongside

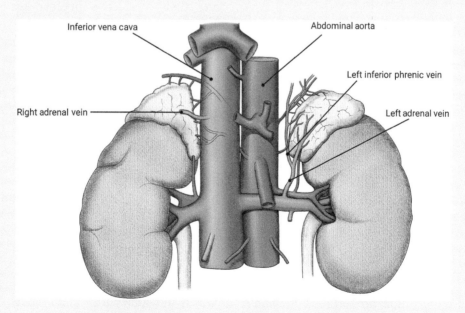

FIGURE 3.5 Vascular supply of the adrenal glands.

(*continued*)

(continued)

branches of the hepatic vein). In contrast, the left adrenal vein connects to the common inferior phrenic vein. Generally, the left adrenal vein is easier to catheterize compared to the right adrenal vein [119].

Approach to Interpreting AVS on Board Exams and in Clinical Practice

Selectivity Index

The selectivity index compares cortisol levels in each adrenal vein to the peripheral cortisol in the inferior vena cava (IVC). While various cutoffs have been suggested, a ratio above 5 on both sides indicates successful cannulation [120].

Lateralization Index

Upon confirming optimal cannulation of both adrenal veins, the next step involves identifying the source of excess aldosterone production. The lateralization index is calculated by determining the aldosterone-to-cortisol levels on each side (A:C ratios for left and right adrenal veins). The higher A:C ratio side (dominant adrenal) is divided by the lower A:C ratio side (nondominant adrenal). A lateralization index of 4 or higher suggests a unilateral source of hyperaldosteronism involving the side with the higher A:C ratio [121].

A lateralization index between 4:1 and 3:1 may indicate either unilateral or bilateral disease, requiring additional testing and consultation with a hyperaldosteronism expert. A lateralization index below 3:1 signifies bilateral disease, and surgery should be deferred in favor of medical therapy [121].

Contralateral Gland Suppression Index

In cases where lateralization to a culprit adrenal gland is apparent, the contralateral suppression index serves as an additional confirmatory step. The aldosterone-to-cortisol ratio of the nondominant adrenal gland (unaffected side) should be lower or equal to the peripheral A:C ratio [122].

3.3 PHEOCHROMOCYTOMAS AND OTHER PARAGANGLIOMA SYNDROMES

3.3.1 Alpha-Blockers

3.3.1.1 Physiology

What Are Catecholamines

Catecholamines, a group of structurally related hormones including epinephrine, norepinephrine, and dopamine, are synthesized in the adrenal medulla. Furthermore, there are additional sources of catecholamine, including the brain, sympathetic nervous system nerve endings, retroperitoneal paraganglia, and chromaffin tissue located at the aortic bifurcation (organ of Zuckerkandl). Structurally, epinephrine, norepinephrine, and dopamine contain a *pyrocatechol ring* in their basic structure, hence their collective name, catecholamines [123].

Metanephrines is a general term for catecholamine metabolites formed when epinephrine, norepinephrine, and dopamine are broken down by specific enzymes in the body. As an example, metanephrine and normetanephrine are examples of metanephrines [124].

The continuous intratumoral conversion of catecholamines (epinephrine and norepinephrine) into their respective metabolites (metanephrine and normetanephrine) by the enzyme catechol-O-methyltransferase (COMT) makes fractionated metanephrines in plasma or urine valuable screening tools for pheochromocytomas and paragangliomas (PPGLs). Since catecholamines (epinephrine, norepinephrine, and dopamine) are released intermittently, screening tests that only use catecholamines may not detect PPGLs [125].

Fractionated metanephrines refer to the metabolites of epinephrine (metanephrine) and norepinephrine (normetanephrine) [124]. A clinically significant elevation of epinephrine or its metabolite, metanephrine, typically indicates the presence of adrenal phenylethanolamine N-methyltransferase (PNMT), a cortisol-induced enzyme. Although PNMT is present in extra-adrenal tissues such as paraganglia, it does not convert norepinephrine into epinephrine in these tissues, as it is not under paracrine stimulation by cortisol [123]. Therefore, the levels of epinephrine or its metabolite, metanephrine, can provide important diagnostic information on the presence of adrenal PNMT and help identify adrenal PPGL (See Figure 3.6) [123].

What Are Adrenergic Receptors?

Adrenergic receptors are a class of G-protein coupled receptors (GPCRs) that play essential roles in the nervous system by mediating the actions of catecholamines, such as adrenaline and noradrenaline [126].

Adrenergic receptors are classified into two main subtypes: alpha (α) and beta (β) receptors, with each subtype further divided into subgroups ($\alpha1$, $\alpha2$, $\beta1$, $\beta2$, and $\beta3$) [127].

1. Alpha-1 ($\alpha1$) receptors: Primarily found on smooth muscle cells. Activation of this receptor subtype leads to vasoconstriction, and increased peripheral resistance, events which result in elevated blood pressure [127].
2. Alpha-2 ($\alpha2$) receptors: These inhibitory receptors are located in both the central and peripheral nervous systems. Their activation reduces sympathetic outflow, which results in a reduction in both blood pressure and pulse rate [128].
3. Beta-1 ($\beta1$) receptors: Predominantly found in the heart. The activation of these receptors increases heart rate and force of myocardial contraction. These effects are essential for maintaining cardiac function and regulating blood pressure [129].
4. Beta-2 ($\beta2$) receptors: These receptors are found in smooth muscle and, when activated, result in bronchodilation, vasodilation, and relaxation of smooth muscles in the uterus and gastrointestinal tract [130].
5. Beta-3 ($\beta3$) receptors: $\beta3$ receptors are mainly found in adipose tissue and are involved in lipolysis, thermogenesis, and regulation of energy expenditure [131].

3.3.1.2 Mechanism of Action

Alpha-adrenergic receptor blockers bind to alpha-adrenergic receptors and prevent their activation by catecholamines like adrenaline and noradrenaline. There are two clinically significant groups of alpha-blockers based on the receptor subtype targeted by these agents.

Firstly, alpha-1 receptors blockers like prazosin, terazosin, and doxazosin antagonize the vasoconstrictive effects of catecholamines. These agents promote vasodilation and a subsequent reduction in peripheral vascular resistance.

On the other hand, phenoxybenzamine is a nonselective alpha-adrenergic receptor blocker that binds irreversibly to alpha-1 and alpha-2 receptors causing a more sustained vasodilation and reduction in blood pressure than the previously described selective alpha-1 blockers.

Practice Pearl(s)

In patients with pheochromocytoma who are being prepared for surgery, alpha-adrenergic blockers should be administered preoperatively for at least 7 days.

This is required to normalize blood pressure and reduce the risk of a hypertensive crisis during surgery. Phenoxybenzamine is administered at doses of 10 mg every 6–12 hours and increased by 30–40 mg every 6 hours to a maximum dose of 240 mg daily [132]. Alternatively, selective alpha-1-adrenergic blockers, like prazosin, terazosin, or doxazosin, may be used for their relatively favorable side-effect profiles (lower incidence of orthostatic hypotension and nasal stuffiness) and lower cost [133].

Blood pressure should be monitored twice daily, targeting low-normal levels. However, the eventual goals should be adjusted based on the patient's age and comorbidities. Encouraging patients to consume a high-sodium diet (>5000 mg daily) to counteract the effects of catecholamine-induced volume contraction and orthostasis associated with alpha-adrenergic blockade is also essential [134].

Initial treatment is usually alpha-blockers. These block alpha-adrenergic receptors and help to control blood pressure. Once an alpha-blocker has controlled symptoms effectively, a beta-blocker can be used to manage any remaining symptoms (See Table 3.4). [135].

Clinical Trial Evidence

The study retrospectively reviewed the efficiency of phenoxybenzamine, prazosin, and doxazosin for preoperative preparation in pheochromocytoma

(continued)

(continued)

patients. Phenoxybenzamine was used in 21 patients, prazosin in 11 patients, and doxazosin in 17 patients. Intraoperative hypertension occurred in 81% of the phenoxybenzamine group, 73% of the prazosin group, and 82% of the doxazosin group, with no significant difference among the groups ($P > 0.05$). No significant differences were found in postoperative blood pressure measurements and volume replacements. The study concluded that pheochromocytoma surgery is safe with any of these preoperative medications [136].

3.3.2   Beta-Blockers

3.3.2.1   Physiology

See Section 3.3.1 for the physiology of adrenergic receptors.

3.3.2.2   Mechanism of Action

Beta-blockers competitively inhibit the binding of catecholamines (epinephrine and norepinephrine) to beta-adrenergic receptors, a process that reduces myocardial contractility and heart rate [137].

The negative inotropic effects of beta-blockers decrease the overall workload on the heart and reduce myocardial oxygen demand. This can benefit pheochromocytoma patients who often experience tachycardia and increased myocardial oxygen demand [138].

Catecholamines can cause arrhythmias by increasing cardiac automaticity and hence altering the electrical conduction within the heart. Beta-blockers, through their negative chronotropic effects, can help mitigate these arrhythmias by suppressing the abnormal electrical activity of the heart [139].

It is important to note that beta-blockers should not be used as the initial means of controlling blood pressure in patients with PPGLs, as they can exacerbate hypertension by causing unopposed alpha-adrenergic receptor stimulation [140]. Consequently, alpha-blockers should be initiated first, and once adequate

alpha-blockade has been achieved and blood pressure stabilized, beta-blocker may be introduced to address tachycardia [141, 142].

Practice Pearl(s)

In managing pheochromocytomas, the alpha-adrenergic blockade is administered 10–14 days before surgery to normalize blood pressure and expand the contracted intravascular volume. Phenoxybenzamine is commonly used, but other short-acting and selective α-1 antagonists, such as prazosin, terazosin, and doxazosin, are suitable alternatives. It is worth noting that careful dose adjustment is required to avoid hypotension in these patients. Furthermore, patients should be encouraged to consume fluids and have liberal salt intake during alpha blockade to prevent severe hypotension. Nonetheless, caution is required in encouraging liberal fluid and salt intake in patients with congestive heart failure or renal failure [142].

Beta-blockers should be initiated cautiously with low doses. Propranolol, a nonselective beta-blocker, should be started at 10 mg every six hours. Alternatively, a selective beta-blocker, metoprolol, should be started at 12.5 mg twice daily. On the second day, it should be converted to a single, long-acting dose and adjusted to control tachycardia, targeting a heart rate of 60–80 beats per minute. Maximum doses typically include 120 mg of propranolol or 200 mg of metoprolol [143].

Clinical Trial Evidence

There is currently no strong evidence to support the preference for one type of beta-blocker therapy over another in patients with pheochromocytomas. Indeed, the two major types of beta-blockers can be used for rate control after adequate alpha-adrenergic blockade is achieved. Consequently, the choice of a specific beta-blocker should depend on factors such as a patient's comorbidities, potential side effects, and clinical response [143].

3.3.3 Chemotherapy

3.3.3.1 Physiology

Pheochromocytomas and paragangliomas, collectively called PPGLs, are rare neuroendocrine tumors originating from chromaffin cells found in the adrenal medulla and sympathetic/parasympathetic paraganglia, respectively [144]. As is known about most neoplasms, PPGLs are formed due to an interplay of various factors, including genetic, epigenetic, and environmental factors [145].

Approximately 30–40% of PPGLs are associated with germline mutations in susceptibility genes, such as SDHx, RET, NF1, and VHL, which can predispose these individuals to the development of these tumors [146,147].

Furthermore, epigenetic changes, such as DNA methylation and histone modification, can lead to altered gene expression and contribute to the development of PPGLs [148]. The tumor microenvironment, including factors like hypoxia and angiogenesis, also plays a critical role in the growth and progression of these tumors [149]. The genetic changes associated with the development of PPGLs are beyond the scope of this text and will, therefore, not be discussed further.

3.3.3.2 Mechanism of Action

Cyclophosphamide, vincristine, and dacarbazine (CVD) therapy is a chemotherapy regimen used in the treatment of PPGLs [150]. The combination of these three drugs targets cancer cells through different mechanisms, disrupting their growth and division, ultimately leading to cell death [151].

Cyclophosphamide is an alkylating agent that forms DNA cross-links, preventing DNA replication and transcription [152]. It works by transferring an alkyl group to the DNA molecule, which disrupts the DNA structure and function. The cross-linking causes DNA strand breaks and leads to the activation of cellular repair mechanisms. If the damage is too severe, the cell undergoes apoptosis (programmed cell death) [153].

Vincristine is a vinca alkaloid that binds to tubulin, a protein that forms microtubules [154]. Microtubules are essential components of the cell's cytoskeleton and play a crucial role in cell division (mitosis). By binding to tubulin, vincristine disrupts microtubule formation, leading to the arrest of mitosis in metaphase [155]. This disruption of cell division eventually leads to cell death.

Dacarbazine is an alkylating agent that works by methylating the purine bases of DNA, particularly guanine [156]. This methylation leads to the formation of abnormal base pairing, ultimately inhibiting DNA replication and RNA synthesis [8].

DNA damage triggers cellular repair mechanisms, and if the damage cannot be repaired, the cell undergoes apoptosis [157].

Practice Pearl(s)

In patients with metastatic pheochromocytoma, the combination of cyclophosphamide, vincristine, and dacarbazine (CVD) is usually recommended as palliative treatment [158]. This regimen has demonstrated some efficacy in reducing tumor size and catecholamine production. Nonetheless, the response to chemotherapy in metastatic pheochromocytoma is variable, and the overall survival benefit remains unclear [159].

Clinical Trial Evidence

In this retrospective study, the authors evaluated the clinical benefits of systemic chemotherapy for patients with metastatic pheochromocytomas or sympathetic paragangliomas. Out of 54 patients treated at The University of Texas MD Anderson Cancer Center, 52 were enrolled in the study. A clinically meaningful response was observed in 17 patients (33%), characterized by decreased blood pressure, reduced antihypertensive medication use, or tumor size reduction. Median overall survival (OS) was 6.4 years (95% CI: 5.2–16.4 years) for responders and 3.7 years (95% CI: 3.0–7.5 years) for nonresponders. Response to chemotherapy significantly impacted OS (hazard ratio: 0.22; 95% CI: 0.05–1.0; $P = 0.05$). All responders received dacarbazine and cyclophosphamide, with 14 receiving vincristine and 12 receiving doxorubicin. The study concluded that chemotherapy might decrease tumor size and improve blood pressure control in approximately 33% of patients with metastatic pheochromocytoma, potentially leading to more prolonged survival [160].

Clinical Pearl

This is a detailed practice guide on the perioperative management of patients of PPGLs (see Table 3.4).

TABLE 3.4 Perioperative management pearls for PPGLs.

Practice question	Recommendation	Pearl(s)
Timing of alpha blockade	For tumors <3 cm in size, start 7 days prior to surgery. For tumors >3 cm, start 10–14 days prior to surgery.	In hospitalized patients, titration can be accelerated in a monitored setting.
Choice of alpha-blocker	Doxazosin 1 mg at bedtime or 1 mg twice daily. Phenoxybenzamine 10 mg daily or 10 mg twice daily.	Phenoxybenzamine's effect tends to plateau at 90 mg/day. Phenoxybenzamine is associated with a significant risk for reflex tachycardia.
Choice of beta-blocker	Propranolol 10 mg every 6–8 h. Metoprolol succinate 25 mg once daily.	This should be started 2–3 days prior to surgery.
What if the patient is already on antihypertensive therapy?	Diuretics should be stopped. ACEi and ARBs may be tapered or even stopped. Continue calcium channel blockers.	Diuretics will counteract the goal of expanding plasma volume. CCBs are associated with decreased mortality and morbidity in this patient population.

Source: Adapted from ref. [161].

3.3.4   Methyltyrosine

3.3.4.1   Physiology

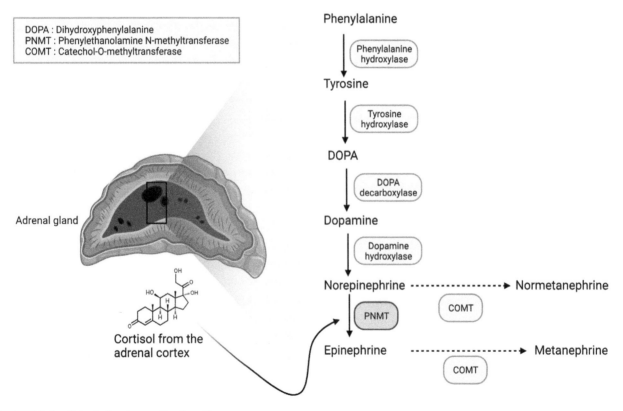

FIGURE 3.6   Catecholamine synthesis pathway.

3.3.4.2   Mechanism of Action

Metyrosine inhibits the enzyme tyrosine hydroxylase (TH), the rate-limiting step in catecholamine synthesis (see Figure 3.6). As you may recall, TH converts L-tyrosine to L-dihydroxyphenylalanine (L-DOPA), and by inhibiting this enzyme, metyrosine effectively reduces the production of catecholamines [161].

> **Practice Pearl(s)**
>
> Metyrosine is used cautiously in pheochromocytoma cases when other agents are ineffective or for patients requiring tumor resection [161]. The Mayo Clinic's short-term pre-procedure protocol involves increasing metyrosine doses (250–1000 mg) every six hours.

> **Clinical Trial Evidence**
>
> This retrospective study compared the outcomes of abdominal surgical resection in pheochromocytoma or paraganglioma patients pretreated with metyrosine (MET) vs. phenoxybenzamine (PBZ). MET was administered in 63 cases, and all patients experienced wide perioperative hemodynamic oscillations. Patients who received MET+PBZ, on the other hand, had lower minimum systolic and diastolic blood pressures (median systolic: 74 vs. 80 mmHg, $P = 0.01$; median diastolic: 42 vs. 46 mmHg, $P = 0.005$) and larger intraoperative blood pressure oscillations than PBZ-only patients. However, no significant differences in postoperative comorbid outcomes were found between the two groups [162].

3.3.5   MIBG

3.3.5.1   Physiology

The mechanism of catecholamine synthesis was reviewed in Section 3.3.4.

3.3.5.2   Mechanism of Action

Metaiodobenzylguanidine (MIBG) is a radiopharmaceutical agent used for the diagnosis and treatment of PPGLs [163]. The mechanism of MIBG action in PPGLs relies on its structural similarity with norepinephrine and its ability to selectively be taken up by neurons that express norepinephrine transporters [163].

MIBG can be labeled radioactively (usually with iodine 123 or 131) for diagnostic purposes. When injected into the patient, the radiolabeled MIBG is taken up by the catecholamine-secreting tumors through the norepinephrine transporters. The tumor can be imaged using a gamma camera, which helps detect and locate PPGLs within the body [164].

The radiolabeled compound used in MIBG therapy is iodine 131, which emits both beta and gamma radiation. The beta radiation emitted by MIBG causes cell damage and ultimately leads to the death of tumor cells. Gamma cameras can detect gamma rays and monitor the therapeutic response [165].

> **Practice Pearl(s)**
>
> High-specific-activity ^{131}I-meta-iodobenzylguanidine HSA-131I-MIBG is a treatment option for patients with inoperable or metastatic pheochromocytoma or paraganglioma who have positive MIBG scans and disease progression or symptoms. The treatment aims to stabilize the disease and control symptoms. The treatment involves dosimetry assessment using HSA-131I-MIBG imaging over three to five days, followed by two doses of 500 mCi (or 8 mCi/kg if weight < 62.5 kg) of HSA-^{131}I-MIBG given at least 90 days apart. Thyroid blockade with stable iodide is mandatory, and a 60-minute infusion time is recommended for pediatric patients aged 12 years and older [166].

FIGURE 3.6   Synthesis of catecholamines. The rate-limiting step in the synthesis of catecholamine occurs at the initial conversion of L-tyrosine into L-3,4-dihydroxyphenylalanine (DOPA) via the tyrosine hydroxylase enzyme. DOPA is then converted to dopamine. Next, dopamine is hydroxylated into L-norepinephrine, which is then converted into epinephrine. The conversion of norepinephrine to epinephrine requires the cortisol-induced enzyme phenylethanolamine-N-methyl transferase (PNMT) [54]. Consequently, epinephrine and its metabolite (metanephrine) are produced exclusively by PNMT-containing tissues such as chromaffin cells in the adrenal gland and the organ of Zuckerkandl (located at the aortic bifurcation). Finally, catecholamines (norepinephrine and epinephrine) are converted into their metabolites, i.e. normetanephrine and metanephrine, respectively, by catechol-O-methyltransferase (COMT) [58].

Clinical Trial Evidence

This is a phase 2 multicenter trial that evaluated the efficacy and safety of high-specific-activity ^{131}I-meta-iodobenzylguanidine (HSA ^{131}I-MIBG) in patients with advanced pheochromocytoma and paraganglioma (PPGL). Of the 68 patients who received at least one therapeutic dose of HSA ^{131}I-MIBG, 25% had a durable reduction in baseline antihypertensive medication use, and 92% had a partial response or stable disease as the best objective response within 12 months. HSA ^{131}I-MIBG also resulted in decreased elevated serum chromogranin levels in 68% of patients. The median overall survival was 36.7 months, and the most common adverse events were nausea, myelosuppression, and fatigue. HSA ^{131}I-MIBG has the potential to provide sustained blood pressure control and tumor response in patients with advanced PPGL, making it a viable treatment option [12].

3.3.6 Calcium Channel Blockers

3.3.6.1 Physiology

Upon depolarization of the chromaffin cell membrane, voltage-gated calcium channels (VGCCs) open, allowing the entry of calcium ions. These calcium ions bind to calmodulin, forming a calcium–calmodulin complex, which subsequently activates myosin light chain kinase [167]. This activation leads to the phosphorylation of myosin light chains. The phosphorylated myosin light chains then interact with actin filaments, resulting in the contraction of the actin cytoskeleton. As a result, the chromaffin granules are propelled toward the plasma membrane. Once the granules dock at the plasma membrane, they undergo fusion, which ultimately leads to the release of catecholamines such as epinephrine and norepinephrine into the bloodstream [167].

3.3.6.2 Mechanism of Action

Calcium channel blockers (CCBs) are a class of medications that block the influx of calcium ions into cells through voltage-dependent L-type calcium channels [168].

In the context of pheochromocytoma, CCBs act to reduce the release of catecholamines, including epinephrine and norepinephrine, from the tumor cells. By blocking calcium channels, CCBs decrease the intracellular calcium concentration, which in turn inhibits the exocytosis of catecholamines from the chromaffin granules [169]. This results in a decrease in blood pressure and a reduction in the severity and frequency of hypertensive crisis and other catecholamine-mediated symptoms such as palpitations, sweating, and anxiety [170, 171].

CCBs prevent the depolarization of cells, resulting in the inhibition of calcium-mediated contraction of smooth muscle cells in blood vessels. This leads to vasodilation and reduced blood pressure. CCBs are often used in combination with alpha and beta-adrenergic blockers for the management of PPGL [143].

Practice Pearl(s)

- Calcium channel blockers such as nicardipine and amlodipine can control blood pressure pre- and intra-operatively [172].
- The starting dose for nicardipine is 30 mg twice daily (sustained-release), and for amlodipine, 2.5–5 mg once daily.

Clinical Trial Evidence

A retrospective study was conducted to evaluate the impact of calcium channel blockers (CCBs) on postoperative morbidity and mortality in patients undergoing surgery for phaeochromocytoma or paraganglioma.

The authors analyzed the medical records of 105 patients who underwent surgery between 1991 and 2002. All patients received nicardipine as the CCB of choice for perioperative blood pressure management.

The study indicated that 61.9% of patients experienced transient intraoperative hypertension, with 13% having systolic blood pressure (SBP) > 220 mmHg and 2.8% having SBP > 180 mmHg for more than 10 minutes. Furthermore, 12.3% of patients had SBP < 80 mmHg for more than 10 minutes, 10.4% of patients developed postoperative complications, and 2.8% died.

The median ICU and hospital length of stay were 1 day and 10 days, respectively. In conclusion, the use of CCBs alone did not prevent all hemodynamic changes, but it was associated with low morbidity (10.4%) and mortality (2.8%) [173].

 Concepts to Ponder

Understanding terminology

The ongoing intratumoral conversion of catecholamines (epinephrine and norepinephrine) into their respective metabolites (metanephrine and normetanephrine) by COMT makes fractionated metanephrines in plasma or urine valuable for screening. However, because catecholamines are released intermittently, screening tests that only use catecholamines might not detect a PPGL [174].

The term "fractionated metanephrines" refers to the metabolites of epinephrine and norepinephrine, specifically metanephrine and normetanephrine [175].

A clinically significant increase in epinephrine or metanephrine (its metabolite) typically indicates the presence of adrenal pheochromocytoma. Although the cortisol-induced enzyme PNMT is present in extra-adrenal tissues such as paraganglia, it does not undergo paracrine stimulation by locally-derived cortisol in these tissues and, therefore, does not convert norepinephrine into epinephrine [176].

3.4 CLASSIC CONGENITAL ADRENAL HYPERPLASIA

3.4.1 Glucocorticoids

3.4.1.1 Physiology

The steroidogenesis pathway illustrates the various enzyme defects in congenital adrenal hyperplasia

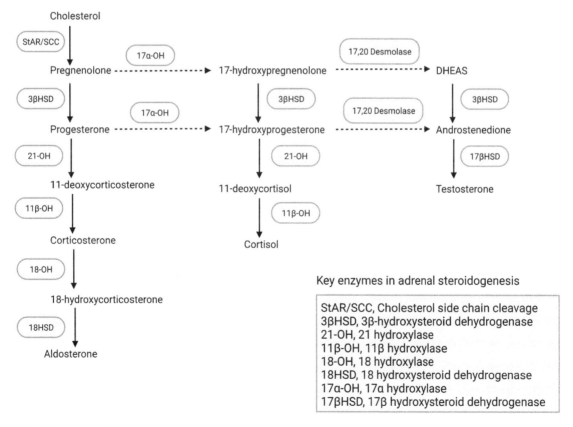

FIGURE 3.7   Adrenal steroidogenesis.

(CAH). Steroidogenic acute regulatory protein (StAR) mobilizes cholesterol from the outer to the inner mitochondrial membrane within the adrenal gland. Cytochrome P450 side-cleavage enzyme (P450scc) in the inner mitochondrial membrane converts cholesterol to pregnenolone, representing the rate-limiting step of adrenal steroidogenesis. Both ACTH and luteinizing hormone (LH) exert trophic stimulation on the downstream effects of StAR [177].

In the zona glomerulosa, pregnenolone is converted to progesterone by 3beta-hydroxysteroid dehydrogenase (3β-HSD). Progesterone then undergoes a series of enzymatic transformations involving 21-hydroxylase (CYP21A2) and aldosterone synthase to produce aldosterone. In the zona fasciculata, pregnenolone is hydroxylated into 17-hydroxypregnenolone by CYP17A1 (17-alpha-hydroxylase enzyme/17,20 lyase). Subsequent reactions involving 3β-HSD, CYP21A2, and CYP11B1 (11 beta-hydroxylase) lead to cortisol production. Finally, in the zona reticularis, CYP17A1 and 3β-HSD participate in the formation of androgen precursors such as DHEA and androstenedione [178] (See Figure 3.7).

Glucocorticoid physiology was reviewed in Section 3.1.1.

3.4.1.2   Mechanism of Action

Classic CAH is primarily caused by a deficiency in the enzyme 21-hydroxylase (21OHD) [15]. This enzyme deficiency reduces the synthesis of both cortisol and aldosterone production while increasing the production of adrenal androgens [179]. The main goals of treatment for CAH include replacing the deficient hormones and suppressing the excess production of adrenal androgens [180].

Glucocorticoids such as hydrocortisone replace the deficient cortisol in patients with CAH [181]. Also, glucocorticoids exert negative feedback control on the hypothalamus and the pituitary gland, leading to a decrease in both corticotropin-releasing hormone (CRH) and adrenocorticotropic hormone (ACTH) production, respectively [182]. Consequently, exogenous steroids suppress adrenal androgen overproduction, reducing the symptoms of androgen excess, such as premature puberty, hirsutism, and acne [183].

Practice Pearl(s)

Patients with 21OHD need to take stress doses of steroids during times of acute stress such as surgery, illness, or labor in order to avoid an adrenal crises [184] (see Table 3.5). It is important that women who are trying to conceive or are pregnant use a glucocorticoid inactivated by the placental 11β-hydroxysteroid dehydrogenase type 2, such as prednisone or prednisolone [186]. This will prevent fetal exposure to excess glucocorticoids that can negatively affect fetal development [187].

TABLE 3.5   Glucocorticoid replacement therapy in congenital adrenal hyperplasia.

Glucocorticoid(s)	Dosing schedule	Practice pearls
Hydrocortisone	Administered in three divided doses totaling 15–30 mg/day	Preferred due to fewer Cushingoid complications
Prednisolone or methylprednisolone	Longer-acting glucocorticoids, usually given twice a day – a larger dose (4–6 mg) in the morning and a smaller dose (1–2.5 mg) at bedtime	
Prednisone	Not applicable	Not preferred since it has to undergo hepatic metabolism into prednisolone.
Dexamethasone	Bedtime administration of 0.25–1 mg.	Effective for ACTH suppression.
Combination therapy	Hydrocortisone during the day and a small dose of a long-acting glucocorticoid at bedtime (1–2 mg prednisolone or methylprednisolone; 0.1–0.25 mg dexamethasone).	Effective in minimizing glucocorticoid exposure and keeping ACTH low

Source: Adapted from ref. [185].

Clinical Trial Evidence

In this pediatric study, the authors evaluated the benefits of one-year treatment with a single morning oral dose of prednisolone (PD) in comparison to traditional thrice-daily (TID) hydrocortisone (HC) administration in 44 patients with 21-hydroxylase deficiency (21OHD). The patients were divided into two age- and sex-matched groups, with one group receiving PD (2.4–3.5 mg/m² body surface area) and the other receiving TID HC (10–15 mg/m² body surface area). After one year, the PD group maintained a stable bone maturation ratio and preserved growth velocity, while the HC group showed a slight increase in both parameters. Additionally, height standard deviation scores for bone age significantly increased in the PD group. The results suggest that patients with 21OHD treated with a single morning dose of PD achieve better clinical and hormonal control than those on TID HC, allowing for a reduction in the replacement dose [188].

3.4.2 Mineralocorticoids

3.4.2.1 Physiology

Also, see Section 3.1.2.

3.4.2.2 Mechanism of Action

In salt-wasting CAH, the adrenal glands are unable to produce adequate amounts of mineralocorticoids, primarily aldosterone, due to a mutation in the CYP21A2 gene, which encodes the enzyme 21-hydroxylase [15].

Aldosterone plays a crucial role in regulating electrolyte balance and maintaining blood pressure [189]. It promotes the reabsorption of sodium and water in the renal tubules and the excretion of potassium [190]. This process helps maintain blood volume and blood pressure and prevents dehydration and electrolyte imbalances [189].

Fludrocortisone acts as a replacement for the deficient aldosterone in patients with salt-wasting CAH [181]. It binds to the MRs in the kidneys, mimicking the effects of aldosterone [191]. As a result, fludrocortisone helps to restore normal sodium and potassium levels, maintain blood pressure, and prevent dehydration [180].

Practice Pearl(s)

Mineralocorticoid therapy in CAH is typically administered as 9-alpha-fludrocortisone acetate to restore normal serum potassium levels, standing blood pressure, and plasma renin activity. Overdosing may lead to hypertension and hypokalemia, while optimal dosing can potentially reduce glucocorticoid dosage. The need for mineralocorticoids generally decreases post-infancy but remains relatively stable in adulthood [180].

Underdosing may result in chronic volume depletion, which could be clinically inapparent or cause chronic fatigue. The usual adult dose of fludrocortisone ranges from 0.1 to 0.2 mg/day, with some patients requiring higher doses to normalize clinical and laboratory parameters [180].

Clinical Trial Evidence

The study authors investigated the effects of 9 alpha-fluorohydrocortisone (9 alpha-F) therapy on growth in salt-losing congenital adrenal hyperplasia (CAH) patients aged 2–12 years. Patients were divided into two groups: group I had an increased 9 alpha-F dosage after 6 months, while group II maintained the same dosage. In group I, the height velocity decreased significantly from baseline. In group II, no significant changes were observed. The results highlight the importance of careful monitoring of 9 alpha-F to maintain proper growth rates in salt-losing CAH patients [192].

 Concepts to Ponder

What are the distinct clinicopathologic phenotypes of congenital adrenal hyperplasia (CAH)?

CAH is primarily caused by a defect in adrenal steroidogenic enzymes, leading to a decrease in serum cortisol levels. This loss of negative feedback

(continued)

(*continued*)

control stimulates the hypothalamic–pituitary–adrenal (HPA) axis, resulting in increased adrenocorticotropic hormone (ACTH) production. ACTH then causes the buildup and diversion of precursor steroids into either androgen or mineralocorticoid synthesis [193].

It is essential to understand the adrenal steroidogenesis pathway to appreciate the various clinicopathologic phenotypes of CAH.

Congenital lipoid hyperplasia (CLH), a severe form of CAH, is caused by an autosomal recessive mutation in the StAR-encoding gene. CLH is characterized by severe adrenal insufficiency (both mineralocorticoid and glucocorticoid deficiencies) and external female genitalia in male infants [194].

3beta-hydroxysteroid dehydrogenase type 2 (3BHSD) deficiency presents with a clinical spectrum ranging from presentations similar to CLH (both mineralocorticoid and glucocorticoid deficiencies) to a less severe subtype without salt-wasting [195].

17-hydroxylase deficiency results from a CYP17A1 gene mutation, affecting steroidogenesis in both adrenal glands and gonads [196]. Genetic females exhibit normal-appearing female genitalia at birth but later present with delayed puberty. Male infants cannot synthesize testosterone, leading to the development of female-appearing external genitalia [197]. Males lack internal Müllerian structures as their anatomic testes still produce anti-Müllerian hormone. Patients with this deficiency rarely experience overt adrenal crises due to the accumulation of precursors like corticosterone and 11-deoxycorticosterone (DOC), which maintain blood pressure and contribute to hypertension [198].

11β-hydroxylase deficiency results from a CYP11B1 gene mutation, causing defective cortisol synthesis due to a nonfunctional 11β-hydroxylase enzyme [199, 200]. The accumulation of proximal precursors like DOC and 11-deoxycortisol leads to hypertension and hypokalemia [201]. Increased proximal steroid production also results in elevated androgen levels (DHEA, DHEA-S, and androstenedione). Genetic males exhibit enlarged penile shafts at birth, while genetic females display ambiguous genitalia due to intrauterine exposure to high serum androgens [202].

21-hydroxylase deficiency results from a CYP21A2 gene mutation, impairing 21-hydroxylation of progesterone (mineralocorticoid synthesis pathway) and 17-hydroxyprogesterone (glucocorticoid synthesis pathway) [203] See Figure 3.7. As a result, proximal steroidogenic precursors are diverted into androgen production. Newborns with more deleterious CYP21A2 mutations are hemodynamically unstable due to impaired glucocorticoid and mineralocorticoid synthesis, and genetic females present with ambiguous genitalia [204].

3.5 NONCLASSIC CONGENITAL ADRENAL HYPERPLASIA

3.5.1 Insulin Sensitizers

3.5.1.1 Physiology

The effect of insulin resistance on adrenal androgen production was reviewed earlier. There is limited data on the role of insulin resistance in nonclassic congenital adrenal hyperplasia (NCCAH) [205].

3.5.1.2 Mechanism of Action

There is limited data on the role of metformin in the management of NCCAH. Metformin is an oral antihyperglycemic medication that is primarily used to treat type 2 diabetes mellitus. It has been studied in the context of polycystic ovary syndrome (PCOS), which shares some symptoms with NCCAH, such as hyperandrogenism and insulin resistance. However, specific studies focusing on the use of metformin in NCCAH are limited [206].

Practice Pearl(s)

For diabetic patients with nonclassic CAH, the starting dose is 500 mg daily, which is gradually uptitrated over 4 weeks to 850–1000 mg three times a day.

Clinical Trial Evidence

This study aimed to investigate the impact of metformin on androgen production in type 2 diabetic patients with nonclassic congenital adrenal hyperplasia (NCCAH), comparing it to the drug's effect in diabetic patients with normal androgen levels. The participants were women aged 30–45 years recently diagnosed with type 2 diabetes and NCCAH. The study found that metformin decreased fasting plasma glucose by 19% ($p < 0.001$) in NCCAH patients and 17% ($p < 0.001$) in those with normal adrenal function. HOMA-IR, a measure of insulin resistance, decreased by 44% ($p < 0.001$) in the NCCAH group and 48% ($p < 0.001$) in the normal adrenal function group [207].

3.5.2   Oral Contraceptive Pills and Antiandrogens

3.5.2.1   Physiology

In NCCAH, the role of androgens is central to the development of symptoms and other clinical manifestations. Due to a partial deficiency of the 21-hydroxylase enzyme caused by mutations in the CYP21A2 gene, cortisol synthesis is impaired, leading to the accumulation of precursor hormones, particularly 17-hydroxyprogesterone (17-OHP) [208].

As a result of increased 17-OHP levels, precursors are shunted toward the androgen synthesis pathway, causing an increase in the production of androgens such as testosterone and androstenedione [209]. See Figure 3.7.

The excess androgens in individuals with NCCAH are associated with premature pubarche (early development of pubic hair), hirsutism (excessive hair growth in females), acne, menstrual irregularities, and infertility [210].

3.5.2.2   Mechanism of Action

Oral contraceptives increase the production of sex hormone-binding globulin (SHBG) in the liver. This increase in SHBG reduces the concentration of free androgens (such as testosterone) in the bloodstream. This is because by binding to androgens, SHBG decreases the biological activity of these hormones and improves the clinical manifestations of androgen excess in NCCAH patients [211].

Also, oral contraceptives inhibit the hypothalamic pituitary ovarian (HPO) axis. By suppressing the production of gonadotropin-releasing hormone (GnRH) from the hypothalamus, oral contraceptives decrease the secretion of LH and follicle-stimulating hormone (FSH) from the pituitary gland. This suppression ultimately results in reduced ovarian androgen production, further contributing to an improvement of hyperandrogenemia in patients with NCCAH [212].

Also, see Section 6.1.2 for the effects of oral contraceptive pills on hirsutism.

Practice Pearl(s)

Alternative approaches to managing androgen excess and menstrual irregularity in nonclassic CAH should be considered for long-term treatment, especially when fertility is not a primary concern. These approaches may include the use of antiandrogens and oral contraceptives [213].

Antiandrogens, such as spironolactone or cyproterone acetate, can effectively block the actions of androgens at the cellular level, mitigating the effects of androgen excess. These medications are particularly helpful in managing symptoms such as hirsutism and acne associated with nonclassic CAH [210].

Oral contraceptives (OCPs) can also play a significant role in the long-term management of nonclassic CAH. OCPs help regulate menstrual cycles, reducing the frequency of irregular periods [210].

Clinical Trial Evidence

This study aimed to compare the effects of combined oral contraceptives (COCs) containing estradiol valerate (EV) and ethinylestradiol (EE) on cortisol and other adrenal steroid hormones. Fifty-nine healthy women participated in the study and were divided into groups using EV + dienogest (DNG), EE + DNG, or DNG only for 9 weeks. The results showed that EE + DNG treatment increased total cortisol and cortisone levels, while no significant changes were observed for the EV + DNG and DNG-only groups. In conclusion, EV had a milder effect on circulating corticosteroid binding globulin (CBG) and adrenal steroid levels than EE in COCs [214].

Concepts to Ponder

What are the genetic differences between NCCAH and classic congenital adrenal hyperplasia?

Table 3.6 summarizes a comparison of CAH and NCCAH.

TABLE 3.6   Comparison of CAH and NCCAH.

CAH	NCCAH
Large gene deletion involving the CYP21A2 gene.	Usually, a point mutation (70% of patients) in the CYP21A2 gene.
Loss of 21-hydroxylase enzyme activity by 95–100%.	Loss of 21-hydroxylase enzyme activity by 20–50%.

Source: Adapted from ref. [215].

PRACTICE-BASED QUESTIONS

1. Interpret this adrenal venous sampling (AVS) report and recommend the next step in this patient's management

Vein	Aldosterone (A), ng/dL	Cortisol (C), mcg/dL	A:C ratio	Aldosterone ratio[a]
Right adrenal vein	9200	470	19.6	65.3
Left adrenal vein	125	410	0.3	
Inferior vena cava	33	10	3.3	

[a] Right adrenal vein A/C ratio divided by the left adrenal vein A/C ratio. This should always be a ratio of the dominant to nondominant side.

a. Perform a left adrenalectomy
b. Perform a right adrenalectomy
c. Perform bilateral adrenalectomy
d. Start spironolactone
e. Incomplete testing, repeat adrenal vein sampling

Correct answer: The correct answer is b (perform a right adrenalectomy)

Explanation:
Q1.) Step A: Calculate the selectivity index

The cortisol level in each adrenal vein is more than five-fold higher than the cortisol in the inferior vena cava.

Step B: Calculate the lateralization index
The A:C ratio of the dominant (right adrenal, 19.6) to nondominant (left adrenal, 0.3) adrenal gland is 65.3. The estimated LI is greater than 4. This is diagnostic for a unilateral source of hyperaldosteronism (from the right adrenal gland).

Step C: Calculate the contralateral suppression index
Evaluation of the contralateral suppression index is required in this patient with a unilateral source of hyperaldosteronism. The A:C ratio in the nondominant adrenal (left adrenal vein, 0.30) is less than the A:C ratio in the periphery (inferior vena cava, 3.3).

This implies the left adrenal gland is not the source of hyperaldosteronemia and confirms the right adrenal gland as the source.

2. A 45-year-old male presents to the emergency department with severe fatigue, abdominal pain, and vomiting. He has a history of primary adrenal insufficiency and is suspected to be in an adrenal crisis. Which glucocorticoid should be administered as the first-line treatment for this patient?

a. Dexamethasone
b. Hydrocortisone
c. Prednisone
d. Methylprednisolone

Correct answer: b) Hydrocortisone. **Explanation:** Hydrocortisone is the preferred glucocorticoid for the treatment of an adrenal crisis because it closely resembles the natural hormone cortisol produced by the adrenal glands, having both glucocorticoid and mineralocorticoid properties. Hydrocortisone is rapidly absorbed and has a relatively short half-life, making it suitable for acute management. It provides the necessary glucocorticoid effects for managing an adrenal crisis and also addresses the mineralocorticoid deficiency that may occur in primary adrenal insufficiency. Dexamethasone, prednisone, and methylprednisolone are not the first choices for stress dosing during an adrenal crisis due to their varying degrees of mineralocorticoid activity and differences in half-life.

3. A 35-year-old female presents with signs of Cushing's syndrome, including central obesity, facial rounding, and easy bruising. Lab results confirm excessive cortisol production. Which enzyme is responsible for amplifying cortisol's effects on various tissues in this condition?

   a. 11β-hydroxysteroid dehydrogenase type 1 (11β-HSD1)
   b. 11β-hydroxysteroid dehydrogenase type 2 (11β-HSD2)
   c. Aldosterone synthase
   d. 21-Hydroxylase

   Correct answer: a) 11β-hydroxysteroid dehydrogenase type 1 (11β-HSD1). **Explanation:** 11β-HSD1 is primarily expressed in the liver and adipose tissue and is responsible for converting the relatively inactive cortisone to the active cortisol. In conditions of excess cortisol production, such as Cushing's syndrome, the activity of 11β-HSD1 can amplify cortisol's effects on various tissues.

4. Which of the following physiological effects is NOT directly related to the action of cortisol?

   a. Maintenance of blood glucose levels
   b. Suppression of the immune system
   c. Regulation of sleep–wake cycle
   d. Increased absorption of dietary calcium in the intestines

   Correct answer: d) Increased absorption of dietary calcium in the intestines. **Explanation:** Cortisol is involved in maintaining blood glucose levels, suppressing the immune system, and regulating the sleep–wake cycle. However, it does not play a direct role in increasing the absorption of dietary calcium in the intestines. This function is mainly carried out by active vitamin D (calcitriol) and parathyroid hormone (PTH).

5. A 55-year-old male presents with symptoms of hypertension and hypokalemia. Laboratory tests reveal increased levels of aldosterone. Which of the following enzymes is primarily responsible for converting angiotensin I to the potent vasoconstrictor angiotensin II?

   a. Renin
   b. Angiotensin-converting enzyme (ACE)
   c. Angiotensin-converting enzyme 2 (ACE2)
   d. 11β-hydroxysteroid dehydrogenase type 1 (11β-HSD1)

   Correct answer: b) Angiotensin-converting enzyme (ACE). **Explanation:** Angiotensin-converting enzyme (ACE) is a peptidase widely expressed in the vascular endothelium of various tissues, including the brain, skeletal muscle, skin, heart, kidneys, and lungs. It is particularly abundant in the pulmonary vasculature endothelium, where it converts the inactive angiotensin I into the potent vasoconstrictor angiotensin II. Angiotensin II is involved in the regulation of blood pressure and stimulation of aldosterone release by the zona glomerulosa of the adrenal cortex.

6. A 63-year-old female presents with hypertension and fluid retention. Investigations reveal a dysregulation of the renin–angiotensin–aldosterone system (RAAS). Which of the following effects is NOT a direct result of AT1 receptor activation by angiotensin II?

   a. Vasoconstriction
   b. Stimulation of aldosterone release
   c. Vasodilation and urinary sodium loss
   d. Promotion of atherosclerosis and vascular smooth muscle proliferation

   Correct answer: c) Vasodilation and urinary sodium loss. **Explanation:** Activation of AT1 receptors by angiotensin II leads to various effects, such as vasoconstriction, stimulation of aldosterone release, promotion of atherosclerosis, and vascular smooth muscle proliferation. In contrast, vasodilation and urinary sodium loss are the result of AT2 receptor activation, which counteracts the effects of AT1 receptor stimulation.

7. What is the primary target of aldosterone in the kidneys?

   a. Proximal convoluted tubule
   b. Loop of Henle
   c. Distal convoluted tubule and collecting ducts
   d. Glomerulus

   Correct answer: c. Distal convoluted tubule and collecting ducts. **Explanation:** Aldosterone, a mineralocorticoid, primarily targets the distal convoluted tubule (DCT) and the collecting ducts (CD) in the kidneys. This is where it binds to mineralocorticoid receptors (MRs), and subsequently modulates the transcription of target genes to regulate electrolyte balance and blood pressure.

8. Which enzyme is responsible for converting adrenal-derived androgens into more potent androgens, such as testosterone or dihydrotestosterone (DHT)?

   a. 3β-hydroxysteroid dehydrogenase (3β-HSD)
   b. 17β-hydroxysteroid dehydrogenase (17β-HSD)
   c. 5α-reductase
   d. Aromatase

   Correct answer: c. 5α-reductase. **Explanation:** The enzyme 5α-reductase is responsible for converting adrenal-derived androgens, such as dehydroepiandrosterone (DHEA) and androstenedione, into more potent androgens like testosterone or dihydrotestosterone (DHT) in peripheral tissues. These potent androgens then bind to androgen receptors (ARs) and regulate various physiological processes, including the development of secondary sexual characteristics and regulation of body composition.

9. What is the primary mechanism of action of aldosterone antagonists in the treatment of primary hyperaldosteronism?

   a. Increasing the production of renin
   b. Inhibition of sodium and water reabsorption in the proximal tubule
   c. Competitive inhibition of mineralocorticoid receptors in the distal tubules and collecting ducts
   d. Direct inhibition of aldosterone synthesis in the adrenal glands

   Correct answer: c. Competitive inhibition of mineralocorticoid receptors in the distal tubules and collecting ducts. **Explanation:** Aldosterone antagonists, such as spironolactone and eplerenone, work by competitively inhibiting the mineralocorticoid receptors in the distal tubules and collecting ducts of the nephron in the kidneys. This prevents aldosterone from exerting its effects on sodium and water reabsorption and potassium excretion, leading to a decrease in blood pressure and the normalization of electrolyte levels.

10. Which of the following side effects is more commonly associated with spironolactone compared to eplerenone in the treatment of primary hyperaldosteronism?

   a. Hyperkalemia
   b. Gynecomastia in males and mastodynia in females
   c. Hypokalemia
   d. Increased blood pressure

   Correct answer: b. Gynecomastia in males and mastodynia in females. **Explanation:** In a multicenter, randomized, double-blind study comparing the efficacy, safety, and tolerability of eplerenone and spironolactone in patients with hypertension associated with primary aldosteronism, spironolactone was associated with a higher incidence of male gynecomastia (21.2 vs. 4.5%) and female mastodynia (21.1 vs. 0.0%). Despite the lower antihypertensive effect of eplerenone, it had fewer antiandrogenic side effects than spironolactone.

11. A patient diagnosed with pheochromocytoma is scheduled for surgery. In the preoperative period, alpha-adrenergic blockers are administered to normalize blood pressure and expand intravascular space. Which of the following is the preferred drug for this purpose?

   a. Prazosin
   b. Terazosin
   c. Doxazosin
   d. Phenoxybenzamine

   Correct answer: d. Phenoxybenzamine. **Explanation:** Phenoxybenzamine is the preferred drug for preoperative administration in patients with pheochromocytoma, as it provides sustained vasodilation and reduced blood pressure, with a longer duration of action compared to selective alpha-1 blockers. Selective alpha-1-adrenergic blockers like prazosin, terazosin, or doxazosin may be used for their favorable side-effect profiles and lower cost, but phenoxybenzamine is the drug of choice.

12. A patient with pheochromocytoma has been treated with alpha-adrenergic blockers to manage hypertension. They are now experiencing tachycardia and arrhythmias. Which of the following medications should be introduced to address these symptoms?

a. *Alpha*-blockers
b. *Beta*-blockers
c. Calcium channel blockers
d. Angiotensin-converting enzyme (ACE) inhibitors

Correct answer: b. *Beta*-blockers. **Explanation:** Beta-blockers should be introduced to address tachycardia and arrhythmias in patients with pheochromocytoma after adequate alpha-blockade has been achieved and blood pressure has been stabilized. Beta-blockers work by competitively inhibiting the binding of catecholamines to beta-adrenergic receptors, preventing their activation and subsequently decreasing the effects of catecholamines on heart rate and contractility. However, it is essential to emphasize that beta-blockers should not be used as the first line of treatment, as they can exacerbate hypertension by causing unopposed alpha-adrenergic receptor activation.

13. What is the primary mechanism of action of vincristine in the treatment of pheochromocytoma and paragangliomas?

    a. Formation of DNA cross-links
    b. Methylation of purine bases in DNA
    c. Inhibition of tyrosine hydroxylase
    d. Disruption of microtubule formation during cell division

    Correct answer: d. Disruption of microtubule formation during cell division. **Explanation:** Vincristine is a vinca alkaloid that binds to tubulin, a protein that forms microtubules, which are essential components of the cell's cytoskeleton and play a crucial role in cell division (mitosis). By binding to tubulin, vincristine disrupts microtubule formation, leading to the arrest of mitosis in the metaphase. This disruption of cell division eventually leads to cell death.

14. What is the mechanism of action of metyrosine in the management of pheochromocytoma?

    a. Inhibition of tyrosine hydroxylase
    b. Blocking voltage-gated calcium channels
    c. Formation of DNA cross-links
    d. Methylation of purine bases in DNA

    Correct answer: a. Inhibition of tyrosine hydroxylase. **Explanation:** Metyrosine, also known as

alpha-methyl-L-tyrosine or α-MT, inhibits the enzyme tyrosine hydroxylase (TH), which is the rate-limiting step in catecholamine synthesis. Tyrosine hydroxylase converts L-tyrosine to L-dihydroxyphenylalanine (L-DOPA). By inhibiting this enzyme, metyrosine effectively reduces the production of dopamine, norepinephrine, and epinephrine, leading to a decrease in catecholamine levels in the tumor and circulation, and a reduction in the symptoms associated with excessive catecholamine release.

15. Which of the following drugs in the CVD therapy regimen is responsible for the methylation of purine bases in DNA?

    a. Cyclophosphamide
    b. Vincristine
    c. Dacarbazine
    d. Metyrosine

    Correct answer: c. Dacarbazine. **Explanation:** Dacarbazine is an alkylating agent that works by methylating the purine bases of DNA, particularly guanine. This methylation leads to the formation of abnormal base pairing, ultimately inhibiting DNA replication and RNA synthesis. The DNA damage triggers cellular repair mechanisms, and if the damage cannot be repaired, the cell undergoes apoptosis.

16. How do calcium channel blockers (CCBs) help in the management of pheochromocytoma symptoms?

    a. Inhibition of tyrosine hydroxylase
    b. Blocking voltage-gated calcium channels
    c. Formation of DNA cross-links
    d. Methylation of purine bases in DNA

    Correct answer: b. Blocking voltage-gated calcium channels. **Explanation:** Calcium channel blockers (CCBs) are a class of medications that block the influx of calcium ions into cells through voltage-dependent L-type calcium channels. In the context of pheochromocytoma, CCBs act to reduce the release of catecholamines, including epinephrine and norepinephrine, from the tumor cells. By blocking calcium channels, CCBs decrease the intracellular calcium concentration, which in turn inhibits the exocytosis of catecholamines from the chromaffin granules. This results in a decrease in blood pressure and a reduction in the severity and frequency of hypertensive crisis and other catecholamine-mediated symptoms such as palpitations, sweating, and anxiety.

17. A 28-year-old female patient with salt-wasting CAH is being treated with fludrocortisone. Which of the following is the primary mechanism of action of fludrocortisone in managing her condition?

   a. Inhibition of 21-hydroxylase enzyme
   b. Mimicking the effects of aldosterone
   c. Blocking the action of androgens
   d. Suppressing the hypothalamic–pituitary–adrenal axis

   Correct answer: b. Mimicking the effects of aldosterone. **Explanation:** Fludrocortisone is a synthetic mineralocorticoid used in the treatment of salt-wasting CAH to replace the deficient aldosterone. It binds to mineralocorticoid receptors in the kidneys, mimicking the effects of aldosterone. This action helps to restore normal sodium and potassium levels, maintain blood pressure, and prevent dehydration in patients with salt-wasting CAH.

18. A 25-year-old woman with nonclassic congenital adrenal hyperplasia (NCCAH) is experiencing symptoms of hyperandrogenism. Which of the following treatment options would be most appropriate for managing her symptoms?

   a. Insulin sensitizers, such as metformin
   b. Oral contraceptives and antiandrogens
   c. Corticosteroid replacement therapy
   d. Mineralocorticoid replacement therapy

   Correct answer: b. Oral contraceptives and antiandrogens. **Explanation:** In NCCAH, symptoms of hyperandrogenism result from increased production of androgens due to a partial deficiency of the 21-hydroxylase enzyme. Oral contraceptives and antiandrogens, such as spironolactone or cyproterone acetate, can help manage these symptoms. Oral contraceptives increase the production of SHBG in the liver, which reduces the levels of free androgens in the bloodstream.

Antiandrogens block the actions of androgens at the cellular level, mitigating the effects of androgen excess.

19. Which of the following can result from the use of mineralocorticoid receptor antagonists during aldosterone-renin ratio (ARR) testing?

   a. A false-negative aldosterone-renin ratio
   b. A false-positive aldosterone-renin ratio
   c. No effect on aldosterone-renin ratio
   d. A false-negative plasma renin activity

   Correct answer: a. A false-negative aldosterone-renin ratio. **Explanation:** Mineralocorticoid receptor antagonists, such as eplerenone and spironolactone, block the mineralocorticoid receptor and inhibit aldosterone from binding to its receptor. This leads to sodium excretion, a decrease in extracellular volume, and an increase in plasma renin levels. An increase in plasma renin levels can result in a false-negative aldosterone-renin ratio, which may cause some cases of primary hyperaldosteronism to be missed.

20. How do ACE inhibitors, Angiotensin Receptor Blockers (ARBs), or direct renin inhibitors affect aldosterone-renin ratio testing?

   a. They increase plasma renin levels, potentially causing a false-negative aldosterone-renin ratio
   b. They decrease plasma renin levels, potentially causing a false-positive aldosterone-renin ratio
   c. They have no effect on plasma renin levels
   d. They cause a false-positive plasma renin activity

   Correct answer: a. They increase plasma renin levels, potentially causing a false-negative aldosterone-renin ratio. **Explanation:** ACE inhibitors, ARBs, and direct renin inhibitors interfere with renin receptor activation, reflexively increasing plasma renin levels. This may result in a falsely negative aldosterone-renin ratio. If plasma renin activity is >1 ng/mL/hr., primary aldosteronism cannot be ruled out without discontinuing these agents. In contrast, if plasma renin activity is <1 ng/mL/hr. while on these agents, it strongly suggests a diagnosis of primary aldosteronism.

REFERENCES

1. Chrousos, G.P. (2009). Stress and disorders of the stress system. *Nat. Rev. Endocrinol.* 5 (7): 374–381.

2. Øksnes, M., Ross, R., and Løvås, K. (2015). Optimal glucocorticoid replacement in adrenal insufficiency. *Best Pract. Res. Clin. Endocrinol. Metab.* 29 (1): 3–15.

3. Elenkov, I.J. and Chrousos, G.P. (1999). Stress hormones, Th1/Th2 patterns, pro/anti-inflammatory cytokines and susceptibility to disease. *Trends Endocrinol. Metab.* 10 (9): 359–368.

4. Lupien, S.J., McEwen, B.S., Gunnar, M.R., and Heim, C. (2009). Effects of stress throughout the lifespan on the brain, behaviour and cognition. *Nat. Rev. Neurosci.* 10 (6): 434–445.

5. Lightman, S.L. and Conway-Campbell, B.L. (2010). The crucial role of pulsatile activity of the HPA axis for continuous dynamic equilibration. *Nat. Rev. Neurosci.* 11 (10): 710–718.

6. Verrey, F., Beron, J., and Spindler, B. (1996). Corticosteroid regulation of renal Na, K-ATPase. *Miner. Electrolyte Metab.* 22 (5–6): 279–292.

7. Oakley, R.H. and Cidlowski, J.A. (2013). The biology of the glucocorticoid receptor: new signaling mechanisms in health and disease. *J. Allergy Clin. Immunol.* 132 (5): 1033–1044.

8. Vandevyver, S., Dejager, L., and Libert, C. (2014). Comprehensive overview of the structure and regulation of the glucocorticoid receptor. *Endocr. Rev.* 35 (4): 671–693.

9. Barnes, P.J. (1998). Anti-inflammatory actions of glucocorticoids: molecular mechanisms. *Clin. Sci. (Lond.)* 94 (6): 557–572.

10. Peng, K., Pan, Y., Li, J. et al. (2016). 11β-hydroxysteroid dehydrogenase type 1(11β-HSD1) mediates insulin resistance through JNK activation in adipocytes. *Sci. Rep.* 6 (1): 37160.

11. Tomlinson, J.W. and Stewart, P.M. (2001). Cortisol metabolism and the role of 11β-hydroxysteroid dehydrogenase. *Best Pract. Res. Clin. Endocrinol. Metab.* 15 (1): 61–78.

12. Chapman, K., Holmes, M., and Seckl, J. (2013). 11β-hydroxysteroid dehydrogenases: intracellular gate-keepers of tissue glucocorticoid action. *Physiol. Rev.* 93 (3): 1139–1206.

13. Bornstein, S.R., Allolio, B., Arlt, W. et al. (2016). Diagnosis and treatment of primary adrenal insufficiency: an endocrine society clinical practice guideline. *J. Clin. Endocrinol. Metab.* 101 (2): 364–389.

14. Hahner, S., Loeffler, M., Fassnacht, M. et al. (2007). Impaired subjective health status in 256 patients with adrenal insufficiency on standard therapy based on cross-sectional analysis. *J. Clin. Endocrinol. Metab.* 92 (10): 3912–3922.

15. White, P.C. and Speiser, P.W. (2000). Congenital adrenal hyperplasia due to 21-hydroxylase deficiency. *Endocr. Rev.* 21 (3): 245–291.

16. Dineen, R., Thompson, C.J., and Sherlock, M. (2019). Adrenal crisis: prevention and management in adult patients. *Ther. Adv. Endocrinol. Metab.* 10: 2042018819848218.

17. Hahner, S., Spinnler, C., Fassnacht, M. et al. (2015). High incidence of adrenal crisis in educated patients with chronic adrenal insufficiency: a prospective study. *J. Clin. Endocrinol. Metab.* 100 (2): 407–416.

18. Peacey, S.R., Guo, C.-Y., Robinson, A.M. et al. (1997). Glucocorticoid replacement therapy: are patients over treated and does it matter? *Clin. Endocrinol.* 46 (3): 255–261.

19. Kobori, H., Nangaku, M., Navar, L.G., and Nishiyama, A. (2007). The intrarenal renin-angiotensin system: from physiology to the pathobiology of hypertension and kidney disease. *Pharmacol. Rev.* 59 (3): 251–287.

20. Phillips, M.I. and Schmidt-Ott, K.M. (1999). The discovery of renin 100 years ago. *Physiology* 14 (6): 271–274.

21. Nguyen, G., Delarue, F., Burcklé, C. et al. (2002). Pivotal role of the renin/prorenin receptor in angiotensin II production and cellular responses to renin. *J. Clin. Invest.* 109 (11): 1417–1427.

22. Skinner, S.L., Mccubbin, J.W., and Page, I.H. (1964). Control of renin secretion. *Circ. Res.* 15: 64–76.

23. Peti-Peterdi, J. (2006). Calcium wave of tubuloglomerular feedback. *American Journal of Physiology-Renal Physiology* 291 (2): F473–F480.

24. Harrison-Bernard, L.M. (2009). The renal renin-angiotensin system. *Adv. Physiol. Educ.* 33 (4): 270–274.

25. DiBona, G.F. (2002). Sympathetic nervous system and the kidney in hypertension. *Curr. Opin. Nephrol. Hypertens.* 11 (2): 197–200.

26. Navar, L.G., Prieto, M.C., Satou, R., and Kobori, H. (2011). Intrarenal angiotensin II and its contribution to the genesis of chronic hypertension. *Curr. Opin. Pharmacol.* 11 (2): 180–186.

27. Tipnis, S.R., Hooper, N.M., Hyde, R. et al. (2000). A human homolog of angiotensin-converting enzyme. Cloning and functional expression as a captopril-insensitive carboxypeptidase. *J. Biol. Chem.* 275 (43): 33238–33243.

28. Donoghue, M., Hsieh, F., Baronas, E. et al. (2000). A novel angiotensin-converting enzyme-related carboxypeptidase (ACE2) converts angiotensin I to angiotensin 1-9. *Circ. Res.* 87 (5): E1–E9.

29. Santos, R.A.S., Sampaio, W.O., Alzamora, A.C. et al. (2018). The ACE2/angiotensin-(1-7)/MAS axis of the renin-angiotensin system: focus on angiotensin-(1-7). *Physiol. Rev.* 98 (1): 505–553.

30. de Gasparo, M., Catt, K.J., Inagami, T. et al. (2000). International union of pharmacology. XXIII. The angiotensin II receptors. *Pharmacol. Rev.* 52 (3): 415–472.

31. Griendling, K.K., Murphy, T.J., and Alexander, R.W. (1993). Molecular biology of the renin-angiotensin system. *Circulation* 87 (6): 1816–1828.

32. Sadoshima, J. and Izumo, S. (1993). Molecular characterization of angiotensin II – induced hypertrophy of cardiac myocytes and hyperplasia of cardiac fibroblasts. Critical role of the AT1 receptor subtype. *Circ. Res.* 73 (3): 413–423.

33. Atlas, S.A. (2007). The renin-angiotensin aldosterone system: pathophysiological role and pharmacologic inhibition. *J. Manag. Care Pharm.* 13 (8 Suppl B): 9–20.

34. Hunyady, L. and Catt, K.J. (2006). Pleiotropic AT1 receptor signaling pathways mediating physiological and pathogenic actions of angiotensin II. *Mol. Endocrinol.* 20 (5): 953–970.

35. Weber, K.T., Brilla, C.G., Campbell, S.E. et al. (1993). Myocardial fibrosis: role of angiotensin II and aldosterone. *Basic Res. Cardiol.* 88 (Suppl 1): 107–124.

36. Ross, R. (1999). Atherosclerosis – an inflammatory disease. *N. Engl. J. Med.* 340 (2): 115–126.

37. Griendling, K.K., Minieri, C.A., Ollerenshaw, J.D., and Alexander, R.W. (1994). Angiotensin II stimulates NADH and NADPH oxidase activity in cultured vascular smooth muscle cells. *Circ. Res.* 74 (6): 1141–1148.

38. Tsutsumi, Y., Matsubara, H., Masaki, H. et al. (1999). Angiotensin II type 2 receptor overexpression activates the vascular kinin system and causes vasodilation. *J. Clin. Invest.* 104 (7): 925–935.

39. Carey, R.M. (2017). Update on angiotensin AT2 receptors. *Curr. Opin. Nephrol. Hypertens.* 26 (2): 91–96.

40. Suzuki, Y., Ruiz-Ortega, M., Lorenzo, O. et al. (2003). Inflammation and angiotensin II. *Int. J. Biochem. Cell Biol.* 35 (6): 881–900.

41. Matavelli, L.C., Huang, J., and Siragy, H.M. (2011). Angiotensin AT2 receptor stimulation inhibits early renal inflammation in renovascular hypertension. *Hypertension* 57 (2): 308–313.

42. Iwai, M. and Horiuchi, M. (2009). Devil and angel in the renin–angiotensin system: ACE–angiotensin II–AT1 receptor axis vs. ACE2–angiotensin-(1–7)–Mas receptor axis. *Hypertens. Res.* 32 (7): 533–536.

43. Funder, J.W. (2006) Minireview: aldosterone and the cardiovascular system: genomic and nongenomic effects. *Endocrinology*, 147 (12), 5564–5567.

44. Xanthakis, V. and Vasan, R.S. (2013). Aldosterone and the risk of hypertension. *Curr. Hypertens. Rep.* 15 (2): 102–107.

45. Frohlich, E.D. (2007). The Salt Conundrum. *Hypertension* 50 (1): 161–166.

46. Connell, J.M.C., MacKenzie, S.M., Freel, E.M. et al. (2008). A lifetime of aldosterone excess: long-term consequences of altered regulation of aldosterone production for cardiovascular function. *Endocr. Rev.* 29 (2): 133–154.

47. Tsilosani, A., Gao, C., and Zhang, W. (2022). Aldosterone-regulated sodium transport and blood pressure. *Front. Physiol.* 13.

48. Verbalis, J.G. (2003). Disorders of body water homeostasis. *Best Pract. Res. Clin. Endocrinol. Metab.* 17 (4): 471–503.

49. Park, K.S. and Yoo, K.Y. (2017). Role of vasopressin in current anesthetic practice. *Korean J. Anesthesiol.* 70 (3): 245–257.

50. Leopold, J.A. (2011). Aldosterone, mineralocorticoid receptor activation, and cardiovascular remodeling. *Circulation* 124 (18): e466–e468.

51. Farquharson, C.A.J. and Struthers, A.D. (2002). Aldosterone induces acute endothelial dysfunction in vivo in humans: evidence for an aldosterone-induced vasculopathy. *Clin. Sci. (Lond.)* 103 (4): 425–431.

52. Brown, N.J. (2008). Aldosterone and vascular inflammation. *Hypertension* 51 (2): 161–167.

53. Caprio, M., Newfell, B.G., la Sala, A. et al. (2008). Functional mineralocorticoid receptors in human vascular endothelial cells regulate intercellular adhesion molecule-1 expression and promote leukocyte adhesion. *Circ. Res.* 102 (11): 1359–1367.

54. Whitworth, J.A., Williamson, P.M., Mangos, G., and Kelly, J.J. (2005). Cardiovascular consequences of cortisol excess. *Vasc. Health Risk Manag.* 1 (4): 291–299.

55. Ferrario, C.M. and Strawn, W.B. (2006). Role of the renin-angiotensin-aldosterone system and proinflammatory mediators in cardiovascular disease. *Am. J. Cardiol.* 98 (1): 121–128.

56. Funder, J.W. (2017). Aldosterone and mineralocorticoid receptors – physiology and pathophysiology. *Int. J. Mol. Sci.* 18 (5).

57. Seccia, T.M., Caroccia, B., Gomez-Sanchez, E.P. et al. (2018). The biology of normal zona glomerulosa and aldosterone-producing adenoma: pathological implications. *Endocr. Rev.* 39 (6): 1029–1056.

58. Subramanya, A.R. and Ellison, D.H. (2014). Distal convoluted tubule. *CJASN* 9 (12): 2147–2163.

59. Charmandari, E., Kino, T., and Chrousos, G.P. (2004). Familial/sporadic glucocorticoid resistance: clinical phenotype and molecular mechanisms. *Ann. N. Y. Acad. Sci.* 1024: 168–181.

60. Pratt, W.B. and Toft, D.O. (1997). Steroid receptor interactions with heat shock protein and immunophilin chaperones. *Endocr. Rev.* 18 (3): 306–360.

61. Faresse, N. (2014). Post-translational modifications of the mineralocorticoid receptor: how to dress the receptor according to the circumstances? *J. Steroid Biochem. Mol. Biol.* 143: 334–342.

62. Yang, J. and Young, M.J. (2009). The mineralocorticoid receptor and its coregulators. *J. Mol. Endocrinol.* 43 (2): 53–64.

63. De Bosscher, K. and Haegeman, G. (2009). Minireview: latest perspectives on antiinflammatory actions of glucocorticoids. *Mol. Endocrinol.* 23 (3): 281–291.

64. Loffing, J. and Korbmacher, C. (2009). Regulated sodium transport in the renal connecting tubule (CNT) via the epithelial sodium channel (ENaC). *Pflugers Arch. - Eur. J. Physiol.* 458 (1): 111–135.

65. Verrey, F., Schaerer, E., Zoerkler, P. et al. (1987). Regulation by aldosterone of Na+, K+-ATPase mRNAs, protein synthesis, and sodium transport in cultured kidney cells. *J. Cell Biol.* 104 (5): 1231–1237.

66. Leroy, V., De Seigneux, S., Agassiz, V. et al. (2009). Aldosterone activates NF-κB in the collecting duct. *J. Am. Soc. Nephrol.* 20 (1): 131–144.

67. Aperia, A. (2007). New roles for an old enzyme: Na,K-ATPase emerges as an interesting drug target. *J. Intern. Med.* 261 (1): 44–52.

68. Arroyo, J.P. and Gamba, G. (2012). Advances in WNK signaling of salt and potassium metabolism: clinical implications. *Am. J. Nephrol.* 35 (4): 379–386.

69. Crowley, S.D. and Coffman, T.M. (2012). Recent advances involving the renin-angiotensin system. *Exp. Cell Res.* 318 (9): 1049–1056.

70. Vallon, V. and Lang, F. (2005). New insights into the role of serum- and glucocorticoid-inducible kinase SGK1 in the regulation of renal function and blood pressure. *Curr. Opin. Nephrol. Hypertens.* 14 (1): 59–66.

71. Mutig, K., Kahl, T., Saritas, T. et al. (2011). Activation of the bumetanide-sensitive Na+,K+,2Cl− cotransporter (NKCC2) is facilitated by Tamm-Horsfall protein in a chloride-sensitive manner. *J. Biol. Chem.* 286 (34): 30200–30210.

72. McCormick, J.A., Bhalla, V., Pao, A.C., and Pearce, D. (2005). SGK1: a rapid aldosterone-induced regulator of renal sodium reabsorption. *Physiology* 20 (2): 134–139.

73. Ceccato, F., Torchio, M., Tizianel, I. et al. (2023). Renin and electrolytes indicate the mineralocorticoid activity of fludrocortisone: a 6 year study in primary adrenal insufficiency. *J. Endocrinol. Investig.* 46 (1): 111–122.

74. El-Tawil, A. (2010). Is the DHEAS/cortisol ratio a potential filter for non-operable constipated cases? *World J. Gastroenterol.* 16 (6): 659–662.

75. Hunt, P.J., Gurnell, E.M., Huppert, F.A. et al. (2000). Improvement in mood and fatigue after dehydroepiandrosterone replacement in Addison's disease in a randomized, double blind trial. *J. Clin. Endocrinol. Metab.* 85 (12): 4650–4656.

76. Arlt, W., Callies, F., van Vlijmen, J.C. et al. (1999). Dehydroepiandrosterone replacement in women with adrenal insufficiency. *N. Engl. J. Med.* 341 (14): 1013–1020.

77. Gurnell, E.M., Hunt, P.J., Curran, S.E. et al. (2008). Long-term DHEA replacement in primary adrenal insufficiency: a randomized, controlled trial. *J. Clin. Endocrinol. Metab.* 93 (2): 400–409.

78. Alkatib, A.A., Cosma, M., Elamin, M.B. et al. (2009). A systematic review and meta-analysis of randomized placebo-controlled trials of DHEA treatment effects on quality of life in women with adrenal insufficiency. *J. Clin. Endocrinol. Metab.* 94 (10): 3676–3681.

79. Arlt, W. (2009). The approach to the adult with newly diagnosed adrenal insufficiency. *J. Clin. Endocrinol. Metab.* 94 (4): 1059–1067.

80. Lebbe, M. and Arlt, W. (2013). What is the best diagnostic and therapeutic management strategy for an Addison patient during pregnancy? *Clin. Endocrinol.* 78 (4): 497–502.

81. Suzuki, R., Morita, H., Nishiwaki, H., and Yoshimura, A. (2010). Adrenal insufficiency in a haemodialysis patient. *NDT Plus* 3 (1): 99–100.

82. Inder, W.J., Meyer, C., and Hunt, P.J. (2015). Management of hypertension and heart failure in patients with Addison's disease. *Clin. Endocrinol.* 82 (6): 789–792.

83. Coluzzi, F., LeQuang, J.A.K., Sciacchitano, S. et al. (2023). A closer look at opioid-induced adrenal insufficiency: a narrative review. *Int. J. Mol. Sci.* 24 (5): 4575.

84. Funder, J.W., Carey, R.M., Mantero, F. et al. (2016). The management of primary aldosteronism: case detection, diagnosis, and treatment: an endocrine society clinical practice guideline. *J. Clin. Endocrinol. Metab.* 101 (5): 1889–1916.

85. Brown, N.J. (2003). Eplerenone: cardiovascular protection. *Circulation* 107 (19): 2512–2518.

86. Handler, J. (2012). Overlapping spironolactone dosing in primary aldosteronism and resistant essential hypertension. *J. Clin. Hypertens. (Greenwich)* 14 (10): 732–734.

87. Pitt, B., Zannad, F., Remme, W.J. et al. (1999). The effect of spironolactone on morbidity and mortality in patients with severe heart failure. Randomized Aldactone Evaluation Study Investigators. *N. Engl. J. Med.* 341 (10): 709–717.

88. Parthasarathy, H.K., Ménard, J., White, W.B. et al. (2011). A double-blind, randomized study comparing the antihypertensive effect of eplerenone and spironolactone in patients with hypertension and evidence of primary aldosteronism. *J. Hypertens.* 29 (5): 980–990.

89. Monticone, S., D'Ascenzo, F., Moretti, C. et al. (2018). Cardiovascular events and target organ damage in primary aldosteronism compared with essential hypertension: a systematic review and meta-analysis. *Lancet Diabetes Endocrinol.* 6 (1): 41–50.

90. Mulatero, P., Monticone, S., Bertello, C. et al. (2013). Long-term cardio- and cerebrovascular events in patients with primary aldosteronism. *J. Clin. Endocrinol. Metab.* 98 (12): 4826–4833.

91. Nishikawa, T., Omura, M., Satoh, F. et al. (2011). Guidelines for the diagnosis and treatment of primary aldosteronism – the Japan Endocrine Society 2009. *Endocr. J.* 58 (9): 711–721.

92. Hung, A., Ahmed, S., Gupta, A. et al. (2021). Performance of the aldosterone to renin ratio as a screening test for primary aldosteronism. *J. Clin. Endocrinol. Metab.* 106 (8): 2423–2435.

93. Young, W.F. Jr. (2019). Diagnosis and treatment of primary aldosteronism: practical clinical perspectives. *J. Intern. Med.* 285 (2): 126–148.

94. Rossi, G.P., Ceolotto, G., Rossitto, G. et al. (2020). Effects of mineralocorticoid and AT1 receptor antagonism on the aldosterone-renin ratio in primary aldosteronism-the EMIRA study. *J. Clin. Endocrinol. Metab.* 105 (6): dgaa080.

95. Hundemer, G.L., Curhan, G.C., Yozamp, N. et al. (2018). Cardiometabolic outcomes and mortality in medically treated primary aldosteronism: a retrospective cohort study. *Lancet Diabetes Endocrinol.* 6 (1): 51–59.

96. Funder, J.W., Carey, R.M., Fardella, C. et al. (2008). Case detection, diagnosis, and treatment of patients with primary aldosteronism: an endocrine society clinical practice guideline. *J. Clin. Endocrinol. Metab.* 93 (9): 3266–3281.

97. Ellison, D.H., Velázquez, H., and Wright, F.S. (1989). Adaptation of the distal convoluted tubule of the rat. Structural and functional effects of dietary salt intake and chronic diuretic infusion. *J. Clin. Invest.* 83 (1): 113–126.

98. Kleyman, T.R. and Cragoe, E.J. (1988). Amiloride and its analogs as tools in the study of ion transport. *J. Membr. Biol.* 105 (1): 1–21.

99. Warnock, D.G., Kusche-Vihrog, K., Tarjus, A. et al. (2014). Blood pressure and amiloride-sensitive sodium channels in vascular and renal cells. *Nat. Rev. Nephrol.* 10 (3): 146–157.

100. Palmer, L.G. and Frindt, G. (1986). Amiloride-sensitive Na channels from the apical membrane of the rat cortical collecting tubule. *Proc. Natl. Acad. Sci. U. S. A.* 83 (8): 2767–2770.

101. Weiner, I.D. and Wingo, C.S. (1997). Hypokalemia – consequences, causes, and correction. *J. Am. Soc. Nephrol.* 8 (7): 1179–1188.

102. Navar, L.G., Kobori, H., Prieto, M.C., and Gonzalez-Villalobos, R.A. (2011). Intratubular renin-angiotensin system in hypertension. *Hypertension* 57 (3): 355–362.

103. Schrier, R.W. (2010). Aldosterone "escape" vs "breakthrough.". *Nat. Rev. Nephrol.* 6 (2): 61.

104. Cataliotti, A., Malatino, L.S., Jougasaki, M. et al. (2001). Circulating natriuretic peptide concentrations in patients with end-stage renal disease: role of brain natriuretic peptide as a biomarker for ventricular remodeling. *Mayo Clin. Proc.* 76 (11): 1111–1119.

105. Pitt, B., Remme, W., Zannad, F. et al. (2003). Eplerenone, a selective aldosterone blocker, in patients with left ventricular dysfunction after myocardial infarction. *N. Engl. J. Med.* 348 (14): 1309–1321.

106. Rossi, G.P., Bernini, G., Caliumi, C. et al. (2006). A prospective study of the prevalence of primary aldosteronism in 1,125 hypertensive patients. *J. Am. Coll. Cardiol.* 48 (11): 2293–2300.

107. Monticone, S., Burrello, J., Tizzani, D. et al. (2017). Prevalence and clinical manifestations of primary aldosteronism encountered in primary care practice. *J. Am. Coll. Cardiol.* 69 (14): 1811–1820.

108. Young, W.F. (2007). Primary aldosteronism: renaissance of a syndrome. *Clin. Endocrinol.* 66 (5): 607–618.

109. Karagiannis, A., Tziomalos, K., Papageorgiou, A. et al. (2008). Spironolactone versus eplerenone for the treatment of idiopathic hyperaldosteronism. *Expert. Opin. Pharmacother.* 9 (4): 509–515.

110. Tetti, M., Monticone, S., Burrello, J. et al. (2018). Liddle syndrome: review of the literature and description of a new case. *Int. J. Mol. Sci.* 19 (3).

111. O'Shaughnessy, K.M. (2015). Gordon Syndrome: a continuing story. *Pediatr. Nephrol.* 30 (11): 1903–1908.

112. Young, W.F. (2016). Chapter 16 – Endocrine hypertension. In: *Williams Textbook of Endocrinology, 13th* (ed. S. Melmed, K.S. Polonsky, P.R. Larsen, and H.M. Kronenberg), 556–588. Philadelphia: Content Repository Only!

113. Armanini, D., Calò, L., and Semplicini, A. (2003). Pseudohyperaldosteronism: pathogenetic mechanisms. *Crit. Rev. Clin. Lab. Sci.* 40 (3): 295–335.

114. Al-Harbi, T. and Al-Shaikh, A. (2012). Apparent mineralocorticoid excess syndrome: report of one family with three affected children. *J. Pediatr. Endocrinol. Metab.* 25 (11–12): 1083–1088.

115. Melby, J.C., Spark, R.F., Dale, S.L. et al. (1967). Diagnosis and localization of aldosterone-producing adenomas by adrenal-vein cateterization. *N. Engl. J. Med.* 277 (20): 1050–1056.

116. Young, W.F., Stanson, A.W., Thompson, G.B. et al. (2004). Role for adrenal venous sampling in primary aldosteronism. *Surgery* 136 (6): 1227–1235.

117. Kempers, M.J.E., Lenders, J.W.M., van Outheusden, L. et al. (2009). Systematic review: diagnostic procedures to differentiate unilateral from bilateral adrenal abnormality in primary aldosteronism. *Ann. Intern. Med.* 151 (5): 329–337.

118. El Ghorayeb, N., Mazzuco, T.L., Bourdeau, I. et al. (2016). Basal and post-ACTH aldosterone and its ratios are useful during adrenal vein sampling in primary aldosteronism. *J. Clin. Endocrinol. Metab.* 101 (4): 1826–1835.

119. Scholten, A., Cisco, R.M., Vriens, M.R. et al. (2013). Variant adrenal venous anatomy in 546 laparoscopic adrenalectomies. *JAMA Surg.* 148 (4): 378–383.

120. Ceral, J., Solar, M., Krajina, A. et al. (2010). Adrenal venous sampling in primary aldosteronism: a low dilution of adrenal venous blood is crucial for a correct interpretation of the results. *Eur. J. Endocrinol.* 162 (1): 101–107.

121. Deipolyi, A.R. and Oklu, R. (2015). Adrenal vein sampling in the diagnosis of aldosteronism. *JVD* 3: 17–23.

122. Rossi, G.P., Auchus, R.J., Brown, M. et al. (2014). An expert consensus statement on use of adrenal vein sampling for the subtyping of primary aldosteronism. *Hypertension* 63 (1): 151–160.

123. Eisenhofer, G., Huynh, T.-T., Pacak, K. et al. (2004). Distinct gene expression profiles in norepinephrine- and epinephrine-producing hereditary and sporadic pheochromocytomas: activation of hypoxia-driven angiogenic pathways in von Hippel-Lindau syndrome. *Endocr. Relat. Cancer* 11 (4): 897–911.

124. Eisenhofer, G., Goldstein, D.S., Walther, M.M. et al. (2003). Biochemical diagnosis of pheochromocytoma: how to distinguish true- from false-positive test results. *J. Clin. Endocrinol. Metab.* 88 (6): 2656–2666.

125. Lenders, J.W.M., Pacak, K., Walther, M.M. et al. (2002). Biochemical diagnosis of pheochromocytoma: which test is best? *JAMA* 287 (11): 1427–1434.

126. Bylund, D.B., Eikenberg, D.C., Hieble, J.P. et al. (1994). International Union of Pharmacology nomenclature of adrenoceptors. *Pharmacol. Rev.* 46 (2): 121–136.

127. Ruffolo, R.R., Nichols, A.J., Stadel, J.M., and Hieble, J.P. (1991). Structure and function of alpha-adrenoceptors. *Pharmacol. Rev.* 43 (4): 475–505.

128. MacDonald, E., Kobilka, B.K., and Scheinin, M. (1997). Gene targeting – homing in on alpha 2-adrenoceptor-subtype function. *Trends Pharmacol. Sci.* 18 (6): 211–219.

129. Brodde, O.E., Michel, M.C., and Zerkowski, H.R. (1995). Signal transduction mechanisms controlling cardiac contractility and their alterations in chronic heart failure. *Cardiovasc. Res.* 30 (4): 570–584.

130. Bond, R.A., Leff, P., Johnson, T.D. et al. (1995). Physiological effects of inverse agonists in transgenic mice with myocardial overexpression of the beta 2-adrenoceptor. *Nature* 374 (6519): 272–276.

131. Granneman, J.G., Lahners, K.N., and Chaudhry, A. (1991). Molecular cloning and expression of the rat beta 3-adrenergic receptor. *Mol. Pharmacol.* 40 (6): 895–899.

132. Ramachandran, R. and Rewari, V. (2017). Current perioperative management of pheochromocytomas. *Indian J Urol* 33 (1): 19–25.

133. Prys-Roberts, C. and Farndon, J.R. (2002). Efficacy and safety of doxazosin for perioperative management of patients with pheochromocytoma. *World J. Surg.* 26 (8): 1037–1042.

134. Yamada, T., Fukuoka, H., Hosokawa, Y. et al. (2020). Patients with pheochromocytoma exhibit low aldosterone renin ratio-preliminary reports. *BMC Endocr. Disord.* 20 (1): 140.

135. Reisch, N., Peczkowska, M., Januszewicz, A., and Neumann, H.P.H. (2006). Pheochromocytoma: presentation, diagnosis and treatment. *J. Hypertens.* 24 (12): 2331–2339.

136. Kocak, S., Aydintug, S., and Canakci, N. (2002). Alpha blockade in preoperative preparation of patients with pheochromocytomas. *Int. Surg.* 87 (3): 191–194.

137. Frishman, W.H. (1988). Beta-adrenergic receptor blockers. Adverse effects and drug interactions. *Hypertension* 11 (3 Pt 2): II21-29.

138. Kinney, M.A.O., Narr, B.J., and Warner, M.A. (2002). Perioperative management of pheochromocytoma. *J. Cardiothorac. Vasc. Anesth.* 16 (3): 359–369.

139. Nazari, M.A., Rosenblum, J.S., Haigney, M.C. et al. (2020). Pathophysiology and acute management of tachyarrhythmias in pheochromocytoma JACC review topic of the week. *J. Am. Coll. Cardiol.* 76 (4): 451–464.

140. Myklejord, D.J. (2004). Undiagnosed pheochromocytoma: the anesthesiologist nightmare. *Clin. Med. Res.* 2 (1): 59–62.

141. Kuok, C.-H., Yen, C.-R., Huang, C.-S. et al. (2011). Cardiovascular collapse after labetalol for hypertensive crisis in an undiagnosed pheochromocytoma during cesarean section. *Acta Anaesthesiol. Taiwanica* 49 (2): 69–71.

142. Azadeh, N., Ramakrishna, H., Bhatia, N.L. et al. (2016). Therapeutic goals in patients with pheochromocytoma: a guide to perioperative management. *Ir. J. Med. Sci.* 185 (1): 43–49.

143. Fang, F., Ding, L., He, Q., and Liu, M. (2020). Preoperative management of pheochromocytoma and paraganglioma. *Front. Endocrinol.* 11.

144. Lenders, J.W.M. and Eisenhofer, G. (2017). Update on modern management of pheochromocytoma and paraganglioma. *Endocrinol Metab (Seoul)* 32 (2): 152–161.

145. Dahia, P.L.M. (2014). Pheochromocytoma and paraganglioma pathogenesis: learning from genetic heterogeneity. *Nat. Rev. Cancer* 14 (2): 108–119.

146. Jochmanova, I. and Pacak, K. (2018). Genomic landscape of pheochromocytoma and paraganglioma. *Trends Cancer* 4 (1): 6–9.

147. Burnichon, N., Rohmer, V., Amar, L. et al. (2009). The succinate dehydrogenase genetic testing in a large prospective series of patients with paragangliomas. *J. Clin. Endocrinol. Metab.* 94 (8): 2817–2827.

148. Björklund, P. and Backman, S. (2018). Epigenetics of pheochromocytoma and paraganglioma. *Mol. Cell. Endocrinol.* 469: 92–97.

149. Martinelli, S., Amore, F., Canu, L. et al. (2023). Tumour microenvironment in pheochromocytoma and paraganglioma. *Front Endocrinol (Lausanne)* 14: 1137456.

150. Huang, H., Abraham, J., Hung, E. et al. (2008). Treatment of malignant pheochromocytoma/paraganglioma with cyclophosphamide, vincristine, and dacarbazine. *Cancer* 113 (8): 2020–2028.

151. Averbuch, S.D., Steakley, C.S., Young, R.C. et al. (1988). Malignant pheochromocytoma: effective treatment with a combination of cyclophosphamide, vincristine, and dacarbazine. *Ann. Intern. Med.* 109 (4): 267–273.

152. Emadi, A., Jones, R.J., and Brodsky, R.A. (2009). Cyclophosphamide and cancer: golden anniversary. *Nat. Rev. Clin. Oncol.* 6 (11): 638–647.

153. Kohn, K.W. (1996). Beyond DNA cross-linking: history and prospects of DNA-targeted cancer treatment – fifteenth Bruce F. Cain Memorial Award Lecture. *Cancer Res.* 56 (24): 5533–5546.

154. Jordan, M.A. and Wilson, L. (2004). Microtubules as a target for anticancer drugs. *Nat. Rev. Cancer* 4 (4): 253–265.

155. Dumontet, C. and Jordan, M.A. (2010). Microtubule-binding agents: a dynamic field of cancer therapeutics. *Nat. Rev. Drug Discov.* 9 (10): 790–803.

156. Tanabe, A., Naruse, M., Nomura, K. et al. (2013). Combination chemotherapy with cyclophosphamide, vincristine, and dacarbazine in patients with

malignant pheochromocytoma and paraganglioma. *Horm Cancer* 4 (2): 103–110.

157. Roos, W.P. and Kaina, B. (2013). DNA damage-induced cell death: from specific DNA lesions to the DNA damage response and apoptosis. *Cancer Lett.* 332 (2): 237–248.

158. Niemeijer, N.D., Alblas, G., van Hulsteijn, L.T. et al. (2014). Chemotherapy with cyclophosphamide, vincristine and dacarbazine for malignant paraganglioma and pheochromocytoma: systematic review and meta-analysis. *Clin. Endocrinol.* 81 (5): 642–651.

159. Asai, S., Katabami, T., Tsuiki, M. et al. (2017). Controlling tumor progression with cyclophosphamide, vincristine, and dacarbazine treatment improves survival in patients with metastatic and unresectable malignant pheochromocytomas/paragangliomas. *HORM CANC* 8 (2): 108–118.

160. Ayala-Ramirez, M., Feng, L., Habra, M.A. et al. (2012). Clinical benefits of systemic chemotherapy for patients with metastatic pheochromocytomas or sympathetic extra-adrenal paragangliomas: insights from the largest single-institutional experience. *Cancer* 118 (11): 2804–2812.

161. Gruber, L.M., Jasim, S., Ducharme-Smith, A. et al. (2021). The role for metyrosine in the treatment of patients with pheochromocytoma and paraganglioma. *J. Clin. Endocrinol. Metab.* 106 (6): e2393–e2401.

162. Butz, J.J., Weingarten, T.N., Cavalcante, A.N. et al. (2017). Perioperative hemodynamics and outcomes of patients on metyrosine undergoing resection of pheochromocytoma or paraganglioma. *Int. J. Surg.* 46: 1–6.

163. Shapiro, B., Copp, J.E., Sisson, J.C. et al. (1985). Iodine-131 metaiodobenzylguanidine for the locating of suspected pheochromocytoma: experience in 400 cases. *J. Nucl. Med.* 26 (6): 576–585.

164. Wieland, D.M., Brown, L.E., Rogers, W.L. et al. (1981). Myocardial imaging with a radioiodinated norepinephrine storage analog. *J. Nucl. Med.* 22 (1): 22–31.

165. Sisson, J.C., Shapiro, B., Beierwaltes, W.H. et al. (1984). Radiopharmaceutical treatment of malignant pheochromocytoma. *J. Nucl. Med.* 25 (2): 197–206.

166. Jha, A., Taïeb, D., Carrasquillo, J.A. et al. (2021). High-specific-activity 131I-MIBG vs 177Lu-DOTATATE targeted radionuclide therapy for metastatic pheochromocytoma and paraganglioma. *Clin. Cancer Res.* 27 (11): 2989–2995.

167. Douglas, W.W. and Rubin, R.P. (1961). The role of calcium in the secretory response of the adrenal medulla to acetylcholine. *J. Physiol.* 159 (1): 40–57.

168. Fleckenstein, A. (1977). Specific pharmacology of calcium in myocardium, cardiac pacemakers, and vascular smooth muscle. *Annu. Rev. Pharmacol. Toxicol.* 17: 149–166.

169. Favre, L., Forster, A., Fathi, M., and Vallotton, M.B. (1986). Calcium-channel inhibition in pheochromocytoma. *Acta Endocrinol.* 113 (3): 385–390.

170. García, M.I.D.O., Palasí, R., Gómez, R.C. et al. (2019). Surgical and pharmacological management of functioning pheochromocytoma and paraganglioma. *Exon Publications* 63–80.

171. Manger, W.M. (2006). An overview of pheochromocytoma: history, current concepts, vagaries, and diagnostic challenges. *Ann. N. Y. Acad. Sci.* 1073: 1–20.

172. Jaiswal, S.K., Memon, S.S., Lila, A. et al. (2021). Preoperative amlodipine is efficacious in preventing intraoperative HDI in pheochromocytoma: pilot RCT. *J. Clin. Endocrinol. Metab.* 106 (8): e2907–e2918.

173. Lebuffe, G., Dosseh, E.D., Tek, G. et al. (2005). The effect of calcium channel blockers on outcome following the surgical treatment of phaeochromocytomas and paragangliomas. *Anaesthesia* 60 (5): 439–444.

174. Grouzmann, E., Drouard-Troalen, L., Baudin, E. et al. (2010). Diagnostic accuracy of free and total metanephrines in plasma and fractionated metanephrines in urine of patients with pheochromocytoma. *Eur. J. Endocrinol.* 162 (5): 951–960.

175. Kim, H.J., Lee, J.I., Cho, Y.Y. et al. (2015). Diagnostic accuracy of plasma free metanephrines in a seated position compared with 24-hour urinary metanephrines in the investigation of pheochromocytoma. *Endocr. J.* 62 (3): 243–250.

176. Kantorovich, V. and Pacak, K. (2010). Pheochromocytoma and paraganglioma. *Prog. Brain Res.* 182: 343–373.

177. King, S.R. and Stocco, D.M. (2011). Steroidogenic acute regulatory protein expression in the central nervous system. *Front. Endocrinol.* 2.

178. Al Alawi, A.M., Nordenström, A., and Falhammar, H. (2019). Clinical perspectives in congenital adrenal hyperplasia due to 3β-hydroxysteroid dehydrogenase type 2 deficiency. *Endocrine* 63 (3): 407–421.

179. Merke, D.P. and Bornstein, S.R. (2005). Congenital adrenal hyperplasia. *Lancet* 365 (9477): 2125–2136.

180. Speiser, P.W., Arlt, W., Auchus, R.J. et al. (2018). Congenital adrenal hyperplasia due to steroid 21-hydroxylase deficiency: an endocrine society clinical practice guideline. *J. Clin. Endocrinol. Metab.* 103 (11): 4043–4088.

181. El-Maouche, D., Arlt, W., and Merke, D.P. (2017). Congenital adrenal hyperplasia. *Lancet* 390 (10108): 2194–2210.

182. Etxabe, J. and Vazquez, J.A. (1994). Morbidity and mortality in Cushing's disease: an epidemiological approach. *Clin. Endocrinol.* 40 (4): 479–484.

183. Auchus, R.J. and Arlt, W. (2013). Approach to the patient: the adult with congenital adrenal hyperplasia. *J. Clin. Endocrinol. Metab.* 98 (7): 2645–2655.

184. Arlt, W., Willis, D.S., Wild, S.H. et al. (2010). Health status of adults with congenital adrenal hyperplasia: a cohort study of 203 patients. *J. Clin. Endocrinol. Metab.* 95 (11): 5110–5121.

185. Yau, M., Gujral, J., and New, M.I. (2000). Congenital adrenal hyperplasia: diagnosis and emergency treatment. In: *Endotext* (ed. K.R. Feingold, B. Anawalt, M.R. Blackman, et al.). South Dartmouth: MDText.com, Inc. https://www.ncbi.nlm.nih.gov/books/NBK279085/.

186. Miller, W.L. and Auchus, R.J. (2011). The molecular biology, biochemistry, and physiology of human steroidogenesis and its disorders. *Endocr. Rev.* 32 (1): 81–151.

187. Kapoor, A., Petropoulos, S., and Matthews, S.G. (2008). Fetal programming of hypothalamic-pituitary-adrenal (HPA) axis function and behavior by synthetic glucocorticoids. *Brain Res. Rev.* 57 (2): 586–595.

188. Caldato, M.C.F., Fernandes, V.T., and Kater, C.E. (2004). One-year clinical evaluation of single morning dose prednisolone therapy for 21-hydroxylase deficiency. *Arq. Bras. Endocrinol. Metabol.* 48 (5): 705–712.

189. Joffe, H.V. and Adler, G.K. (2005). Effect of aldosterone and mineralocorticoid receptor blockade on vascular inflammation. *Heart Fail. Rev.* 10 (1): 31–37.

190. Kwon, T.-H., Frøkiær, J., and Nielsen, S. (2013). Regulation of aquaporin-2 in the kidney: a molecular mechanism of body-water homeostasis. *Kidney Res Clin Pract* 32 (3): 96–102.

191. Gomez-Sanchez, E. and Gomez-Sanchez, C.E. (2014). The multifaceted mineralocorticoid receptor. *Compr. Physiol.* 4 (3): 965–994.

192. Lopes, L.A., Dubuis, J.M., Vallotton, M.B., and Sizonenko, P.C. (1998). Should we monitor more closely the dosage of 9 alpha-fluorohydrocortisone in salt-losing congenital adrenal hyperplasia? *J. Pediatr. Endocrinol. Metab.* 11 (6): 733–737.

193. Baranowski, E.S., Arlt, W., and Idkowiak, J. (2018). Monogenic disorders of adrenal steroidogenesis. *Horm. Res. Paediatr.* 89 (5): 292–310.

194. Kim, C.J. (2014). Congenital lipoid adrenal hyperplasia. *Ann Pediatr Endocrinol Metab* 19 (4): 179–183.

195. Leka-Emiri, S., Taibi, L., Mavroeidi, V. et al. (2022). 3β-hydroxysteroid dehydrogenase type 2 (3βHSD2) deficiency due to a novel compound heterozygosity of a missense mutation (p.Thr259Met) and frameshift deletion (p.Lys273ArgFs*7) in an under-virilized infant male with salt wasting. *Sex. Dev.* 16 (1): 64–69.

196. Xu, S., Hu, S., Yu, X. et al. (2017). 17α-hydroxylase/17,20-lyase deficiency in congenital adrenal hyperplasia: a case report. *Mol. Med. Rep.* 15 (1): 339–344.

197. Kim, S.M. and Rhee, J.H. (2015). A case of 17 alpha-hydroxylase deficiency. *Clin. Exp. Reprod. Med.* 42 (2): 72–76.

198. Ammar, R., and Ramadan, A. (2020) Incidental diagnosis of 17 alpha-hydroxylase deficiency: a case report. *Oxford Medical Case Reports*, 2020 (12), omaa108.

199. Nimkarn, S. and New, M.I. (2008). Steroid 11beta-hydroxylase deficiency congenital adrenal hyperplasia. *Trends Endocrinol. Metab.* 19 (3): 96–99.

200. Alsanea, M.N., Al-Agha, A., and Shazly, M.A. Classical 11β-hydroxylase deficiency caused by a novel homozygous mutation: a case study and literature review. *Cureus* 14 (1): e21537.

201. Bulsari, K. and Falhammar, H. (2017). Clinical perspectives in congenital adrenal hyperplasia due to 11β-hydroxylase deficiency. *Endocrine* 55 (1): 19–36.

202. Menabò, S., Polat, S., Baldazzi, L. et al. (2014). Congenital adrenal hyperplasia due to 11-beta-hydroxylase deficiency: functional consequences of four CYP11B1 mutations. *Eur. J. Hum. Genet.* 22 (5): 610–616.

203. Burdea, L. and Mendez, M.D. (2023). 21 Hydroxylase deficiency. In: *StatPearls*. Treasure Island (FL): StatPearls Publishing https://www.ncbi.nlm.nih.gov/books/NBK493164/.

204. Nimkarn, S., Gangishetti, P.K., Yau, M., and New, M.I. (1993). 21-Hydroxylase-deficient congenital

adrenal hyperplasia. In: *GeneReviews®* (ed. M.P. Adam, G.M. Mirzaa, R.A. Pagon, et al.). Seattle: University of Washington, Seattle.

205. Speiser, P.W., Serrat, J., New, M.I., and Gertner, J.M. (1992). Insulin insensitivity in adrenal hyperplasia due to nonclassical steroid 21-hydroxylase deficiency. *J. Clin. Endocrinol. Metab.* 75 (6): 1421–1424.

206. Gambineri, A., Fanelli, F., Prontera, O. et al. (2013). Prevalence of hyperandrogenic states in late adolescent and young women: epidemiological survey on italian high-school students. *J. Clin. Endocrinol. Metab.* 98 (4): 1641–1650.

207. Krysiak, R. and Okopien, B. (2014). The effect of metformin on androgen production in diabetic women with non-classic congenital adrenal hyperplasia. *Exp. Clin. Endocrinol. Diabetes* 122 (10): 568–571.

208. Witchel, S.F. and Azziz, R. (2010). Nonclassic congenital adrenal hyperplasia. *Int. J. Pediatr. Endocrinol.* 2010.

209. Jha, S. and Turcu, A.F. (2021). Non-classic congenital adrenal hyperplasia: what do endocrinologists need to know? *Endocrinol. Metab. Clin. N. Am.* 50 (1): 151–165.

210. Livadas, S. and Bothou, C. (2019). Management of the female with non-classical congenital adrenal hyperplasia (NCCAH): a patient-oriented approach. *Front. Endocrinol.* 10.

211. Zimmerman, Y., Eijkemans, M.J.C., Coelingh Bennink, H.J.T. et al. (2014). The effect of combined oral contraception on testosterone levels in healthy women: a systematic review and meta-analysis. *Hum. Reprod. Update* 20 (1): 76–105.

212. Nordenström, A. and Falhammar, H. (2019). Management of endocrine disease: diagnosis and management of the patient with non-classic CAH due to 21-hydroxylase deficiency. *Eur. J. Endocrinol.* 180 (3): R127–R145.

213. Martin, K.A., Anderson, R.R., Chang, R.J. et al. (2018). Evaluation and treatment of hirsutism in premenopausal women: an endocrine society clinical practice guideline. *J. Clin. Endocrinol. Metab.* 103 (4): 1233–1257.

214. Kangasniemi, M.H., Arffman, R.K., Haverinen, A. et al. (2022). Effects of estradiol- and ethinylestradiol-based contraceptives on adrenal steroids: a randomized trial. *Contraception* 116: 59–65.

215. Trapp, C.M. and Oberfield, S.E. (2012). Recommendations for treatment of nonclassic congenital adrenal hyperplasia (NCCAH): an update. *Steroids* 77 (4): 342–346.

216. Schimmer, B.P. and Funder, J.W. (2015). ACTH, adrenal steroids, and pharmacology of the adrenal cortex. In: *Goodman & Gilman's: The Pharmacological Basis of Therapeutics, 12th* (ed. L.L. Brunton, B.A. Chabner, and B.C. Knollmann), 1215–1216. New York: McGraw-Hill Education.

CHAPTER 4

Pancreatic Gland Therapies

4.1 DIABETES MELLITUS

4.1.1 Insulin

4.1.1.1 Physiology

Structure of Insulin

Insulin is a 51 amino acid peptide hormone that consists of two chains (A and B) linked by a pair of disulfide bonds. The A (21 amino acids) and B (30 amino acids) chains of insulin are linked by an intervening sequence of amino acids known as the connecting peptide (c-peptide) [1]. The gene that encodes human insulin produces an mRNA transcript that is translated into a large 110 amino acid polypeptide sequence known as **preproinsulin**. Preproinsulin then undergoes further processing in the lumen of the rough endoplasmic reticulum to produce proinsulin. Proinsulin is then ferried into the Golgi apparatus, where it is subsequently cleaved into the native insulin peptide and c-peptide [2]. Along with these products of proinsulin processing, amylin and other intermediate peptides are packaged into secretory granules by the pancreatic beta cell [3].

Regulation of Blood Glucose

Glucose homeostasis depends on the action of insulin and a host of other counterregulatory hormones. This fine-tuned system depends on the action of hormones, neural stimuli, and other regulatory cytokines working together in various organs to control plasma glucose. In fact, the pancreatic beta cell is crucial in directing the orchestra of this complex homeostatic system [4].

During the fasting state, the relative decrease in insulin levels results in the oxidation of fatty acids in adipose tissue, making fatty acids a primary source of energy in the fasting state. For example, the liver uses fatty acids for gluconeogenesis during a prolonged fast. On the contrary, the brain has obligatory glucose requirements, which makes it necessary to have alternative sources of energy supply during a fast. The liver serves as a valuable source of glucose during a prolonged fast. Glucagon is released by alpha cells of the pancreas during fasting and promotes hepatic gluconeogenesis and glycogenolysis, thus maintaining plasma glucose concentration within a physiological range.

In contrast, during the postprandial state, glucose sensing by the pancreatic beta cell results in insulin release. Insulin then exerts its metabolic action through various processes, including the inhibition of hepatic glucose output (reduced glycogenolysis and gluconeogenesis), the promotion of glucose uptake by peripheral tissues (muscle and adipose tissue), and a reduction in lipolysis (adipose tissue) [5]. Next, we will explore the effects of insulin on various tissues, including skeletal muscle, adipose tissue, and liver.

The Effects of Insulin on Various Tissues

Skeletal muscle relies on glucose and free fatty acids as energy sources in the postprandial and fasting states, respectively.

Endocrinology: Pathophysiology to Therapy, First Edition. Akuffo Quarde.
© 2024 John Wiley & Sons Ltd. Published 2024 by John Wiley & Sons Ltd.

Skeletal muscle serves as the primary site of glucose uptake after ingestion of a meal (postprandial period), with insulin being the primary hormone responsible for this function. An increase in serum glucose after meal intake is sensed by pancreatic beta cells, which subsequently release insulin. Insulin then binds to the insulin receptor (IR) and initiates a signaling cascade that results in the ferrying of glucose transporter 4 (also known as GLUT 4) from the sarcoplasm to the plasma membrane of skeletal muscle [6, 7] through a process of exocytosis [7]. GLUT-4 then mediates glucose uptake by the skeletal muscle.

When glucose enters the myocyte of skeletal muscles, it is phosphorylated by the hexokinase enzyme to glucose-6-phosphate, which can be channeled into either glycogen synthesis (and storage) or used in the glycolytic pathway. A substantial amount of glucose entering the glycolytic pathway is oxidized to produce energy, with only 10% being channeled into lactate production [8].

On the other hand, during the fasting state, relatively low insulin levels impair the usual anti-lipolytic action of insulin in white adipose tissue. Consequently, increased lipolysis in white adipose tissue results in the production of fatty acids. These free fatty acids become the primary source of fuel for skeletal muscle [9].

Also, during fasting, the liver serves as the main source of endogenous glucose production. This allows cells that can only utilize glucose as a primary source of energy, such as neurons, red blood cells, and renal medulla cells, to function optimally. The liver achieves this goal by increasing glycogenolysis, gluconeogenesis, and glycogen synthesis in the postabsorptive period. This complex system requires the interaction of various hormones (insulin, glucagon, catecholamines, glucocorticoids), substrates (glucose, glycerol), and allosteric factors (acetyl CoA, glucose, and glucose-6-phosphate) [10] beyond the scope of this text.

In the postprandial period, insulin mediates various processes that suppress glucose production by the liver.

1. Through its antilipolytic action, insulin suppresses the breakdown of triglycerides into free fatty acids in white adipose tissue. Consequently, free fatty acid, a substrate for gluconeogenesis in the liver, is reduced, resulting in the suppression of hepatic glucose production [10, 11].
2. Glucagon stimulates hepatic glycogenolysis (increased hepatic glucose production). The presence of high levels of circulating insulin after a meal inhibits the release of glucagon by alpha cells of the pancreas which consequently reduces hepatic glucose output [11].

Insulin Receptor

The IR has an extracellular portion composed of two alpha subunits and a transmembrane section comprising two beta subunits. In normal physiology, alpha subunits inhibit the intrinsic tyrosine kinase activity of beta subunits [12].

When insulin binds to the alpha subunit of the IR, it suppresses the ability of the alpha subunit to inhibit the beta subunit. Consequently, insulin binding to IR promotes the phosphorylation of intracellular proteins required for various downstream signaling cascades in different tissues [13]. See Figure 4.1.

4.1.1.2 Mechanism of Action

The mechanism of insulin action was reviewed earlier in Section 4.1.1.

Insulin resistance is central to our understanding of persistent hyperglycemia in patients with type 2 diabetes mellitus (see Table 4.1). It is characterized by an inability of normal plasma insulin to exert its glucose-lowering effects in the fed state (postprandial). Consequently, increased hepatic glucose output, increased lipolysis, and impaired peripheral glucose uptake lead to hyperglycemia [16].

Practice Pearl(s)

Insulin therapy may be either adjunctive or utilized primarily in managing type 2 diabetes mellitus. However, insulin therapy is required to prevent life-threatening ketoacidosis for patients with either anatomic or functional pancreatic insufficiency (e.g. type 1 diabetes mellitus).

Although guided by clinical evidence, the recommendations for insulin use in type 2 diabetes mellitus vary significantly across various clinical practice guidelines. It is, however, generally accepted that insulin should be initiated in patients with anticipated beta-cell failure and worsening hyperglycemia despite adherence to optimized doses of non-insulin therapies [17, 18].

Patients with type 1 diabetes mellitus require both basal and prandial insulin if they are on multiple daily insulin injections. The usual starting total daily

(continued)

(continued)

dose of insulin (TDDi) is 0.5 units per kg body per day. The TDDi is split up into basal (40–60%) and bolus (40–60%) insulin. Furthermore, patients with optimal carbohydrate counting skills may use a carbohydrate ratio to estimate the amount of bolus insulin [19].

 Pathophysiology Pearl

Ketosis is a physiological state characterized by an elevated concentration of ketone bodies in the bloodstream. This condition could originate from various situations, such as diabetic ketoacidosis (DKA), alcoholic ketoacidosis, or starvation. Diabetic ketoacidosis is commonly observed among patients with type 1 diabetes mellitus and might occur either as the primary presenting feature of diabetes mellitus or as a secondary outcome of an intercurrent illness such as an infection or myocardial infarction.

In terms of pathophysiology, insulin deficiency in patients with type 1 diabetes mellitus impedes glucose uptake by cells, thereby preventing its utilization for glycolysis or glycogenesis. Concurrently, a surge in circulating glucagon levels is observed due to a perceived cellular glucose requirement. Consequently, beta-oxidation is facilitated by hormones such as glucagon, adrenaline, and cortisol.

The rapid turnover of fatty acids due to accelerated beta-oxidation produces large quantities of acetyl-CoA, which, when in excess, are converted into ketones, culminating in ketosis. As the concentration of ketones in the blood escalate, diabetic ketoacidosis sets in.

In a scenario where acetoacetic acid accrues, a portion is transformed into acetone. Given its volatile nature, acetone is exhaled in the breath of the patient, resulting in the characteristic sweet, fruity breath odor associated with DKA.

The therapeutic approach for DKA primarily involves a constant-rate insulin infusion and rigorous intravenous rehydration to reinstate circulating volume, rectify acidosis, and promote glucose uptake by cells. Recognizing the necessity of supplementing the infusion fluid with potassium is crucial, as insulin administration will encourage cellular potassium uptake and result in hypokalemia.

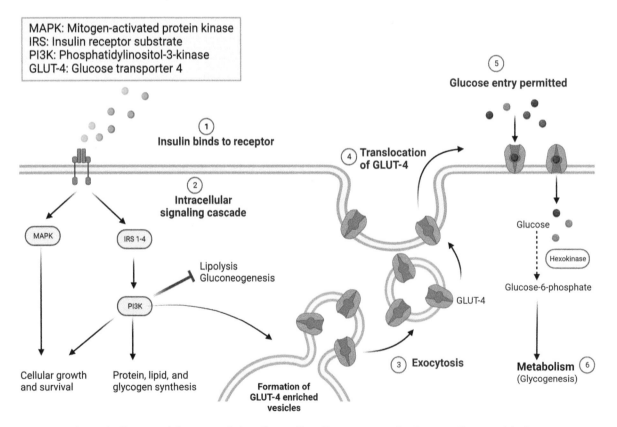

FIGURE 4.1   Schematic diagram of the intracellular effects of insulin receptor activation. Insulin-to-IR binding promotes intracellular effects, including increased glycogen, protein, and lipid synthesis. Lipolysis and gluconeogenesis are, however, inhibited. Insulin further promotes the recruitment of glucose transporter channels on peripheral tissues (e.g. skeletal muscle).

TABLE 4.1 Mechanisms of insulin resistance in type 2 diabetes mellitus.

Tissue	Pathophysiologic defect	Result
Skeletal muscle	Impaired translocation of GLUT4 to the plasma membrane of myocytes. Defective tyrosine phosphorylation of various proximal insulin receptor substrates.	Reduction in glucose uptake by skeletal muscle [5].
Adipose tissue	Reduced sensitivity of adipose to tissue to the anti-lipolytic action of insulin (an unknown underlying mechanism). Release of adipokines associated with insulin resistance.	Increased lipolysis [14].
Liver	Adipokines and free fatty acids (adipose tissue-derived) impair insulin signaling in the liver.	Impaired suppression of hepatic glucose output, which results in persistent hyperglycemia [15].

TABLE 4.2 Pharmacodynamic profile of various insulins.

Type	Onset	Peak	Duration
Long-acting			
Detemir U100	1–2 h	Mild effect at 4 h	<24 h
Glargine U100	1 h	None	24 h
Glargine U300	6 h	None	24–36 h
Degludec U100/U200	1 h	None	42 h
Intermediate-acting			
NPH insulin U100	1–2 h	4–14 h	4–14 h
Bolus insulin			
Lispro, Aspart, Glulisine U100 (rapid-acting)	5–15 min	0.5–1.5 h	3–5 h
Fiasp (ultra-rapid acting)	2.5–5 min	1 h	3–5 h
Regular human insulin (short-acting)	30–60 min	2–4 h	6–12 h

TABLE 4.2 (Continued)

Type	Onset	Peak	Duration
Concentrated insulin Humulin R U500			6–10 h
Inhaled insulin			
Afreeza	5–15 min	50 min	3 h
Oral insulin			
ORMD-0801[a]	–	–	–

U100 refers to 100 units of insulin in 1 mL of liquid.
U200 refers to 200 units of insulin in 1 mL of liquid.
U300 refers to 300 units of insulin in 1 mL of liquid.
[a] ORMD-0801 is a potential oral insulin therapy for the management of type 2 diabetes. There are ongoing phase 3 trials of this medication [20].
Source: Adapted from refs. [19, 21, 22].

TABLE 4.3 Pharmacokinetic profile of exogenous insulin.

Pharmacokinetic factor	Characteristics
Absorption	SC administration of exogenous insulin results in direct absorption into the bloodstream. The T50% has an intraindividual variability of 50% and an interindividual variability of 25%.
Distribution	The volume of distribution is dependent of the extracellular space.
Metabolism and elimination	Degradation of exogenous insulin occurs in the kidney (~60%) and liver (~40%) after SC administration.

SC, Subcutaneous.
T50% Coefficient of variation of absorption of 50% (Time for 50% of the administered dose to be absorbed).
Endogenous insulin (50% of insulin delivered into the portal vein by the pancreas is metabolized in the liver).
Source: Adapted from refs. [23–26].

The pharmacodynamic profile of various insulins used in treating diabetes mellitus is summarized in Table 4.2.

Refer to Table 4.3 for the pharmacokinetic profile of exogenous insulin, after subcutaneous administration.

Insulin analogs are produced as a result of amino acid substitutions or additions to the human insulin amino acid sequence (Figure 4.2).

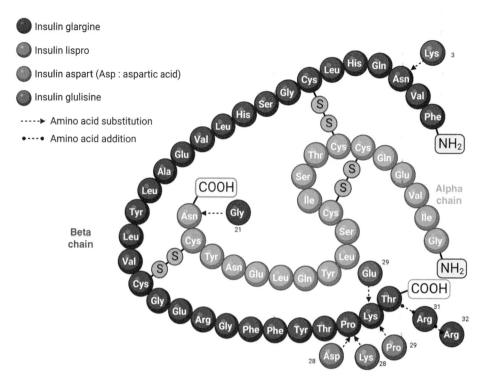

FIGURE 4.2 A schematic diagram of the amino acid sequence of human insulin. Various amino acid substitutions or additions to recombinant human insulins are shown (color-coded).

 Clinical Pearl

What are the factors associated with improved absorption of insulin administered subcutaneously?

1. Exercise of a limb will improve insulin absorption within an hour of injection.

2. Rubbing or massaging the site of the injection.

3. Warm compresses, hot shower, or bath improves and accelerates insulin absorption.

4. Site of injection: absorption is faster if insulin is injected into abdominal subcutaneous tissue than at alternative sites.

Clinical Trial Evidence

(Refer to Table 4.4)

TABLE 4.4 Important trials of long-acting insulin therapies.

Study	Population	Intervention	Outcome
Comparison of insulin degludec and glargine.	T2DM, mean body mass index was 25 kg/m². The mean level of glycated hemoglobin (HbA1c) was 8.5% (n = 435).	Patients were randomized (2 : 1) to degludec or glargine, with each treatment administered once daily along with one or more oral antidiabetic drugs.	The study concluded that initiating insulin therapy with IDeg provides similar long-term glycemic control to IGlar, but with a significantly lower rate of overall confirmed hypoglycemia once stable glycemic control and insulin dosing are achieved; RR 0.63, 95% CI 0.42 to 0.94, P = 0.02)[27].
Comparison of insulin glargine and human NPH insulin in addition to oral therapy.	T2DM, HbA1C >7.5% on or two oral agents for diabetes (n = 756).	Patients received bedtime glargine insulin or NPH insulin once daily with dose titration using a predefined algorithm to aim for fasting capillary glucose of ≤100 mg/dl (5.5 mmol/l).	Mean fasting glucose and HbA1C were similar in both groups; however, documented nocturnal hypoglycemia was less in the glargine compared to the NPH arm, 26.7% vs. 33.2%, P value <0.05) [28].

Pathophysiology Pearl

What is the challenge in administering insulin via the oral route?

Endogenous insulin is secreted via either high-frequency pulses every 5–15 minutes or low-frequency ultradian pulses every 80–120 minutes. After an oral glucose challenge, about 40–80% of insulin released into the portal vein undergoes first-pass metabolism in the liver.

This phase of hepatic metabolism enables insulin to exert various effects on glucose metabolism, such as the promotion of glycogenolysis, inhibition of glycogenesis, increased gluconeogenesis, and a reduction in glucagon secretion [25].

Of all the routes of potential insulin administration (pulmonary, subcutaneous, rectal, ocular, vaginal), the oral route is the closest to mimicking the portal-systemic blood insulin gradient seen with endogenous insulin. This is because orally administered insulin is delivered into the portal vein after absorption. Thus, oral insulin administration mimics what exists physiologically. Unfortunately, insulin is a peptide hormone; hence, it is subject to degradation in the harsh acidic pH of the stomach. Also, additional hindrances to oral insulin absorption, such as enzymatic degradation, efflux pumps, and epithelial barriers, contribute to its poor bioavailability [29].

The pharmaceutical industry has attempted various means of delivering oral insulin. This has, however, remained a persistent challenge due to the reasons outlined above [20].

4.1.2 Biguanides

4.1.2.1 Physiology

Glucose Metabolism

Glucose is the central source of energy for all cells in the human. Plasma glucose is therefore kept within a very narrow physiologic range of 64.8–104.4 mg/dl, independent of dietary intake [30]. To achieve this, various adaptive processes that prevent hypoglycemia and hyperglycemia coexist in a delicate balance.

The processes for preventing a significant decline in plasma glucose (hypoglycemia) during a fast state include the synthesis of glucose from noncarbohydrate sources (gluconeogenesis) and the breakdown of glycogen stores (glycogenolysis) [31].

On the other hand, synthesizing glycogen from glucose (glycogenesis) [32] and converting glucose to triacylglycerol (fats) helps mitigate significant hyperglycemia in the postprandial period [33, 34].

Ultimately, plasma glucose is ferried to various tissues and metabolized based on prevailing conditions – dependent on fasting or a postprandial state [5].

Gluconeogenesis

The normal human body requires, on average, about 160 g of glucose per day [35], of which 75% is utilized primarily by the central nervous system for energy production [36].

There are, however, very limited stores of readily accessible glucose in humans. Indeed, only 20 g of glucose is present in body fluids, with almost 190 g present in a stored form known as glycogen [37].

Depending on the level of energy expenditure by an individual, additional sources of glucose may be required. Furthermore, survival beyond 24 hours without extra dietary glucose intake would be impossible since most of these reserves would be depleted [38]. This makes **gluconeogenesis** a critical process for producing valuable glucose molecules needed for energy production. Gluconeogenesis generates glucose endogenously from mainly non-glucose precursors such as pyruvate, lactate, glycerol, and amino acids (see Table 4.5). It occurs mainly in

TABLE 4.5 Sources of glucose precursors required for gluconeogenesis.

Glucose precursor	Source
Lactate	It is produced by anaerobic respiration in skeletal muscle. Lactate is then transformed into pyruvate by lactate dehydrogenase in the liver.
Glycerol	It is produced by the breakdown of triglycerides in adipose tissues. Glycerol is then converted into dihydroxyacetone phosphate (DHAP) in readiness for gluconeogenesis.
Amino acids	Hydrolysis of protein in food or skeletal muscle generates amino acids, which are converted either into pyruvate or DHAP.

Source: Adapted from ref. [39].

hepatocytes and renal tissue, with these sites accounting for 75% and 25% of glucose produced through gluconeogenesis, respectively [40, 41].

The first two steps of gluconeogenesis aim to convert pyruvate into phosphoenolpyruvate (PEP), with oxaloacetate being an intermediate product. These steps required ATP and carbon dioxide [42] (see Figure 4.3).

Once PEP is formed, a series of sequential enzymatic steps results in the formation of **fructose 1,6 bisphosphate**.

Fructose 1,6 bisphosphate is hydrolyzed into fructose 6-phosphate under the influence of the allosteric enzyme, fructose 1,6 bisphosphate.

Subsequently, fructose 6-phosphate then undergoes an isomerization step which produces glucose-6-phosphate mediated by phosphoglucose isomerase. The fate of glucose-6-phosphate varies significantly by the tissue in which it is formed. Unlike glucose, glucose-6-phosphate cannot permeate cellular membranes, thus making it an easily accessible substrate for further metabolic processes.

In **skeletal muscle,** for example, glucose-6-phosphate can be turned into either glycogen (a storage form of glucose) or pyruvate to be utilized in energy production (glycolysis) [40, 43].

Conversely, in **hepatocytes** and **renal cells,** glucose-6-phosphate is converted to glucose in the presence of the enzyme glucose-6-phosphatase. Since cellular membranes contain glucose transporters, glucose can readily leave these primary sites of gluconeogenesis in order to be transported to other cells in the human body [44].

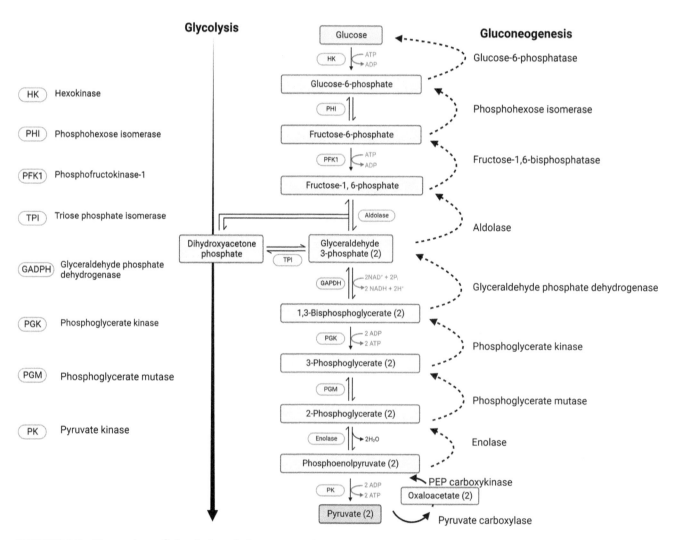

FIGURE 4.3   Comparison of glycolysis and gluconeogenesis.

Glycolysis

Glycolysis involves a sequence of reactions that ultimately changes glucose into two pyruvate molecules, two ATP, two NADH, and two water molecules [45]. See Figure 4.3.

Glucose is converted to glucose-6-phosphate via the enzyme hexokinase. The formation of glucose-6-phosphate destabilizes the glucose molecule and traps it inside the cell. Phosphoglucose isomerase then facilitates an isomerization step that converts glucose-6-phosphate to fructose-6-phosphate. Phosphofructokinase then promotes the phosphorylation of fructose-6-phosphate into fructose-1,6-bisphosphate. Sequential enzymatic steps ultimately result in the formation of pyruvate [45].

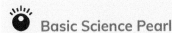

Basic Science Pearl

Glycolysis is the anaerobic metabolic breakdown of glucose into lactate and pyruvate.

Glycogenesis

Glycogenesis is the process of the formation of glycogen molecules (a storage form of glucose). After ingesting a meal rich in carbohydrates, plasma glucose levels rise. Pancreatic beta cells detect this increase in plasma glucose and, in turn, release insulin. Insulin then travels through the bloodstream to hepatocytes, binding to its corresponding IR and initiating a signal transduction pathway that activates various protein kinases in the cytoplasm [46].

These protein kinases inactivate glycogen synthase kinase (an enzyme that is responsible for the inactivation of glycogen synthase). Consequently, glycogen formation is promoted due to the loss of inhibition of the key regulatory enzyme, glycogen synthase [47]. See Figure 4.4.

Upon insulin binding to its receptor, a signaling cascade is initiated, involving the activation of insulin receptor substrate (IRS) and phosphatidylinositol 3-kinase (PI3K). This leads to the activation of Akt (protein kinase B), which inhibits glycogen synthase

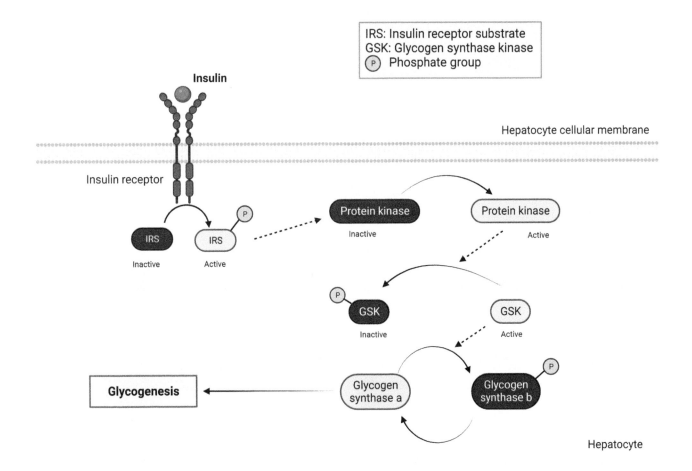

FIGURE 4.4   Insulin-mediated glycogen synthesis.

kinase-3 (GSK-3). The inhibition of GSK-3 promotes the conversion of inactive glycogen synthase b to its active form, glycogen synthase a, facilitating glycogen synthesis and storage [48]. Glycogen synthase ultimately catalyzes the elongation of glycogen by sequentially attaching glucose monomers via alpha 1,4 glycosidic bonds [32].

Glycogenolysis

Glycogen breakdown or degradation (glycogenolysis) involves various enzymes, which result in the liberation of glucose from the glycogen molecule [49]. There is an initial phosphorolysis step that requires glycogen phosphorylase. This is followed by a glycogen remodeling step which requires a transferase and alpha 1,6-glucosidase enzymes. This remodeled glycogen molecule then releases glucose which is transformed by the hexokinase enzyme into **glucose-1-phosphate**. Glucose 1 phosphate is then acted upon by phosphoglucomutase in order to change it into **glucose-6-phosphate**.

As was previously discussed, the fate of glucose-6-phosphate is dependent on its location. In skeletal muscle, it will be utilized in glycolysis and energy (ATP) production. However, in hepatocytes, **glucose-6-phosphate** will be converted into glucose which is subsequently released into the systemic circulation [50].

Glycogen degradation and **glycogen synthesis** do not occur simultaneously in normal physiology. Indeed, cells have a unique mechanism that regulates both metabolic processes reciprocally [51].

The role of insulin in the fed state in promoting glycogen synthesis was described earlier. Glucagon, on the other hand, is required for glycogen degradation.

Glucagon binds to the glucagon receptor and initiates a cascade of downstream processes, which results in the formation of cyclic AMP (a second messenger) that binds to regulatory sites on Protein Kinase A. Activated PKA ultimately inhibits glycogen synthase (involved in glycogenesis), while conversely activating glycogen phosphorylase (involved in glycogenolysis) [5, 50].

4.1.2.2   Mechanism of Action

Metformin, a biguanide, exerts its pharmacotherapeutic effects at various sites involved in the pathogenesis of type 2 diabetes mellitus.

- Decreases hepatic gluconeogenesis [52].
- Improves glucose uptake in skeletal muscle and adipose tissue [53].

TABLE 4.6   Mechanisms and sites of action of metformin.

Site of action	Cellular effects	Glycemic outcome
Mitochondria (hepatocyte)	Inhibits complex I of the ETC, which reduces ATP production (increased ADP: ATP and AMP: ATP ratios). A deficit in cellular ATP is detected by the "*cellular energy sensor*" AMPK. AMPK then promotes catabolic processes[A], which generate ATP and inhibits anabolic processes[β] that consume ATP.	Reduced hepatic glucose output.
Cytoplasm (hepatocyte)	Inhibition of fructose 1,6 bisphosphatase (gluconeogenic enzyme) by the high AMP: ATP ratio (AMPK-independent pathway).	Reduced hepatic glucose output.
Gastrointestinal tract (colonic enterocyte)	Increases anaerobic glucose metabolism in enterocytes.	
Skeletal muscle	Glucose uptake by glucose transporters (GLUT-4).	

Catabolic processes[A]: Glycolysis and oxidation of fatty acids.
Anabolic processes[β]: Fatty acid synthesis, glycogen synthesis, protein synthesis, gluconeogenesis.
Source: Adapted from refs. [55, 56].

- Improves insulin sensitivity by enhancing intracellular IRS signaling pathways [54].

Refer to Table 4.6 for a summary of proposed mechanisms of action of metformin in type 2 diabetes mellitus.

Practice Pearl(s)

Metformin is a synthetic derivative of natural guanidine isolated from the French lilac plant (*Galega officinalis*) [57, 58]. Interestingly, this plant was used in medieval Europe for the treatment of an ailment characterized by "sweet tasting urine" – now known as diabetes mellitus.

The recommended starting dose is 500 mg daily, which can be slowly titrated upwards in increments of 500 mg per week to a typical maintenance dose of 1000 mg twice daily [59].

Metformin is associated with significant gastrointestinal discomfort and diarrhea, which is mitigated by a slow up-titration in dose at the time of medication initiation.

Due to the risk of *metformin-associated lactic acidosis* (MALA), the dose of metformin should be adjusted in patients with chronic kidney disease [60] (see Table 4.7).

TABLE 4.7   Adjustment of metformin dose in chronic kidney disease.

Estimated GFR	Dose adjustment
> 60 mL per minute per body surface area	None, monitor renal function annually
>45–<60 mL per minute per body surface area	None, monitor renal function every three to six months
30–45 mL per minute per body surface area	Reduce to 500 mg per day. Do not initiate metformin in treatment-naïve patients
<30 mL per minute per body surface area	Contraindicated

Source: Adapted from ref. [61].

Clinical Trial Evidence

In the multicenter **Metformin Study Group (MSG) trial**, the efficacy of metformin in patients with non-insulin-dependent diabetes mellitus was evaluated [62].

Inclusion Criteria of the MSG Trial

- Fasting plasma glucose >140 mg/dL
- Age of 40–70 years
- Body weight of 120–170% of ideal body weight

TABLE 4.8   The metformin study group outcomes.

Study protocol	Intervention	Outcome
I	Metformin (n = 143) or placebo (n = 146)	FPG concentration decreased by 52 ± 5 mg per deciliter (2.9 ± 0.3 mmol per liter) in the metformin arm and increased by 6 ± 5 mg per deciliter (0.3 ± 0.3 mmol per liter) in the placebo group (P < 0.001).
II	Metformin (n = 210), glyburide (n = 209) or metformin + glyburide (n = 213)	FPG decreased by 63 ± 5 mg per deciliter (3.5 ± 0.3 mmol per liter) in the combination-therapy group, increased by 14 ± 4 mg per deciliter (0.8 ± 0.2 mmol per liter) in the glyburide-only group decreased by 1 ± 5 mg per deciliter (0.1 ± 0.3 mmol per liter) in the metformin group, (P < 0.001 for the comparison of combination therapy with glyburide).

Fasting Plasma Glucose (FPG).
Source: Adapted from ref. [62].

A summary of the study outcomes is shown in Table 4.8.

4.1.3   Meglitinides

4.1.3.1   Physiology

Phases of Insulin Release After a Meal

Insulin acts to lower high blood glucose levels by simultaneously promoting the uptake of glucose into cells and inhibiting the liver's production of glucose. Insulin release is a complex process that occurs in a biphasic manner (two distinct phases), known as the first and second phases of insulin release [63].

First Phase of Insulin Release: The first phase of insulin release occurs within minutes of a meal and is a rapid, short-lived response (lasting approximately 10 minutes) to an increase in arterial glucose concentration [64]. The rapid release of preformed secretory granules of insulin accounts for this phase. This initial surge of insulin is thought to be triggered by the stimulation of the beta cells in the pancreas by glucose and other nutrients in the meal. The first phase of insulin release helps to quickly lower blood glucose levels by promoting the uptake of glucose into cells while inhibiting hepatic glucose production [65].

Second Phase of Insulin Release: The second phase of insulin release occurs several minutes to several hours after the first phase and is a slower, sustained response to elevated blood glucose levels [3]. This phase of insulin release is thought to be regulated by the release of other hormones, such as incretins, that are produced in response to a meal. The second phase of insulin release helps to maintain stable blood glucose levels for several hours after a meal by promoting the uptake of glucose into cells and inhibiting the liver's production of glucose [3, 66].

Various circulating factors, including glucose, incretins, amino acids, ketone bodies, lactic acid, and fatty acids, facilitate the release of insulin by pancreatic beta cells. Furthermore, glucose-induced insulin release plays a predominant role in determining the concentration of extracellular insulin in both the fasting and postprandial state. Glucose enters pancreatic beta cells through the active glucose transporter 2 (GLUT-2) transporter (see Figure 4.5). Glucokinase then catalyzes the metabolism of glucose into glucose-6-phosphate, which then results in the generation of intracellular ATP through the process of glycolysis. NADH and $FADH_2$ produced from glycolysis are further incorporated into the mitochondrial electron transport chain to augment intracellular ATP levels [67]. Consequently, the high ATP to ADP ratio in the pancreatic beta cell inhibits the ATP-sensitive potassium (KATP) channels in the plasma membrane [68]. This results in the depolarization of the plasma membrane, the opening of voltage-gated calcium channels, and the influx of calcium via the L-type voltage-gated calcium channels [69, 70]. A rise in intracellular calcium then facilitates the fusion of insulin secretory granules with the pancreatic plasma membrane. Finally, insulin, c peptide, proinsulin, and other secretory products are released through the process of exocytosis [3].

GLUT-2 channels ferry glucose into the pancreatic beta cell (see Figure 4.5). This is followed by the phosphorylation of glucose into glucose-6-phosphate by glucokinase. ATP generated as a consequence of glycolysis blocks potassium channels on pancreatic cell membranes, consequently depolarizing the cell membrane. Depolarization of the pancreatic beta-cell membrane activates pancreatic L-type voltage-gated calcium channels, which funnels calcium into the pancreatic beta cell. Increased intracellular calcium leads to the liberation of endocytic stores of insulin into systemic circulation [71].

Additionally, fatty acids are an alternative insulin secretagogue. Fatty acids undergo beta-oxidation and oxidative phosphorylation in pancreatic beta cells. ATP produced as a consequence then inhibits the ATP-dependent or sensitive potassium channels, which results in the eventual release of insulin via exocytosis (previously described as glucose-mediated insulin release) [72]. Furthermore fatty acids in the gut stimulate the release of incretins. Incretins then augment the release of insulin by pancreatic beta cells [66] (see Section 4.1.7).

4.1.3.2   Mechanism of Action

Meglitinides stimulate early-phase insulin release by blocking the ATP-dependent potassium channels (KATP) of the pancreatic beta cell directly [73]. This occurs independent of the intracellular ATP to ADP ratio (see Figure 4.5). Inhibition of the potassium channels results in the depolarization of the cell membrane, the opening of voltage-gated calcium channels, an influx of calcium, and finally, the exocytosis of insulin-laden granules [74].

Refer to Table 4.9 for a summary of the pharmacokinetic profile of meglitinides.

Practice Pearl(s)

1. Repaglinide (Prandin) is administered orally, between 0.5 and 4 mg twice to three times a day (maximum daily dose of 16 mg). It should be taken about half an hour to an anticipated meal. Patients should be advised to skip a scheduled dose of repaglinide if a meal is skipped due to the risk of hypoglycemia. The time to its onset of action is about 30 minutes, with a duration of action of 4–6 hours [76]. One of the advantages of repaglinide is that it has a quick onset and offset of action, which makes it effective in controlling post-meal glucose spikes [77].

2. Being an insulin secretagogue, repaglinide, like sulfonylureas, is associated with weight gain. Other side effects include rhinosinusitis, diarrhea, and joint pain [78].

3. Repaglinide is excreted primarily through the biliary system, making it a suitable alternative to metformin and sulfonylureas in patients with **chronic kidney disease** [77].

4. Repaglinide is contraindicated in patients taking clopidogrel or gemfibrozil [79].

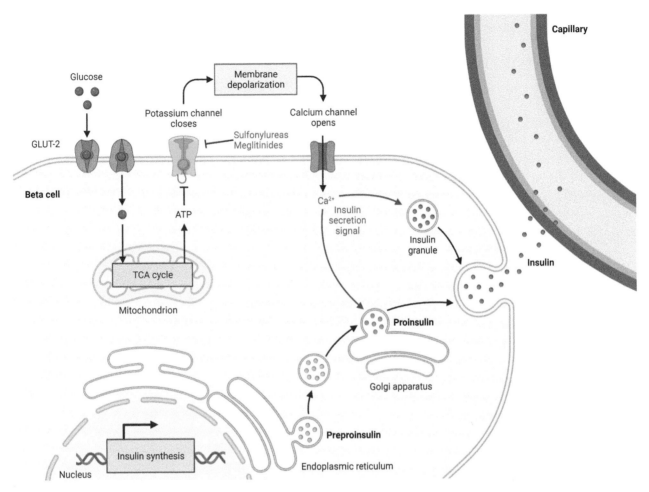

FIGURE 4.5 Schematic representation of insulin release from the pancreatic beta cell.

TABLE 4.9 Pharmacokinetic profile of meglitinides.

Pharmacokinetic factor	Repaglinide	Nateglinide
Absorption	Peak plasma concentration 30–60 min after oral administration.	Peak plasma concentration within 1 hour after oral administration.
Distribution	98% is bound to plasma albumin.	98% is bound to plasma albumin.
Metabolism and elimination	Metabolized by hepatic CYP450(CYP3A4) and eliminated through the biliary system (90% biliary tract, 8% renal system, 2% unchanged) [74].	Metabolized by hepatic CYP450 (CYP3A4). It is eliminated primarily by the renal system (85% renal, 15% unchanged) [75].

CYP450, Cytochrome P450.
Source: Adapted from refs. [74, 75].

Clinical Trial Evidence

The efficacy of repaglinide in the treatment of type 2 diabetes mellitus, either as monotherapy or add-on therapy, has been evaluated in various clinical trials.

Table 4.10 summarizes selected clinical trials evaluating the efficacy of meglitinide therapy in type 2 diabetes mellitus.

(continued)

(*continued*)

TABLE 4.10   Clinical trials evaluating the efficacy of repaglinide in type 2 diabetes mellitus.

Study	Population	Intervention	Outcome
Comparison with sulfonylureas [80]	T2DM with no known ASCVD (n = 124)	Repaglinide (RPG) 1 mg per day (n = 62) or glimepiride (GMP) 1 mg per day (n = 62). The dose was optimized over a 2-month titration period. 12-month study.	Change in HbA1c from baseline was −1.2 (95% CI 6.2 to −0.48), P < 0.01 in the RPG arm. Change in HbA1C from baseline was-1.1 (95% CI −5.6 to −0.54) in the GMP arm. Change in PPG from baseline was −46 (95% CI −64 to −12) in the RPG arm; −21 (95% CI −48 to −13) in the GMP arm, P < 0.05 comparing RPG to GMP.
Comparison with metformin [81]	T2DM, treatment naïve, diet managed with an HbA1C > 7%. No known ASCVD (n = 112)	RPG 1 mg per day (n = 56) or metformin 1000 mg per day(n = 56). The dose was optimized over a 2-month titration period. 12-month study.	There was no statistically significant difference between the RPG and MET arms when mean changes in HbA1c and FPG were compared. The reduction in PPG was greater in the RPG compared to the MET group (P < 0.05).
Comparison with pioglitazone [82]	T2DM, treatment-experienced with HbA1C 7.0–12%, BMI <45 kg/m² (n = 246)	Randomized to RPG (n = 61), PGZ (n = 62), or a combination of both (n = 123).	The combination therapy of repaglinide and pioglitazone was more effective in improving glycemic parameters than either drug alone. The mean reduction in HbA(1c) was −1.76% for the combination therapy, compared to −0.18% for repaglinide alone and an increase of +0.32% for pioglitazone alone.

PPG, Postprandial glucose; HbA1C, glycated hemoglobin A1C; FPG, fasting plasma glucose; RPG, repaglinide; PGZ, pioglitazone; MET, metformin.
Source: Adapted from refs. [80–82].

4.1.4   Sulfonylureas

4.1.4.1   Physiology

The physiology of insulin release was reviewed in Section 4.1.3.

4.1.4.2   Mechanism of Action

The KATP channel typically regulates insulin secretion in response to changes in glucose levels. When plasma glucose levels are low, the KATP channel is open, which hyperpolarizes the beta-cell membrane and reduces insulin secretion [83]. See Figure 4.5.

When glucose levels in the blood increase, glucose enters the beta cells of the pancreas and is metabolized to produce ATP. The increase in intracellular ATP levels leads to the closure of the KATP channel, which in turn depolarizes the cell membrane and leads to an influx of calcium ions through voltage-gated calcium channels. The rise in intracellular calcium concentration stimulates the exocytosis of insulin granules, which releases insulin into the bloodstream [84].

Sulfonylureas work by binding to and inhibiting the function of the SUR1 subunit of the KATP channels, which are predominantly expressed in pancreatic beta cells. It is worth noting that the SUR1 subunit is one of two subunits that make up the KATP channel, the other being the Kir6.2 subunit [85].

By inhibiting the KATP channel, sulfonylureas prevent it from opening and hyperpolarizing the cell membrane in response to decreases in glucose levels. This maintains membrane depolarization and the influx of calcium ions, leading to increased insulin secretion [86].

In addition to inhibiting the KATP channel, sulfonylureas may also enhance insulin release by increasing the sensitivity of beta cells to glucose. This may involve activating intracellular signaling pathways that promote insulin secretion or increasing the expression of other proteins involved in insulin exocytosis [87, 88].

The different sulfonylurea drugs vary in their binding affinity for the SUR1 subunit and in their duration of action. For example, glyburide and glimepiride have a higher binding affinity for SUR1 and a longer duration of action than tolbutamide and glipizide, which have lower binding affinities and shorter durations of action [89].

Practice Pearl(s)

Glipizide is metabolized by the liver into several inactive metabolites, which means that its clearance and elimination half-life remain unaffected despite any reduction in the estimated glomerular filtration rate (GFR). It is considered the sulfonylurea of choice for this patient population [90].

Both glibenclamide and glyburide are metabolized by the liver but are eliminated equally through bile and urine. However, in individuals with an estimated GFR of less than 60 mL/min, the use of these drugs is contraindicated [91, 92].

Glimepiride undergoes hepatic metabolism, resulting in two main metabolites, one of which has hypoglycemic activity [93]. In CKD, the metabolites may accumulate, and the drug is contraindicated in individuals with an estimated GFR of less than 60 mL/min. Compared to glyburide, glimepiride causes less hypoglycemia [90].

Gliclazide is metabolized into inactive metabolites, which are primarily eliminated through urine (80%). This drug presents a lower risk of hypoglycemia than glibenclamide and glimepiride [94].

Table 4.11 summarizes the pharmacokinetic profile of selected sulfonylureas.

Sulfonylureas carry an increased risk for hypoglycemia (especially among the elderly and people living with chronic kidney disease), weight gain, and progressive pancreatic beta-cell exhaustion.

Also, there may be cardiovascular safety concerns with sulfonylureas; therefore, they should be used cautiously among this population of patients. The DIGAMI trial (Diabetes Mellitus, Insulin Glucose Infusion in Acute Myocardial Infarction) was an iconic clinical trial conducted during the 90s that assessed intensive glucose regulation using insulin therapy on type 2 diabetic patients who had experienced an acute myocardial infarction (AMI). Trial participants included 620 patients with type 2 diabetes who had experienced an AMI. They were randomly assigned to either an intensive insulin treatment group or conventional treatment group, with intensive insulin treatment proving less successful with regards to cardiovascular outcomes than conventional therapy [98]. Interestingly, the SUR2 subtype of the KATP is present in cardiomyocytes. Impaired coronary vasodilation due to interference with potassium conductance predisposes ischemic cardiomyocytes to arrhythmia [99].

The cardiovascular safety of sulfonylureas, a class of medications commonly used to treat type 2 diabetes, has been a topic of interest and investigation in recent years. While early studies suggested that sulfonylureas may be associated with an increased risk of cardiovascular events, more recent evidence suggests that the cardiovascular safety of these medications may be comparable to other commonly used diabetes medications.

CAROLINA (Cardiovascular Outcome Study of Linagliptin vs. Glimepiride in Patients with Type 2 Diabetes) was a randomized, controlled trial designed to directly compare cardiovascular safety and efficacy of

---

TABLE 4.11 Pharmacokinetic profile of sulfonylureas.

Drug name (Trade name)	Dose range	Maximum daily dose	Frequency	Onset of action	Duration of action
Glimepiride (Amaryl)	1–2 mg daily	8 mg	Once or twice daily	2–3 h	24 h
Glipizide (Glucotrol)	2.5–5 mg daily	20 mg	Once daily	1–3 h	12–24 h
Glipizide (Glucotrol XL)	20 mg daily	20 mg	Daily	6–12 h	12–24 h
Glyburide (Glynase)	1.25–5 mg daily	20 mg	Once or twice daily	2–4 h	≤24 h
Glyburide, micronized (Glynase)	0.75–3 mg daily	12 mg	Once or twice daily	2–4 h	≤24 h

Source: Adapted from refs. [95–97].

both linagliptin and glimepiride among 6033 participants with type 2 diabetes and high cardiovascular risk. The primary endpoint was defined as cardiovascular death, nonfatal myocardial infarction, and stroke rates among all subjects randomly allocated. Results of CAROLINA showed that both treatments were noninferior in terms of cardiovascular outcomes among both groups, with similar rates being achieved for their primary endpoint outcomes among both groups (the results showed similarity of rates among both groups) [100].

Clinical Trial Evidence

Metformin has historically been the first-line drug for the treatment of type 2 diabetes mellitus. However, the choice of add-on therapy to metformin for patients with uncontrolled diabetes has been based on expert opinion. The GRADE (Glycemia Reduction in Type 2 Diabetes – Glycemic Outcomes) study evaluated the efficacy of various add-on therapies to metformin (see Table 4.12).

TABLE 4.12 Summary of the GRADE study.

Study	Population	Intervention	Outcome
GRADE	Type 2 diabetes mellitus, duration of diabetes <10 years, HbA1c 6.8–8.5% on metformin monotherapy.	Patients were assigned to four groups, glimepiride, liraglutide, sitagliptin, or glargine insulin ($n = 5047$).	The primary outcome of an estimated HbA1c >7.5% differed significantly across all groups ($P < 0.001$). The rate of the primary outcome was 26.5 per 100 participant years for glargine and 26.1 for liraglutide, which was similar but lower than those with glimepiride (30.4) and sitagliptin (38.1). Glimepiride was associated with the highest risk for hypoglycemia.

GRADE, Glycemia Reduction in Type 2 Diabetes – Glycemic Outcomes.
Source: Adapted from ref. [101].

4.1.5 Dopaminergic Agonists

4.1.5.1 Physiology

There are dopaminergic receptors in various tissues, including central and peripheral sites. Dopaminergic receptors exist in the basal ganglia, frontal cortex, anterior pituitary gland, kidneys, pancreas, and vascular system [102].

Under physiologic conditions, increased sympathetic tone promotes hyperglycemia, lipolysis (which increases free fatty acids), and an increased appetite. Dopamine activates central dopamine type 2 receptors (D2R), reducing noradrenaline secretion (sympatholytic effect), which, consequently, has favorable effects on glucose homeostasis [103].

Also, the activation of dopaminergic receptors on islet cells of the pancreas inhibits insulin secretion [104].

4.1.5.2 Mechanism of Action

Bromocriptine, a **sympatholytic D2-dopamine agonist**, exerts its hypoglycemic effects through two proposed mechanisms.

1. **Inhibition of excessive sympathetic tone within the CNS:** Bromocriptine inhibits sympathetic tone within the CNS, reducing post-meal plasma glucose levels due to the inhibition of hepatic glucose production [105].
2. **Reduction of plasma glucose, triglyceride, and FFA levels:** Bromocriptine reduces plasma glucose, triglyceride, and FFA levels due to its ability to reduce insulin secretion [105, 106].

Practice Pearl(s)

Bromocriptine in a quick-release (QR) formulation is approved by the US Food and Drug Administration (FDA) as an adjunct to diet and exercise in patients with type 2 diabetes mellitus. The quick-release formulation (cycloset®) has a different pharmacokinetic profile from the more conventional bromocriptine (parlodel®) used to treat hyperprolactinemia. Bromocriptine QR has a high bioavailability, approximately 95%, reaching a peak plasma concentration within an hour after oral administration [107].

The starting dose of bromocriptine QR is 0.8 mg daily which can be slowly uptitrated to a maximum total daily dose of 4.8 mg. It should ideally be dosed within two hours of awakening. This is because patients with type 2 diabetes have a low level of central dopaminergic activity in the morning, which increases central sympathetic tone and promotes hyperglycemia (*refer to the physiology of dopamine in glucose regulation*) [106].

Clinical Trial Evidence

In the Cycloset Safety Trial, 3095 patients with type 2 diabetes were randomly assigned to either quick-release bromocriptine or placebo in a ratio of 2:1. The study found that 8.6% of patients in the bromocriptine-QR group reported serious adverse events, while 9.6% of patients in the placebo group reported similar adverse events (HR 1.02 [96% one-sided CI 1.27]).

Furthermore, the frequency of cardiovascular disease (CVD) endpoint in the bromocriptine-QR group was 1.8%, compared to 3.2% in the placebo group (HR 0.60 [95% CI 0.35–0.96]). This suggests that the use of bromocriptine-QR may have a beneficial effect on cardiovascular outcomes in patients with type 2 diabetes, with the most commonly reported adverse event in the bromocriptine-QR group being nausea [108].

4.1.6 PPAR-Gamma Agonists

4.1.6.1 Physiology

Peroxisome proliferator-activated receptors (PPARs) are transcription factors belonging to the nuclear receptor superfamily. This large superfamily of nuclear hormone receptors includes the *thyroid hormone receptor, steroid hormone receptors, vitamin D3 receptor (VDR), retinoid acid receptor (RAR)*, and *PPARs*. The three isoforms of the PPARs (α, δ, and γ) act on various DNA response elements present on the nuclear retinoic acid receptor [109].

For example, PPAR-α transcription factors are found in the kidney, cardiomyocytes, intestinal

TABLE 4.13   Physiologic effects of PPAR activation.

PPAR subtype	Physiologic effects
PPARα	Stimulates beta-oxidation of fatty acids (lipid catabolism). Controls vascular integrity.
PPARδ	Increases glucose uptake and glycogenesis in skeletal muscle.
PPARγ	Increases fatty acid oxidation in skeletal muscle, liver, and adipose tissue. Augments insulin-stimulated glucose uptake by adipocytes, skeletal muscles, and hepatocytes. Increases HDL cholesterol and reduced triglycerides.

Source: Adapted from ref. [111].

mucosa, and brown adipose tissue. Activation of the PPAR alpha receptor modulates fatty acid metabolism, leading to the lowering of lipid levels. PPAR-δ is found throughout the body and can also promote fatty acid oxidation and lipid uptake when activated. Finally, PPAR-γ is found in adipose tissue(both white and brown), intestines, and immune cells. Its activation stimulates adipocyte differentiation and triglyceride storage [110] (see Table 4.13).

The mechanism of gene transcription by PPARs involves the formation of PPAR-RXR (Retinoid X Receptor) heterodimers. This step involves PPARs binding to specific ligands, such as fatty acids, which induce a conformational change in the PPAR protein, allowing it to form a heterodimer with RXR [112].

Once the PPAR-RXR heterodimer is recruited to the promoter region, it binds to specific DNA sequences called peroxisome proliferator response elements (PPREs) located upstream of the target gene. The PPAR-RXR heterodimer interacts with other transcription factors and coactivators to initiate the transcription of the target gene. Additionally, PPAR-RXR heterodimers can compete with other transcription factors for binding to identical DNA sequences and inhibit the expression of specific genes [113].

It is important to note that the regulation of gene transcription by PPAR-RXR heterodimers plays a critical role in regulating metabolic pathways and other biological processes. The transcription of the target gene is completed with pre-mRNA formation and subsequent mRNA processing, leading to the production of functional proteins involved in metabolism.

4.1.6.2 Mechanism of Action

Pioglitazone binds to PPARs found in adipose tissue, liver, and skeletal muscle. PPARs are crucial in controlling glucose and lipid metabolism by regulating the transcription of genes involved in glucose utilization, fat storage, and insulin sensitivity [114].

Pioglitazone improves insulin sensitivity by increasing glucose uptake and utilization in adipose tissue, skeletal muscle, and liver tissue – ultimately leading to better glycemic control as more glucose enters cells for energy use [115]. Furthermore, pioglitazone decreases the hepatic gluconeogenesis rate, reducing the incidence of fasting hyperglycemia [114].

Also, pioglitazone can increase insulin sensitivity by encouraging preadipocyte differentiation and proliferation, which in turn increases adipose tissue mass. This adipose tissue repository is critical for storing glucose and fat and improving insulin sensitivity [116].

Practice Pearl(s)

Pioglitazone improves insulin resistance, maintains the function of beta cells of the pancreas in patients with type 2 diabetes mellitus, improves lipid profile, and reverses steatosis in patients with nonalcoholic fatty liver disease [117].

A review of the mechanism of pioglitazone-mediated side effects is shown in Table 4.14.

TABLE 4.14   Mechanism of cardinal side effects associated with pioglitazone.

Side effect	Mechanism
Weight gain	Stimulates PPAR gamma receptors in adipocytes which induces adipogenesis [118].
Fluid retention	Promotes peripheral vasodilation and enhances renal sodium conservation [119].
Fragility fractures	Unclear.
Bladder cancer	Unclear.

Source: Adapted from refs. [118, 119].

Clinical Trial Evidence

The cardiovascular safety of pioglitazone is shown in Table 4.15.

TABLE 4.15   Studies evaluating the cardiovascular safety of pioglitazone.

Study	Population	Intervention	Outcome
IRIS	Recent ischemic stroke or TIA with insulin resistance (n = 3676).	Pioglitazone to a target dose of 45 mg/d (n = 1939) or placebo (n = 1937).	Primary outcome of fatal or nonfatal stroke or MI was 9.0% in the pioglitazone arm and 11.8% in the placebo arm, HR 0.76 (95% CI of 0.62–0.93, P = 0.007) [120].
PROactive Study	Recent macrovascular disease and T2DM (n = 5238).	Pioglitazone titrated to 45 mg/d (n = 2605) or matching placebo (n = 2633).	The secondary endpoint of all-cause mortality, nonfatal MI, and stroke was 301 patients in the pioglitazone arm and 358 patients in the placebo arm, HR 0.84 (95% CI of 0.72–0.98, P = 0.027) [121].

IRIS, Insulin Resistance Intervention after Stroke; MI, myocardial infarction; PROactive, PROspective pioglitAzone Clinical Trial In macroVascular Events; T2DM, Type 2 diabetes mellitus.
Source: Adapted from refs. [120, 121].

4.1.7 GLP-1 Agonists

4.1.7.1 Physiology

What Is the Incretin Effect

Incretins are gut-derived hormones that are secreted in response to food intake. Two essential incretin hormones are *glucagon-like peptide-1 (GLP-1)* and *glucose-dependent insulinotropic polypeptide (GIP)* [122], which are produced by selective post-translational modification of proglucagon, a 160-residue peptide expressed by the α-cells of the pancreas, K and L cells of the small intestine. K cells from the upper intestine are responsible for the production of GIP, while L cells of the lower intestine produce GLP-1 [123].

The effects of these hormones on glucose metabolism are mediated through their interactions with specific G protein-coupled receptors (GPCRs) present on pancreatic beta cells. The activation of GPCRs by incretin hormones initiates intracellular cyclic AMP formation and the eventual activation of protein kinase A. Protein kinase A is then involved in promoting various sequential intracellular processes, which result in augmented insulin secretion by the beta cells of the pancreas [124].

The *"incretin effect"* is described as enhanced insulin secretion in response to an oral glucose load (two to threefold increase in insulin release) compared with intravenous glucose administration [123].

Effects of Incretins on Metabolism

GLP-1 and GIP stimulate insulin secretion from pancreatic beta cells in a glucose-dependent manner, which means they increase insulin secretion in response to an elevation in plasma glucose. This glucose-dependent insulinotropic effect of incretins helps to maintain glucose homeostasis, especially in the postabsorptive period.

In addition to their insulinotropic effects, incretins also inhibit glucagon secretion from pancreatic alpha cells, which helps to reduce hepatic glucose production.

Furthermore, GLP-1 and GIP promote beta-cell growth and survival. These effects of incretins on beta cells are significant in the context of type 2 diabetes, where there is impaired beta-cell function [125].

Incretins also have extrapancreatic effects that contribute to their glucose-lowering effects. For example, GLP-1 and GIP can slow gastric emptying, which helps reduce the nutrient absorption rate and improve glycemic control. They can also promote early satiety, contributing to weight loss and improved glycemic control [125, 126].

In summary, incretins play a critical role in glucose metabolism by stimulating insulin secretion, inhibiting glucagon secretion, promoting beta-cell function and survival, and reducing appetite and food intake.

4.1.7.2 Mechanism of Action

GLP-1 receptor agonists, such as semaglutide and liraglutide, and dipeptidyl peptidase-4 (DPP-4) inhibitors, such as sitagliptin and saxagliptin (see Section 4.1.9), are two classes of drugs that are commonly used in clinical practice (see Figure 4.6).

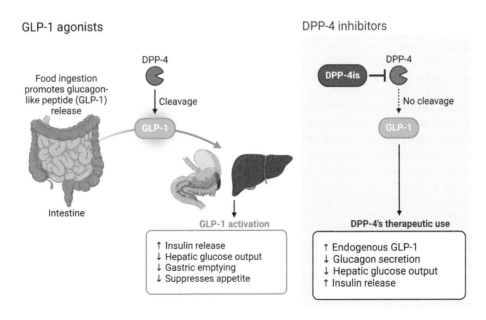

FIGURE 4.6 Mechanism of action of incretin mimetics.

GLP-1 receptor agonists mimic the effects of GLP-1 by activating the GLP-1 receptor, whereas DPP-4 inhibitors increase the half-life of endogenous GLP-1 by inhibiting its degradation. Both of these drug classes can improve glycemic control and have additional benefits, such as weight loss and cardiovascular risk reduction [127].

Practice Pearl(s)

Here is a detailed summary of the starting and titrating doses of GLP-1 agonists:

- Victoza (liraglutide): The initial dose of Victoza is 0.6 mg subcutaneously once daily, which can be titrated up to 1.2 mg subcutaneously once daily after a week. If further glycemic control is necessary, the dose can be increased to 1.8 mg subcutaneously once daily [128].
- Semaglutide (Ozempic): The initial dose of Semaglutide is 0.25 mg subcutaneously once weekly for the first month, followed by an increase to 0.5 mg subcutaneously once weekly. If additional glycemic control is needed, the dose can be increased to 1 mg and eventually 2 mg (maximum dose for diabetes treatment) subcutaneously once weekly [129].
- Bydureon (exenatide extended-release): Bydureon is administered in a fixed 2 mg subcutaneous dose once weekly [130].
- Byetta (exenatide immediate-release): The initial dose of Byetta is 5 mcg subcutaneously twice daily, and it can be titrated up to 10 mcg subcutaneously twice daily after one month [131].

- Rybelsus (semaglutide oral): The starting dose of Rybelsus is 3 mg once daily for the first month, followed by an increase to 7 mg once daily for the next two months. If additional glycemic control is needed, the dose can be increased to 14 mg orally once daily [132].
- Trulicity (dulaglutide): The initial dose of Mounjaro is 0.75 mg subcutaneously once weekly, and it can be titrated up to 1.5 mg subcutaneously once weekly after four weeks if necessary. Additional doses include 3 mg and 4.5 mg once weekly [133].
- Mounjaro (tirzepatide): A starting dose of 5 mg subcutaneously once weekly, followed by a weekly titration up to 15 mg or 20 mg, depending on the patient's response and tolerability [134].

Patients should be closely monitored during treatment for adverse effects, such as gastrointestinal side effects, hypoglycemia, and injection site reactions. Additionally, GLP-1 agonists should be cautiously administered in patients with a history of pancreatitis or thyroid C-cell tumors, as these medications may increase the risk of these conditions.

Clinical Trial Evidence

Cardiovascular Outcome Trials (CVOTs) for diabetes are clinical trials designed to assess the cardiovascular safety of medications used for treating this condition. Their purpose is to establish whether any particular drug increases risk factors like myocardial infarction, stroke, or cardiovascular death [135].

Since 2008, the US Food and Drug Administration (FDA) has mandated that new medications for treating diabetes undergo cardiovascular risk assessment trials before being approved for use [136]. The requirement was issued due to concerns that certain diabetes medications could increase cardiovascular event risks, according to studies and observations [137]. These trials have led to important shifts in the treatment of diabetes, with greater focus placed on cardiovascular risk reduction beyond the previous management goal of controlling blood glucose levels [138].

CVOTs are large-scale randomized, double-blind, placebo-controlled trials conducted to assess cardiovascular outcomes in type 2 diabetes patients with established disease or high cardiovascular risk [139]. They usually last several years and seek to demonstrate whether an investigational drug is non-inferior to placebo in terms of cardiovascular safety or provides additional cardiovascular benefits that go beyond controlling glycemia [140] (see Table 4.16).

TABLE 4.16 Summary of landmark CVOTs for incretin mimetics.

Study	Population	Intervention	Outcome
LEADER	Patients with T2DM and HbA1c >7% and at least one CV condition[a] (n = 9340).	Liraglutide titrated to 1.8 mg daily or the maximum tolerated dose (n = 4668) vs matching placebo (n = 4672).	Primary composite outcome of death from CV causes, nonfatal MI or nonfatal stroke occurred in fewer patients in the liraglutide arm 13% than in the placebo arm 14.9% HR, 0.87; 95% CI, 0.78–0.97; $P < 0.001$ for noninferiority; $P = 0.01$ for superiority [128].
SUSTAIN-6	Patients with T2DM and HbA1c >7% and at least one CV conditio[‡] (n = 3297).	Semaglutide 0.5 mg weekly (n = 826), semaglutide 1 mg weekly (n = 822), matching placebo 0.5 mg (n = 824) or matching placebo (n = 825) assigned in a 1 : 1 : 1 : 1 ratio.	Primary composite outcome of death from CV causes, nonfatal MI or nonfatal stroke occurred in fewer patients in the semaglutide arm 6.6% than in the placebo arm 8.9% HR, 0.74; 95% CI, 0.58–0.95; $P < 0.001$ for noninferiority; $P = 0.02$ for superiority [141].
REWIND	Patients with T2DM and HbA1c ≤ 9.5% with either a previous cardiovascular event or cardiovascular risk factors (n = 9901).	Dulaglutide 1.5 mg weekly (n = 4949) or matching placebo (n = 4952).	Primary composite outcome of vascular death, nonfatal MI or nonfatal stroke occurred in fewer patients in the dulaglutide arm 12.0% than in the placebo arm 13.4% HR, 0.88; 95% CI, 0.79–0.99; $P = 0.026$ [133].
ELIXA	T2DM with recent MI or hospitalization for unstable angina within the previous 180 days (n = 6068).	Once daily SC lixisenatide 10 mcg daily (n = 3034) or matching placebo (n = 3034).	Composite primary outcome of CV death, nonfatal MI, nonfatal stroke or hospitalization for unstable angina occurred in 13.4% of patients in the lixisenatide arm and 13.2% in the placebo arm, HR 1.02 with 95% CI of 0.89–1.17; $P < 0.001$ for noninferiority and $P = 0.81$ for superiority[Δ] [142].
SURPASS-4	T2DM with established CV disease or at high risk for CV events (n = 3045).	Tirzepatide 5 mg weekly(n = 329), tirzepatide 10 mg weekly(n = 328), tirzepatide 15 mg weekly(n = 338), or glargine insulin (n = 1000) assigned in a 1 : 1 : 1 : 3 ratio.	Composite 4-point MACE occurred in 3% of patients in the tirzepatide arm and 4% of patients in the glargine arm, HR 0.74 with 95% CI of 0.51–1.08. Tirzepatide was not associated with an excess CV risk based on this study [143].

[a] CV, Conditions included coronary artery disease, cerebrovascular disease, peripheral vascular disease, chronic kidney disease III or more, chronic heart failure of New York Heart Association class II or III for those ≥50 years of age. For those ≥60 years of age: persistent microalbuminuria, left ventricular hypertrophy, left ventricular dysfunction (either systolic or diastolic), or an ankle brachial pressure index <0.9.
[b] Lixisenatide did not change the rates of CV outcomes in this study.
MACE (cardiovascular death, myocardial infarction, stroke, and hospitalization for unstable angina).
Source: Adapted from refs. [128, 133, 141–143].

CVOTs go beyond simply evaluating cardiovascular safety to also evaluate potential cardiovascular benefits from medications. For example, some CVOTs have shown that certain diabetes medications can reduce the risk of major cardiovascular events, such as empagliflozin and canagliflozin, which belong to the class of sodium-glucose cotransporter-2 (SGLT2) inhibitors [138].

Overall, CVOTs are an integral component of drug development processes for new diabetes medications and provide valuable information regarding the cardiovascular safety and efficacy of these treatments. Their role ensures patients with diabetes receive safe and effective care while also offering vital insights into the complex relationship between diabetes, cardiovascular disease, and drug therapy [135].

Pathophysiology Pearl

What are the mechanisms of the cardiovascular benefit of GLP-1 agonists

The major consequences of uncontrolled type 2 diabetes include deposition of atherosclerotic plaque, endothelial dysfunction, cardiac myocyte hypertrophy, and myocardial fibrosis – each having negative impacts on ventricular function as well as myocardial perfusion [144]. GLP-1 receptor agonists have demonstrated cardiovascular protection through reduced inflammation, improved left ventricular function, increased plaque stability, and amelioration of ischemic injury. Furthermore, these agents induce vasodilation and modify atherosclerotic processes while decreasing infarct size by increasing glucose uptake by myocardial cells [145].

4.1.8   SGLT-2 Inhibitors

4.1.8.1   Physiology

Plasma glucose is filtered through the glomerulus and reabsorbed in the proximal tubule through a complex process mediated by various transporters. Most glucose reabsorption in the proximal tubule is facilitated by the sodium-glucose cotransporter 2 (SGLT2) protein, primarily expressed in the apical membrane of the S1 and S2 segments the proximal tubule.

The sodium-glucose cotransporter 1 (SGLT1) protein reabsorbs the remaining glucose in the apical membrane of the S3 segment of the proximal tubule [146, 147]. The reabsorption of glucose and sodium is driven by the electrochemical potential gradient of sodium, which is maintained by the Na^+/K^+ pump in the basolateral membrane. The accumulated glucose in the epithelium is then transported into the blood through the GLUT2 protein located in the basolateral membrane [148]. See Figure 4.7.

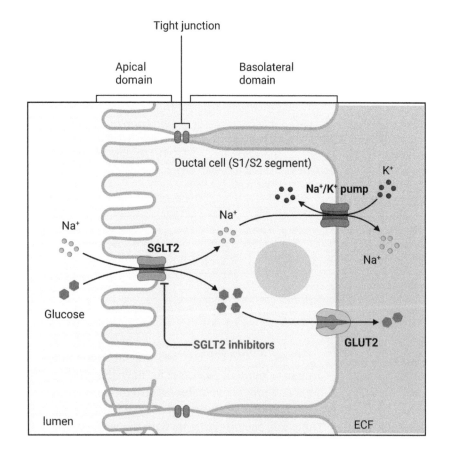
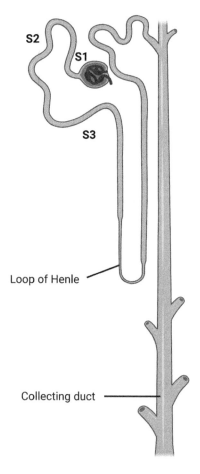

FIGURE 4.7   Mechanism of action of SGLT2 inhibitors.

4.1.8.2   Mechanism of Action

The mechanism of action of SGLT-2 inhibitors involves the inhibition of the SGLT-2 protein in the kidneys, which is primarily responsible for the reabsorption of glucose from the glomerular ultrafiltrate. SGLT-2 inhibitors block the function of SGLT-2, which leads to increased urinary glucose excretion and decreased blood glucose levels [149].

SGLT-2 inhibitors, such as dapagliflozin, canagliflozin, and empagliflozin, primarily inhibit glucose reabsorption in the S1 and S2 segments of the proximal tubule, where SGLT-2 is primarily expressed [150]. The S3 segment of the proximal tubule, where SGLT-1 is primarily expressed, is responsible for reabsorbing the remaining glucose from the glomerular filtrate. However, because SGLT-1 has a lower glucose transport capacity than SGLT-2, its inhibition by SGLT-2 inhibitors is considered clinically insignificant [146].

Overall, the inhibition of SGLT-2 by these medications reduces the amount of glucose that is reabsorbed into the bloodstream, leading to a decrease in blood glucose levels [151].

Practice Pearl(s)

Here is a summary of the dosing recommendations for some common SGLT2 inhibitors:

Dapagliflozin (Farxiga): The recommended starting dose is 5 mg once daily (The maximum dose is 10 mg once daily).

Canagliflozin (Invokana): The recommended starting dose is 100 mg once daily. (The maximum dose is 300 mg once daily).

Empagliflozin (Jardiance): The recommended starting dose is 10 mg once daily (Maximum dose is 25 mg once daily).

Ertugliflozin (Steglatro): The recommended starting dose is 5 mg once daily (The maximum dose is 15 mg once daily).

SGLT2 inhibitors are generally safe and effective medications for the treatment of type 2 diabetes. However, like all medications, they can have side effects and precautions that should be considered. Some common side effects and precautions associated with SGLT2 inhibitors include urinary tract infections, dehydration, and diabetic ketoacidosis (DKA) [152].

Clinical Trial Evidence

The cardiovascular outcome trials (CVOTs) for SGLT-2 inhibitors have shown consistent benefits in reducing the risk of major adverse cardiovascular events, hospitalization for heart failure, and progression of kidney disease in patients with type 2 diabetes (Table 4.17).

TABLE 4.17   Summary of landmark CVOTs for SGLT2 inhibitors.

Study	Population	Intervention	Outcome
EMPA-REG OUTCOME	T2DM at a high risk for CVD (n = 7020).	Empagliflozin 10 mg or 25 mg once a day (n = 4687), or matching placebo (n = 2333).	Composite primary outcome of CV mortality, nonfatal MI or nonfatal stroke occurred in 10.5% of the empagliflozin arm and 12.1% of the placebo arm, HR 0.86; 95% CI 0.74–0.99, P = 0.04 for superiority) [138].
CANVAS	T2DM with an A1C ≥7% to ≤10.5% and at a high risk for CVD (n = 10 142).	Canagliflozin 100 mg or 300 mg once a day (n = 5795) or matching placebo (n = 4347).	The composite primary outcome of CV mortality, nonfatal MI or nonfatal stroke was lower in the canagliflozin arm (26.9 events per 1000 person-years) compared to the placebo arm (31.5 events per 1000 person-years), HR 0.86; 95% CI 0.75–0.97, P = 0.02 for superiority [153].

(continued)

(*continued*)

TABLE 4.17   (Continued)

Study	Population	Intervention	Outcome
DECLARE-TIMI 58	T2DM with established ASCVD or at risk for ASCVD (n = 17,160).	Dapagliflozin 10 mg daily (n = 8574) or matching placebo (n = 8569).	CV death or hospitalization for heart failure occurred in less patients on dapagliflozin (4.9%) compared to those on placebo (5.8%), HR 0.83; 0.73–0.95, P = 0.005 for superiority [154].

ASCVD, Atherosclerotic cardiovascular disease.

4.1.9   DPP-4 Inhibitors

4.1.9.1   Physiology

DPP-4 is a multifunctional enzyme expressed on the surface of many cell types, including immune cells, epithelial cells, and endothelial cells. DPP4 plays a crucial role in several physiological processes, including glucose metabolism, immune regulation, and inflammation [155, 156].

In glucose metabolism, DPP4 regulates insulin secretion by cleaving incretin hormones such as GLP-1 and GIP. GLP-1 and GIP are hormones released from the gut in response to food intake that stimulate insulin secretion and decrease glucagon secretion, leading to improved glycemic control [157]. By cleaving these hormones, DPP4 reduces their activity and may contribute to impaired insulin secretion [156, 158].

4.1.9.2   Mechanism of Action

DPP-4 inhibitors block the activity of DPP4, an enzyme that degrades incretin hormones such as GLP-1 and GIP [159].

DPP4 inhibitors block the degradation of GLP-1 and GIP by DPP4, resulting in increased levels of these hormones in the blood. Incretins can then exert their physiological effects of increasing insulin secretion and decreasing glucagon secretion, which ultimately lowers blood glucose levels [160].

Practice Pearl(s)

The DPP-4 inhibitor class exhibits structural heterogeneity, resulting in varying pharmacokinetic (PK) and pharmacodynamic (PD) profiles among members.

Sitagliptin is primarily eliminated unchanged in the urine, while vildagliptin is mainly metabolized in the kidneys to inactive metabolites, with 25% being excreted unchanged in the urine [161]. Saxagliptin is primarily metabolized in the liver to an active metabolite that is eliminated via the urine [162].

In contrast, linagliptin is the only DPP-4 inhibitor that is entirely eliminated through the biliary system [163]. Due to this unique elimination pathway, linagliptin is the preferred DPP-4 inhibitor for patients with all stages of kidney failure, as no dose adjustments are required [164].

A summary of the pharmacokinetic profiles of various DPP4 inhibitors is shown in Table 4.18.

TABLE 4.18   Pharmacokinetic profile of DPP4 inhibitors.

Drug name (Trade name)	Dose range	Maximum daily dose	Frequency	Onset of action	Duration of action
Sitagliptin (Januvia)	25–100 mg daily	100 mg	Once daily	1–4 h	24 h
Linagliptin (Tradjenta)	5 mg daily	5 mg	Once daily	1.5 h	24 h
Saxagliptin (Onglyza)	2.5–5 mg daily	5 mg	Once daily	2 h	24 h
Alogliptin (Nesina)	12.5–25 mg daily	25 mg	Once daily	2–3 h	24 h

DPP4 inhibitors are generally well tolerated and have a favorable safety profile [165, 166].

Clinical Trial Evidence

See Table 4.19 for a summary of selected landmark CVOTs for DPP4 inhibitors.

TABLE 4.19   Summary of landmark CVOTs for DPP4 inhibitors.

Study	Population	Intervention	Outcome
EXAMINE	T2DM with either an acute MI or unstable angina requiring hospitalization (n = 5380).	Alogliptin 6.25 mg daily, 12.5 mg or 25 mg daily vs placebo.	Primary composite outcome of 11.3% in the alogliptin arm and 11.8% in the placebo arm, HR 0.96, upper limit one-sided CI of 1.16 $P < 0.001$ for noninferiority [167].
CARMELINA	T2DM at high risk for CV and renal outcomes (n = 6979).	Linagliptin 5 mg once daily (n = 3494) or matching placebo (n = 3485).	Primary composite outcome of CV death, nonfatal MI or nonfatal stroke occurred in 12.4% of the linagliptin arm and 12.1% of the placebo arm, HR 1.02; 95% CI of 0.89–1.17 $P < 0.001$ for noninferiority [100].
TECOS	T2DM with established cardiovascular disease.	Sitagliptin 50 mg daily, 100 mg daily (n = 7257) or matching placebo(n = 7266).	Primary composite outcome occurred in 11.4% of patients in the sitagliptin arm and 11.6% of the placebo arm, HR in the ITT analysis was 0.98; 95% CI 0.89–1.08 $P = 0.65$ for superiority [168].

ITT, Intention to treat.

4.1.10   Alpha-Glucosidase Inhibitors

4.1.10.1   Physiology

Alpha-glucosidases are enzymes located in the brush border of the small intestine required for the digestion and absorption of carbohydrates. These enzymes are responsible for the hydrolysis of alpha-glycosidic bonds of disaccharides and oligosaccharides to produce absorbable monosaccharides, such as glucose.

The two main types of alpha-glucosidases found in the small intestine are **sucrase-isomaltase** and **maltase-glucoamylase** [169]. Sucrase-isomaltase, hydrolyzes the alpha-1,4-glycosidic bonds in sucrose, which yields glucose [170]. Maltase-glucoamylase hydrolyzes the alpha-1,4-glycosidic bonds in maltose and oligosaccharides, producing glucose as the primary product [171].

4.1.10.2   Mechanism of Action

Alpha-glucosidase inhibitors (AGIs) are compounds that act as pseudocarbohydrates in the intestine, competing with ingested carbohydrates for the alpha-glucosidase enzymes located in the brush border of the gut epithelium. As mentioned earlier, these enzymes are responsible for breaking down complex carbohydrates, such as oligosaccharides and polysaccharides, into easily absorbable monosaccharides.

Acarbose, a pseudo-tetrasaccharide, contains nitrogen between its first and second glucose molecule, which gives it a high affinity for the alpha-glucosidase enzyme. Acarbose exerts competitive inhibition with ingested carbohydrates for the alpha-glucosidase enzyme. Acarbose and other AGIs delay carbohydrate digestion and glucose absorption, leading to improved postprandial glycemic control in patients with diabetes [172, 173].

Practice Pearl(s)

It is recommended to administer acarbose with the first bite of a meal to maximize its effect on postprandial hyperglycemia. The starting dose for acarbose is typically 25 mg three times daily, which can be titrated to a maximum of 100 mg three times daily [174–176].

Acarbose may cause some gastrointestinal side effects such as bloating, flatulence, and diarrhea, which can limit its tolerability by patients. These side effects may be managed with a lower dose and gradual titration. Hypoglycemia is not a significant concern when acarbose is used alone but can occur when it is used in combination with insulin or other hypoglycemic agents [174].

Clinical Trial Evidence

A summary of the acarbose on cardiovascular and diabetes outcomes in patients with coronary heart disease and impaired glucose tolerance (ACE) study is shown in Table 4.20.

TABLE 4.20   Evaluation of the efficacy of acarbose in type 2 diabetes mellitus.

Study	Population	Intervention	Outcome
ACE	Patients with coronary heart disease and impaired glucose tolerance evaluated at outpatient clinics in China (n = 6522).	Acarbose 50 mg three times a day (n = 3272) or matching placebo (n = 3250).	The primary outcome[a] occurred in 14% of patients in the acarbose arm and 15% of those in the placebo arm, HR 0.98; 95% CI 0.86–1.11 P = 0.73) [177].

[a] Primary outcome was defined as a composite of cardiovascular death, nonfatal myocardial infarction, nonfatal stroke, hospital admission for unstable angina, and hospital admission for heart failure.

4.1.11   Amylin Agonists

4.1.11.1   Physiology

Amylin is a pancreatic peptide hormone that plays an important role in the regulation of glucose metabolism. It is co-secreted with insulin by beta cells of the pancreas in response to food ingestion. Amylin works to slow gastric emptying and suppress postprandial glucagon secretion, resulting in a reduction in glucose release from the liver, and thereby helping to control postprandial hyperglycemia [178, 179].

4.1.11.2   Mechanism of Action

Amylin analogs, such as pramlintide, have a similar mode of action to natural amylin, a hormone that is co-secreted with insulin by pancreatic β-cells. These analogs have been developed to mimic the effects of amylin in regulating glucose metabolism.

Pramlintide acts by slowing the rate at which food is digested, which leads to a delay in the absorption of glucose into the bloodstream. By inhibiting the secretion of glucagon after a meal, pramlintide also helps to reduce the levels of glucose produced by the liver. Furthermore, pramlintide works on the satiety center of the brain to suppress appetite, leading to a reduction in food intake and body weight [180].

Pramlintide is administered subcutaneously before meals after which it is rapidly absorbed with a peak effect within 30 minutes of administration. The duration of its action is around 3–4 hours, making it suitable for administration prior to each meal [181].

Practice Pearl(s)

Pramlintide (Symlin) is an amylin analog that is administered as a subcutaneous injection before meals [182]. The initial dose is typically 15 mcg, and it can be increased to 30 or 60 mcg based on individual response.

The dose of prandial insulin would need to be titrated downwards in patients starting amylin mimetics, this is because these agents reduce the degree of postprandial hyperglycemia.

Clinical Trial Evidence

A 52-week, double-blind, placebo-controlled, multicenter study involved 480 patients with type 1 diabetes mellitus randomized to receive preprandial injections of placebo or 30 micrograms of pramlintide q.i.d., in addition to their insulin treatment. Pramlintide treatment led to a mean reduction in HbA1c of 0.67% from baseline to week 13 that was significantly greater than the reduction in HbA1c in the placebo arm (0.16%). This significant treatment difference was sustained through week 52.

The greater HbA1c reduction was associated with an average weight loss and was not accompanied by an increased risk of severe hypoglycemia. The open-label extension of the study revealed that pramlintide treatment improved glycemic control without inducing weight gain or increasing the overall risk of severe hypoglycemia in patients with type 1 diabetes.

The most common adverse events reported were mild nausea and anorexia, which dissipated over time. The findings of this study suggest that pramlintide treatment may be a viable option for long-term glycemic control in patients with type 1 diabetes [183].

 Concepts to Ponder Over

The "ominous octet" is a term introduced by Dr. Ralph A. DeFronzo, an eminent diabetes researcher, to describe the eight crucial pathophysiological mechanisms implicated in the development of type 2 diabetes mellitus. These mechanisms include insulin resistance, incretin deficiency, glucagon excess, increased hepatic glucose production, adipokine dysregulation, inflammation, neurotransmitter dysfunction, and increased renal glucose reabsorption (see Figure 4.8).

Important trials in diabetes care every diabetes care specialist should know

The diabetes prevention program study

The Diabetes Prevention Program (DPP), approved by the National Institute of Health, set out to explore whether specific interventions might prevent or delay diabetes in 27 locations across America, randomly assigning participants one of four treatment

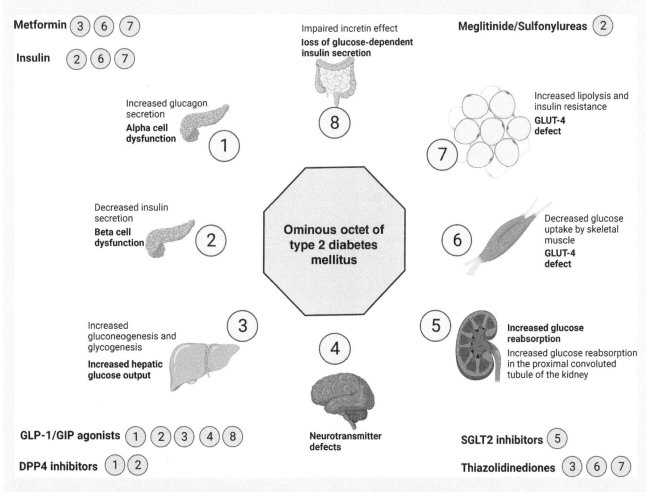

FIGURE 4.8   Pathophysiologic defects of T2DM and the medications addressing the defects.

(continued)

(continued)

strategies – lifestyle changes and behavioral modifications, metformin therapy, troglitazone therapy (a previously discontinued thiazolidinedione), or placebo.

3234 participants aged 25 or above participated in this study and all met criteria for prediabetes: elevated fasting plasma glucose and impaired glucose tolerance.

The lifestyle intervention group was offered extensive education and counseling about diet, physical activity, and behavioral modification. This group's aim was to achieve sustained weight loss of at least 7% through lower fat and caloric consumption and an aerobic exercise routine of 150 minutes each week. The metformin group was given two doses of 850 mg metformin twice daily, while the placebo group received inert pills twice daily. Patients in the metformin and placebo groups also received basic lifestyle education but without intensive counseling services. Troglitazone group participants initially received daily doses of 400 mg; however, due to concerns of liver toxicity from troglitazone, they were removed from this arm of research but continued being monitored; troglitazone was eventually withdrawn from US markets in 2000.

The outcomes of the Diabetes Prevention Program were encouraging. Participants who successfully lost modest amounts through diet modification and physical activity greatly decreased their risks of diabetes; similarly, metformin group demonstrated decreased risks as well, though to a lesser degree [184].

The diabetes complication and control trial

Studies have demonstrated the significance of maintaining near euglycemia as a way to protect individuals with diabetes from severe microvascular complications. According to the Diabetes Complication and Control Trial (DCCT), which examined traditional and intensive approaches in managing type 1 diabetes complications, 1441 participants were randomized to traditional and intensive therapies.

Trial results demonstrated that intensive glycemic control significantly lowered the risk of microvascular complications among type 1 diabetic patients. Patients in a high-intensity treatment group, with an average hemoglobin A1c level around 7%, experienced about 60% fewer diabetes-related eye, kidney, or nerve diseases as compared with standard treatment groups with average HbA1cs around 9% over a period of 6.5 years [185].

Following the conclusion of the Diabetes Control and Complication Trial in 1993, researchers initiated the Epidemiology of Diabetes Interventions and Complications (EDIC), a long-term follow-up study that continued to monitor over 90% of DCCT participants [186].

United Kingdom Prospective Diabetes Study

The United Kingdom Prospective Diabetes Study (UKPDS), conducted between 1977 and 1997, followed on the research conducted by DCCT by studying newly diagnosed type 2 diabetes patients. This study divided patients into two groups, the conventional therapy or the while intensive therapy arm.

Results from the 10-year follow-up study of UKPDS participants revealed that those randomized to the intensive therapy arm during the trial experienced lower risks of myocardial infarction and death than their conventional therapy counterparts, despite HbA1c levels becoming equal soon after the conclusion of the research study [187].

4.2   NEUROENDOCRINE TUMORS

4.2.1   Telotristat

4.2.1.1   Physiology

Synthesis of Serotonin

Neuroendocrine cells of the gastrointestinal tract, such as enterochromaffin cells, have long been recognized for producing serotonin, also referred to as 5-hydroxytryptamine (5-HT). Serotonin can be produced using amino acids like tryptophan. Initial steps involve the uptake of tryptophan from the bloodstream via carrier-mediated transport. Subsequently, tryptophan is converted to 5-hydroxytryptophan (5-HTP) through tryptophan hydroxylase (TPH) enzyme activity – this being the rate-limiting step in serotonin synthesis. Next, 5-HTP is decarboxylated using aromatic L-amino acid decarboxylase (AADC) to produce serotonin. Once synthesized, serotonin is transported into vesicles via vesicular monoamine transporter (VMAT) for storage until being released in response to nerve impulses. Serotonin is secreted via exocytosis and interacts with receptors on postsynaptic neurons. Once released, serotonin is then metabolized by monoamine oxidase (MAO) and aldehyde dehydrogenase (ALDH), producing 5-hydroxyindoleacetaldehyde (5-HIAA), which is excreted via urine [188] (see Figure 4.9).

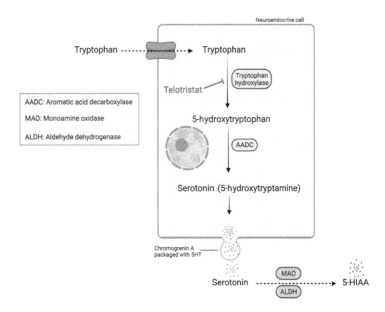

FIGURE 4.9 Biosynthesis of serotonin by neuroendocrine cells. Tryptophan hydroxylase is the rate-limiting step in the series of enzymatic reactions which converts tryptophan to 5HT.

4.2.1.2   Mechanism of Action

Telotristat is a tryptophan hydroxylase inhibitor that irreversibly binds to the active site of TPH, thereby preventing the conversion of tryptophan to 5-HTP, the precursor to serotonin. Through its inhibitory action on TPH, telotristat ultimately results in a decrease in the synthesis and release of serotonin in the gastrointestinal tract, which leads to a reduction in the symptoms of carcinoid syndrome [189].

Practice Pearl(s)

Telotristat is typically administered orally and is generally well tolerated. It is often used in combination with somatostatin analogs, which are another class of medications used in the treatment of carcinoid syndrome [190] (see Table 4.21). For the treatment of carcinoid syndrome related-diarrhea, the recommended starting dose of telotristat ethyl is 250 mg three times daily with food [191].

TABLE 4.21   Summary of the TELESTAR and TELECAST studies.

Study	Population	Intervention	Outcome
TELESTAR	Patients with well-differentiated NETs complicated by carcinoid syndrome and not adequately controlled with somatostatin analogs (n = 135).	Telotristat 250 mg (n = 45) or 500 mg (n = 45) three times a day or matching placebo (n = 45) for up to 12 weeks. This was followed by a 36 week open label extension.	The estimated difference in bowel movement frequency per day compared to placebo was −0.81 for telotristat ethyl 250 mg (P < 0.001) and − 0.69 for telotristat ethyl 500 mg (P < 0.001) [191].
TELECAST	Patients with well-differentiated NETs complicated by carcinoid syn-drome and not ad-equately controlled with somatostatin analogs (n = 76).	Telotristat 250 mg (n = 25) or 500 mg (n = 25) three times a day or matching pla-cebo (n = 26).	At the 12-week mark, a significant decrease in u5-HIAA levels from baseline was observed in both the 250 mg and 500 mg telotristat ethyl groups. The treatment differences from placebo were −54.0% (95% confidence limits −85.0%, −25.1%) for the 250 mg group and − 89.7% (95% confidence limits −113.1%, −63.9%) for the 500 mg group (P < 0.001 for both groups compared to placebo) [192].

4.2.2   Acid-Lowering Drugs

4.2.2.1   Physiology

Secretion of Gastric Acid

Gastric acid secretion is regulated by a complex interplay of endocrine and paracrine signaling pathways involving various cells in the stomach (see Figure 4.10).

G cells, which are located in the antrum of the stomach, secrete the hormone gastrin largely in response to stimuli such as the presence of food. Gastrin is responsible for the release of hydrochloric acid (HCl) from parietal cells, which are located in the body and fundus of the stomach.

Furthermore, histamine, which is released from the enterochromaffin-like (ECL) cells in response to gastrin and other stimuli, also stimulates HCl secretion from the parietal cells. Histamine acts on the H2 receptors located on the parietal cells to stimulate the production of cyclic AMP, which in

turn activates the proton pump on the surface of the parietal cells.

Acetylcholine, which is released from the vagus nerve and from local enteric neurons, also stimulates HCl secretion from the parietal cells. Acetylcholine acts on the M3 receptors located on the parietal cells to increase intracellular calcium, which activates the proton pump. The proton pump, located on the apical surface of the parietal cells, is responsible for the final step in gastric acid secretion. It actively transports H+ ions into the lumen of the stomach in exchange for K+ ions, a process that establishes a highly acidic environment (pH 1.5–3.5) necessary for the digestion of food and the activation of various digestive enzymes [193].

Islet Cells of the Pancreas

The islets of Langerhans, or islet cells, are a group of pancreatic endocrine cells embedded within a rich background of acinar exocrine tissue. These endocrine cells make up roughly 2% of the pancreatic volume, with most islets located in the tail of the pancreas [194]. The islets of Langerhans contain various types of cells, including beta, alpha, delta, PP, epsilon, G, and EC cells [195] (see Table 4.22).

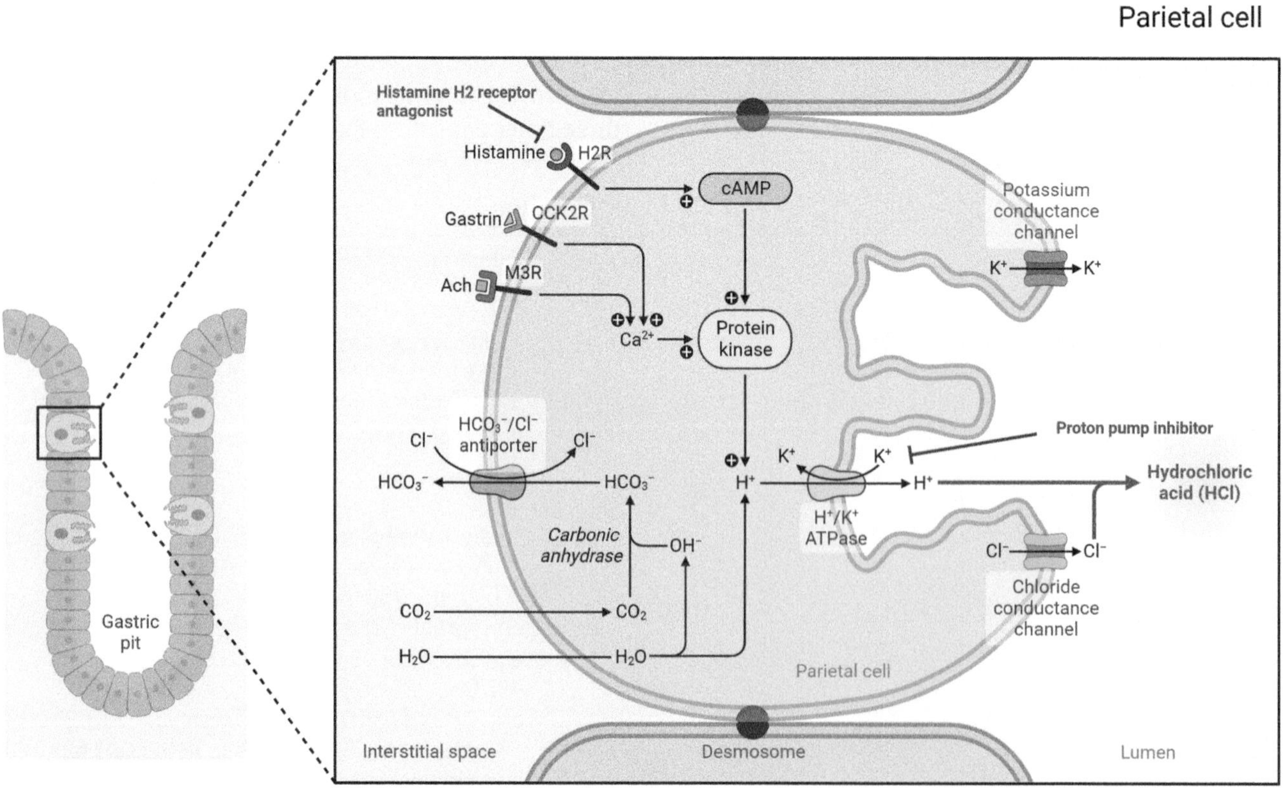

FIGURE 4.10   Regulation of gastric acid production by the parietal cell.

TABLE 4.22 Hormones produced by islets cells.

Islet cell (frequency)	Hormone produced	Effects(s)
Beta cells (50–70%)	Insulin and amylin	Insulin enhances peripheral glucose uptake and inhibits hepatic gluconeogenesis and glycogenolysis [195, 196]. Amylin slows gastric emptying and stimulates early satiety [197].
Alpha cells (20–30%)	Glucagon	Promotes both hepatic gluconeogenesis and glycogenolysis. Glucagon stimulates hepatic ketogenesis during a prolonged fast [198, 199].
Delta cells (10%)	Somatostatin	Inhibits the secretion of insulin, glucagon, and pancreatic polypeptide [195].
PP cells (2%)	Pancreatic polypeptide	Inhibits the secretion of glucagon by alpha cells and also promotes early satiety [195].
Epsilon cells (1%)	Ghrelin	Inhibits the incretin effect (insulin release after an oral glucose load). Stimulates the secretion of growth hormone and is also called the "hunger hormone" [200].
G cells (absent)	Gastrin	Pancreatic gastrin-producing cells are present during embryonic development but undergo involution in adults. Re-expression of gastrin occurs in pancreatic neuroendocrine tumors (Zollinger–Ellison syndrome) [201].
EC cells (rare)	Serotonin	Carcinoid syndrome [202, 203].

A typical adult pancreas is comprised of approximately one million islet cells [204], with beta cells being polyhedral in shape and evenly dispersed throughout the pancreas [205]. Alpha cells are columnar in shape and primarily found in the body and tail of the pancreas [206], while the distribution of delta cells is more variable and characterized by dendritic processes. PP cells are present in the head and uncinate process of the pancreas [196] (see Figure 4.11).

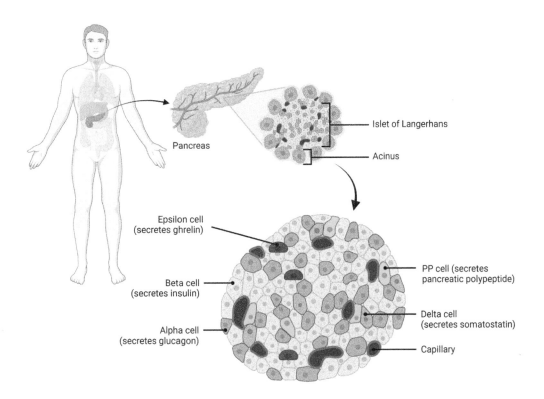

Islet of Langerhans

FIGURE 4.11 Pancreatic islet cells. The distribution of various islet cells and their corresponding hormones.

4.2.2.2   Mechanism of Action

Proton pump inhibitors (PPIs) are commonly used in the treatment of gastric acid-related disorders, including gastroesophageal reflux disease (GERD), peptic ulcers, and Zollinger–Ellison syndrome (ZES), which is caused by gastrinomas, a type of neuroendocrine tumor.

Gastrinomas are rare tumors that produce large amounts of gastrin, a hormone that stimulates gastric acid production. Excessive gastric acid production can lead to complications such as peptic ulcers, diarrhea, and abdominal pain [207]. PPIs work by irreversibly binding to and inhibiting the H^+/K^+-ATPase proton pump located on the apical surface of the parietal cells in the stomach. This inhibits the final step in gastric acid secretion, accounting for a significant reduction in the amount of acid produced by the parietal cells [208].

Clinical Trial Evidence

Intravenous pantoprazole is an effective option for controlling gastric acid hypersecretion in conditions such as Zollinger–Ellison syndrome or idiopathic gastric acid hypersecretion when oral medications are not feasible. This study evaluated the efficacy and safety of 15-minute infusions of pantoprazole (80–120 mg every 8–12 hours) in controlling gastric acid output for up to 7 days. The study found that all patients had effective control of gastric acid output within the first hour of treatment, and 81% of patients had effective control for up to 7 days with doses of 80 mg every 12 hours. Some patients required upward dose titration. No serious adverse events were observed. Intravenous pantoprazole is a safe and effective option for perioperative control of gastric acid hypersecretion in conditions such as ZES [209].

Practice Pearl(s)

The management of gastrinomas, a type of neuroendocrine tumor that causes hypergastrinemia, typically involves the use of acid-lowering medications, such as proton pump inhibitors (PPIs) [209].

The use of gastric resection surgery for peptic ulcers has diminished with the advent of H2 blockers and PPIs. This is due to the fact that PPIs are capable of nearly fully suppressing acid secretion in the stomach, thereby preventing complications such as duodenal ulcer perforation, severe esophagitis, and frequent diarrhea. As a result, gastrectomy is no longer required for gastrinoma patients [210]. However, while PPIs can prevent the development of complications from hyperacidity, they are not effective in halting the progression and growth of gastrinomas. The following are the usual adult doses for some of the commonly used PPIs:

Omeprazole: 20–40 mg once daily
Lansoprazole: 15–30 mg once daily
Esomeprazole: 20–40 mg once daily
Pantoprazole: 40 mg once daily
Rabeprazole: 20 mg once daily

4.2.3   Somatostatin Analogs

4.2.3.1   Physiology

Somatostatin, an inhibitory peptide hormone produced by delta cells of the pancreas and neuroendocrine cells throughout the body, exerts wide-ranging inhibitory effects on endocrine function. A summary of its effects may include these:

1. Somatostatin works within the digestive tract by targeting G cells of the stomach to inhibit gastrin release and ultimately lower acid secretion [211].
2. Somatostatin acts to block serotonin release, an essential hormone in controlling intestinal motility that may also contribute to pathogenic conditions like carcinoid syndrome [212].
3. Somatostatin inhibits insulin and glucagon release from beta and alpha cells of the pancreas, respectively. [213].
4. Somatostatin plays an integral part in regulating endocrine health and can even block GHRH secretions from the hypothalamus, thus lowering the secretion of growth hormone from the pituitary gland [213] (see Chapter 1).

Thus, Somatostatin is integral in managing our endocrine systems while acting as an effective therapeutic target against various related disorders [214].

4.2.3.2 Mechanism of Action

Somatostatin analogs are synthetic compounds designed to replicate the inhibitory effects of somatostatin on hormone secretion. As part of their treatment for carcinoid syndrome, somatostatin analogs such as octreotide and lanreotide may help decrease symptoms caused by excessive hormone production, such as diarrhea, flushing, and abdominal pain. At 90–120 minutes, Octreotide's half-life far exceeds that of endogenous somatostatin. When administered subcutaneously, it inhibits hormone secretion [215].

Octreotide has physiological actions similar to somatostatin by binding to somatostatin receptor subtypes 2 and 5, which are highly expressed in neuroendocrine tumors [216].

Somatostatin analogs not only promote hormone secretion but can also have antiproliferative properties against neuroendocrine tumors. By inhibiting secretions of growth factors and angiogenic factors, they may slow growth rates of neuroendocrine tumors as well as possibly lead to tumor regression in some cases [217].

Practice Pearl(s)

Practical guidelines for the use of somatostatin analogs were reviewed in Chapter 1.

Clinical Trial Evidence

Refer to Table 4.23 for a summary of clinical trials evaluating the role of somatostatin analogs in NETs.

TABLE 4.23   Trials evaluating the efficacy of somatostatin analogs in NETs.

Study	Population	Intervention	Outcome
CLARINET	Patients with advanced, well-differentiated or moderately differentiated, nonfunctioning, somatostatin receptor-positive neuroendocrine tumors of grade 1 or 2, and disease-progression status (n = 204).	Randomized, double-blind, placebo-controlled study of lanreotide (120 mg) or placebo once every 28 days for 96 weeks.	Lanreotide significantly prolonged progression-free survival. The 24-month progression-free survival rates were 65.1% (lanreotide) vs 33.0% (placebo). No significant differences in quality of life or overall survival. Most common treatment-related adverse event: diarrhea (26% lanreotide, 9% placebo) [218].
PROMID	Treatment-naive patients with well-differentiated metastatic midgut NETs (n = 85).	Placebo-controlled, double-blind, phase IIIB study with patients randomly assigned to receive either placebo or octreotide LAR 30 mg intramuscularly in monthly intervals until tumor progression or death.	Octreotide LAR significantly prolonged time to tumor progression (median 14.3 months) compared to placebo (6 months) (HR = 0.34; 95% CI, 0.20–0.59; P = 0.000072). After 6 months, stable disease was observed in 66.7% of octreotide LAR group and 37.2% of placebo group. HR for overall survival was 0.81 (95% CI, 0.30–2.18) [219].

Source: Adapted from refs. [218, 219].

Concepts to Ponder Over

How does chronic achlorhydria lead to the formation of carcinoid tumors?

Ingestion of food triggers the activation of G cells in the stomach, leading to the release of gastrin by the gastric antrum. Gastrin binds to CCK receptors on gastric enterochromaffin-like (ECL) cells, inducing histamine release. The released histamine binds to H2 receptors on gastric parietal cells, producing hydrochloric acid, which is essential in creating an acidic environment in the gut. The acidic environment then triggers the release of somatostatin by delta cells of the pancreas, providing negative feedback inhibition of gastrin release from G cells. However, in cases of achlorhydria, such as pernicious anemia, this negative feedback loop is impaired, resulting in the uncontrolled release of gastrin from G cells. This uncontrolled release of gastrin, apart from promoting increased histamine production by gastric ECL cells, also leads to their unchecked proliferation, which can eventually result in tumorigenesis (carcinoid formation) [220].

4.3 HYPOGLYCEMIA SYNDROMES

4.3.1 Somatostatin Analogs

4.3.1.1 Physiology

Somatostatin, also known as growth hormone-inhibiting hormone (GHIH), regulates insulin secretion by inhibiting the release of several hormones, including insulin, glucagon, and growth hormone. Somatostatin is produced by pancreatic delta cells, and it binds to specific receptors on beta cells in the islets of Langerhans, where insulin is produced. When somatostatin binds to its receptors on beta cells, it inhibits insulin release by decreasing the amount of calcium that enters the cell in response to glucose. This ultimately leads to decreased insulin secretion from beta cells [221].

4.3.1.2 Mechanism of Action

Somatostatin analogs have a role in the treatment of hypoglycemia syndromes, including insulinoma, which is a rare pancreatic neuroendocrine tumor associated with hyperinsulinemia. By binding to somatostatin receptor subtypes, somatostatin analogs

TABLE 4.24 Distribution of the density of somatostatin receptors in insulinomas.

Somatostatin receptor	Benign insulinoma	Malignant insulinoma
SSTR2	Low	High
SSTR4	High	High
SSTR5	Low	High

Source: Adapted from refs. [224].

can inhibit insulin secretion and decrease hypoglycemic episodes in patients with insulinoma [222, 223]. The response of insulinomas to treatment with somatostatin analogs is dependent on their SSTR density (see Table 4.24).

Practice Pearl(s)

Treatment of symptomatic benign insulinomas can begin with the short-acting subcutaneous form of octreotide, administered at a dosage of 100–600 mcg per day in 2–4 divided doses for a two-week period. This is then followed by slowly transitioning from short-acting to long-acting formulations. To achieve this, two weeks of continued treatment with short-acting insulin is recommended after the first dose of the long-acting form (initially 100–200 mcg, with subsequent dosage adjustments). If the response to treatment is appropriate, long-acting forms such as octreotide 20–30 mg I.M. every 4 weeks or lanreotide 30 mg I.M. every 2 weeks can be considered. An alternative option is the use of lanreotide 60–120 mg subcutaneously every 4 weeks [225].

Clinical Trial Evidence

The rarity of insulinomas has led to a limited number of well-powered clinical studies investigating the role of somatostatin analogs in their treatment.

 Pathophysiology Pearl

Protective mechanisms against hypoglycemia

Hypoglycemia occurs when glucose utilization from the circulation, primarily by the brain but also by other tissues, exceeds the sum of glucose delivery into the circulation from ingested carbohydrates and hepatic and renal glucose production. As blood glucose levels decrease within the physiological range, the body initiates a sequence of responses. First, there is a decrease in insulin secretion, followed by an increase in glucagon secretion and an increase in epinephrine secretion in the absence of glucagon. To defend against prolonged hypoglycemia, the body finally increases cortisol and growth hormone secretion. However, if these defenses fail, plasma glucose levels continue to fall, leading to severe hypoglycemia [226].

4.3.2   Diazoxide and Diuretics

4.3.2.1   Physiology

See Sections 4.1.3 and 4.1.4 (mechanism of insulin secretion by beta cells of the pancreas).

4.3.2.2   Mechanism of Action

KATP channels are membrane-spanning proteins that regulate insulin secretion by controlling electrical activity within cells; when open, they lead to hyperpolarization of the beta-cell membrane, which inhibits insulin secretion [227].

Diazoxide works by binding to a specific site on the sulfonylurea receptor, a subunit of KATP channels, and stabilizing them in their open position – this results in decreased insulin secretion and an increase in blood glucose levels [228].

Practice Pearl(s)

The therapeutic dosage for adults is 3–8 mg/kg per day divided into two or three equal doses, and higher dosages may be required for refractory cases. Treatment should start with a daily dose of 150–200 mg, administered in two or three divided doses to maintain glycemic control [225].

Diazoxide is a relatively safe drug, but it can cause adverse effects such as fluid retention and hypertrichosis. It is contraindicated in patients with a history of heart failure or pulmonary

---

hypertension. Due to the risk of fluid retention, thiazide diuretics are recommended at the time of initiation of diazoxide [229].

Clinical Trial Evidence

The rarity of insulinomas has led to a limited number of well-powered clinical studies investigating the role of diazoxide in their treatment.

4.3.3   Calcium Channel Blockers

4.3.3.1   Physiology

The role of calcium in insulin secretion (see Figure 4.5).

4.3.3.2   Mechanism of Action

Verapamil is a calcium channel blocker, acting by inhibiting calcium from entering pancreatic beta cells – leading to reduced levels of insulin. Verapamil may also inhibit glucagon secretion, although its exact mechanism remains unknown. Case reports and small studies have reported its use for managing insulinomas; however, more research needs to be conducted into its efficacy and safety [230, 231].

Practice Pearl(s)

There are no standardized dosing guidelines for the use of verapamil in the management of insulinoma.

Clinical Trial Evidence

The rarity of insulinomas has led to a limited number of well-powered clinical studies investigating the role of verapamil in their treatment.

4.3.4   mTOR Inhibitors

4.3.4.1   Physiology

The mammalian target of rapamycin (mTOR) signaling pathway plays an important role in the regulation of cellular metabolism, growth, and proliferation. In particular, mTOR signaling has been implicated in the regulation of insulin production and glucose homeostasis [232, 233].

4.3.4.2   Mechanism of Action

In insulinoma, mTOR inhibitors, such as everolimus and temsirolimus, have been studied as potential therapeutic option. These drugs work by inhibiting mTOR signaling, which reduces cell proliferation and induces cell death [234, 235].

Practice Pearl(s)

The starting dose of everolimus is usually 10 mg/day, and adjustments may be made based on the individual patient's response and tolerance [236].

Clinical Trial Evidence

The rarity of insulinomas has led to a limited number of well-powered clinical studies investigating the role of everolimus in their treatment.

Refractory hypoglycemia is a significant cause of morbidity and mortality in patients with metastatic insulinoma. In this retrospective, multicenter study conducted, everolimus was evaluated as a potential therapeutic option for these patients. The study aimed to determine the time to the first recurrence of symptomatic hypoglycemia after everolimus initiation, as well as to assess ongoing hyperglycemic medical options, tumor response, and safety information.

The study included 12 patients with metastatic insulinoma and refractory hypoglycemia who were treated with everolimus. Everolimus was administered at a starting dose of 10 mg/day (except for one patient who received 5 mg/day) after a median of four failed therapeutic approaches. The medication was given with the aim of normalizing blood glucose levels. After a median duration of 6.5 months (range 1–35 months), the median time to the first recurrence of symptomatic hypoglycemia was 6.5 months (range 0–35 months). This occurred in 11 of the 12 patients.

Of the 12 patients, three discontinued everolimus due to cardiac or pulmonary adverse events at

1, 1.5, and 7 months after initiation, which led to two deaths. Another three patients discontinued everolimus because of tumor progression at 2, 3, and 10 months after initiation, without recurrence of hypoglycemia.

The study's findings suggest that everolimus is an effective treatment for patients with metastatic insulinoma and refractory hypoglycemia. However, tolerance should be carefully monitored, as adverse events were observed in some patients [237].

4.3.5   Phenytoin

4.3.5.1   Physiology

The role of calcium in insulin secretion (see Figure 4.5).

4.3.5.2   Mechanism of Action

Phenytoin has been suggested as an effective treatment option for insulinoma-related hypoglycemia due to its ability to inhibit insulin secretion. Phenytoin may work by blocking calcium channels on beta cells in the pancreas that play an integral part in insulin secretion [238, 239].

Practice Pearl(s)

Phenytoin should only be considered an occasional option to treat insulinoma-associated hypoglycemia due to a lack of research on its safety or efficacy; diazoxide or octreotide treatments tend to be preferred and should be seen as first-line therapies in such instances.

Clinical Trial Evidence

The rarity of insulinomas has led to a limited number of well-powered clinical studies investigating the role of phenytoin in their treatment.

Concepts to Ponder Over

Interpretation of the 72-hour fast

A thorough evaluation is warranted in most cases of fasting hypoglycemia in nondiabetic patients, as it is an extremely rare occurrence. It is important to understand the following pathophysiologic concepts when interpreting a 72-hour fast result. Rote memorization will likely lead to errors on a board examination and in real-life practice.

- When the plasma glucose concentration reaches a mean of approximately 55 mg/dl (3.0 mmol/l), symptoms that prompt the behavioral defense of food ingestion usually develop. At this glucose level and lower, insulin secretion is almost completely suppressed, resulting in plasma insulin levels below 3 U/ml (18 pmol/l), C-peptide levels below 0.6 ng/ml (0.2 nmol/l), and proinsulin levels below 5.0 pmol/l.
- Insulin or insulin-like action inhibits ketogenesis (this results in a low beta-hydroxybutyrate level).
- C-peptide, an essential component of insulin precursors, is present in the setting of endogenous insulin production (either due to an insulinoma or insulin secretagogue).

- Exogenous insulin contains only the alpha and beta chains; as such, c-peptide will remain undetectable among patients who inject insulin surreptitiously.
- In normal physiology, glycogen stores are expected to be depleted after a 72-hour fast. As a result, glucose will fail to increase appreciably (that is, >25 mg/dl) at the end of a fast, except in patients with persistent endogenous hyperinsulinemia.
- In essence, if there is excess insulin (or insulin-like action), glycogen stores will never be completely depleted. These patients will therefore mount an appropriate increase in serum glucose (that is, >25 mg/dl) after glucagon administration.
- Finally, insulin is expected to be appropriately low for normal persons with severe hypoglycemia at the end of a 72-hour fast. Indeed, a relative decline in insulin levels will promote ketogenesis due to the action of multiple counterregulatory hormones.

Now apply these concepts in interpreting differential diagnosis of fasting hypoglycemia (see Table 4.25).

TABLE 4.25   Interpretation of the 72 h fast.

Glucose (mg/dl)	Insulin (micro U/ml)	C-peptide (nmol/L)	Proinsulin (pmol/L)	Beta-hydroxybutyrate (mmol/L)	Glucose increase after glucagon (mg/dl)	Diagnosis
<55	<3	<0.2	<5	>2.7	<25	Normal
<55	>>3	<0.2	<5	<2.7 or normal	>25	Exogenous insulin
<55	>3 or normal	>0.2 or normal	>5 or normal	<2.7 or normal	>25	Insulinoma or NIPHS
<55	>3 or normal	>0.2 or normal	>5 or normal	<2.7 or normal	>25	Oral hypoglycemic agent
<55	>>3	>>0.2	>>5 or normal	<2.7 or normal	>25	Autoimmune: agonist antibodies to the insulin
<55	<3	<0.2	<5	<2.7 or normal	>25	IGF-II mediated
<55	>3	<0.2	<5	<2.7 or normal	>25	Autoimmune: insulin receptor antibodies

NIPHS, Non-insulinoma pancreatogenous hypoglycemia syndrome.
Source: Adapted from ref. [240].

Can these principles be applied to patients who experience postprandial hypoglycemia, such as patients with hypoglycemia after bariatric surgery?

The interpretation of endogenous insulin production for postprandial or reactive hypoglycemia can be challenging. This is because C-peptide, which is a marker of insulin secretion, has a half-life of approximately 30 minutes. As a result, C-peptide levels may remain detectable even if insulin (half-life of a few minutes) is appropriately suppressed during postprandial hypoglycemia [240].

PRACTICE-BASED QUESTIONS

1. Insulin is a peptide hormone that consists of how many amino acid chains?

   a. One
   b. Two
   c. Three
   d. Four
   e. Five

   Answer: b. Two. Insulin consists of two chains (A and B) that are linked by disulfide bonds.

2. During the postprandial state, what is the primary hormone responsible for glucose uptake by skeletal muscle?

   a. Glucagon
   b. Epinephrine
   c. Insulin
   d. Cortisol
   e. Growth hormone

   Answer: c. Insulin. Insulin is the primary hormone responsible for glucose uptake by skeletal muscle during the postprandial state.

3. What is the main source of glucose production during the fasting state?

   a. Skeletal muscle
   b. Adipose tissue
   c. Liver
   d. Pancreas
   e. Kidneys

   Answer: c. Liver. The liver serves as the main source of endogenous glucose production during the fasting state.

4. Which tissue is primarily responsible for lipolysis during the fasting state?

   a. Skeletal muscle
   b. Adipose tissue
   c. Liver
   d. Pancreas
   e. Kidneys

   Answer: b. Adipose tissue. Adipose tissue is primarily responsible for lipolysis during the fasting state.

5. What is the principal pathophysiologic defect in skeletal muscle that leads to insulin resistance in type 2 diabetes?

   a. Impaired translocation of GLUT4 to plasma membrane of myocytes
   b. Defective tyrosine phosphorylation of various proximal insulin receptor substrates
   c. Release of adipokines associated with insulin resistance

   Answer: a. Insulin resistance in skeletal muscle is characterized by impaired translocation of GLUT4 to the plasma membrane of myocytes.

6. What is the mechanism of action of meglitinides?

   a. Inhibit the ATP-dependent potassium channels of the pancreatic beta cell
   b. Increase the expression of other proteins involved in insulin exocytosis
   c. Increase the sensitivity of beta cells to glucose
   d. Block the function of the SUR1 subunit of the ATP-sensitive potassium channels

   Answer: a) Inhibit the ATP-dependent potassium channels of the pancreatic beta cell. Meglitinides stimulate early-phase insulin release by blocking the ATP-dependent potassium channels of the pancreatic beta cell directly. This occurs independent of intracellular ATP to ADP ratio and results in depolarization of the cell membrane, opening of voltage-gated calcium channels, an influx of calcium, and finally, the exocytosis of insulin-laden granules.

7. Which of the following sulfonylureas is considered the drug of choice for individuals with chronic kidney disease?

   a. Glipizide
   b. Glibenclamide

c. Glyburide

d. Glimepiride

Answer: a) Glipizide. Glipizide is metabolized by the liver into several inactive metabolites, which means that its clearance and elimination half-life remain unaffected despite any reduction in estimated glomerular filtration rate (GFR). In individuals with chronic kidney disease (CKD), there is no need for dosage adjustments when using glipizide, as it is considered the sulfonyl-urea of choice for this patient population.

8. What is the main function of incretins in insulin release?

   a. Stimulates the release of insulin by pancreatic beta cells

   b. Inhibits the liver's production of glucose

   c. Promotes the uptake of glucose into cells

   d. Inhibits the ATP-dependent potassium channels of the pancreatic beta cell

   Answer: a) Stimulate the release of insulin by pancreatic beta cells. Incretins are hormones produced by the gastrointestinal tract in response to food intake. They stimulate the release of insulin by pancreatic beta cells, helping to lower blood glucose levels after a meal.

9. What is the mechanism of action of bromocriptine in type 2 diabetes mellitus?

   a. It increases insulin secretion

   b. It activates alpha-adrenergic receptors

   c. It inhibits sympathetic tone within the CNS

   d. It reduces insulin resistance

   Answer: c) It inhibits sympathetic tone within the CNS. **Explanation:** Bromocriptine inhibits sympathetic tone within the CNS, reducing post-meal plasma glucose levels due to the inhibition of hepatic glucose production. It also reduces plasma glucose, triglyceride, and FFA levels.

10. What is the mechanism of action of pioglitazone?

   a. It activates the PPAR gamma receptors in adipocytes, inducing adipogenesis

   b. It increases insulin secretion

   c. It decreases glucose uptake and utilization

   d. It reduces adipose tissue mass

Answer: a) It activates the PPAR gamma receptors in adipocytes, inducing adipogenesis. **Explanation:** The mechanism of action of pioglitazone involves binding to peroxisome proliferator-activated receptors (PPARs) found in adipose tissue, liver, and skeletal muscle. PPARs are nuclear receptors that play a crucial role in the regulation of genes involved in glucose and lipid metabolism. By activating the PPARs, pioglitazone stimulates the transcription of genes involved in glucose uptake and utilization, fatty acid storage, and insulin sensitivity.

11. What is the incretin effect?

   a. Enhanced insulin secretion in response to an oral glucose load compared to intravenous glucose administration

   b. Enhanced glucagon secretion in response to an oral glucose load compared to intravenous glucose administration

   c. Enhanced glucose uptake and utilization in response to an oral glucose load compared to intravenous glucose administration

   d. Enhanced lipolysis in response to an oral glucose load compared to intravenous glucose administration

   Answer: a) Enhanced insulin secretion in response to an oral glucose load compared to intravenous glucose administration. **Explanation:** The incretin effect is described as enhanced insulin secretion in response to an oral glucose load (two to threefold increase) compared with intravenous glucose administration.

12. How do GLP-1 agonists improve glycemic control?

   a. By promoting hepatic glucose production

   b. By inhibiting insulin secretion

   c. By reducing appetite and food intake

   d. By promoting glucagon secretion

   Answer: c) By reducing appetite and food intake. **Explanation:** GLP-1 and GIP can slow gastric emptying, which helps to reduce the rate of nutrient absorption and improve glycemic control. They can also reduce appetite and food intake, which may contribute to weight loss and improved glycemic control.

13. What is the mechanism of action of DPP-4 inhibitors?

   a. They activate the GLP-1 receptor
   b. They increase the half-life of endogenous GLP-1 by inhibiting its degradation
   c. They promote beta-cell growth and survival
   d. They inhibit hepatic glucose production

   Answer: b) They increase the half-life of endogenous GLP-1 by inhibiting its degradation. **Explanation:** DPP-4 inhibitors increase the half-life of endogenous GLP-1 by inhibiting its degradation. This leads to enhanced incretin signaling and improved glycemic control.

14. Which protein is primarily responsible for the majority of glucose reabsorption in the proximal tubule?

   a. SGLT-1
   b. SGLT-2
   c. GLUT2
   d. Na+/K+ pump

   Answer: b) SGLT-2. SGLT-2 is primarily responsible for the majority of glucose reabsorption in the proximal tubule, which is mediated by various transporters.

15. Which of the following is a medication used in the treatment of carcinoid syndrome?

   a. Telotristat
   b. Metformin
   c. Losartan
   d. Atorvastatin

   Answer: a) Telotristat. **Explanation:** Telotristat is a medication used in the treatment of carcinoid syndrome, a group of symptoms that occur in some people with neuroendocrine tumors. It is a tryptophan hydroxylase inhibitor that works by irreversibly binding to the active site of TPH, thereby preventing the conversion of tryptophan to 5-hydroxytryptophan (5-HTP), the precursor to serotonin. This results in a decrease in the synthesis and release of serotonin in the gastrointestinal tract, which leads to a reduction in the symptoms of carcinoid syndrome.

16. Which of the following cells in the pancreas are responsible for the production of insulin?

   a. Delta cells
   b. PP cells
   c. Alpha cells
   d. Beta cells

   Answer: d) Beta cells. **Explanation:** Beta cells are a type of islet cell in the pancreas responsible for the production of insulin, which enhances peripheral glucose uptake and inhibits hepatic gluconeogenesis and glycogenolysis.

17. Which of the following classes of medications works by inhibiting the H+/K+-ATPase proton pump on the surface of the parietal cells in the stomach?

   a. Somatostatin analogs
   b. H2 blockers
   c. Telotristat
   d. Proton pump inhibitors (PPIs)

   Answer: d) Proton pump inhibitors (PPIs). **Explanation:** Proton pump inhibitors (PPIs) are a class of acid-lowering drugs commonly used in the treatment of gastric acid-related disorders, including gastroesophageal reflux disease (GERD), peptic ulcers, and Zollinger–Ellison syndrome. PPIs work by irreversibly binding to and inhibiting the H+/K+-ATPase proton pump located on the apical surface of the parietal cells in the stomach, which inhibits the final step in gastric acid secretion, leading to a reduction in the amount of acid produced by the parietal cells.

18. Which of the following hormones is produced by delta cells in the pancreas?

   a. Somatostatin
   b. Glucagon
   c. Insulin
   d. Amylin

   Answer: a) Somatostatin. **Explanation:** Somatostatin is a peptide hormone that has a broad range of inhibitory effects on the endocrine system. It is produced by the delta cells in the pancreas and other neuroendocrine cells throughout the body. Somatostatin inhibits the secretion of various hormones, including serotonin, gastrin, insulin, glucagon, growth hormone, and thyroid-stimulating hormone.

19. Which cells in the stomach secrete gastrin in response to food stimuli?

    a. Parietal cells
    b. Delta cells
    c. G cells
    d. EC cells

    Answer: c) G cells. G cells located in the antrum of the stomach secrete the hormone gastrin in response to stimuli such as the presence of food.

20. What is the final step in gastric acid secretion?

    a. Release of gastrin by G cells
    b. Secretion of histamine by ECL cells
    c. Activation of the proton pump on the surface of the parietal cells
    d. Stimulation of M3 receptors on the parietal cells

    Answer: c) Activation of the proton pump on the surface of the parietal cells. The proton pump is responsible for the final step in gastric acid secretion. It actively transports H+ ions into the lumen of the stomach in exchange for K+ ions, creating a highly acidic environment that is necessary for the digestion of food and the activation of digestive enzymes.

21. Which hormone is produced by delta cells in the pancreas?

    a. Glucagon
    b. Insulin
    c. Somatostatin
    d. Pancreatic polypeptide

    Answer: c) Somatostatin. Delta cells in the pancreas produce somatostatin, which inhibits the secretion of various hormones, including serotonin, gastrin, insulin, glucagon, growth hormone, and thyroid-stimulating hormone. Somatostatin analogs are synthetic compounds that mimic the inhibitory effects of somatostatin on hormone secretion and can be used in the treatment of various endocrine disorders.

REFERENCES

1. Steiner, D.F., Park, S.-Y., Støy, J. et al. (2009). A brief perspective on insulin production. *Diabetes Obes. Metab.* 11 (Suppl 4): 189–196.

2. Davidson, H.W. (2004). (Pro)Insulin processing: a historical perspective. *Cell Biochem. Biophys.* 40: 143–158.

3. Fu, Z., Gilbert, E.R., and Liu, D. (2013). Regulation of insulin synthesis and secretion and pancreatic beta-cell dysfunction in diabetes. *Curr. Diabetes Rev.* 9: 25–53.

4. Norton, L., Shannon, C., Gastaldelli, A., and DeFronzo, R.A. (2022). Insulin: the master regulator of glucose metabolism. *Metabolism* 129: 155142.

5. Petersen, M.C. and Shulman, G.I. (2018). Mechanisms of insulin action and insulin resistance. *Physiol. Rev.* 98: 2133–2223.

6. Ramos, P.A., Lytle, K.A., Delivanis, D. et al. (2021). Insulin-stimulated muscle glucose uptake and insulin signaling in lean and obese humans. *J. Clin. Endocrinol. Metab.* 106: 1631–1646.

7. Chang, L., Chiang, S.-H., and Saltiel, A.R. (2004). Insulin signaling and the regulation of glucose transport. *Mol. Med.* 10: 65–71.

8. Wasserman, D.H. (2022). Insulin, muscle glucose uptake, and hexokinase: revisiting the road not taken. *Physiology* 37: 115–127.

9. Abdul-Ghani, M.A. and DeFronzo, R.A. (2010). Pathogenesis of insulin resistance in skeletal muscle. *J. Biomed. Biotechnol.* 2010: 476279.

10. Petersen, M.C., Vatner, D.F., and Shulman, G.I. (2017). Regulation of hepatic glucose metabolism in health and disease. *Nat. Rev. Endocrinol.* 13: 572–587.

11. Lewis, G.F., Carpentier, A.C., Pereira, S. et al. (2021). Direct and indirect control of hepatic glucose production by insulin. *Cell Metab.* 33: 709–720.

12. Boucher, J., Kleinridders, A., and Kahn, C.R. (2014). Insulin receptor signaling in normal and insulin-resistant states. *Cold Spring Harb. Perspect. Biol.* 6: a009191.

13. Belfiore, A., Malaguarnera, R., Vella, V. et al. (2017). Insulin receptor isoforms in physiology and disease: an updated view. *Endocr. Rev.* 38: 379–431.

14. Morigny, P., Houssier, M., Mouisel, E., and Langin, D. (2016). Adipocyte lipolysis and insulin resistance. *Biochimie* 125: 259–266.

15. Meshkani, R. and Adeli, K. (2009). Hepatic insulin resistance, metabolic syndrome and cardiovascular disease. *Clin. Biochem.* 42: 1331–1346.

16. Lee, S.-H., Park, S.-Y., and Choi, C.S. (2022). Insulin resistance: from mechanisms to therapeutic strategies. *Diabetes Metab. J.* 46: 15–37.

17. Aschner, P. (2020). Insulin therapy in type 2 diabetes. *Am. J. Ther.* 27: e79–e90.

18. Meneghini, L.F. (2013). Insulin therapy for type 2 diabetes. *Endocrine* 43: 529–534.

19. Janež, A., Guja, C., Mitrakou, A. et al. (2020). Insulin therapy in adults with type 1 diabetes mellitus: a narrative review. *Diabetes Ther* 11: 387–409.

20. King Hamad University Hospital, Bahrain. (2021). A double-blinded, placebo-controlled, phase 3 study to evaluate the efficacy and safety of ORMD-0801 in uncontrolled type 2 DM subjects on diet control alone, metformin monotherapy, or two or three oral glucose-lowering agents. `clinicaltrials.gov`

21. Lamos, E.M., Younk, L.M., and Davis, S.N. (2016). Concentrated insulins: the new basal insulins. *Ther. Clin. Risk Manag.* 12: 389–400.

22. (2015). An inhaled insulin (Afrezza). *JAMA* 313: 2176–2177.

23. Duckworth, W.C., Bennett, R.G., and Hamel, F.G. (1998). Insulin degradation: progress and potential. *Endocr. Rev.* 19: 608–624.

24. Rabkin, R., Ryan, M.P., and Duckworth, W.C. (1984). The renal metabolism of insulin. *Diabetologia* 27: 351–357.

25. Matteucci, E., Giampietro, O., Covolan, V. et al. (2015). Insulin administration: present strategies and future directions for a noninvasive (possibly more physiological) delivery. *Drug Des. Devel. Ther.* 9: 3109–3118.

26. Turnheim, K. and Waldhäusl, W.K. (1988). Essentials of insulin pharmacokinetics. *Wien. Klin. Wochenschr.* 100: 65–72.

27. Onishi, Y., Iwamoto, Y., Yoo, S.J. et al. (2013). Insulin degludec compared with insulin glargine in insulin-naïve patients with type 2 diabetes: a 26-week, randomized, controlled, Pan-Asian, treat-to-target trial. *J Diabetes Investig* 4: 605–612.

28. Riddle, M.C., Rosenstock, J., Gerich, J., and on behalf of the Insulin Glargine 4002 Study Investigators (2003). The treat-to-target trial: randomized addition of glargine or human NPH insulin to oral therapy of type 2 diabetic patients. *Diabetes Care* 26: 3080–3086.

29. Chen, M.-C., Sonaje, K., Chen, K.-J., and Sung, H.-W. (2011). A review of the prospects for polymeric nanoparticle platforms in oral insulin delivery. *Biomaterials* 32: 9826–9838.

30. La Rotta, H.C.E., Ciniciato, G.P.M.K., and González, E.R. (2011). Triphenylmethane dyes, an alternative for mediated electronic transfer systems in glucose oxidase biofuel cells. *Enzym. Microb. Technol.* 48: 487–497.

31. Marks, V. (2005). GLUCOSE | Metabolism and maintenance of blood glucose level*. In: *Encyclopedia of Human Nutrition*, 2nde (ed. B. Caballero), 398–404. Oxford: Elsevier.

32. Adeva-Andany, M.M., González-Lucán, M., Donapetry-García, C. et al. (2016). Glycogen metabolism in humans. *BBA Clin* 5: 85–100.

33. Glimcher, L.H. and Lee, A.-H. (2009). From sugar to fat. *Ann. N. Y. Acad. Sci.* 1173: E2–E9.

34. Flatt, J.P. (1970). Conversion of carbohydrate to fat in adipose tissue: an energy-yielding and, therefore, self-limiting process. *J. Lipid Res.* 11: 131–143.

35. Vallon, V. and Thomson, S.C. (2017). Targeting renal glucose reabsorption to treat hyperglycaemia: the pleiotropic effects of SGLT2 inhibition. *Diabetologia* 60: 215–225.

36. Mergenthaler, P., Lindauer, U., Dienel, G.A., and Meisel, A. (2013). Sugar for the brain: the role of glucose in physiological and pathological brain function. *Trends Neurosci.* 36: 587–597.

37. (2021). Gluconeogenesis- Reaction and regulation. `https://chem.libretexts.org/@go/page/234035`. Accessed 11 May 2023

38. Sanvictores, T., Casale, J., and Huecker, M.R. (2023). *Physiology, Fasting*. StatPearls.

39. Hanson, R.W. and Owen, O.E. (2013). Gluconeogenesis. In: *Encyclopedia of Biological Chemistry*, 2nde (ed. W.J. Lennarz and M.D. Lane), 381–386. Waltham: Academic Press.

40. Hatting, M., Tavares, C.D.J., Sharabi, K. et al. (2018). Insulin regulation of gluconeogenesis. *Ann. N. Y. Acad. Sci.* 1411: 21–35.

41. Gerich, J.E., Meyer, C., Woerle, H.J., and Stumvoll, M. (2001). Renal gluconeogenesis: its importance in human glucose homeostasis. *Diabetes Care* 24: 382–391.

42. Martin-Requero, A., Ayuso, M.S., and Parrilla, R. (1986). Rate-limiting steps for hepatic gluconeogenesis. Mechanism of oxamate inhibition of mitochondrial pyruvate metabolism. *J. Biol. Chem.* 261: 13973–13978.

43. Pilkis, S.J. and Granner, D.K. (1992). Molecular physiology of the regulation of hepatic gluconeogenesis and glycolysis. *Annu. Rev. Physiol.* 54: 885–909.

44. van Schaftingen, E. and Gerin, I. (2002). The glucose-6-phosphatase system. *Biochem. J.* 362: 513–532.

45. Bolaños, J.P., Almeida, A., and Moncada, S. (2010). Glycolysis: a bioenergetic or a survival pathway? *Trends Biochem. Sci.* 35: 145–149.

46. Cohen, P., Nimmo, H.G., and Proud, C.G. (1978). How does insulin stimulate glycogen synthesis? *Biochem. Soc. Symp.* 69–95.

47. Fang, X., Yu, S.X., Lu, Y. et al. (2000). Phosphorylation and inactivation of glycogen synthase kinase 3 by protein kinase A. *Proc. Natl. Acad. Sci. U. S. A.* 97: 11960–11965.

48. Patel, S., Doble, B., and Woodgett, J.R. (2004). Glycogen synthase kinase-3 in insulin and Wnt signalling: a double-edged sword? *Biochem. Soc. Trans.* 32: 803–808.

49. Paredes-Flores, M.A. and Mohiuddin, S.S. (2023). *Biochemistry, Glycogenolysis*. StatPearls.

50. Jiang, G. and Zhang, B.B. (2003). Glucagon and regulation of glucose metabolism. *Am J Physiol-Endocrinol Metab* 284: E671–E678.

51. Roach, P.J. (2002). Glycogen and its metabolism. *Curr. Mol. Med.* 2: 101–120.

52. Pernicova, I. and Korbonits, M. (2014). Metformin – mode of action and clinical implications for diabetes and cancer. *Nat. Rev. Endocrinol.* 10: 143–156.

53. LaMoia, T.E. and Shulman, G.I. (2021). Cellular and molecular mechanisms of metformin action. *Endocr. Rev.* 42: 77–96.

54. Gunton, J.E., Delhanty, P.J.D., Takahashi, S.-I., and Baxter, R.C. (2003). Metformin rapidly increases insulin receptor activation in human liver and signals preferentially through insulin-receptor substrate-2. *J. Clin. Endocrinol. Metab.* 88: 1323–1332.

55. Hardie, D.G., Ross, F.A., and Hawley, S.A. (2012). AMPK - a nutrient and energy sensor that maintains energy homeostasis. *Nat. Rev. Mol. Cell Biol.* 13: 251–262.

56. Rena, G., Hardie, D.G., and Pearson, E.R. (2017). The mechanisms of action of metformin. *Diabetologia* 60: 1577–1585.

57. Yendapally, R., Sikazwe, D., Kim, S.S. et al. (2020). A review of phenformin, metformin, and imeglimin. *Drug Dev. Res.* 81: 390–401.

58. Zhou, J., Massey, S., Story, D., and Li, L. (2018). Metformin: an old drug with new applications. *Int. J. Mol. Sci.* 19: 2863.

59. Davidson, M.B. and Peters, A.L. (1997). An overview of metformin in the treatment of type 2 diabetes mellitus. *Am. J. Med.* 102: 99–110.

60. Blough, B., Moreland, A., and Mora, A. (2015). Metformin-induced lactic acidosis with emphasis on the anion gap. *Proc. (Baylor Univ. Med. Cent.)* 28: 31–33.

61. Hur, K.Y., Kim, M.K., Ko, S.H. et al. (2020). Metformin treatment for patients with diabetes and chronic kidney disease: a Korean diabetes association and korean society of nephrology consensus statement. *Diabetes Metab. J.* 44: 3–10.

62. DeFronzo, R.A. and Goodman, A.M. (1995). Efficacy of metformin in patients with non-insulin-dependent diabetes mellitus. *N. Engl. J. Med.* 333: 541–549.

63. Rorsman, P., Eliasson, L., Renström, E. et al. (2000). The cell physiology of biphasic insulin secretion. *Physiology* 15: 72–77.

64. Gerich, J.E. (2002). is reduced first-phase insulin release the earliest detectable abnormality in individuals destined to develop type 2 diabetes? *Diabetes* 51: S117–S121.

65. Meier, J.J. (2016). Chapter 32 - Insulin secretion. In: *Endocrinology: Adult and Pediatric*, 7the (ed. J.L. Jameson, L.J. De Groot, D.M. de Kretser, et al.), 546–555.e5. Philadelphia: W.B. Saunders.

66. Rorsman, P. and Ashcroft, F.M. (2018). Pancreatic β-cell electrical activity and insulin secretion: of mice and men. *Physiol. Rev.* 98: 117–214.

67. Keane, K. and Newsholme, P. (2014). Metabolic regulation of insulin secretion. *Vitam. Horm.* https://doi.org/10.1016/B978-0-12-800174-5.00001-6.

68. Wiederkehr, A. and Wollheim, C.B. (2006). Minireview: implication of mitochondria in insulin secretion and action. *Endocrinology* 147: 2643–2649.

69. Rorsman, P. and Braun, M. (2013). Regulation of insulin secretion in human pancreatic islets. *Annu. Rev. Physiol.* 75: 155–179.

70. Taguchi, N., Aizawa, T., Sato, Y. et al. (1995). Mechanism of glucose-induced biphasic insulin release: physiological role of adenosine triphosphate-sensitive K+ channel-independent glucose action. *Endocrinology* 136: 3942–3948.

71. Henquin, J.C. (2009). Regulation of insulin secretion: a matter of phase control and amplitude modulation. *Diabetologia* 52: 739–751.

72. Ježek, P., Jabůrek, M., Holendová, B., and Plecitá-Hlavatá, L. (2018). Fatty acid-stimulated insulin secretion vs. Lipotoxicity. *Mol J Synth Chem Nat Prod Chem* 23: 1483.

73. Scott, L.J. (2012). Repaglinide: a review of its use in type 2 diabetes mellitus. *Drugs* 72: 249–272.

74. Guardado-Mendoza, R., Prioletta, A., Jiménez-Ceja, L.M. et al. (2013). The role of nateglinide and repaglinide, derivatives of meglitinide, in the treatment of type 2 diabetes mellitus. *Arch. Med. Sci.* 9: 936–943.

75. Weaver, M.L., Orwig, B.A., Rodriguez, L.C. et al. (2001). Pharmacokinetics and metabolism of nateglinide in humans. *Drug Metab. Dispos.* 29: 415–421.

76. Culy, C.R. and Jarvis, B. (2001). Repaglinide: a review of its therapeutic use in type 2 diabetes mellitus. *Drugs* 61: 1625–1660.

77. Hatorp, V. (2002). Clinical pharmacokinetics and pharmacodynamics of repaglinide. *Clin. Pharmacokinet.* 41: 471–483.

78. Milner, Z. and Akhondi, H. (2023). *Repaglinide.* StatPearls.

79. Pakkir Maideen, N.M., Manavalan, G., and Balasubramanian, K. (2018). Drug interactions of meglitinide antidiabetics involving CYP enzymes and OATP1B1 transporter. *Ther. Adv. Endocrinol. Metab.* 9: 259–268.

80. Derosa, G., Mugellini, A., Ciccarelli, L. et al. (2003). Comparison between repaglinide and glimepiride in patients with type 2 diabetes mellitus: a one-year, randomized, double-blind assessment of metabolic parameters and cardiovascular risk factors. *Clin. Ther.* 25: 472–484.

81. Derosa, G., Mugellini, A., Ciccarelli, L. et al. (2003). Comparison of glycaemic control and cardiovascular risk profile in patients with type 2 diabetes during treatment with either repaglinide or metformin. *Diabetes Res. Clin. Pract.* 60: 161–169.

82. Jovanovic, L., Hassman, D.R., Gooch, B. et al. (2004). Treatment of type 2 diabetes with a combination regimen of repaglinide plus pioglitazone. *Diabetes Res. Clin. Pract.* 63: 127–134.

83. Bennett, K., James, C., and Hussain, K. (2010). Pancreatic β-cell KATP channels: hypoglycaemia and hyperglycaemia. *Rev. Endocr. Metab. Disord.* 11: 157–163.

84. Panten, U., Schwanstecher, M., and Schwanstecher, C. (1996). Sulfonylurea receptors and mechanism of sulfonylurea action. *Exp Clin Endocrinol Diabetes Off J Ger Soc Endocrinol Ger Diabetes Assoc* 104: 1–9.

85. Principalli, M.A., Dupuis, J.P., Moreau, C.J. et al. (2015). Kir6.2 activation by sulfonylurea receptors: a different mechanism of action for SUR1 and SUR2A subunits via the same residues. *Physiol. Rep.* 3: e12533.

86. Proks, P., Reimann, F., Green, N. et al. (2002). Sulfonylurea stimulation of insulin secretion. *Diabetes* 51: S368–S376.

87. Ashcroft, F.M. (1996). Mechanisms of the glycaemic effects of sulfonylureas. *Horm Metab Res Horm Stoffwechselforschung Horm Metab* 28: 456–463.

88. Panten, U., Schwanstecher, M., and Schwanstecher, C. (1996). Mode of action of sulfonylureas. In: *Oral Antidiabetics* (ed. J. Kuhlmann and W. Puls), 129–159. Berlin, Heidelberg: Springer.

89. Gopalakrishnan, M., Molinari, E.J., Shieh, C.-C. et al. (2000). Pharmacology of human sulphonylurea receptor SUR1 and inward rectifier K+ channel Kir6.2 combination expressed in HEK-293 cells. *Br. J. Pharmacol.* 129: 1323–1332.

90. Ioannidis, I. (2014). Diabetes treatment in patients with renal disease: is the landscape clear enough? *World J. Diabetes* 5: 651–658.

91. Luzi, L. and Pozza, G. (1997). Glibenclamide: an old drug with a novel mechanism of action? *Acta Diabetol.* 34: 239–244.

92. Feldman, J.M. (1985). Glyburide: a second-generation sulfonylurea hypoglycemic agent. History, chemistry, metabolism, pharmacokinetics, clinical use and adverse effects. *Pharmacotherapy* 5: 43–62.

93. Szoke, E., Gosmanov, N.R., Sinkin, J.C. et al. (2006). Effects of glimepiride and glyburide on glucose counterregulation and recovery from hypoglycemia. *Metab. Clin. Exp.* 55: 78–83.

94. Betônico, C.C.R., Titan, S.M.O., Correa-Giannella, M.L.C. et al. (2016). Management of diabetes mellitus in individuals with chronic kidney disease: therapeutic perspectives and glycemic control. *Clinics* 71: 47–53.

95. Sola, D., Rossi, L., Schianca, G.P.C. et al. (2015). Sulfonylureas and their use in clinical practice. *Arch. Med. Sci.* 11: 840–848.

96. KnowledgeDose (2019). *Sulfonylureas: Site of Action, Pharmacokinetics & Dose Conversion.* KnowledgeDose https://www.knowledgedose.com/sulfonylureas-site-of-action-pharmacokinetics-dose-conversion/.

97. Skillman, T.G. and Feldman, J.M. (1981). The pharmacology of sulfonylureas. *Am. J. Med.* 70: 361–372.

98. Malmberg, K. (1997). Prospective randomised study of intensive insulin treatment on long term survival after acute myocardial infarction in patients with diabetes mellitus. DIGAMI (Diabetes Mellitus, Insulin Glucose Infusion in Acute Myocardial Infarction) Study Group. *BMJ* 314: 1512–1515.

99. Terao, Y., Ayaori, M., Ogura, M. et al. (2011). Effect of sulfonylurea agents on reverse cholesterol transport in vitro and vivo. *J. Atheroscler. Thromb.* 18: 513–530.

100. Rosenstock, J., Kahn, S.E., Johansen, O.E. et al. (2019). Effect of linagliptin vs glimepiride on major adverse cardiovascular outcomes in patients with

type 2 diabetes: the Carolina randomized clinical trial. *JAMA* 322: 1155–1166.

101. GRADE Study Research Group, Nathan, D.M., Lachin, J.M. et al. (2022). Glycemia reduction in type 2 diabetes - glycemic outcomes. *N. Engl. J. Med.* 387: 1063–1074.

102. Lopez Vicchi, F., Luque, G.M., Brie, B. et al. (2016). Dopaminergic drugs in type 2 diabetes and glucose homeostasis. *Pharmacol. Res.* 109: 74–80.

103. Cincotta, A.H., Meier, A.H., and Cincotta, M. (1999). Bromocriptine improves glycaemic control and serum lipid profile in obese Type 2 diabetic subjects: a new approach in the treatment of diabetes. *Expert Opin. Investig. Drugs* 8: 1683–1707.

104. Rubí, B., Ljubicic, S., Pournourmohammadi, S. et al. (2005). Dopamine D2-like receptors are expressed in pancreatic beta cells and mediate inhibition of insulin secretion*. *J. Biol. Chem.* 280: 36824–36832.

105. Shivaprasad, C. and Kalra, S. (2011). Bromocriptine in type 2 diabetes mellitus. *Indian J Endocrinol Metab* 15: S17–S24.

106. DeFronzo, R.A. (2011). Bromocriptine: a sympatholytic, D2-dopamine agonist for the treatment of type 2 diabetes. *Diabetes Care* 34: 789–794.

107. Valiquette, G. (2011). Bromocriptine for diabetes mellitus type II. *Cardiol. Rev.* 19: 272.

108. Gaziano, J.M., Cincotta, A.H., O'Connor, C.M. et al. (2010). Randomized clinical trial of quick-release bromocriptine among patients with type 2 diabetes on overall safety and cardiovascular outcomes. *Diabetes Care* 33: 1503–1508.

109. Jay, M.A. and Ren, J. (2007). Peroxisome proliferator-activated receptor (PPAR) in metabolic syndrome and type 2 diabetes mellitus. *Curr. Diabetes Rev.* 3: 33–39.

110. Ferré, P. (2004). The biology of peroxisome proliferator-activated receptors: relationship with lipid metabolism and insulin sensitivity. *Diabetes* 53: S43–S50.

111. Grygiel-Górniak, B. (2014). Peroxisome proliferator-activated receptors and their ligands: nutritional and clinical implications - a review. *Nutr. J.* 13: 17.

112. Viswakarma, N., Jia, Y., Bai, L. et al. (2010). Coactivators in PPAR-regulated gene expression. *PPAR Res.* 2010: e250126.

113. Leonardini, A., Laviola, L., Perrini, S. et al. (2010). Cross-Talk between PPAR and Insulin Signaling and Modulation of Insulin Sensitivity. *PPAR Res.* 2009: 818945.

114. Smith, U. (2001). Pioglitazone: mechanism of action. *Int. J. Clin. Pract. Suppl.* September (121): 13–18.

115. Kobayashi, M., Iwanishi, M., Egawa, K., and Shigeta, Y. (1992). Pioglitazone increases insulin sensitivity by activating insulin receptor kinase. *Diabetes* 41: 476–483.

116. McLaughlin, T.M., Liu, T., Yee, G. et al. (2010). Pioglitazone increases the proportion of small cells in human abdominal subcutaneous adipose tissue. *Obes Silver Spring Md* 18: 926–931.

117. DeFronzo, R.A., Inzucchi, S., Abdul-Ghani, M., and Nissen, S.E. (2019). Pioglitazone: the forgotten, cost-effective cardioprotective drug for type 2 diabetes. *Diab. Vasc. Dis. Res.* 16: 133–143.

118. Wang, Y.-X. (2010). PPARs: diverse regulators in energy metabolism and metabolic diseases. *Cell Res.* 20: 124–137.

119. Mudaliar, S., Chang, A.R., and Henry, R.R. (2003). Thiazolidinediones, peripheral edema, and type 2 diabetes: incidence, pathophysiology, and clinical implications. *Endocr Pract Off J Am Coll Endocrinol Am Assoc Clin Endocrinol* 9: 406–416.

120. Kernan, W.N., Viscoli, C.M., Furie, K.L. et al. (2016). Pioglitazone after ischemic stroke or transient ischemic attack. *N. Engl. J. Med.* 374: 1321–1331.

121. Dormandy, J.A., Charbonnel, B., Eckland, D.J.A. et al. (2005). Secondary prevention of macrovascular events in patients with type 2 diabetes in the PROactive study (PROspective pioglitAzone clinical trial in macrovascular events): a randomised controlled trial. *Lancet Lond Engl* 366: 1279–1289.

122. Mari, A., Bagger, J.I., Ferrannini, E. et al. (2013). Mechanisms of the incretin effect in subjects with normal glucose tolerance and patients with type 2 diabetes. *PLoS ONE* 8: e73154.

123. Nauck, M.A. and Meier, J.J. (2018). Incretin hormones: their role in health and disease. *Diabetes Obes. Metab.* 20: 5–21.

124. Drucker, D.J. (2006). The biology of incretin hormones. *Cell Metab.* 3: 153–165.

125. Nauck, M.A., Quast, D.R., Wefers, J., and Pfeiffer, A.F.H. (2021). The evolving story of incretins (GIP and GLP-1) in metabolic and cardiovascular disease: a pathophysiological update. *Diabetes Obes. Metab.* 23: 5–29.

126. Holst, J.J. (2019). The incretin system in healthy humans: the role of GIP and GLP-1. *Metabolism* 96: 46–55.

127. Gilbert, M.P. and Pratley, R.E. (2020). GLP-1 analogs and DPP-4 inhibitors in type 2 diabetes therapy: review of head-to-head clinical trials. *Front. Endocrinol.* 11: 178.

128. Marso, S.P., Daniels, G.H., Brown-Frandsen, K. et al. (2016). Liraglutide and cardiovascular outcomes in type 2 diabetes. *N. Engl. J. Med.* 375: 311–322.

129. Ahrén, B., Masmiquel, L., Kumar, H. et al. (2017). Efficacy and safety of once-weekly semaglutide versus once-daily sitagliptin as an add-on to metformin, thiazolidinediones, or both, in patients with type 2 diabetes (SUSTAIN 2): a 56-week, double-blind, phase 3a, randomised trial. *Lancet Diabetes Endocrinol.* 5: 341–354.

130. Athauda, D., Maclagan, K., Skene, S.S. et al. (2017). Exenatide once weekly versus placebo in Parkinson's disease: a randomised, double-blind, placebo-controlled trial. *Lancet Lond Engl* 390: 1664–1675.

131. DeFronzo, R.A., Ratner, R.E., Han, J. et al. (2005). Effects of exenatide (exendin-4) on glycemic control and weight over 30 weeks in metformin-treated patients with type 2 diabetes. *Diabetes Care* 28: 1092–1100.

132. Semenya, A.M. and Wilson, S.A. (2020). Oral semaglutide (rybelsus) for the treatment of type 2 diabetes mellitus. *Am. Fam. Physician* 102: 627–628.

133. Gerstein, H.C., Colhoun, H.M., Dagenais, G.R. et al. (2019). Dulaglutide and cardiovascular outcomes in type 2 diabetes (REWIND): a double-blind, randomised placebo-controlled trial. *Lancet Lond Engl* 394: 121–130.

134. Frias, J.P., Nauck, M.A., Van, J. et al. (2020). Efficacy and tolerability of tirzepatide, a dual glucose-dependent insulinotropic peptide and glucagon-like peptide-1 receptor agonist in patients with type 2 diabetes: a 12-week, randomized, double-blind, placebo-controlled study to evaluate different dose-escalation regimens. *Diabetes Obes. Metab.* 22: 938–946.

135. Davies, M.J., Drexel, H., Jornayvaz, F.R. et al. (2022). Cardiovascular outcomes trials: a paradigm shift in the current management of type 2 diabetes. *Cardiovasc. Diabetol.* 21: 144.

136. (2008). Guidance for industry on diabetes mellitus-evaluating cardiovascular risk in new antidiabetic therapies to treat type 2 diabetes. Availability. In: Fed. Regist. https://www.federalregister.gov/documents/2008/12/19/E8-30086/guidance-for-industry-on-diabetes-mellitus-evaluating-cardiovascular-risk-in-new-antidiabetic.

137. Nissen, S.E. and Wolski, K. (2007). Effect of rosiglitazone on the risk of myocardial infarction and death from cardiovascular causes. *N. Engl. J. Med.* 356: 2457–2471.

138. Zinman, B., Wanner, C., Lachin, J.M. et al. (2015). Empagliflozin, cardiovascular outcomes, and mortality in type 2 diabetes. *N. Engl. J. Med.* 373: 2117–2128.

139. Holman, R.R., Sourij, H., and Califf, R.M. (2014). Cardiovascular outcome trials of glucose-lowering drugs or strategies in type 2 diabetes. *Lancet Lond Engl* 383: 2008–2017.

140. Schnell, O., Standl, E., Catrinoiu, D. et al. (2018). Report from the 3rd cardiovascular outcome trial (CVOT) summit of the diabetes & cardiovascular disease (D&CVD) EASD study group. *Cardiovasc. Diabetol.* 17: 30.

141. Marso, S.P., Bain, S.C., Consoli, A. et al. (2016). Semaglutide and cardiovascular outcomes in patients with type 2 diabetes. *N. Engl. J. Med.* 375: 1834–1844.

142. Pfeffer, M.A., Claggett, B., Diaz, R. et al. (2015). Lixisenatide in patients with type 2 diabetes and acute coronary syndrome. *N. Engl. J. Med.* 373: 2247–2257.

143. Prato, S.D., Kahn, S.E., Pavo, I. et al. (2021). Tirzepatide versus insulin glargine in type 2 diabetes and increased cardiovascular risk (SURPASS-4): a randomised, open-label, parallel-group, multicentre, phase 3 trial. *Lancet* 398: 1811–1824.

144. Cox, E.J., Alicic, R.Z., Neumiller, J.J., and Tuttle, K.R. (2020). *Clinical Evidence and Proposed Mechanisms for Cardiovascular and Kidney Benefits from Glucagon-Like Peptide-1 Receptor Agonists.* US Endocrinol.

145. Ussher, J.R. and Drucker, D.J. (2023). Glucagon-like peptide 1 receptor agonists: cardiovascular benefits and mechanisms of action. *Nat. Rev. Cardiol.* 20 (7): 463–474.

146. Ghezzi, C., Loo, D.D.F., and Wright, E.M. (2018). Physiology of renal glucose handling via SGLT1, SGLT2 and GLUT2. *Diabetologia* 61: 2087–2097.

147. Ferrannini, E. (2017). Sodium-glucose co-transporters and their inhibition: clinical physiology. *Cell Metab.* 26: 27–38.

148. Wright, E.M. (2021). SGLT2 inhibitors: physiology and pharmacology. *Kidney360* 2: 2027–2037.

149. Nair, S. and Wilding, J.P.H. (2010). Sodium glucose cotransporter 2 inhibitors as a new treatment for diabetes mellitus. *J. Clin. Endocrinol. Metab.* 95: 34–42.

150. Fonseca-Correa, J.I. and Correa-Rotter, R. (2021). Sodium-glucose cotransporter 2 inhibitors mechanisms of action: a review. *Front. Med.* 8: 777861.

151. Vallon, V. and Verma, S. (2021). Effects of SGLT2 inhibitors on kidney and cardiovascular function. *Annu. Rev. Physiol.* 83: 503–528.

152. Padda, I.S., Mahtani, A.U., and Parmar, M. (2023). *Sodium-Glucose Transport Protein 2 (SGLT2) Inhibitors*. StatPearls.

153. Neal, B., Perkovic, V., Mahaffey, K.W. et al. (2017). Canagliflozin and cardiovascular and renal events in type 2 diabetes. *N. Engl. J. Med.* 377: 644–657.

154. Wiviott, S.D., Raz, I., Bonaca, M.P. et al. (2019). Dapagliflozin and cardiovascular outcomes in type 2 diabetes. *N. Engl. J. Med.* 380: 347–357.

155. Röhrborn, D., Wronkowitz, N., and Eckel, J. (2015). DPP4 in Diabetes. *Front. Immunol.* 6: 386.

156. Deacon, C.F. (2019). Physiology and pharmacology of DPP-4 in glucose homeostasis and the treatment of type 2 diabetes. *Front. Endocrinol.* 10: 80.

157. Gallwitz, B. (2019). Clinical use of DPP-4 inhibitors. *Front. Endocrinol.* 10: 389.

158. Godinho, R., Mega, C., Teixeira-de-Lemos, E. et al. (2015). The place of dipeptidyl peptidase-4 inhibitors in type 2 diabetes therapeutics: a "me too" or "the special one" antidiabetic class? *J. Diabetes Res.* 2015: e806979.

159. Nielsen, L.L. (2005). Incretin mimetics and DPP-IV inhibitors for the treatment of type 2 diabetes. *Drug Discov. Today* 10: 703–710.

160. Farngren, J. and Ahrén, B. (2019). Incretin-based medications (GLP-1 receptor agonists, DPP-4 inhibitors) as a means to avoid hypoglycaemic episodes. *Metabolism* 99: 25–31.

161. Herman, G.A., Stevens, C., Van Dyck, K. et al. (2005). Pharmacokinetics and pharmacodynamics of sitagliptin, an inhibitor of dipeptidyl peptidase IV, in healthy subjects: results from two randomized, double-blind, placebo-controlled studies with single oral doses. *Clin. Pharmacol. Ther.* 78: 675–688.

162. Boulton, D.W. (2017). Clinical pharmacokinetics and pharmacodynamics of saxagliptin, a dipeptidyl peptidase-4 inhibitor. *Clin. Pharmacokinet.* 56: 11–24.

163. Fuchs, H., Runge, F., and Held, H.-D. (2012). Excretion of the dipeptidyl peptidase-4 inhibitor linagliptin in rats is primarily by biliary excretion and P-gp-mediated efflux. *Eur J Pharm Sci Off J Eur Fed Pharm Sci* 45: 533–538.

164. Yagoglu, A.I., Dizdar, O.S., Erdem, S. et al. (2020). The effect of linagliptin on renal progression in type-2 diabetes mellitus patients with chronic kidney disease: a prospective randomized controlled study. *Nefrologia* 40: 664–671.

165. Béliard Veillard, R. and Pinto, B. (2018). *DPP-IV Inhibitors*. Johns Hopkins Diabetes Guide `https://www.hopkinsguides.com/hopkins/view/Johns_Hopkins_Diabetes_Guide/547042/all/DPP_IV_Inhibitors`.

166. Alogliptin. `https://go.drugbank.com/drugs/DB06203`.

167. White, W.B., Cannon, C.P., Heller, S.R. et al. (2013). Alogliptin after acute coronary syndrome in patients with type 2 diabetes. *N. Engl. J. Med.* 369: 1327–1335.

168. Green, J.B., Bethel, M.A., Armstrong, P.W. et al. (2015). Effect of sitagliptin on cardiovascular outcomes in type 2 diabetes. *N. Engl. J. Med.* 373: 232–242.

169. Sim, L., Willemsma, C., Mohan, S. et al. (2010). Structural basis for substrate selectivity in human maltase-glucoamylase and sucrase-isomaltase N-terminal domains. *J. Biol. Chem.* 285: 17763–17770.

170. Gericke, B., Schecker, N., Amiri, M., and Naim, H.Y. (2017). Structure-function analysis of human sucrase-isomaltase identifies key residues required for catalytic activity. *J. Biol. Chem.* 292: 11070–11078.

171. Kuttel, M.M. and Naidoo, K.J. (2005). Free energy surfaces for the alpha(1 --> 4)-glycosidic linkage: implications for polysaccharide solution structure and dynamics. *J. Phys. Chem. B* 109: 7468–7474.

172. DiNicolantonio, J.J., Bhutani, J., and O'Keefe, J.H. (2015). Acarbose: safe and effective for lowering postprandial hyperglycaemia and improving cardiovascular outcomes. *Open Heart* 2: e000327.

173. Altay, M. (2022). Acarbose is again on the stage. *World J. Diabetes* 13: 1–4.

174. Coniff, R. and Krol, A. (1997). Acarbose: a review of US clinical experience. *Clin. Ther.* 19: 16–26. discussion 2-3.

175. Rosak, C., Nitzsche, G., König, P., and Hofmann, U. (1995). The effect of the timing and the administration of acarbose on postprandial hyperglycaemia. *Diabet Med J Br Diabet Assoc* 12: 979–984.

176. Jenney, A., Proietto, J., O'Dea, K. et al. (1993). Low-dose acarbose improves glycemic control in

NIDDM patients without changes in insulin sensitivity. *Diabetes Care* 16: 499–502.

177. Holman, R.R., Coleman, R.L., Chan, J.C.N. et al. (2017). Effects of acarbose on cardiovascular and diabetes outcomes in patients with coronary heart disease and impaired glucose tolerance (ACE): a randomised, double-blind, placebo-controlled trial. *Lancet Diabetes Endocrinol.* 5: 877–886.

178. Ludvik, B., Kautzky-Willer, A., Prager, R. et al. (1997). Amylin: history and overview. *Diabet Med J Br Diabet Assoc* 14 (Suppl 2): S9–S13.

179. Kiriyama, Y. and Nochi, H. (2018). Role and cytotoxicity of amylin and protection of pancreatic islet β-cells from amylin cytotoxicity. *Cell* 7: 95.

180. Padhi, S., Nayak, A.K., and Behera, A. (2020). Type II diabetes mellitus: a review on recent drug based therapeutics. *Biomed. Pharmacother.* 131: 110708.

181. McQueen, J. (2005). Pramlintide acetate. *Am J Health-Syst Pharm AJHP Off J Am Soc Health-Syst Pharm* 62: 2363–2372.

182. Ramkissoon, C.M., Aufderheide, B., Bequette, B.W., and Palerm, C.C. (2014). A model of glucose-insulin-pramlintide pharmacokinetics and pharmacodynamics in type I diabetes. *J. Diabetes Sci. Technol.* 8: 529–542.

183. Whitehouse, F., Kruger, D.F., Fineman, M. et al. (2002). A randomized study and open-label extension evaluating the long-term efficacy of pramlintide as an adjunct to insulin therapy in type 1 diabetes. *Diabetes Care* 25: 724–730.

184. Diabetes Prevention Program (DPP) - NIDDK. In: Natl. Inst. Diabetes Dig. Kidney Dis. https://www.niddk.nih.gov/about-niddk/research-areas/diabetes/diabetes-prevention-program-dpp.

185. Diabetes Control and Complications Trial Research Group, Nathan, D.M., Genuth, S. et al. (1993). The effect of intensive treatment of diabetes on the development and progression of long-term complications in insulin-dependent diabetes mellitus. *N. Engl. J. Med.* 329: 977–986.

186. Epidemiology of Diabetes Interventions and Complications (EDIC) Research Group (1999). Epidemiology of diabetes interventions and complications (EDIC). Design, implementation, and preliminary results of a long-term follow-up of the diabetes control and complications trial cohort. *Diabetes Care* 22: 99–111.

187. Holman, R.R., Paul, S.K., Bethel, M.A. et al. (2008). 10-year follow-up of intensive glucose control in type 2 diabetes. *N. Engl. J. Med.* 359: 1577–1589.

188. Frazer, A. and Hensler, J.G. (1999). Chapter 13 – Serotonin. In: *Basic Neurochemistry: Molecular, Cellular and Medical Aspects*, 6ee (ed. G.J. Siegel, B.W. Agranoff, R.W. Albers, et al.). Philadelphia: Lippincott-Raven https://www.ncbi.nlm.nih.gov/books/NBK20375/.

189. Lyseng-Williamson, K.A. (2018). Telotristat ethyl: a review in carcinoid syndrome diarrhoea. *Drugs* 78: 941–950.

190. Kasi, P.M. (2018). Telotristat ethyl for the treatment of carcinoid syndrome diarrhea not controlled by somatostatin analogues. *Drugs Today (Barc.)* 54: 423–432.

191. Kulke, M.H., Hörsch, D., Caplin, M.E. et al. (2016). Telotristat ethyl, a tryptophan hydroxylase inhibitor for the treatment of carcinoid syndrome. *J. Clin. Oncol.* 35: 14–23.

192. Pavel, M., Gross, D.J., Benavent, M. et al. (2018). Telotristat ethyl in carcinoid syndrome: safety and efficacy in the TELECAST phase 3 trial. *Endocr. Relat. Cancer* 25: 309–322.

193. Zippi M, Fiorino S, Budriesi R, Micucci M, Corazza I, Pica R, Biase D de, Gallo CG, Hong W (2021). Paradoxical relationship between proton pump inhibitors and COVID-19: a systematic review and meta-analysis. *World J. Clin. Cases* 9:2763–2777

194. Paniccia, A. and Schulick, R.D. (2017). Chapter 4 - Pancreatic physiology and functional assessment. In: *Blumgart's Surgery of the Liver, Biliary Tract and Pancreas, 2-Volume Set*, 6the (ed. W.R. Jarnagin), 66–76.e3. Philadelphia: Elsevier.

195. Da Silva, X.G. (2018). The cells of the islets of langerhans. *J. Clin. Med.* https://doi.org/10.3390/jcm7030054.

196. Brereton, M.F., Vergari, E., Zhang, Q., and Clark, A. (2015). Alpha-, Delta- and PP-cells. *J. Histochem. Cytochem.* 63: 575–591.

197. Kiriyama, Y. and Nochi, H. (2018). Role and cytotoxicity of amylin and protection of pancreatic islet β-cells from amylin cytotoxicity. *Cells.* https://doi.org/10.3390/cells7080095.

198. Briant, L., Salehi, A., Vergari, E. et al. (2016). Glucagon secretion from pancreatic α-cells. *Ups. J. Med. Sci.* 121: 113–119.

199. Iki, K. and Pour, P.M. (2007). Distribution of pancreatic endocrine cells including IAPP-expressing

cells in non-diabetic and type 2 diabetic cases. *J Histochem Cytochem Off J Histochem Soc* 55: 111–118.

200. Napolitano, T., Silvano, S., Vieira, A. et al. (2018). Role of ghrelin in pancreatic development and function. *Diabetes Obes. Metab.* 20 (Suppl 2): 3–10.

201. Smith, J.P., Fonkoua, L.K., and Moody, T.W. (2016). The role of gastrin and CCK receptors in pancreatic cancer and other malignancies. *Int. J. Biol. Sci.* 12: 283–291.

202. Tsoukalas, N., Chatzellis, E., Rontogianni, D. et al. (2017). Pancreatic carcinoids (serotonin-producing pancreatic neuroendocrine neoplasms). *Medicine (Baltimore)* `https://doi.org/10.1097/MD.0000000000006201`.

203. La Rosa, S., Franzi, F., Albarello, L. et al. (2011). Serotonin-producing enterochromaffin cell tumors of the pancreas: clinicopathologic study of 15 cases and comparison with intestinal enterochromaffin cell tumors. *Pancreas* 40: 883–895.

204. Tomita, T. (2002). New markers for pancreatic islets and islet cell tumors. *Pathol. Int.* 52: 425–432.

205. Geron, E., Boura-Halfon, S., Schejter, E.D., and Shilo, B.-Z. (2015). The edges of pancreatic islet β cells constitute adhesive and signaling microdomains. *Cell Rep.* 10: 317–325.

206. Mikami, S. and Mutoh, K. (1971). Light- and electron-microscopic studies of the pancreatic islet cells in the chicken under normal and experimental conditions. *Z Für Zellforsch Mikrosk Anat* 116: 205–227.

207. Rossi, R.E., Elvevi, A., Citterio, D. et al. (2021). Gastrinoma and Zollinger Ellison syndrome: a roadmap for the management between new and old therapies. *World J. Gastroenterol.* 27: 5890–5907.

208. Shin, J.M. and Sachs, G. (2008). Pharmacology of proton pump inhibitors. *Curr. Gastroenterol. Rep.* 10: 528–534.

209. Lew, E.A., Pisegna, J.R., Starr, J.A. et al. (2000). Intravenous pantoprazole rapidly controls gastric acid hypersecretion in patients with Zollinger–Ellison syndrome. *Gastroenterology* 118: 696–704.

210. Imamura, M., Komoto, I., and Taki, Y. (2022). How to treat gastrinomas in patients with multiple endocrine neoplasia type1: surgery or long-term proton pump inhibitors? *Surg. Today* `https://doi.org/10.1007/s00595-022-02627-z`.

211. Liu, Y., Vosmaer, G.D.C., Tytgat, G.N.J. et al. (2005). Gastrin (G) cells and somatostatin (D) cells in patients with dyspeptic symptoms: helicobacter pylori associated and non-associated gastritis. *J. Clin. Pathol.* 58: 927–931.

212. Wängberg, B., Nilsson, O., Theodorsson, E. et al. (1991). The effect of a somatostatin analogue on the release of hormones from human midgut carcinoid tumour cells. *Br. J. Cancer* 64: 23–28.

213. Hindmarsh, P.C., Brain, C.E., Robinson, I.C. et al. (1991). The interaction of growth hormone releasing hormone and somatostatin in the generation of a GH pulse in man. *Clin. Endocrinol.* 35: 353–360.

214. Modlin, I.M., Pavel, M., Kidd, M., and Gustafsson, B.I. (2010). Review article: somatostatin analogues in the treatment of gastroenteropancreatic neuroendocrine (carcinoid) tumours. *Aliment. Pharmacol. Ther.* 31: 169–188.

215. Costa, F. and Gumz, B. (2014). Octreotide – a review of its use in treating neuroendocrine tumours. *Eur Endocrinol* 10: 70–74.

216. Enzler, T. and Fojo, T. (2017). Long-acting somatostatin analogues in the treatment of unresectable/metastatic neuroendocrine tumors. *Semin. Oncol.* 44: 141–156.

217. Stueven, A.K., Kayser, A., Wetz, C. et al. (2019). Somatostatin analogues in the treatment of neuroendocrine tumors: past, present and future. *Int. J. Mol. Sci.* 20: 3049.

218. Caplin, M.E., Pavel, M., Ćwikła, J.B. et al. (2014). Lanreotide in metastatic enteropancreatic neuroendocrine tumors. *N. Engl. J. Med.* 371: 224–233.

219. Rinke, A., Müller, H.-H., Schade-Brittinger, C. et al. (2009). Placebo-controlled, double-blind, prospective, randomized study on the effect of octreotide LAR in the control of tumor growth in patients with metastatic neuroendocrine midgut tumors: a report from the PROMID Study Group. *J. Clin. Oncol. Off. J. Am. Soc. Clin. Oncol.* 27: 4656–4663.

220. Hou, W. and Schubert, M.L. (2007). Treatment of gastric carcinoids. *Curr Treat Options Gastroenterol* 10: 123–133.

221. Bertherat, J., Tenenbaum, F., Perlemoine, K. et al. (2003). Somatostatin receptors 2 and 5 are the major somatostatin receptors in insulinomas: an in vivo and in vitro study. *J. Clin. Endocrinol. Metab.* 88: 5353–5360.

222. Peltola, E., Vesterinen, T., Leijon, H. et al. Immunohistochemical somatostatin receptor expression in insulinomas. *APMIS* `https://doi.org/10.1111/apm.13297`.

223. Haris, B., Saraswathi, S., and Hussain, K. (2020). Somatostatin analogues for the treatment of hyperinsulinaemic hypoglycaemia. *Ther. Adv. Endocrinol. Metab.* 11: 2042018820965068.

224. Portela-Gomes, G.M., Stridsberg, M., Grimelius, L. et al. (2007). Differential expression of the five somatostatin receptor subtypes in human benign and malignant insulinomas - predominance of receptor subtype 4. *Endocr. Pathol.* 18: 79–85.

225. Matej, A., Bujwid, H., and Wroński, J. (2016). Glycemic control in patients with insulinoma. *Hormones* 15: 489–499.

226. Sprague, J.E. and Arbeláez, A.M. (2011). Glucose counterregulatory responses to hypoglycemia. *Pediatr Endocrinol Rev PER* 9: 463–475.

227. Newman-Lindsay, S., Lakshminrusimha, S., and Sankaran, D. (2022). Diazoxide for neonatal hyperinsulinemic hypoglycemia and pulmonary hypertension. *Child Basel Switz* 10: 5.

228. Yasuda, A., Seki, T., Kitajima, N. et al. (2020). A case of insulinoma effectively treated with low-dose diazoxide. *Clin Case Rep* 8: 1884–1889.

229. Baudin, E., Caron, P., Lombard-Bohas, C. et al. (2013). Malignant insulinoma: recommendations for characterisation and treatment. *Ann. Endocrinol.* 74: 523–533.

230. Ulbrecht, J.S., Schmeltz, R., Aarons, J.H., and Greene, D.A. (1986). Insulinoma in a 94-year-old woman: long-term therapy with verapamil. *Diabetes Care* 9: 186–188.

231. Taye, A. and Libutti, S.K. (2015). Diagnosis and management of insulinoma: current best practice and ongoing developments. *Res Rep Endocr Disord* 5: 125–133.

232. Lamberti, G., Brighi, N., Maggio, I. et al. (2018). The role of mTOR in neuroendocrine tumors: future cornerstone of a winning strategy? *Int. J. Mol. Sci.* 19: 747.

233. Vinik, A.I. (2014). Advances in diagnosis and treatment of pancreatic neuroendocrine tumors. *Endocr. Pract.* 20: 1222–1230.

234. Zhan, H.-X., Cong, L., Zhao, Y.-P. et al. (2012). Activated mTOR/P70S6K signaling pathway is involved in insulinoma tumorigenesis. *J. Surg. Oncol.* 106: 972–980.

235. Bollard, J., Patte, C., Massoma, P. et al. (2018). Combinatorial treatment with mTOR inhibitors and streptozotocin leads to synergistic in vitro and in vivo antitumor effects in insulinoma cells. *Mol. Cancer Ther.* 17: 60–72.

236. Baratelli, C., Brizzi, M.P., Tampellini, M. et al. (2014). Intermittent everolimus administration for malignant insulinoma. *Endocrinol. Diabetes Metab. Case Rep.* 2014: 140047.

237. Bernard, V., Lombard-Bohas, C., Taquet, M.-C. et al. (2013). Efficacy of everolimus in patients with metastatic insulinoma and refractory hypoglycemia. *Eur. J. Endocrinol.* 168: 665–674.

238. Mathur, A., Gorden, P., and Libutti, S.K. (2009). Insulinoma. *Surg. Clin. North Am.* 89: 1105–1121.

239. Aderka D, Shaklai M, Doron M, Laron Z, Pinkhas J, Vries A de (1975). Phenytoin in metastatic insulinoma. *JAMA* 234:1119

240. Cryer, P.E., Axelrod, L., Grossman, A.B. et al. (2009). Evaluation and management of adult hypoglycemic disorders: an Endocrine Society Clinical Practice Guideline. *J. Clin. Endocrinol. Metab.* 94: 709–728.

CHAPTER 5

Parathyroid Gland and Bone Therapies

5.1 PRIMARY HYPERPARATHYROIDISM

5.1.1 Calcimimetics

5.1.1.1 Physiology

Regulation of Serum Calcium and Phosphorus

The regulation of serum calcium and phosphorus is dependent on an intricate relationship between parathyroid hormone (PTH), $1\alpha,25$ dihydroxyvitamin D ($1\alpha,25$ [OH]$_2$D), and fibroblast growth factor 23 (FGF23). The skeleton, gastrointestinal tract, and kidneys are the principal sites of action of these key regulators of serum calcium and phosphorus [1]. The skeleton serves as an extensive repository of total body calcium and phosphorus. It is worth noting that bone comprises calcium and phosphorus-containing hydroxyapatite crystals ($Ca_{10}(PO_4)_6(OH)_2$), collagenous and noncollagenous proteins. Indeed, approximately 99% (about 1 kg in a healthy adult) [2] and 85% (about 700 g) of total body calcium and phosphorus are present in bone, respectively [2, 3]. Consequently, only 0.1% of calcium and about 1% of phosphorus exist in the extracellular fluid compartment [2].

Parathyroid hormone facilitates calcium reabsorption and phosphate excretion via the kidneys. PTH is also critical in the hydroxylation of 25 hydroxyvitamin D (25-OHD) at its 1α position, resulting in calcitriol formation ($1\alpha,25(OH)_2$D). Calcitriol subsequently promotes intestinal calcium and phosphate conservation (see Section 5.2.2) [4]. Additionally, PTH indirectly activates osteoclasts responsible for the liberation of calcium and phosphorus from the skeleton (see Section 5.1.2) [5].

FGF23 inhibits both renal phosphate conservation and calcitriol formation, which results in a net effect of a reduced level of serum calcium and phosphorus (see Section 5.4.2) [6].

Calcitonin, a less characterized hormone in calcium physiology, reduces calcium resorption from skeletal stores and also inhibits renal reabsorption of calcium [7]. This explains the utility of calcitonin in the acute treatment of hypercalcemia (see Section 5.3.2) [8].

Calcium Sensing and PTH Regulation

Calcium is required for various bodily functions, including hormonal secretion, muscle contraction, coagulation, neural transmission, to mention a few [9, 10]. Calcium exists in several forms in extracellular fluid. These include its free or ionized form (about 50% of circulating calcium), albumin-bound (~40%), and complexed form (~10% bound to anions such as bicarbonate, citrate, phosphates, and citrate) [11].

The calcium-sensing receptor (CaSR), a G-protein-coupled receptor expressed by chief cells of the

Endocrinology: Pathophysiology to Therapy, First Edition. Akuffo Quarde.
© 2024 John Wiley & Sons Ltd. Published 2024 by John Wiley & Sons Ltd.

parathyroid gland [12], C cells of the thyroid, and renal tubules, plays a pivotal role in regulating serum calcium. The activation of CaSR inhibits the synthesis and eventual release of PTH by the parathyroids, augments calcitonin release by C cells of the thyroid [13] (see Section 5.3.2), and finally inhibits renal calcium reabsorption (independent of PTH action) [14] (see Section 5.2.2).

At the level of the parathyroid glands, CaSR activation by ionized calcium (an extracellular first messenger) results in downstream processes (Phospholipase C-Inositol triphosphate-diacylglycerol pathway), which increases the liberation of calcium from its stores in the endoplasmic reticulum [15, 16]. Increased intracellular calcium inhibits the fusion of PTH-containing vesicles with the plasma membrane, which results in reduced secretion of PTH. Additionally, the transcription and translation of PTH are regulated by $1\alpha,25(OH)_2D$ (binding of active vitamin D to

vitamin D response elements in the promoter region of the PTH gene promotes PTH synthesis) (not shown) [17, 18]. Similarly, magnesium, another relevant extracellular divalent cation, can also activate the CaSR and impair PTH synthesis [15].

5.1.1.2 Mechanism of Action

Calcimimetics promote the sensitivity of the CaSR to serum calcium by lowering the set point for activation of the receptor. This, in effect, leads to the activation of the CaSR even at lower levels of ionized calcium, a process that inhibits PTH release [19]. In contrast to divalent cations (calcium and magnesium), which bind the amino-terminal domain of the CaSR, calcimimetics bind to the 7-transmembrane domain of the receptor (see Figure 5.1). Calcimimetics promote a conformational change in the CaSR, resulting in increased receptor sensitivity to extracellular calcium

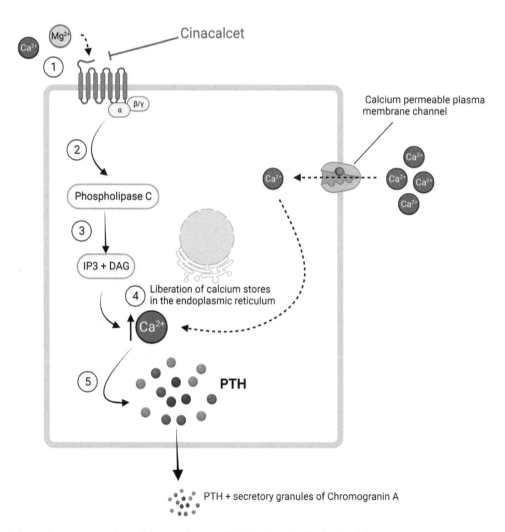

FIGURE 5.1 Schematic representation of the regulation of PTH release by ionized calcium.

(a positive allosteric effect) [20, 21]. Ultimately, these agents reduce serum calcium by inhibiting PTH secretion and promote renal calcium excretion [21]. Cinacalcet is a prototypical calcimimetic utilized in the medical management of primary hyperparathyroidism [22, 23].

Practice Pearl(s)

- Serum calcium should be checked within a week of a dose change of cinacalcet *(sensipar).*
- Hypotension and arrhythmias are possible severe reactions. Nausea and diarrhea are, however, more likely side effects [24].
- Indications for cinacalcet use in PHPT include poor surgical candidates (or refusal of surgery) and those with hypercalcemia refractory to curative parathyroidectomy [25].

Clinical Trial Evidence

Cinacalcet is FDA-approved for the management of significant hypercalcemia in primary hyperparathyroidism.

Key Message

Cinacalcet can lead to >1 mg/dL decline in serum calcium from baseline in patients with primary hyperparathyroidism.

In this phase three, double-blind, multicenter randomized placebo-controlled trial, 140 subjects were randomized to either cinacalcet or placebo. Inclusion criteria included total corrected serum calcium between 11.3 and 12.5 mg/dl, failed parathyroidectomy, or poor surgical candidates. The primary outcome (normalization of serum calcium) was assessed at 28 weeks, after which subjects in both arms were enrolled in an open-label extension phase of the study. The primary outcome occurred in 84.8% of subjects in the intervention arm and 5.9% in the placebo arm. This was statistically significant. Interestingly, adverse events (nausea and muscle spasms) were similar between both arms of the study [26].

Clinical Pearl

What is "von Recklinghausen's disease of bone"?

Osteitis fibrosa cystica (OFC), also known as "von Recklingshausen's disease of bone," was first reported in 1891 [27]. However, the association between this condition and a parathyroid tumor was clearly demonstrated by Dr. Felix Mandl in 1925 after the removal of a parathyroid tumor in a patient with radiographic features consistent with OFC, which resulted in a dramatic resolution of hypercalciuria and bone pain [28]. Primary hyperparathyroidism (PHPT) is a cause of hypercalcemia and has a highly variable reported incidence rate. However, there are no population-based estimates of the prevalence of this condition [29]. It is characterized by hypercalcemia in the setting of elevated or inappropriately normal serum intact parathyroid hormone. Autonomous parathyroid hormone production, either in a single parathyroid adenoma or multiple adenomas, accounts for manifestations of this condition. Kidney stones, fragility fractures (osteoporosis), and symptomatic hypercalcemia are known complications. The indications for surgical treatment in primary hyperparathyroidism include the following, age < 50 years, serum calcium greater than 1 mg/dl above the upper limit of normal, osteoporosis, estimated glomerular filtration rate < 60 ml/min/1.73 m², and nephrolithiasis/urolithiasis [23]. Medical therapy may serve as a bridge to surgery or a reasonable alternative to surgery in special circumstances. For example, patients not deemed optimal surgical candidates may be managed with medical therapy [22].

5.1.2 Bisphosphonates

5.1.2.1 Physiology

PTH-Mediated Osteoclastogenesis

PTH has a dual effect on bone remodeling (resorption-formation sequence), depending on whether the skeleton is continuously or intermittently exposed to PTH. Chronic and persistent exposure of the skeleton to elevated levels of PTH typical of PHPT results in bone resorption, while intermittent exposure (for example, treatment of osteoporosis with PTH analogs) promotes bone formation (see Section 5.5.3) [30, 31].

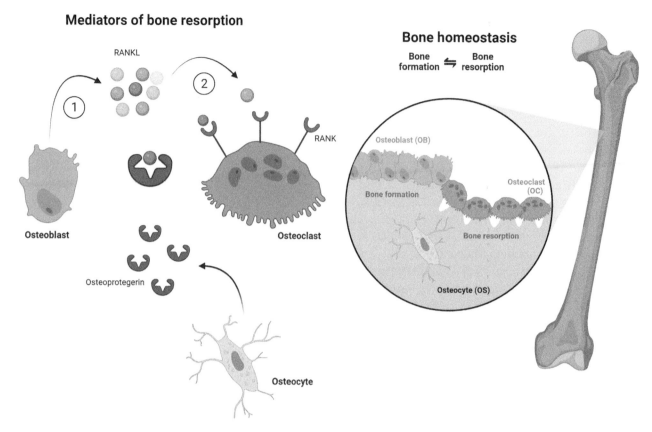

Mediators of bone resorption

Bone homeostasis

FIGURE 5.2   The role of PTH in osteoblast–osteoclast interaction.

Osteoblasts are the primary target for PTH action in bone. The role of PTH in bone resorption will be reviewed next (see Figure 5.2).

PTH binds to its cognate PTH-1R receptor on osteoblasts (derived from mesenchymal stem cells), thereby initiating the process of bone resorption. Consequently, osteoblast surface-bound *receptor activator of nuclear factor kappa-B ligand* (RANK-L) will bind to the RANK receptor present on osteoclasts (derived from hematopoietic stem cells) [32]. This results in the activation and differentiation of a precursor osteoclast into a matured osteoclast. The liberation of calcium and phosphorus from hydroxyapatite crystals by matured osteoclasts occurs in bone resorption pits. OPG, a decoy receptor (alternate binding site) for RANK-L, reduces osteoclast activation [33, 34].

Cholesterol Synthesis in Osteoclasts

Cholesterol synthesis is required for the maintenance of cellular membrane integrity and function in various tissues, including the skeleton. In osteoclasts, farnesyl pyrophosphate synthase (FPPS) plays a critical role in the mevalonic acid-cholesterol synthesis pathway [35].

5.1.2.2   Mechanism of Action

Nitrogen-containing bisphosphonates inhibit FPPS in osteoclasts [36]. Although the enzyme FPPS is present in several tissues, its inhibition by bisphosphonates occurs selectively at the level of the skeleton. This is due to the preferential deposition of bisphosphonates in hydroxyapatite crystals present in the skeleton [37]. Activated osteoclasts dissolve bisphosphonate-laden hydroxyapatite crystals during bone resorption and consequently ingest bisphosphonates. Impaired lipid synthesis in osteoclasts promotes their eventual apoptosis (inhibition of bone resorption) [35]. A schematic representation of the mechanism of action of bisphosphonates is shown in Figure 5.3.

Practice Pearl(s)

The exact duration of treatment with bisphosphonate therapy is unclear in PHPT. Also, see Sections 5.3.1 and 5.5.1.

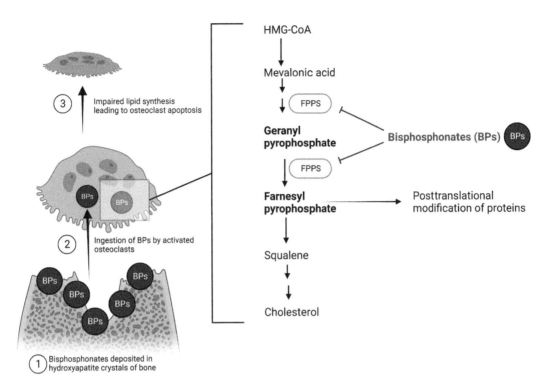

FIGURE 5.3   The mechanism of action of nitrogen-containing bisphosphonates in osteoclasts. The steps involved include an initial deposition of bisphosphonates in hydroxyapatite crystals, followed by their ingestion by activated osteoclasts and final osteoclast apoptosis due to impaired synthesis of cholesterol.

Clinical Trial Evidence
Bisphosphonates can lower serum calcium acutely, although they do not lead to a sustained normalization of serum calcium over an extended period of time [38].

Key Message

Bisphosphonates promote bone mineral density (BMD) at mainly trabecular sites (lumbar spine and hip), although their effect on fracture incidence in patients with PHPT remains unclear.

In this randomized, double-blind, placebo-controlled trial, patients with asymptomatic PHPT who did not meet the criteria for surgery or refused surgery were randomized to 10 mg of oral alendronate daily or placebo for 12 months. There was an additional 12-month phase after the first year, where both arms received alendronate. After 24 months of therapy, subjects in the alendronate arm experienced a statistically significant increase in bone mineral density at the lumbar spine and hip, compared to placebo [39].

 Concepts to Ponder Over

What is pseudohyperparathyroidism?

Pseudohyperparathyroidism is a benign cause of hypercalcemia in pregnant or lactating mothers. It is characterized by hypercalcemia, an appropriately suppressed serum PTH and high serum parathyroid hormone-related protein (PTHrp) in the absence of

(continued)

(continued)

malignancy [40]. Although PTHrp is typically associated with humoral hypercalcemia of malignancy, it can also be secreted by the placenta and breast tissue as part of a normal physiologic state (see Section 5.5.4) [41].

Discuss the effects of either medical therapy or curative parathyroidectomy on cortical and trabecular bone in primary hyperparathyroidism.

Although PHPT promotes the loss of cortical bone (distal third radius) to a greater extent than it does trabecular bone (hip and lumbar), medical treatment with a bisphosphonate or curative parathyroidectomy does not necessarily lead to an appreciable increase in BMD at the third distal radius at the expense of trabecular sites [42–44]. It is worth noting that classically, the rate of bone turnover at the distal third radius is relatively slow; thus, antiresorptive therapy is expected to cause a very minimal change in BMD at this site [39]. Also, PHPT expands the remodeling space of trabecular bone to a greater degree than it does cortical bone. This makes the trabecular site of

bone an ideal location for remineralization after surgery or bisphosphonate therapy [31, 42].

The human skeleton consists of cortical and trabecular compartments, representing 80% and 20% of total bone mass, respectively. Trabecular bone is principally composed of marrow and fat (~80%) and only 20% bone; nonetheless, its unique microarchitecture facilitates the transfer of mechanical stressors from the articular to the cortical surface of bone critical in maintaining bone function (see Section 5.5.1; Table 5.1) [47].

TABLE 5.1   Comparison of the percentage of cortical and trabecular at the femoral neck, lumbar spine, and distal radius.

Bone location	Cortical bone (%)	Trabecular bone (%)
Femoral neck	75	25
Lumbar spine	34	66
Distal radius	95	5

Source: Adapted from Refs. [45, 46].

5.2   HYPOPARATHYROIDISM

5.2.1   Thiazide Diuretics

5.2.1.1   Physiology

The distal convoluted tubule (DCT) is a critical site of renal calcium regulation and is responsible for the absorption of ~10% of filtered calcium in the nephron. In contrast to other sections of the nephron, which absorb calcium through largely paracellular routes, the DCT exclusively conserves calcium through active transcellular transporters [48]. The additional sites of renal calcium handling include the proximal convoluted tubule (PCT) (60–70% of filtered calcium) and the thick ascending limb of the loop of Henle (about 25% of filtered calcium) [1]. Active transcellular transport in the DCT is regulated by parathyroid hormone and calcitonin. Conversely, passive paracellular transport in the TALH and PCT is facilitated through non-hormone-dependent processes [49, 50] (see Section 5.2.2). The role of the thiazide-sensitive sodium chloride cotransporter will be reviewed next (see Figure 5.4).

Calcium influx across the apical membrane (i.e. from the glomerular ultrafiltrate into the cytosol of the DCT) is an active transport process mediated by the transient receptor potential vanilloid 5 (TRPV5) protein. Afterward, calbindin-D28K (a calcium-binding protein not depicted in the figure) ferries intracytosolic calcium through the cytosol to the basolateral membrane of the DCT. At this stage, ionized calcium will be pumped into the peritubular capillary fluid by the type 1 sodium-calcium exchanger (NCX1) and type 1 plasma membrane calcium ATPase protein (PMCA1) [50, 51]. Source: Adapted from [51].

The role of calcitriol and calcitonin is described in Section 5.2.2.

5.2.1.2   Mechanism of Action

1. Inhibition of the thiazide-sensitive Sodium-chloride cotransporter NCC by thiazide diuretics promotes the loss of sodium and chloride (see Figure 5.4). As a result, there is a compensatory increase in sodium reabsorption at the proximal tubule with the aim of restoring extracellular volume [52]. Sodium conservation at the level of the proximal tubule consequently

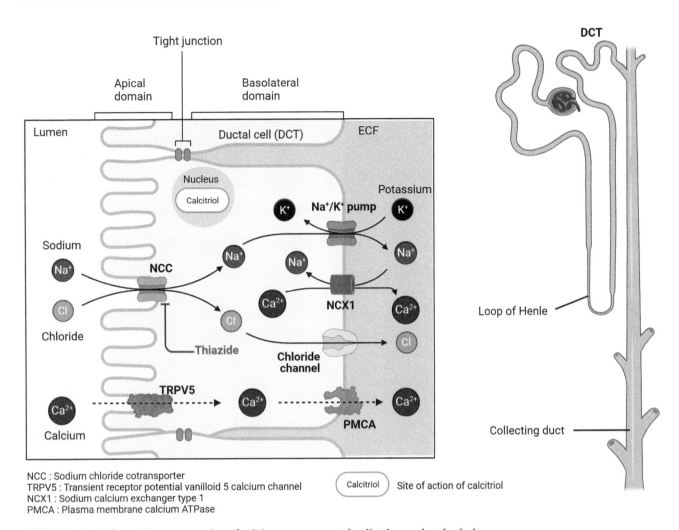

NCC : Sodium chloride cotransporter
TRPV5 : Transient receptor potential vanilloid 5 calcium channel
NCX1 : Sodium calcium exchanger type 1
PMCA : Plasma membrane calcium ATPase

(Calcitriol) Site of action of calcitriol

FIGURE 5.4   Schematic representation of calcium transport at the distal convoluted tubule.

leads to calcium conservation as well (coupling of sodium and water conservation to calcium reabsorption) [52, 53]. This accounts for the hypocalciuric effect of thiazide diuretics [51].

2. The blood pressure-lowering effect of thiazides activates the renin–angiotensin–aldosterone system, which then drives sodium (and calcium) conservation at the proximal tubule [51].

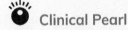 **Clinical Pearl**

Hypoparathyroidism is a relatively rare endocrine condition compared to PHPT. The biochemical profile of patients with this disorder includes serum calcium below the lower limit of the normal reference range and either an undetectable or inappropriately low serum PTH. Hypoparathyroidism in up to 75% of patients can be attributed to neck surgery. Chronic management of this condition includes the use of calcium supplements, vitamin D analogs, thiazide diuretics, and recombinant human PTH(1–84) [54].

These are the general management goals of hypoparathyroidism

(continued)

(*continued*)

24-hour urine calcium should be in the normal reference range. For patients with hypercalciuria, reduce sodium and calcium intake and start a thiazide diuretic.

- The serum calcium-phosphate product <55 mg^2/dL^2.
- Serum magnesium and 25-OHD should be within normal.

- Serum calcium should be either close to the low normal range or no more than 0.5 mg/dL below the lower limit of normal.
- Phosphate binders or a low phosphate diet is recommended for patients with serum phosphorus >6.5 mg/dL [55].

Practice Pearl(s)

Thiazide diuretics are indicated in patients with severe hypercalciuria, although the risk for diuretic-induced renal losses of potassium and magnesium should be borne in mind [54, 56].

Clinical Trial Evidence

There are no available long-term randomized controlled studies on the use of thiazide diuretics in hypoparathyroidism.

 Pathophysiology Pearl

Furosemide-induced hypercalciuria

Furosemide is utilized in the acute treatment of hypercalcemia. This is dependent on furosemide's effect on the paracellular transport of calcium at the TALH [57] (Figure 5.5).

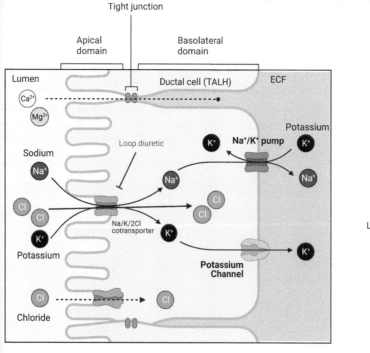
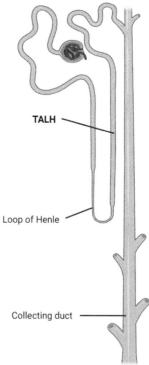

Na/K/2Cl cotransporter: Sodium potassium chloride symporter

FIGURE 5.5   Mechanism of action of furosemide at the TALH.

Maintenance of a positive luminal transepithelial voltage gradient is required to facilitate the paracellular transport of divalent cations (calcium and magnesium) from the ultrafiltrate into peritubular capillaries. The apical Na/K/2Cl cotransporter and renal outer medullary potassium K$^+$ (ROMK) are required to generate the necessary voltage gradient necessary for the sustenance of divalent cation transport [57]. Furosemide inhibits the Na$^+$/K$^+$/2Cl$^-$ symporter on the apical membrane of the TALH, which consequently impairs the positive transepithelial voltage gradient required for calcium and magnesium reabsorption [50, 51].

5.2.2 Active Vitamin D

5.2.2.1 Physiology

1 alpha, 25 dihydroxyvitamin D (1α,25(OH)$_2$D), also referred to as calcitriol (active vitamin D), plays a central role in the handling of renal and intestinal calcium.

Renal Calcium Absorption

See Figure 5.6.

Calcitriol diffuses through the basolateral membranes of the DCT and subsequently engages its cognate cytosolic vitamin D receptor (VDR). The calcitriol–VDR complex then traverses the nuclear membrane to bind to hormone response elements (HREs) present in DNA. As a result, there is an increase in the transcription and translation of calcium channels and pumps, including TRPV5, NCX1, and PMCA1 [58, 59] (also see Figure 5.4).

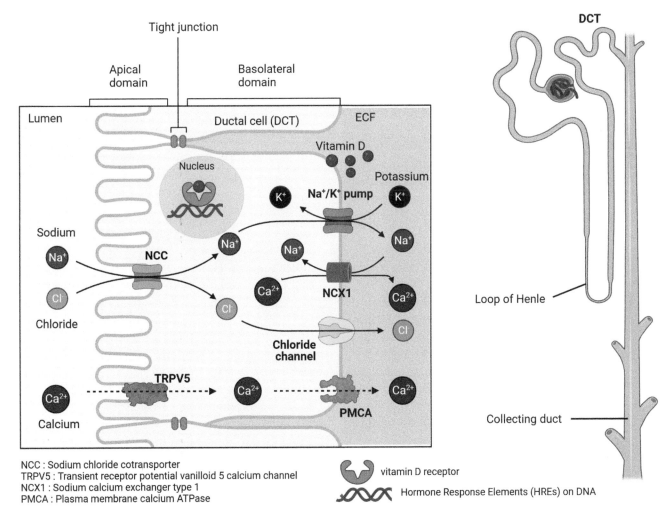

NCC : Sodium chloride cotransporter
TRPV5 : Transient receptor potential vanilloid 5 calcium channel
NCX1 : Sodium calcium exchanger type 1
PMCA : Plasma membrane calcium ATPase

vitamin D receptor

Hormone Response Elements (HREs) on DNA

FIGURE 5.6 Mechanism of action of calcitriol at the distal renal tubular cell.

Intestinal Calcium Absorption

Intestinal calcium absorption involves both passive paracellular transport through tight junctions and active transcellular transport across enterocytes, involving TRPV6 channels, calbindin proteins, PMCA, and NCX. Paracellular transport refers to the movement of calcium ions through the spaces between epithelial cells, which are regulated by tight junctions. This process does not require energy and occurs passively due to a concentration gradient [60].

Tight junctions, made up of proteins such as claudins and occludins, form barriers between cells that regulate the passage of ions and solutes [61]. The permeability of these tight junctions to calcium ions depends on the extracellular calcium concentration and the presence of CaSR. When activated by high extracellular calcium levels, CaSR can increase the permeability of tight junctions, allowing more calcium ions to pass through. Transcellular transport involves the movement of calcium ions across the enterocytes (intestinal epithelial cells) from the apical (luminal) side to the basolateral (blood-facing) side.

Calcium ions enter the enterocytes through channels called TRPV6 (transient receptor potential vanilloid 6) present in the apical membrane. TRPV6 channels are highly selective for calcium ions and facilitate their influx from the intestinal lumen into the cells [62].

Once inside the enterocytes, calcium ions are bound to cytoplasmic proteins, mainly calbindin-D9k and calbindin-D28k. These proteins serve as intracellular calcium buffers and shuttle calcium ions across the cell toward the basolateral membrane. This prevents an increase in free cytosolic calcium concentrations, which could otherwise lead to toxic effects [63].

The calcium ions are then actively transported across the basolateral membrane into the bloodstream. This is facilitated by the plasma membrane calcium ATPase (PMCA) and the sodium-calcium exchanger (NCX). PMCA uses ATP to pump calcium ions out of the cell against their concentration gradient, while NCX utilizes the sodium gradient to extrude calcium ions in exchange for sodium ions. Both transporters work together to maintain low intracellular calcium concentrations and ensure efficient calcium absorption [64] (Figure 5.7).

Calcitriol diffuses into the intestinal epithelial cell. The binding of calcitriol to the nuclear VDR leads to the transcription of NCX1, TRPV6 (ubiquitously expressed in the intestine), and calbindin. These

calcium channels and exchangers facilitate the translocation of calcium from the intestinal lumen into the intestinal capillary network [65].

5.2.2.2 Mechanism of Action

Calcitriol, by increasing both intestinal and renal calcium conservation, increases serum calcium in the setting of hypoparathyroidism.

Practice Pearl(s)

Calcitriol has a short half-life ($t_{1/2}$) of 4–6 hours. Consequently, it has a quick onset of action (1–3 days) and offset of action [66].

Although not previously discussed in this chapter, 25-OHD undergoes conversion to $1\alpha,25(OH)_2D$ at nonrenal sites by 1α-hydroxylase (a PTH-independent process) [66]. Supplementation with either ergocalciferol (vitamin D2) or cholecalciferol (vitamin D3) is, therefore, reasonable even in hypoparathyroidism [67].

Clinical Trial Evidence

Alfacalcidol and calcitriol are routinely utilized in the care of patients with hypoparathyroidism in Europe and North America, respectively [54].

Key Message

Active vitamin D (alfacalcidol or calcitriol) leads to the maintenance of normocalcemia in hypoparathyroidism. However, this therapeutic benefit occurs at the expense of an increased risk of hyperphosphatemia and hypercalciuria.

In this open-label, randomized-controlled, single-center study, a total of 45 subjects with hypoparathyroidism were treated with either alfacalcidol (1-hydroxycholecalciferol) or calcitriol. The between-group difference in serum calcium at six months was not statistically significant. Serum calcium was 8.7 mg/dL in the alfacalcidol group and 8.9 mg/dL in the calcitriol group. More importantly, events of clinically significant hypercalciuria and hyperphosphatemia were no different between both arms of the study [68].

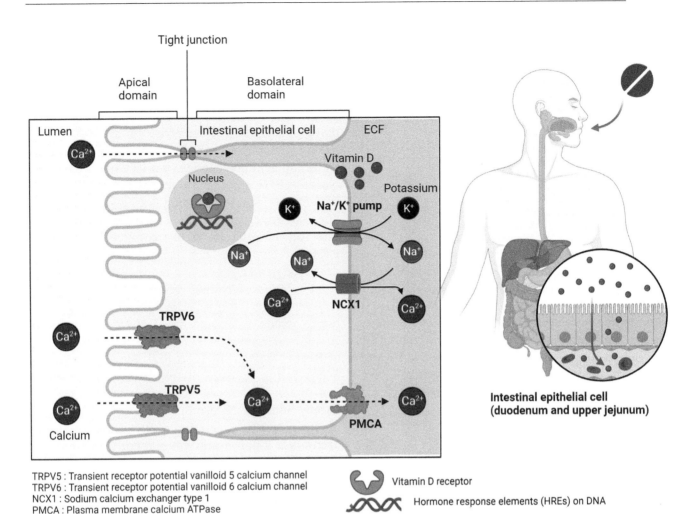

TRPV5 : Transient receptor potential vanilloid 5 calcium channel
TRPV6 : Transient receptor potential vanilloid 6 calcium channel
NCX1 : Sodium calcium exchanger type 1
PMCA : Plasma membrane calcium ATPase

Vitamin D receptor

Hormone response elements (HREs) on DNA

FIGURE 5.7 Intestinal handling of calcium. *Source:* Adapted from [65].

5.2.3 Calcium

5.2.3.1 Physiology

The role of serum calcium in regulating PTH release was discussed earlier in Section 5.1.1 The relationship between serum-ionized calcium and PTH is shown in Figure 5.8.

The activation of CaSR on parathyroid glands by ionized calcium reduces PTH secretion (described in Section 5.1.1). The steep slope of the sigmoidal curve highlights the degree of responsiveness of parathyroid glands to changes in serum calcium within the physiologic range (narrow band) See Figure 5.8. At extremes of serum calcium, either below or above the normal range of serum calcium, the curve flattens out. The setpoint depicted by the arrow is the amount of serum-ionized calcium that results in 50% of the maximum PTH secretory potential of the parathyroid glands [69]. PTH secretion is inhibited by elevated ionized calcium above the set point of the CaSR. Conversely, low ionized calcium below the set point of the CaSr promotes the release of PTH [70].

5.2.3.2 Mechanism of Action

The role of calcium in various bodily functions was described in Section 5.1.1.

Practice Pearl(s)

- Dairy products, although a rich source of calcium, have concomitantly high levels of phosphorus (hypoparathyroid glands ism is characterized by hyperphosphatemia at baseline).
- Calcium carbonate contains about 40% elemental calcium by weight. It is, however, limited by the need for normal gastric acidity and its significant constipating effect.

(continued)

(continued)

- Calcium citrate is a suitable alternative to calcium carbonate because it does not require normal gastric acidity and is not generally associated with constipation. It contains about 21% elemental calcium by molecular weight [54].

Clinical Trial Evidence

In this retrospective cohort study, a total of 14 patients with chronic hypoparathyroidism were switched from daily oral calcium (median intake of calcium carbonate was 3750 mg/day) to an alternate daily regimen with a median intake of 1500 mg/day. Symptomatic hypocalcemic events were compared between the preintervention (three months) and postintervention (three months) periods. There was a statistically significant decline in symptomatic hypocalcemic events leading to emergency room visits, from 21 to 3 visits during the study period [71].

Key Message

Calcium carbonate administered via an alternate daily schedule (every other day) can improve compliance and reduce episodes of symptomatic hypocalcemia.

5.2.4   Recombinant Human PTH

5.2.4.1   Physiology

The initial messenger RNA (ribonucleic acid) transcript produced by the PTH gene is a 115 amino acid polypeptide precursor referred to as pre-proPTH. Pre-proPTH is then processed into an intermediate 90 amino acid polypeptide (pro-PTH) [72]. The final bioactive PTH, an 84 amino acid peptide is co-secreted with chromogranin A (a ubiquitous glycoprotein produced by endocrine cells) via secretory vesicles [73]. The role of calcium in mediating the process of PTH secretion by the parathyroid glands was described earlier.

The amino terminal (N-terminal) end of PTH is responsible for the biological action of PTH at target organs expressing the PTH-1R receptor [74]. In contrast, the carboxy-terminal (C-terminal) end of PTH is biologically inert [75]. Bioactive PTH has a circulating half-life of approximately 4 minutes and rapidly undergoes metabolism in the liver and kidney into its N-terminal and C-terminal fragments [72, 76]. Clearance of the C-terminal end occurs via kidneys and consequently accumulates in chronic renal insufficiency. The liver is responsible for the clearance of the N-terminal end of PTH [74, 76].

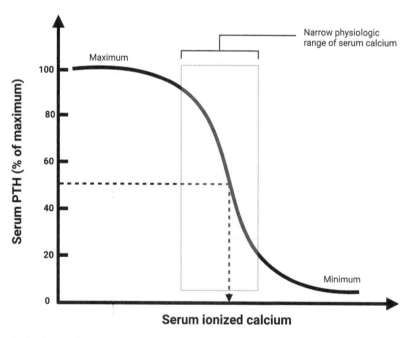

FIGURE 5.8   The sigmoidal relationship between serum ionized calcium and parathyroid hormone secretion.

5.2.4.2 Mechanism of Action

Recombinant human (rh) parathyroid hormone rhPTH(1–84) regulates calcium and phosphorus homeostasis through various mechanistic pathways.

1. PTH promotes phosphaturia by inhibiting the function of sodium-phosphate cotransporters in the proximal renal tubule, which promotes the normalization of serum phosphate in hypoparathyroidism (see Section 5.4.1) [77].
2. PTH promotes calcium reabsorption from the kidneys and intestines due to its pivotal role in the formation of $1\alpha,25(OH)_2D$ (see Section 5.2.2) [77].

rhPTH(1–84) has a pharmacokinetic profile that allows for once-daily administration, making it an ideal agent in managing hypoparathyroidism. In contrast, PTH(1–34) is approved for the management of osteoporosis but not hypoparathyroidism. This is because the shorter half-life of PTH(1–34) (a truncated form of endogenous PTH) results in suboptimal maintenance of normocalcemia with once-daily administration [72].

Practice Pearl(s)

- Musculoskeletal complaints are the most common adverse side effect of rhPTH (1–84) [78].

Clinical Trial Evidence

In the landmark REPLACE trial, a double-blind, placebo-controlled study, patients with confirmed hypoparathyroidism were randomized in a 2:1 assignment ratio to either 50 micrograms(mcg) (titrated by protocol to 75 or 100 mcg) of rhPTH(1–84) or matching placebo. The primary outcome was defined as the proportion of subjects who experienced a 50% or greater reduction in the total daily dose of calcium or active vitamin D, while sustaining eucalcemia. 53% of subjects in the intervention arm compared to 2% in the placebo arm experienced the primary outcome(percentage difference in groups of 51.1%, 95% CI 39.9–62.3; $p < 0.0001$) [79].

Key Message

Long-term therapy with rhPTH(1–84) results in significant reductions in the need for calcium, calcitriol, or thiazide diuretics (ameliorates hypercalciuria) [78, 79].

 Concepts to Ponder Over

What is pseudohypoparathyroidism?

This condition is characterized by hypocalcemia, hyperphosphatemia, and a paradoxically high serum PTH (resistance to PTH action) [80]. It occurs because of a loss-of-function mutation in the *guanine nucleotide-binding protein, alpha stimulating polypeptide* (GNAS) gene, which encodes the alpha subunit of the stimulatory G protein responsible for the downstream effects of PTH to PTH-1R receptor interaction. The classic clinical features of this condition include short stature, brachydactyly, obesity, and round facies [80, 81].

Furthermore, resistance to PTH action in the proximal renal tubule leads to hypocalcemia and hyperphosphatemia, similar to what would be found in isolated hypoparathyroidism patients. Patients, however, show paradoxical elevations of serum PTH levels; hence the name *pseudohypoparathyroidism* [80].

The guanine nucleotide-binding protein alpha stimulating (GNAS) gene plays an essential role in the transcription of stimulatory G protein (Gsα). Gsα is expressed biallelically across tissues – this means there are distinct paternal and maternal alleles required for its expression. Consequently, clinical and biochemical features depend on which parent gave rise to a mutant allele [82].

Normal paternal Gsα gene expression does not occur in proximal renal tubules, pituitary glands, or gonadal tissue. Therefore, this gene does not play any role in renal electrolyte handling (calcium and phosphorus). The paternal Gsα gene expression occurs primarily in skeletal tissue [83]. Hence, a child who inherits an altered paternal Gsα gene will present with pseudopseudohypoparathyroidism (PPHP) (i.e. short stature

(continued)

(continued)

without apparent biochemical or hormonal perturbations) [84].

Maternal Gsa gene expression determines most of the downstream effects of Gsa-coupled receptors in extra-skeletal tissues, including the pituitary gland, kidneys, and gonadal tissues. Furthermore, both maternal and paternal Gsα genes are expressed in skeletal tissue. Consequently, a mutation in the maternal Gsα gene results in classic Pseudohypoparathyroidism type 1A phenotype [85, 86].

Pseudohypoparathyroidism type 1B (PHP1B) occurs when there is an imprinting (methylation) defect in the maternal GNAS gene; unlike PHP1A, however, there is no mutation present [87].

Recall that a mutation in the paternal Gsα gene causes pseudopseudohypoparathyroidism. The second "pseudo" refers to the absence of PTH resistance (low calcium and high phosphorus expected in this condition) in a patient with short stature (Table 5.2).

What are the skeletal effects of hypoparathyroidism?

PTH plays an essential role in bone remodeling. Suppressed bone turnover due to hypoparathyroidism causes an increase in bone mineral density compared to age- and sex-matched controls. Studies on fragility fracture risk are, however, unavailable [91].

TABLE 5.2 Comparison of the clinical features of inactivating PTH/PTHrp signaling disorders.

iPPSD	AHO	Other hormone resistance states	PTH resistance
PPHP	Present	Absent	Absent [88, 89]
PHP1A	Present	Present	Present [85, 86]
PHP1B	Absent	Infrequent	Present [87]
PHP1C	Present	Present	Present [90]

iPPSD, inactivating PTH/PTHrp signaling disorders;
AHO, Albright's hereditary osteodystrophy.
Other hormone resistance states, LH and TSH resistance.
PTH resistance, low calcium, high phosphorus, and a paradoxically high PTH.
PHP1C, Pseudohypoparathyroidism type 1C.
Source: Adapted from Refs. [85–90].

5.3   PAGET'S DISEASE OF BONE

5.3.1   Bisphosphonates

5.3.1.1   Physiology

Pathophysiology of osteoclastogenesis has been described in Section 5.1.2.

5.3.1.2   Mechanism of Action

1. Inhibition of osteoclast activity (see Figure 5.3).
2. Healing of osteolytic bone lesions and restoration of normal bone histology [92].

 Clinical Pearl

Paget's disease of bone (PDB) is a rare bone disease that was first described by James Paget in the 1870s [93]. It presents with disordered bone remodeling. A focal area of increased bone resorption heralds this condition. This is then followed by an accelerated bone formation which results in disorganized bone being laid down. Consequently, the affected bones can be deformed or, worst still, fractured under mechanical stress. PDB is primarily a silent disease in up to 70% of affected individuals [94].

Practice Pearl(s)

Remission is best assessed through the measurement of bone remodeling markers. The therapeutic goal is defined as marker levels at or below the mid-reference range [95]. A single infusion of IV zoledronate can lead to a prolonged period of remission of PDB (including the normalization of ALP levels and symptom relief) [95].

When should bisphosphonate therapy be initiated in the management of PDB?

- In symptomatic patients with bone pain.
- Pagetic lesions involving weight-bearing bones, peri-articular areas, or associated with nerve compression.
- Prophylaxis against perioperative bone loss in patients scheduled for orthopedic procedures involving pagetic bones.
- Hypercalcemia [95, 96].

Clinical Trial Evidence

In this large metanalysis of over 205 subjects with PDB and bone pain, bisphosphonate therapy significantly reduced bone pain compared to placebo. The relative risk for complete resolution of bone pain when bisphosphonates were compared to placebo (31% versus 9%) was 3.42 with a 95% CI of 1.31–8.90) [97].

5.3.2   Calcitonin

5.3.2.1   Physiology

Calcitonin is a 32 amino acid peptide secreted by the parafollicular or C cells of the thyroid gland. Procalcitonin, a 116 amino acid peptide, is the precursor to calcitonin. Under normal physiologic conditions, it is largely produced by the C cells of the thyroid; however, in the setting of significant bacterial sepsis, the calcitonin gene is induced in several extra-thyroidal sites [98]. Calcitonin secretion is dependent on levels of serum calcium. Hypercalcemia induces the production of calcitonin. On the other hand, hypocalcemia inhibits the release of calcitonin [8]. The calcitonin receptor (CTR) is a G-protein coupled receptor that activates various intracellular processes (cyclic adenosine monophosphate/protein kinase A pathway) upon its activation by calcitonin [99]. In summary, activation of CTR at the level of the osteoclast impairs osteoclast cell adhesion, ion transport, and enzyme activity, all critical processes in bone resorption [7]. Inhibition of bone resorption impairs the liberation of calcium from hydroxyapatite crystals and ultimately restores serum calcium in the setting of hypercalcemia [98].

Human calcitonin has a half-life of approximately 5 minutes [100]. Salmon calcitonin, which differs from human calcitonin, is more potent, is cleared more slowly, and has a stronger affinity for the CTR than human calcitonin [101].

5.3.2.2   Mechanism of Action

The role of calcitonin in inhibiting osteoclast activity makes it a suitable agent for PDB. It is, however, seldom prescribed for this purpose due to the significant potency and efficacy of bisphosphonates (pamidronate and zoledronate) [97].

Practice Pearl(s)

Nausea and facial flushing are common side effects.

Neutralizing antibodies may reduce the efficacy of salmon-derived calcitonin in about 20% of patients [102].

Clinical Trial Evidence

Calcitonin has been shown in several studies to have the following therapeutic effects [103, 104]:

- Reduction in the incidence of fractures in PDB.
- Reduce bone remodeling markers such as alkaline phosphatase and urinary hydroxyproline.
- Relief of bone pain in PDB.

 Concepts to Ponder Over

When should osteosarcoma be suspected in PDB?

- New onset bone pain and/or swelling [105].
- Fracture at a previous pagetic site [105].

Why do patients with PDB develop osteosarcoma?

In PDB, there is an imbalance between bone resorption by osteoclasts and bone formation by osteoblasts, leading to disorganized and weak bone structure [93, 106].

This aberrant bone remodeling process has been linked to the activation of several signaling pathways, such as the RANK/RANKL/OPG pathway and the Wnt/β-catenin pathway, which contribute to the increased osteoclastogenesis and abnormal osteoblast differentiation [107]. These dysregulated cellular processes can increase the risk of malignant transformation of bone cells and the development of osteosarcoma [108].

Additionally, PDB patients have been found to have increased levels of various growth factors, such as transforming growth factor-β (TGF-β) and insulin-like growth factor-1 (IGF-1) [109], which can promote cell proliferation and contribute to the development of osteosarcoma [110].

5.4   X-LINKED HYPOPHOSPHATEMIA

X-linked hypophosphatemia (XLH), previously classified as vitamin D-resistant rickets, is a genetic disease characterized by renal phosphate wasting, rickets, short stature, and dental abscesses [111].

5.4.1   Phosphorus

5.4.1.1   Physiology

Renal and Intestinal Phosphate Handling

Inorganic phosphate is a ubiquitous element critical in various biological functions. Phosphate is an integral component of adenosine and guanosine triphosphates (ATP, GTP), phospholipid bilayers, and bone (as part of hydroxyapatite crystals) [112] (Figure 5.9).

Approximately 80–90% of the filtered renal phosphate load is conserved through proximal renal tubular reabsorption (see Figure 5.9). The amount of renal

phosphate lost is offset by intestinal phosphate reabsorption (dietary sources of phosphate are approximately 700 mg) [113].

The sodium-potassium pump (Na-K ATPase) present on the basolateral membrane of the proximal tubular cell facilitates an electrochemical gradient required to reabsorb both sodium and inorganic phosphate from the ultrafiltrate. Sodium phosphate cotransporter 2a and 2c (Npt2a and Npt2c) on the apical membrane transport ferries both sodium and inorganic phosphate from the ultrafiltrate into the proximal tubular cell. A yet-to-be-fully characterized phosphate transporter on the basolateral membrane moves inorganic phosphate from the tubular cell into peritubular capillaries [50].

Intestinal phosphate handling is yet to be fully elucidated. There is, however, evidence that a sodium phosphate cotransporter facilitates the transepithelial transport of inorganic phosphate. Calcitriol upregulates the expression of this transporter leading to the conservation of ingested phosphate [114].

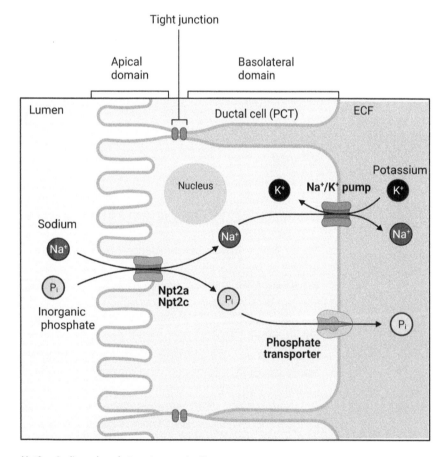

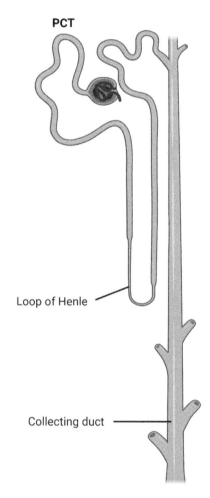

Npt2a : Sodium phosphate cotransporter 2a
Npt2c : Sodium phosphate cotransporter 2c

FIGURE 5.9   Reabsorption of phosphate at the proximal renal tubule. *Source:* Adapted from [50].

5.4.1.2   Mechanism of Action

XLH is associated with significant phosphaturia, a defect that contributes to poor skeletal growth and mineralization. Oral phosphate administered multiple times a day is required to improve serum phosphate and bone mineralization [115].

Practice Pearl(s)

Adults with XLH typically require oral phosphate salts 700–1200 mg/day (in two to three divided doses). Treatment aims to improve symptoms and not to normalize serum phosphate levels [116].

Oral phosphate should be administered along with active vitamin D since phosphate monotherapy promotes secondary hyperparathyroidism and further exacerbates phosphaturia [117].

Clinical Trial Evidence

A small study of 24 pediatric subjects with confirmed XLH treated with conventional therapy (phosphate and vitamin D) was followed up for a

---

median of 3 years. 13 patients experienced a statistically significant increase in height compared to baseline. However, this came at an increased risk for nephrocalcinosis (79% of study participants) [118].

5.4.2   Burosumab (FGF-23 Monoclonal Antibody)

5.4.2.1   Physiology

Phosphate Regulating Gene with **H**omologies to the **E**ndopeptidase on the **X** chromosome (PHEX), an endopeptidase that is constitutively expressed in osteocytes and odontoblasts, plays a critical role in regulating the circulating levels of FGF23 [119] (see Figure 5.10).

FGF23, a 251 amino acid peptide, is secreted by various bone cells (including osteocytes, osteoblasts, and osteoclasts) [120] and is inactivated by PHEX in normal physiology. Along with its cofactor, alpha klotho, FGF-23 reduces the expression of renal sodium phosphate transporters (Npt2a, Npt2c), which results in increased renal phosphate losses. In addition, FGF-23 inhibits the synthesis of calcitriol by upregulating 24-hydroxylase and downregulating

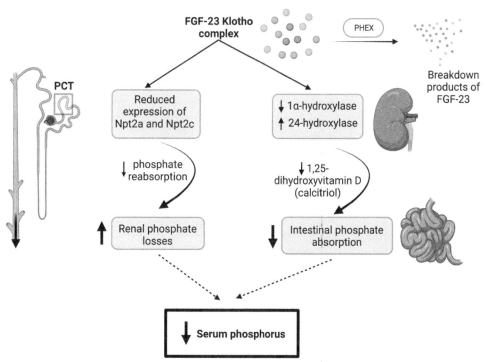

PHEX : **P**hosphate Regulating Gene with **H**omologies to the **E**ndopeptidase on the **X** chromosome

FIGURE 5.10   FGF-23 and phosphate regulation.

1 alpha-hydroxylase expression. Low serum calcitriol impairs intestinal phosphate conservation. The net effect is a reduction in serum phosphate [50].

5.4.2.2   Mechanism of Action

XLH occurs due to a loss of function mutation in the PHEX gene, which leads to defective inactivation of FGF-23. Excess FGF-23, consequently drives the manifestations of this debilitating condition.

Burosumab *(Crysvita®)* is a recombinant human monoclonal immunoglobulin G antibody that prevents the binding of FGF-23 to its receptor [116]. By inhibiting the action of FGF-23, serum phosphorus levels can be increased in XLH [121, 122] (see Figure 5.10).

Practice Pearl(s)

Burosumab should only be started in patients with fasting phosphate below the reference range for age. Conventional therapy (oral phosphate and active vitamin D) should not be given along with burosumab due to the risk of iatrogenic hyperphosphatemia [123].

Clinical Trial Evidence

In this multinational, randomized, double-blind, placebo-controlled trial, 134 adults aged 18–65 years with XLH were randomized to burosumab or placebo in a 1:1 fashion. Burosumab 1 mg/kg or matching placebo was administered subcutaneously at 4-week intervals for a total of 24 weeks. This was followed by an open-label phase of burosumab for a further 24 weeks. Burosumab resulted in serum phosphate levels above the lower limit of normal in 94.1% of subjects, compared to 7.6% of subjects on placebo. Also, 43.1% (burosumab) and 7.7% (placebo) of participants with active fractures at baseline showed complete healing at the end of the study [124].

5.4.3   Calcitriol

5.4.3.1   Physiology

Vitamin D3 is synthesized in the skin from 7-dehydrocholesterol through the direct effects of UV light. Vitamin D2 (ergocalciferol) is an alternative source of vitamin D derived from a plant sterol (ergosterol) [125, 126]. These sources of vitamin D undergo hydroxylation in the liver, leading to the formation of 25-OHD. The 1 alpha-hydroxylase enzyme subsequently converts 25-OHD to 1,25-dihydroxy vitamin D. This final hydroxylation step which leads to the formation of active vitamin D occurs in the kidneys (see Figure 5.11) [127]. Active vitamin D is a hormone that exerts its effects by binding to the ubiquitous vitamin D receptor (VDR) in various tissues. It is noteworthy that VDR is indeed a transcription factor that in conjunction with other modulators, regulates gene transcription in various tissues [128].

Active vitamin D is inactivated by the 24 hydroxylase enzyme into 24,25-dihydroxy vitamin D. FGF23 promotes the inhibitory action of the 24 hydroxylase enzyme on active vitamin D. In addition, FGF-23 inhibits 1 alpha-hydroxylase activity. The net effect is a reduction in circulating levels of active vitamin D [120]. FGF-23 also inhibits renal phosphate conservation by downregulating the expression of renal sodium phosphate transporters.

5.4.3.2   Mechanism of Action

See Figure 5.10 for the effects of calcitriol on phosphate conservation.

Practice Pearl(s)

Calcitriol or alfacalcidol is usually prescribed for adults with XLH. It is imperative that vitamin D deficiency be corrected in patients with XLH [117].

Clinical Trial Evidence

See Section 5.4.1.

 Concepts to Ponder Over

What is the difference between osteoporosis and osteomalacia?

(See Table 5.3)

TABLE 5.3 Comparison of osteoporosis and osteomalacia.

Clinical feature	Osteoporosis	Osteomalacia
25-OH vitamin D	Normal, low or high vitamin D	Usually low
Vertebral fractures	May be present	Usually absent
Volume of osteoid	Normal or decreased	Increased
Symptoms	Silent disease	Symptomatic (muscle pain, muscle weakness, increased fall risk and bone pain).
Biochemical picture	Usually normal calcium, phosphate and bone-specific alkaline phosphatase.	Associated with hypocalcemia, hypophosphatemia and a high alkaline phosphatase.

25-OH vitamin D, 25 hydroxyvitamin D.
Source: Adapted from Ref. [129].

5.5 OSTEOPOROSIS

5.5.1 Bisphosphonates

5.5.1.1 Physiology

The Structure of Bone

Bone is composed of a firm outer covering called cortical bone and an inner meshwork of trabecular bone (Figure 5.12). Both components contribute to maintaining the strength of bone and depending on the location, the proportion of cortical and trabecular bone may vary significantly [131] (see Section 5.1.2).

Cortical bone is comprised of three surfaces – the endosteum, which forms the innermost shell; intra-cortical pores dispersed throughout the cortical bone; and periosteum, which serves as an outermost covering [130]. In contrast, trabecular bone has unique plate-like and rod-like components which serve as supporting struts [131, 132]. Source: Adapted and modified from [131].

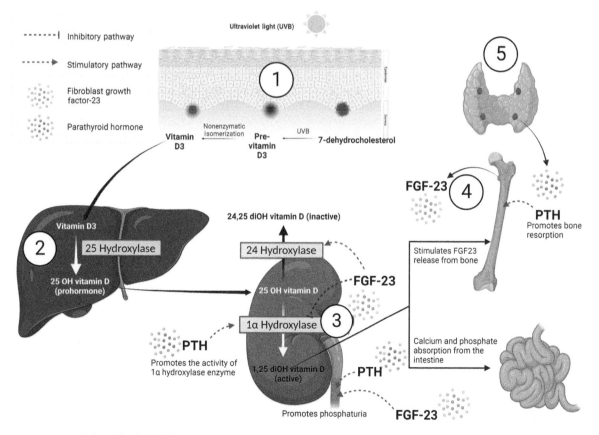

FIGURE 5.11 Regulation of calcitriol by FGF-23.

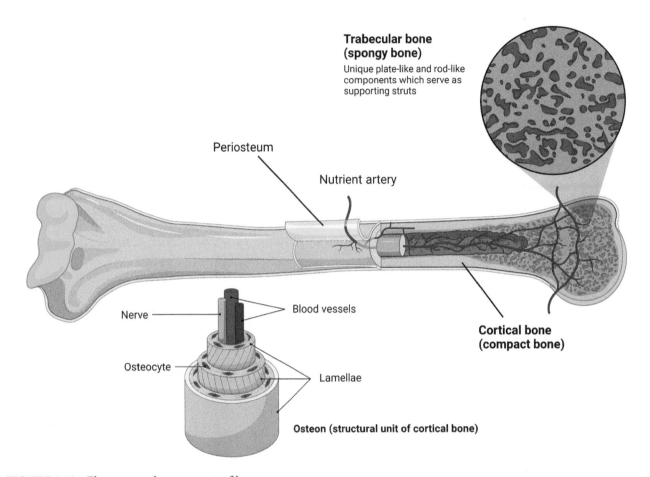

FIGURE 5.12 The structural components of bone.

Bone Cells

Bone is living tissue and is composed of various cells required for maintaining the function of bone. Osteoblasts and osteoclasts are primarily present on the surface of the bone and comprise 4–6% and 1–2%, respectively, of all bone cells [133]. The majority of bone cells are indeed osteocytes (90–95%) deeply embedded in the mineralized bone matrix [134].

Osteoblasts are formed from mesenchymal progenitor cells involved in the formation of chondrocytes, fat, and muscle cells. They mediate the process of both bone mineralization and matrix protein deposition (i.e. bone formation) [135]. Osteoblasts may live up to 200 days before undergoing programmed cell death. However, some may end up either as osteocytes (entombed in the bone matrix) or lining cells (present on quiescent bone surfaces) [136].

Osteoclasts are derivatives of progenitor cells from the hematopoietic-monocyte–macrophage lineage, involved in bone resorption [137]. These cells live a relatively short life compared to osteoblasts and osteocytes, undergoing apoptosis after about 25 days [136].

Finally, osteocytes, the most ubiquitous cells in the bone, are previous osteoblasts trapped in the mineralized bone matrix. They possess mechanoreceptors and hormone receptors which facilitate their role as coordinators of osteoclast and osteoblast function [138].

Bone Remodeling and Modeling

Bone remodeling is characterized by a sequential process of osteoclasts and osteoblasts working together to either maintain or cause a decline in bone mass [139]. Activation of these cells leads to a sequence of bone resorption followed by bone formation. In effect, remodeling results in the replacement of old bone by new bone and occurs mainly at trabecular (also known as cancellous) bone sites [133]. Conversely, bone modeling is defined as a process by which osteoclasts and osteoblasts independently promote a change in the shape of bone. Unlike remodeling, bone modeling causes a net increase in bone mass and predominantly involves periosteal surfaces of cortical bone [39, 99]. Modeling involves the activation of osteoblasts on

TABLE 5.4   Comparison of bone modeling and remodeling.

Feature	Bone remodeling	Bone modeling
Aim	Bone renewal leads to either a decline or maintenance in bone mass.	Reshaping of bone (increase in bone mass),
Mechanism	A sequence of bone resorption followed by formation.	Bone formation or resorption occurs independently.
Location	Periosteal, endocortical, intracortical, and trabecular surfaces.ᵃ	Periosteal, endocortical, or trabecular surfaces,
Timing	10% of the skeleton is remodeled every year throughout adult life.	It occurs predominantly in childhood but also is present throughout life.

ᵃ BMU, *basic multicellular unit* refers to osteoblasts, osteoclasts, and associated blood vessels working in concert to promote bone remodeling.
Source: Adapted and modified from [46, 140, 141].

bone surfaces, resulting in bone formation or activation of osteoclasts, leading to bone resorption [46] (see Table 5.4).

5.5.1.2   Mechanism of Action

The mechanism of action of bisphosphonates was discussed in Section 5.1.2. Bisphosphonates are deposited at sites of active bone remodeling, thus exert their effects to a greater extent at cancellous (trabecular) bone surfaces, resulting in bone formation or activation compared to cortical sites [142]. By inhibiting bone resorption, unopposed bone formation eventually promotes an increase in bone mass. This is referred to as *remodeling-based bone formation* [143]. Remodeling-based bone formation is initiated by osteoclasts, leading to the formation of a scalloped cement line. Consequently, osteoblasts lay new bone over the previous resorption sites, increasing bone mass. On the other hand, modeling-based bone resorption involves the process of osteoblasts independently laying down new bone in the absence of a resorption-formation sequence [143]

Practice Pearl(s)

1. Bisphosphonates are primarily excreted via the kidneys and are therefore not recommended in patients with creatinine clearance below 30 mL/min [144].
2. Oral bisphosphonates are poorly absorbed with limited bioavailability. They are best taken on an empty stomach and well separated from divalent cations (for example, calcium), antacids, and iron [145].
3. Acute phase response (severe bone pain) after intravenous bisphosphonate infusions can be managed by administering peri-infusion NSAIDs [146].
4. Osteonecrosis of the jaw and atypical femoral fractures are rare side effects of bisphosphonates and are more likely in patients exposed to more than 8–10 years of therapy. For these reasons, a drug holiday is recommended after either 5 years of oral alendronate or three years of intravenous zoledronic acid treatment [147].

Clinical Trial Evidence

In the Health Outcomes and Reduced Incidence with Zoledronic Acid Once Yearly (HORIZON) trial, the effects of zoledronic acid on fragility fracture risk were assessed. Postmenopausal women with osteoporosis were randomized to either once yearly infusions of zoledronic acid (5 mg) ($n = 3889$ subjects) or placebo ($n = 3876$ subjects), over a three-year period. Zoledronic acid resulted in a statistically significant reduction in both vertebral and nonvertebral fractures.

Morphometric vertebral fractures occurred in 3.3% of subjects in the zoledronic acid group and 10.9% in the placebo group (relative risk of 0.30; 95% confidence interval of 0.24–0.38, p-value <0.001). Hip fractures occurred in 1.4% of subjects in the zoledronic acid group and 2.5% in the placebo group (hazard ratio of 0.59; 95% confidence interval of 0.42–0.83, p-value 0.002) [148] (Table 5.5).

(continued)

(continued)

TABLE 5.5   Selected trials of bisphosphonates approved for the treatment of osteoporosis.

Bisphosphonate	Trial	Population	Results
Alendronate	Fracture Intervention Trial (FIT)	Postmenopausal women (n = 2027)	Alendronate reduced vertebral fractures by 47% and hip fractures by 51%, compared to placebo [149].
Risedronate	Vertebral Efficacy with Risedronate (VERT)	Postmenopausal women with at least one vertebral fracture (n = 2458)	Risedronate reduced vertebral fractures by 41% and nonvertebral fractures by 39% compared to placebo [150].
Ibandronate	BONE study	Postmenopausal women (n = 2946)	Daily and intermittent ibandronate reduced vertebral fractures by 62% and 50%, respectively, compared to placebo [151].

Source: Adapted from [149–151].

5.5.2   RANK-L Inhibitors

5.5.2.1   Physiology

The role of PTH in bone resorption was introduced in Section 5.1.2.

5.5.2.2   Mechanism of Action

By binding to RANK-L, denosumab, a monoclonal antibody, prevents the interaction of RANK-L (on osteoblasts) with its corresponding osteoclast-bound RANK receptor [152].

Denosumab exerts its anti-fracture efficacy by inhibiting the activity of osteoclasts during bone remodeling [153]. Osteoblasts consequently refill the resorption pits left by the now suppressed osteoclasts, further increasing bone mass [46].

Although denosumab is classified as an anti-resorptive (promotes remodeling-based bone formation), there is evidence that it also promotes *modeling-based bone formation* (see Figure 5.14) [143]. This explains the increase in bone mass observed at predominantly cortical sites among patients treated with this potent antiresorptive agent [46, 143].

Practice Pearl(s)

Discontinuation of denosumab promotes a rapid decline in bone mineral density to pretreatment levels. In contrast to bisphosphonates, drug holidays are not recommended for patients on denosumab. Furthermore, transitioning to bisphosphonate therapy prevents this rapid bone loss seen after inadvertent discontinuation of denosumab [154].

Clinical Trial Evidence

The landmark Fracture Reduction Evaluation of Denosumab in Osteoporosis Every Six Months (FREEDOM) clinical trial led to the approval of denosumab for postmenopausal osteoporosis by the Food and Drugs Administration(FDA). 7868 women with menopause were randomized to either 60 mg of denosumab or placebo, administered subcutaneously over a three-year period. Compared to placebo, denosumab reduced vertebral, hip, and nonvertebral fractures by 68%, 40%, and 20%, respectively [153].

5.5.3   PTH Analogs

5.5.3.1   Physiology

PTH serves a dual role in bone metabolism by promoting both bone resorption and formation. The role of PTH in bone resorption was reviewed earlier (see Section 5.1.2). Indeed, continuous administration of PTH promotes bone resorption, while intermittent exposure of the skeleton to PTH promotes bone formation [155]. Persistent high-amplitude pulses of

PTH promote the activation of PTH-1R receptors on osteoblasts which in turn increase the expression of RANKL. Consequently, RANKL–RANK interaction promotes further activation of osteoclasts, thus facilitating bone resorption. PTH, in effect, exerts its resorptive effects by indirectly activating osteoblasts [156] (see Figure 5.2).

PTH, when released in low-amplitude pulses, as might occur with daily subcutaneous injections, promotes bone formation [157]. In normal physiology, low-amplitude pulses of PTH secretion occur when CaSRs on the chief cells of the parathyroid glands are stimulated. The effect of endogenous PTH, however, tends to be brief due to its short circulating half-life.

When stimulated by PTH, osteocytes reduce the expression of a unique glycoprotein known as sclerostin, a potent inhibitor of bone formation [158]. The stimulation of PTH-1R receptors on osteocytes by PTH inhibits their expression of sclerostin, a potent inhibitor of the canonical Wnt (the mammalian homolog of wingless in drosophila) signaling pathway in osteoblasts [159]. In normal physiology, activation of the Wnt signaling pathway in osteoblasts promotes osteoblastogenesis and inhibits osteoblast apoptosis [160]. In effect, either sclerostin antibodies [161] or genetic conditions associated with the reduced expression of sclerostin, for example, van Buchem's disease [162] and sclerosteosis [163], lead to progressive bone formation.

5.5.3.2   Mechanism of Action

Teriparatide (also known as PTH 1–34, *forteo®*), a PTH analog, is a truncated form of PTH and shares structural homology with the first 34 of 84 amino acids (N terminal end) of endogenous PTH [164].

The binding of PTH 1–34 (just like endogenous PTH) to its PTH-1R on osteoblasts promotes the formation of a ternary complex composed of PTH, PTH-1R, and low-density lipoprotein receptor-related proteins 5 and 6 (LRP5/6, a co-receptor of Wnt) [165]. Formation of the ternary complex, in turn, leads to rapid phosphorylation of LRP5/6 and subsequent stabilization of β-catenin in the cytosol of the osteoblast [166]. β-catenin then directs the transcription and translation of Wnt target genes which mediate the anabolic effects of osteoblasts (Wnt signaling pathway) [159]. Furthermore, PTH-1R (a G protein-coupled receptor) activation by its ligand increases intracytosolic cyclic adenosine monophosphate (cAMP) in osteoblasts. Subsequently, cAMP mediates various intracellular processes (protein kinase A activation),

which promotes bone formation [167, 168]. Also, PTH 1–34 and PTH-1R receptor interaction on osteocytes decreases the expression of sclerostin (a potent inhibitor of Wnt signaling), a process that promotes bone formation. Interestingly, osteocyte activation increases RANK-L and simultaneously reduces OPG leading to increased bone resorption (see Section 5.1.2) [159]. In effect, teriparatide promotes *remodeling-based bone formation* to a greater extent than *modeling-based bone formation*, leading ultimately to net bone formation [169].

Practice Pearl(s)

- Nausea, headaches, and arthralgia are frequent side effects of teriparatide [170, 171].
- Patients should be reminded of the importance of keeping teriparatide in a refrigerator throughout its duration of use [172, 173]. It, unfortunately, becomes rapidly inactivated if left outside a refrigerated environment for more than 24 hours.
- Although osteosarcoma is a frequently cited risk of treatment with teriparatide, the Forteo Patient Registry based on a total of more than 200,000 person-years of exposure did not show an increased incidence of this rare bone tumor in patients [174].
- Asymptomatic hypercalcemia may occur in patients treated with teriparatide, although it is unlikely after six months of treatment [171].
- Teriparatide is not recommended in patients at an increased risk for bone cancer, history of irradiation, patients with an open epiphysis, hyperparathyroidism with hypercalcemia, Paget's disease, or unexplained alkaline phosphatase elevation [172].

 Clinical Pearl

What are the approved indications for teriparatide? [175]

1. Postmenopausal osteoporosis and at high risk for fracture.
2. Glucocorticoid-induced osteoporosis.
3. Men with either primary or hypogonadal osteoporosis are at high risk for fragility fractures.

Clinical Trial Evidence

In the landmark fracture prevention trial of PTH(1–34), 1637 postmenopausal women with a history of prior vertebral fractures were randomized to placebo, 20 or 40 mcg of PTH(1–34). The median duration of follow-up was 21 months. The relative risk for new vertebral fractures in the 20mcg and 40mcg groups, compared to placebo, was 0.35 (95% CI 0.22–0.55) and 0.31 (95% CI 0.19–0.50), respectively [171].

5.5.4 PTHrp Analogs

5.5.4.1 Physiology

Parathyroid hormone-related peptide (PTHrp) is secreted by the placenta, growth plate, and mammary tissue [176] under the influence of various factors, including prolactin and placental lactogen [177]. Of note, PTHrp and PTH share some structural similarities within their first 34 amino acid sequence, which explains why PTHrp serves as a ligand for the PTH-1R receptor [178, 179].

PTHrp is typically not present in the circulation in normal physiology; however, during gestation and postpartum states, PTHrp may increase and impact bone metabolism [40]. Lactating women may develop a physiologic increase in serum calcium as a consequence of increased serum PTHrp. Indeed, transient amelioration of hypoparathyroidism-induced hypocalcemia has been reported in lactating parturients [180].

5.5.4.2 Mechanism of Action

Abaloparatide (tymlos®), recombinant PTHrp(1–34), is an analog of endogenous PTHrp. Indeed, the first 22 amino acids of the N terminal end of both polypeptides are identical. Furthermore, significant changes in amino acids from position 23–34 of the native PTHrp polypeptide confer a significant anabolic effect on abaloparatide [181].

The PTH-1R receptor exists in two subtypes known as the R^G and R^O conformations. As previously mentioned, continuous stimulation of the PTH-1R favors bone resorption, while transient or intermittent stimulation promotes bone formation. Notably, the R^O isoform, when stimulated by its ligand, leads to sustained downstream responses (bone resorption),

while stimulation of the R^G isoform promotes transient downstream effects (bone formation). PTHrp (1–34) binds the R^G isoform to a greater extent than R^O isoform, while PTH (1–34) binds the R^G to a lesser extent than R^O isoform [182]. Abaloparatide, therefore, leads to more significant bone formation than teriparatide [183].

Practice Pearl(s)

- Abaloparatide is packaged in a prefilled multidose device that should be stored in a refrigerator between (2–8°C) before first use but may be kept at room temperature (20–25°C) for no more than 30 days [184].
- The usual practice of switching from antiresorptive agents (bisphosphonates) to anabolic agents (teriparatide or abaloparatide) in "poor responders" leads to unintended consequences. It is worth noting that bone mineral density at the hip may transiently decline within the first 12 months of switching to anabolic agents [185].
- Treatment with abaloparatide and teriparatide had previously been restricted to a duration of no more than 24 months (risk of osteosarcoma from mouse model experiments) [186]. This black box warning has recently been removed by the FDA. More importantly, antiresorptive agents are recommended in all patients who have completed a course of osteoanabolic therapy (to maintain bone mineral density) [147].

Clinical Trial Evidence

In the landmark *Abaloparatide Comparator Trial In Vertebral Endpoints* (ACTIVE) double-blind, multinational, randomized controlled trial, nearly 2500 postmenopausal women with osteoporosis received abaloparatide (80 mcg), placebo, or open-label teriparatide(20 mcg) subcutaneously. The primary outcome of new morphometric vertebral fractures occurred in 0.58% and 4.22% of the abaloparatide and placebo arms, respectively. Abaloparatide compared to placebo had a relative risk of 0.14 (95% confidence interval of 0.05–0.39, *P*-value <0.001) for new morphometric vertebral fractures [187].

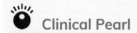 **Clinical Pearl**

What are the types of turnover markers?

Bone turnover markers (BTMs) are biochemical indicators used to quantify bone resorption/formation processes and can measure their rates, utilizing blood or urine samples. BTMs may be employed in both clinical research studies as well as practice settings to monitor treatment responses or predict fracture risks [188, 189].

There are two primary forms of bone turnover markers.

Bone Resorption Markers (BRMs): When bone resorption takes place, certain markers are released into the bloodstream. Examples are C-terminal Telopeptide of Type I Collagen (CTX), N-Terminal Telopeptide of Type I Collagen (NTX), and Deoxypyridinoline (DPD) [190].

Bone Formation Markers: When new bone is created, markers for its development, such as Procollagen type I N propeptide (PINP), Procollagen Type C Propeptide (PICP), and Osteocalcin are released [191].

Bone resorption markers [192]

- CTX – C-terminal telopeptide of type 1 collagen
- NTX – N-terminal telopeptide of type 1 collagen
- PYD and DPD – pyridinoline and deoxypyridinoline
- TRACP-5b – tartrate-resistant acid phosphatase 5b

Bone formation markers [192]

- P1NP – N-propeptide of type 1 collagen
- P1CP – C-propeptide of type 1 collagen
- BSAP – bone-specific alkaline phosphatase
- OC – osteocalcin

Clinical application of bone turnover markers

CTX represents fragments of type I collagen containing cross-linking regions, released into the systemic circulation during bone resorption [193]. Intact P1NP is a procollagen molecule produced by osteoblasts [194].

Serum CTX and P1NP levels provide useful indicators of response to oral bisphosphonate therapy.

Reference intervals help interpret single values of these bone markers by comparing them to the median premenopausal reference interval (treatment target for antiresorptive therapies). Also, serum CTX and P1NP are widely considered the preferred bone turnover markers (BTMs) in clinical practice, though not for use across all clinical situations [195].

Do not use bone turnover markers for the following. . .

- Diagnose osteoporosis
- Predict the risk of ONJ
- Determine whether to initiate treatment with antiresorptive vs. anabolic
- Predict the rate of bone loss in individual patients
- Predict fracture risk in individual patients

When can bone turnover markers be potentially helpful?

1. To monitor for bone resorption during a bisphosphonate holiday. It can also be useful for monitoring increased bone resorption after discontinuation of denosumab therapy, especially after patients have been transitioned to zoledronate [196].
2. To monitor treatment effect with bisphosphonates, teriparatide or abaloparatide [195].
3. To assess adherence to therapy and absorption of oral bisphosphonate therapy [195].

What are the sources of variability in bone turnover markers?

As with most analytical methods in endocrinology, these can be grouped into pre-analytical and analytical factors. Pre-analytical factors include age, sex, ethnicity, time of day, and timing in relation to meals and exercise [191].

Analytic factors include the intrinsic precision of the analytical method used (assay) and the method of processing the sample [192].

5.5.5   Anti-Sclerostin Inhibitors

5.5.5.1   Physiology

Sclerostin (encoded by the SOST gene) is secreted by mature osteocytes embedded in bone [197, 198]. Sclerostin plays a dual role in bone metabolism by negatively regulating osteoblast differentiation (inhibition of bone formation) while promoting osteoclast formation (promotion of bone resorption) [199]. By binding to LRP5/6, sclerostin inhibits the Wnt/β-catenin signaling pathway, leading to impaired bone formation (see Figure 5.13) [197]. Furthermore, sclerostin upregulates RANK-L and downregulates OPG synthesis, which increases bone resorption (see Figure 5.2) [199].

5.5.5.2   Mechanism of Action

Romosozumab (Evenity®) is a humanized monoclonal antibody to endogenous sclerostin, which lifts the inhibition of the Wnt/β-catenin signaling pathway by sclerostin (Figure 5.13).

In normal physiology, the Wnt ligand binds to its cognate receptor, the LRP5/6 complex, on the plasma membrane of osteoblasts. The activated LRP5/6 complex subsequently activates an intracytosolic protein called Disheveled (DSH) [200]. Consequently, DSH turns off glycogen synthase kinase 3β (GSK-3β), an inactivating system for β-catenin. This ultimately allows β-catenin to escape proteosomal degradation in the cytosol of the osteoblast. β-catenin then enters the nucleus, promoting the transcription

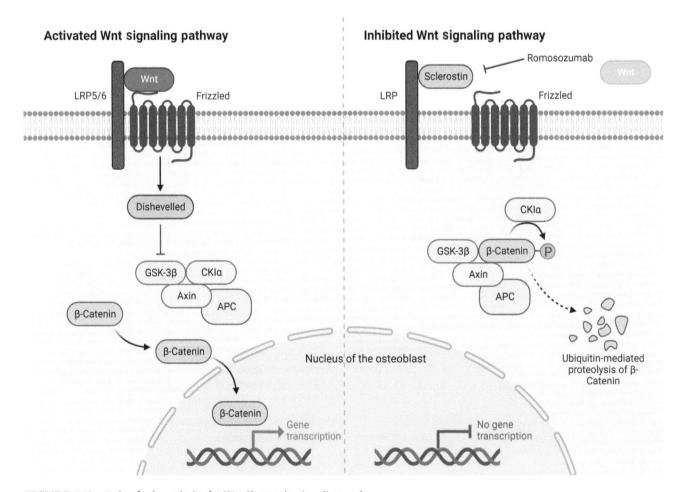

FIGURE 5.13   Role of sclerostin in the Wnt/β-catenin signaling pathway.

and translation of Wnt target genes critical in osteoblast differentiation and activation [201, 202]. Furthermore, sclerostin occupies the Wnt binding site on LRP5/6, inhibiting downstream processes critical in protecting β-catenin. The presence of sclerostin, therefore, inhibits bone formation. Romosozumab promotes bone formation by inhibiting sclerostin [202].

Practice Pearl(s)

Romosozumab plays a dual role in bone metabolism by inhibiting bone resorption (reduces bone resorption markers) and promoting bone formation (increases bone formation markers) within a few weeks of treatment. In contrast to abaloparatide and teriparatide, which promote both resorption and formation, romosozumab is an actual osteoanabolic agent (simultaneously promoting bone formation and inhibiting bone resorption) [200].

Clinical Trial Evidence

In the landmark Fracture Study in Postmenopausal Women with Osteoporosis (FRAME) clinical trial, 7180 postmenopausal women with T scores of −2.5 to −3.5 were randomized to romosozumab (210 mg) or placebo administered subcutaneously over 12 months. Subsequently, both arms of the study received denosumab (subcutaneous, 60 mg) every six months for an additional 12 months (open-label phase). Patients treated with romosozumab had a 75% lower risk for vertebral fractures compared to the placebo arm.

5.5.6 Selective Estrogen Receptor Modulators

5.5.6.1 Physiology

There are estrogen receptors in bone cells, including osteoblasts, osteoclasts, and osteocytes [203]. ERα and ERβ, isoforms of the estrogen receptor, are expressed at different levels depending on the bone compartment. The ERα isoform is disproportionately higher in cortical bone compared to trabecular bone. In contrast, the ERβ isoform is expressed to a greater extent in trabecular bone compared to

cortical bone [204]. Furthermore, ERα is expressed by most osteocytes in cortical bone and osteoblasts on the periosteal and endosteal surfaces of bone [205]. By acting on these receptors, estrogen exerts various pleiotropic effects in bone, including stimulating osteoclast apoptosis while suppressing osteoblast and osteocyte apoptosis [206].

Estrogen (17β-estradiol) binds to ERα in osteoblasts and induces the expression of OPG, a decoy receptor for RANK-L required in negatively regulating bone resorption (inhibition of bone resorption). Also, estrogen decreases the ability of osteoclasts to exert their effects in bone resorption pits by decreasing the synthesis of factors required for creating an acidic environment critical for bone resorption [207].

The processes involved in estrogen–estrogen receptor interaction in both bone and other tissues are explored in Section 6.4.1.

5.5.6.2 Mechanism of Action

Selective estrogen receptor modulators(SERMs) represent a class of compounds that exert variable effects on traditional estrogen receptors (ERα and ERβ) in a tissue-specific manner (that is, either agonist or antagonist effects) [208]. An ideal SERM will be a compound that exerts pro-estrogenic effects in bone, anti-estrogenic effects in breast tissue, and a neutral effect in the uterus [208, 209] (Table 5.6).

TABLE 5.6   Effects of SERMS in various tissues.

SERM	Breast	Endometrium	Bone
Tamoxifen [209]	−	++	+
Raloxifene [210]	−	N	+
Bazedoxifene [210]	−	N	+
Lasofoxifene [211]	−	N	+

−, Estrogen receptor antagonist effects; +, Estrogen receptor agonist effects; N, Neutral effects.
Source: Adapted from [209–211].

Practice Pearl(s)

SERMs maintain bone mineral density only for as long as patients remain on treatment. It is also worth noting that SERMs are effective for preventing mainly vertebral fractures [212].

Clinical Trial Evidence

(Refer to Table 5.7)

TABLE 5.7   Effects of various SERMS on osteoporotic fractures or bone mineral density.

SERM	Dose	Comparison	Outcome
Tamoxifen [213]	10 mg bid (PO)	Placebo	Lumbar spine BMD increased by 0.61% per year, decreased by 1.00% in the placebo group ($P < 0.001$).
Raloxifene [214]	60 mg daily (PO)	Placebo	The mean difference in BMD between treatment and control arms was 2.4% at the lumbar spine ($P < 0.001$).
Bazedoxifene [215]	20 mg or 40 mg daily (PO)	Raloxifene, Placebo	Relative risk reductions in new vertebral fractures of 42% (BZD, 20 mg), 32% (BZD, 40 mg), and 42% (RLF, 42%), respectively, compared to placebo.

PO, per os (by mouth); bid, twice daily; BMD, bone mineral density; BZD, bazedoxifene; RLF, raloxifene.

5.5.7   Hormone Replacement Therapy (Estrogen)

5.5.7.1   Physiology

The role of estrogen and SERMs in bone metabolism was introduced in Section 5.5.6. Estrogen plays a pivotal role in regulating both the accrual and loss of bone throughout life. Indeed, estrogen promotes the acquisition of bone mineral density until peak bone mass is achieved around the third decade of life in both sexes [216]. Subsequently, estrogen maintains bone mineral density until menopause (in women), at which point a physiologic decline in its circulating levels results in accelerated bone loss in the first decade after the onset of menopause [217]. A steady decline in bone density subsequently follows this initial phase of accelerated bone loss [218].

5.5.7.2   Mechanism of Action

Estrogens inhibit bone loss by stimulating estrogen receptors in bone. Estrogens have a more significant effect in improving bone mineral density compared to SERMs. The partial antagonist effect of SERMs on the estrogen receptor may explain this difference. Indeed, a combination of conjugated estrogen with a SERM (bazedoxifene) is referred to as *tissue-selective estrogen complex* (TSEC) therapy. This novel combination therapy promotes the effects of estrogen (by improving vasomotor symptoms and preventing bone loss) while reducing the proliferative effects of estrogen in breast and endometrial tissue [219, 220].

Practice Pearl(s)

In postmenopausal women with a history of hysterectomy and deemed at high risk for fractures, estrogen-only therapy may be considered for fracture prevention. Selected patients should have the following characteristics [147]:

- Less than 60 years or within ten years of the onset of menopause.
- Significant vasomotor symptomatology.
- Low risk for venous thrombosis.
- No history of myocardial infarction, stroke, or breast cancer.
- More conventional therapies such as denosumab or bisphosphonates are inappropriate.

Clinical Trial Evidence

In the landmark Women's Health Initiative (WHI) Estrogen-Alone study, 10,739 postmenopausal women between 50 and 79 years and without a uterus were randomized to either conjugated equine estrogen (CEE, 0.625 mg) or placebo, daily. The hazard ratio for hip fracture (fragility fracture) was 0.61 (95% CI 0.41–0.91), comparing CEE to placebo. There was, however, a statistically significant increase in the risk for stroke for patients exposed to CEE.

Pathophysiology Pearl

What is a selective tissue estrogenic activity regulator (STEAR)?

STEARs are a unique class of estrogen receptor modulators that have profound advantages over other medications that stimulate the estrogen receptor, such as SERMs and estrogen. Tibolone is a prototypical STEAR [221]. Tibolone is converted into three metabolites (two estrogenic and another with both progestogenic and androgenic effects). Most of the estrogen metabolites of tibolone exist in an inactive sulfated form which has to be converted into an active metabolite by the *sulfatase-sulfotransferase enzyme system* [222]. The availability of this enzyme system in local tissue, be it breast, endometrium, or bone, ultimately determines the effects of tibolone [223].

Tibolone has an estrogenic effect in bone and an antiestrogenic effect in breast and endometrial tissue [224].

5.5.8 Calcitonin

5.5.8.1 Physiology

See Section 5.3.2.

5.5.8.2 Mechanism of Action

See Section 5.3.2.

Practice Pearl(s)

Nasal calcitonin should be reserved for patients who cannot tolerate more conventional osteoporosis treatments (denosumab, bisphosphonates, SERMs, or anabolic agents) [147].

Clinical Trial Evidence

In the *Prevent Recurrence of Osteoporotic Fractures* (PROOF) study, a total of 1255 participants were randomized to either placebo or variable doses of salmon calcitonin nasal spray (100, 200, or 400 IU), administered daily. The 200 IU dose of nasal calcitonin led to a 33% reduction in the risk of vertebral fractures compared to placebo. The relative risk for vertebral fractures was 0.67 (95% CI 0.47–0.97) when 200 IU of calcitonin was compared to placebo [225].

 Clinical Pearl

What are the approaches for monitoring bone markers in osteoporosis?

The mean serum CTX in a healthy premenopausal woman is approximately 280 ng/L. The least significant change in CTX is 100 ng/L. For patients on antiresorptive therapy, the optimal treatment response is defined as a decrease in CTX of more than 100 ng/L to below 280 ng/L after six months of treatment [226].

The mean serum P1NP in a healthy premenopausal woman is approximately 35 mcg/L [194]. The least significant change in P1NP is 10 mcg/L. The optimal treatment of response to antiresorptive therapy is a decrease of more than 10 mcg/L to below 35 mcg/L at 6 months of treatment. Conversely, for patients on osteoanabolic therapy, the optimal treatment response is an increase of more than 10 mcg/L above 35 mcg/L at 6 months [227].

5.5.9 Calcium and Vitamin D

5.5.9.1 Physiology

The role of vitamin D in calcium homeostasis (see Section 5.2.2).

5.5.9.2 Mechanism of Action

It has been demonstrated that an increase in serum PTH and bone resorption due to inadequate calcium intake with or without vitamin D deficiency accounts for bone loss in the elderly. Calcium supplementation reduces age-related decline in bone mineral density through a reduction in serum PTH [228].

Practice Pearl(s)

The combination of calcium and vitamin D should be used as an adjunctive treatment for patients with osteoporosis. This is because most landmark studies of current treatments for osteoporosis include the combination of calcium and vitamin D [147]. Since the placebo groups in these studies were also treated with a combination of calcium and vitamin D, it can be safely assumed that these supplements do not necessarily improve the anti-fracture efficacy of more conventional osteoporotic therapies [229].

Clinical Trial Evidence

There has been significant clinical equipoise regarding the anti-fracture efficacy of calcium, vitamin D, or the two in combination. In a meta-analysis including over 39000 participants, combined supplementation with vitamin D (daily doses between 400 and 800 IU) and calcium (daily doses between 1000 and 1200 mg) resulted in a 6% reduction in fracture at any site compared to placebo. Also, there was a 16% reduction in the risk for hip fractures [230].

 Concepts to Ponder Over

What is an ideal anabolic agent for the management of osteoporosis?

The ideal osteoanabolic agent is one that optimizes bone formation and either impairs or has no effect on concomitant bone resorption [231, 232]. Based on these features, romosozumab can be perceived as an "ideal osteoanabolic agent" for osteoporosis [232].

What is the anabolic window in the management of osteoporosis?

The anabolic window refers to a conceptual timeframe within which anabolic agents exert their net maximum osteoanabolic effect. In effect, an osteoanabolic favoring bone formation over bone resorption widens this window, translating into greater bone mineral density accrual [233] (Table 5.8).

TABLE 5.8 Comparison of the anabolic window of various anabolic agents.

Osteoanabolic	Bone formation	Bone resorption	Anabolic window
Teriparatide	++	–	+
Abaloparatide	+	– –	++
Romosozumab	+++	– – –	+++

+ refers to either the extent of stimulation (of bone formation) or width of the anabolic window; – refers to the extent of inhibition of bone resorption.

What is the interplay between osteocytes, osteoblasts, and osteoclasts in the pathogenesis of osteoporosis?

Osteoporosis is a devastating bone disorder characterized by decreased bone mass, compromised microarchitecture and an increased risk of fractures. Osteocytes, osteoblasts, and osteoclasts all play an essential role in maintaining bone health; their dysregulation contributes directly to the pathogenesis of osteoporosis [234].

Osteocytes are one of the most abundant cells found in bone, having evolved from mature osteoblasts. They reside within the matrix and play an essential role in sensing mechanical forces, maintaining mineral homeostasis, and communicating with other bone cells. Osteocytes also secrete factors which regulate osteoblast and osteoclast activity as well as ultimately coupling bone formation with resorption [235].

Osteoblasts are bone-forming cells derived from mesenchymal stem cells. Osteoblasts produce and secrete bone matrix proteins such as type I collagen, osteocalcin, and osteopontin which contribute to mineralizing the bone matrix. Osteoblasts also secrete factors like RANKL that stimulate osteoclast differentiation and activity [236].

Osteoclasts are multinucleated cells derived from hematopoietic stem cells and responsible for bone resorption, with their activity controlled through a complex network of signaling pathways. Osteoclasts release acid and proteases into the bone matrix to dissolve it, freeing calcium ions into circulation [237].

Healthy bone maintains a dynamic equilibrium between bone formation and resorption, managed through interactions among osteocytes, osteoblasts and osteoclasts. Unfortunately, in osteoporosis, this balance becomes disrupted as bone resorption outpaces bone formation [238].

Postmenopausal women may experience lower estrogen levels which is linked to an increase in osteoclast activity and bone resorption, leading to decreased bone mass and an increased risk of fractures. Treatment strategies for osteoporosis aim to restore balance between bone formation and resorption through medications that inhibit osteoclast activity, promote osteoblast function or encourage differentiation of mesenchymal stem cells into osteoblasts [239].

A summary of common anti-resorptive and osteoanabolic agents utilized in the treatment of postmenopausal osteoporosis is shown in Figure 5.14.

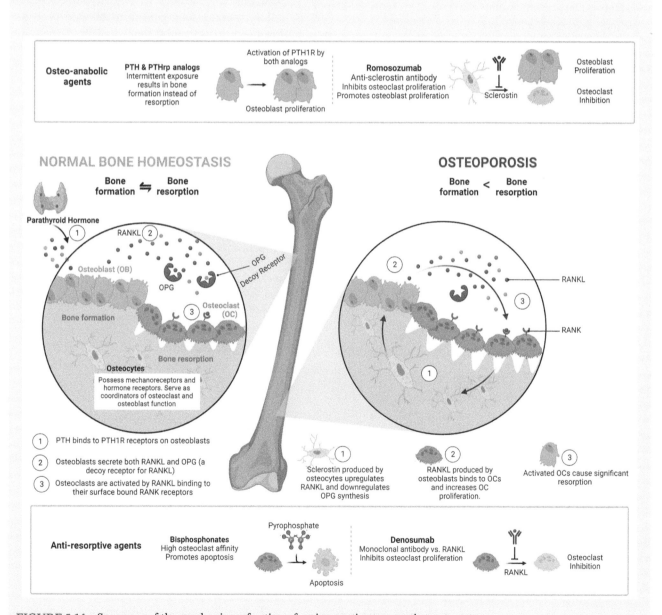

FIGURE 5.14 Summary of the mechanism of action of various anti-osteoporotic treatments.

PRACTICE-BASED QUESTIONS

1. Which of the following is a known complication of primary hyperparathyroidism (PHPT)?

   a. Hypocalcemia
   b. Osteomalacia
   c. Anemia
   d. Fragility fractures

   Answer: d) Fragility fractures are a known complication of PHPT. PHPT causes increased bone resorption, leading to osteoporosis and increased risk of fractures.

2. What is the mechanism of action of calcimimetics?

   a. Directly inhibits osteoclast activity
   b. Promotes bone formation
   c. Lowers the set point for activation of the calcium-sensing receptor (CaSR)
   d. Inhibits renal calcium excretion

   Answer: c) Calcimimetics promote the sensitivity of the CaSR to serum calcium by lowering the set point for activation of the receptor. This leads to the activation of the CaSR even at lower levels of ionized calcium, inhibiting PTH release and ultimately reducing serum calcium.

3. What is the role of PTH in bone remodeling?

   a. PTH promotes bone resorption
   b. PTH promotes bone formation
   c. PTH has no effect on bone remodeling
   d. PTH inhibits both bone resorption and formation

   Answer: a) PTH promotes bone resorption. In the setting of PHPT, persistent exposure to elevated levels of PTH results in bone resorption, leading to osteoporosis.

4. What is the effect of bisphosphonates on bone mineral density (BMD)?

   a. Bisphosphonates promote BMD at mainly cortical sites
   b. Bisphosphonates promote BMD at mainly trabecular sites
   c. Bisphosphonates have no effect on BMD
   d. Bisphosphonates decrease BMD

   Answer: b) Bisphosphonates promote BMD at mainly trabecular sites, such as the lumbar spine and hip. However, their effect on fracture incidence in patients with PHPT remains unclear.

5. Which of the following is a known indication for surgical treatment in PHPT?

   a. Age > 50 years
   b. Serum calcium within normal range
   c. Estimated glomerular filtration rate > 60 mL/min/1.73m²
   d. Nephrolithiasis/urolithiasis

   Answer: d) Nephrolithiasis/urolithiasis is an indication for surgical treatment in PHPT. Other indications include age < 50 years, serum calcium greater than 1 mg/dl above the upper limit of normal, and osteoporosis.

6. What is the biochemical profile of patients with hypoparathyroidism?

   a. Serum calcium above the upper limit of the normal reference range and low serum PTH
   b. Serum calcium below the lower limit of the normal reference range and low or undetectable serum PTH
   c. Serum calcium within the normal reference range and high serum PTH
   d. Serum calcium within the normal reference range and low serum PTH

   Answer: b) Serum calcium below the lower limit of the normal reference range and low or undetectable serum PTH.

   Hypoparathyroidism is characterized by low or undetectable serum PTH and serum calcium levels below the lower limit of the normal reference range.

7. What is the recommended serum calcium level for chronic management of hypoparathyroidism?

   a. Above the upper limit of the normal reference range
   b. Within the normal reference range
   c. Close to the low normal range
   d. No more than 0.5 mg/dL above the upper limit of the normal reference range

   Answer: c) Close to the low normal range. The recommended serum calcium level for chronic management of hypoparathyroidism is close to the low normal range or no more than 0.5 mg/dL below the lower limit of normal.

8. What is the role of thiazide diuretics in the management of hypoparathyroidism?

   a. Increase serum calcium levels
   b. Decrease serum calcium levels
   c. Increase serum phosphorus levels
   d. Decrease serum phosphorus levels

   Answer: a) Increase serum calcium levels. Thiazide diuretics are indicated in patients with severe hypercalciuria, as they decrease urinary calcium excretion and can help maintain serum calcium levels in patients with hypoparathyroidism. However, they can also increase the risk of diuretic-induced renal losses of potassium and magnesium.

9. What is the primary outcome measure in the REPLACE trial?

   a. Reduction in bone pain
   b. Increased bone mineral density
   c. Reduction in total daily dose of calcium or active vitamin D while sustaining eucalcemia
   d. Reduction in serum phosphate levels

   Answer: c) Reduction in total daily dose of calcium or active vitamin D while sustaining eucalcemia. The primary outcome measure in the REPLACE trial was defined as the proportion of subjects who experienced a 50% or greater reduction in the total daily dose of calcium or active vitamin D, while sustaining eucalcemia.

10. Which part of the PTH molecule is biologically active?

   a. N-terminal end
   b. C-terminal end
   c. Intermediate 90 amino acid polypeptide
   d. Pre-proPTH, a 115 amino acid polypeptide precursor

   Answer: a) N-terminal end. The N-terminal end of PTH is responsible for the biological action of PTH at target organs expressing the PTH-1R receptor, while the C-terminal end of PTH is biologically inert.

11. What is the mechanism of action of bisphosphonates?

   a. Inhibition of osteoclast activity
   b. Promotion of calcium reabsorption from the kidneys and intestines
   c. Inhibition of sodium-phosphate cotransporters in the proximal renal tubule
   d. Activation of CTR at the level of the osteoclast

   Answer: a) Inhibition of osteoclast activity. Bisphosphonates inhibit osteoclast activity, which leads to the healing of osteolytic bone lesions and restoration of normal bone histology.

12. What is the genetic basis of X-linked hypophosphatemia?

   a. Loss-of-function mutation in the PHEX gene
   b. Gain-of-function mutation in the GNAS gene
   c. Loss-of-function mutation in the guanine nucleotide-binding protein alpha stimulating polypeptide (GNAS) gene
   d. Mutation in the calcitonin receptor (CTR) gene

   Answer: a) Loss-of-function mutation in the PHEX gene. X-linked hypophosphatemia is caused by a loss-of-function mutation in the PHEX gene, which leads to defective inactivation of FGF-23.

13. What is the role of FGF-23 in regulating phosphate homeostasis?

   a. Increases the expression of renal sodium-phosphate transporters
   b. Inhibits the synthesis of calcitriol
   c. Promotes calcium reabsorption from the kidneys and intestines
   d. Increases bone turnover and resorption

   Answer: b) Inhibits the synthesis of calcitriol. FGF-23 reduces the expression of renal sodium-phosphate transporters, which results in increased renal phosphate losses. In addition, FGF-23 inhibits the synthesis of calcitriol by upregulating 24-hydroxylase and downregulating 1 alpha-hydroxylase expression. Low serum calcitriol impairs intestinal phosphate conservation, leading to a reduction in serum phosphate.

14. What is the role of PTH in bone metabolism?

   a. Promoting only bone resorption
   b. Promoting only bone formation
   c. Promoting both bone resorption and formation
   d. None of the above

Answer: c) Promoting both bone resorption and formation. PTH serves a dual role in bone metabolism by promoting both bone resorption and formation.

15. What is the mechanism of action of bisphosphonates?

    a. By binding to RANK-L, denosumab prevents the interaction of RANK-L with its corresponding osteoclast-bound RANK receptor
    b. By inhibiting bone resorption, unopposed bone formation eventually promotes an increase in bone mass
    c. By promoting the formation of a ternary complex composed of PTH, PTH-1R, and low-density lipoprotein receptor-related proteins 5 and 6 (LRP5/6)
    d. None of the above

    Answer: b) By inhibiting bone resorption, unopposed bone formation eventually promotes an increase in bone mass. Bisphosphonates are deposited at sites of active bone remodeling, thus exert their effects to a greater extent at cancellous (trabecular) compared to cortical sites. By inhibiting bone resorption, unopposed bone formation eventually promotes an increase in bone mass.

16. Which of the following clinical trials led to the approval of denosumab for postmenopausal osteoporosis by the FDA?

    a. Fracture Intervention Trial (FIT)
    b. DATA-SWITCH study
    c. BONE study
    d. Fracture Reduction Evaluation of Denosumab in Osteoporosis Every Six Months (FREEDOM)

    Answer: d) Fracture Reduction Evaluation of Denosumab in Osteoporosis Every Six Months (FREEDOM). The landmark FREEDOM clinical trial led to the approval of denosumab for postmenopausal osteoporosis by the FDA.

17. Which of the following is true about the mechanism of action of romosozumab?

    a. It promotes osteoclast formation.
    b. It inhibits bone formation.
    c. It inhibits sclerostin, thereby promoting bone formation.

    d. It upregulates RANK-L, increasing bone resorption.

    Answer: c. Romosozumab is a humanized monoclonal antibody to endogenous sclerostin, which lifts the inhibition of the Wnt/β-catenin signaling pathway by sclerostin. This results in increased bone formation.

18. Which of the following is true about the role of estrogen in bone metabolism?

    a. Estrogen inhibits osteoclast apoptosis.
    b. Estrogen promotes bone loss.
    c. Estrogen decreases the ability of osteoclasts to exert their effects in bone resorption pits.
    d. Estrogen has a minimal effect on bone mineral density compared to SERMs.

    Answer: c. By acting on estrogen receptors, estrogen exerts various pleiotropic effects in bone, including stimulating osteoclast apoptosis and suppressing osteoblast and osteocyte apoptosis. Estrogen decreases the ability of osteoclasts to exert their effects in bone resorption pits by decreasing the synthesis of factors required for creating an acidic environment critical for bone resorption.

19. Which of the following is an ideal SERM for osteoporosis treatment?

    a. Tamoxifen
    b. Raloxifene
    c. Bazedoxifene
    d. Lasofoxifene

    Answer: c. An ideal SERM will be a compound that exerts pro-estrogenic effects in bone, anti-estrogenic effects in breast tissue, and a neutral effect in the uterus. Bazedoxifene satisfies these criteria, making it an ideal SERM for osteoporosis treatment.

20. Which of the following is true about the combination of calcium and vitamin D in the management of osteoporosis?

    a. It improves the anti-fracture efficacy of more conventional osteoporotic therapies.
    b. It is not necessary as the placebo groups in landmark studies were also treated with it.
    c. It is only recommended for patients who cannot tolerate more conventional osteoporosis treatments.

d. It reduces age-related decline in bone mineral density through a reduction in serum PTH.

Answer: d. Calcium supplementation reduces age-related decline in bone mineral density through a reduction in serum PTH. The combination of calcium and vitamin D should be used as an adjunctive treatment for patients with osteoporosis.

REFERENCES

1. Felsenfeld, A., Rodriguez, M., and Levine, B. (2013). New insights in regulation of calcium homeostasis. *Curr. Opin. Nephrol. Hypertens.* 22: 371–376.

2. Moorthi, R.N. and Moe, S.M. (2011). CKD–mineral and bone disorder: core curriculum 2011. *Am. J. Kidney Dis.* 58: 1022–1036.

3. Vorland, C.J., Stremke, E.R., Moorthi, R.N., and Hill Gallant, K.M. (2017). Effects of excessive dietary phosphorus intake on bone health. *Curr. Osteoporos. Rep.* 15: 473–482.

4. Adams, J.S. and Hewison, M. (2010). Update in vitamin D. *J. Clin. Endocrinol. Metabol.* 95: 471–478.

5. Summers, R. and Macnab, R. (2017). Thyroid, parathyroid hormones and calcium homeostasis. *Anaesthesia & Intensive Care Medicine* 18: 522–526.

6. Martin, A., David, V., and Quarles, L.D. (2012). Regulation and function of the FGF23/klotho endocrine pathways. *Physiol. Rev.* 92: 131–155.

7. Davey, R.A. and Findlay, D.M. (2013). Calcitonin: physiology or fantasy? *J. Bone Miner. Res.* 28: 973–979.

8. Felsenfeld, A.J. and Levine, B.S. (2015). Calcitonin, the forgotten hormone: does it deserve to be forgotten? *Clin. Kidney J.* 8: 180–187.

9. Pu, F., Chen, N., and Xue, S. (2016). Calcium intake, calcium homeostasis and health. *Food Sci. Human Wellness* 5: 8–16.

10. Bagur, R. and Hajnóczky, G. (2017). Intracellular Ca2+ sensing: role in calcium homeostasis and signaling. *Mol. Cell* 66: 780–788.

11. Bushinsky, D.A. and Monk, R.D. (1998). Calcium. *Lancet* 352: 306–311.

12. Chen, R.A. and Goodman, W.G. (2004). Role of the calcium-sensing receptor in parathyroid gland physiology. *Am. J. Physiol. Renal Physiol.* 286: F1005–F1011.

13. Rajala, M.M., Klee, G.G., and Heath, H. (1991). Calcium regulation of parathyroid and C cell function in familial benign hypercalcemia. *J. Bone Miner. Res.* 6: 117–124.

14. Jeon, U.S. (2008). Kidney and calcium homeostasis. *Electrolyte Blood Press* 6: 68–76.

15. Tfelt-Hansen, J. and Brown, E.M. (2005). The calcium-sensing receptor in normal physiology and pathophysiology: a review. *Crit. Rev. Clin. Lab. Sci.* 42: 35–70.

16. Goodman, H.M. (2009). Chapter 10 - Hormonal regulation of calcium balance. In: *Basic Medical Endocrinology*, 4the (ed. H.M. Goodman), 197–218. San Diego: Academic Press.

17. Kumar, R. and Thompson, J.R. (2011). The regulation of parathyroid hormone secretion and synthesis. *J. Am. Soc. Nephrol.* 22: 216–224.

18. Goltzman, D., Mannstadt, M., and Marcocci, C. (2018). Physiology of the calcium-parathyroid hormone-vitamin D axis. *Front. Horm. Res.* 50: 1–13.

19. Pereira, L., Meng, C., Marques, D., and Frazão, J.M. (2018). Old and new calcimimetics for treatment of secondary hyperparathyroidism: impact on biochemical and relevant clinical outcomes. *Clin. Kidney J.* 11: 80–88.

20. Jensen, A.A. and Bräuner-Osborne, H. (2007). Allosteric modulation of the calcium-sensing receptor. *Curr. Neuropharmacol.* 5: 180–186.

21. Nemeth, E.F. (2013). Allosteric modulators of the extracellular calcium receptor. *Drug Discov. Today Technol.* 10: e277–e284.

22. Ng, C.H., Chin, Y.H., Tan, M.H.Q. et al. (2020). Cinacalcet and primary hyperparathyroidism: systematic review and meta regression. *Endocr. Connect.* 9: 724–735.

23. Bilezikian, J.P. (2018). Primary hyperparathyroidism. *J. Clin. Endocrinol. Metabol.* 103: 3993–4004.

24. Luque-Fernández, I., García-Martín, A., and Luque-Pazos, A. (2013). Experience with cinacalcet in primary hyperparathyroidism: results after 1 year of treatment. *Ther. Adv. Endocrinol. Metab.* 4: 77–81.

25. Marcocci, C., Bollerslev, J., Khan, A.A., and Shoback, D.M. (2014). Medical management of primary hyperparathyroidism: proceedings of the fourth international workshop on the management of asymptomatic primary hyperparathyroidism. *J. Clin. Endocrinol. Metabol.* 99: 3607–3618.

26. Khan, A., Bilezikian, J., Bone, H. et al. (2015). Cinacalcet normalizes serum calcium in a double-blind randomized, placebo-controlled study in patients with primary hyperparathyroidism with contraindications to surgery. *Eur. J. Endocrinol.* 172: 527–535.

27. Misiorowski, W. and Bilezikian, J.P. (2020). Osteitis fibrosa cystica. *JBMR Plus* 4: e10403.

28. Mandl, F. (1947). Hyperparathyroidism; a review of historical developments and the present state of knowledge on the subject. *Surgery* 21: 394–440.

29. Clarke, B.L. (2013). Epidemiology of primary hyperparathyroidism. *J. Clin. Densitom.* 16: 8–13.

30. Lewiecki, E.M. and Miller, P.D. (2013). Skeletal effects of primary hyperparathyroidism: bone mineral density and fracture risk. *J. Clin. Densitom.* 16: 28–32.

31. Marcocci, C., Cianferotti, L., and Cetani, F. (2012). Bone disease in primary hyperparathyrodism. *Ther Adv Musculoskelet Dis* 4: 357–368.

32. Ikeda, K. and Takeshita, S. (2016). The role of osteoclast differentiation and function in skeletal homeostasis. *J. Biochem.* 159: 1–8.

33. McClung, M.R., Lewiecki, E.M., Cohen, S.B. et al. (2006). Denosumab in postmenopausal women with low bone mineral density. *N. Engl. J. Med.* 354: 821–831.

34. Udagawa, N., Koide, M., Nakamura, M. et al. (2021). Osteoclast differentiation by RANKL and OPG signaling pathways. *J. Bone Miner. Metab.* 39: 19–26.

35. Drake, M.T., Clarke, B.L., and Khosla, S. (2008). Bisphosphonates: mechanism of action and role in clinical practice. *Mayo Clin. Proc.* 83: 1032–1045.

36. Tsoumpra, M.K., Muniz, J.R., Barnett, B.L. et al. (2015). The inhibition of human farnesyl pyrophosphate synthase by nitrogen-containing bisphosphonates. Elucidating the role of active site threonine 201 and tyrosine 204 residues using enzyme mutants. *Bone* 81: 478–486.

37. Russell, R.G.G. (2007). Bisphosphonates: mode of action and pharmacology. *Pediatrics* 119: S150–S162.

38. Leere, J.S., Karmisholt, J., Robaczyk, M., and Vestergaard, P. (2017). Contemporary medical management of primary hyperparathyroidism: a systematic review. *Front Endocrinol (Lausanne)* 8: 79.

39. Khan, A.A., Bilezikian, J.P., Kung, A.W.C. et al. (2004). Alendronate in primary hyperparathyroidism: a double-blind, randomized, placebo-controlled trial. *J. Clin. Endocrinol. Metab.* 89: 3319–3325.

40. Sato, K. (2008). Hypercalcemia during pregnancy, puerperium, and lactation: review and a case report of hypercalcemic crisis after delivery due to excessive production of PTH-related protein (PTHrP) without malignancy (humoral hypercalcemia of pregnancy). *Endocr. J.* 55: 959–966.

41. Lepre, F., Grill, V., Ho, P.W.M., and Martin, T.J. (1993). Hypercalcemia in pregnancy and lactation associated with parathyroid hormone-related protein. *N. Engl. J. Med.* 328: 666–667.

42. Makras, P. and Anastasilakis, A.D. (2018). Bone disease in primary hyperparathyroidism. *Metabolism* 80: 57–65.

43. Mosekilde, L. (2008). Primary hyperparathyroidism and the skeleton. *Clin. Endocrinol.* 69: 1–19.

44. Bandeira, F., Cusano, N.E., Silva, B.C. et al. (2014). Bone disease in primary hyperparathyroidism. *Arq. Bras. Endocrinol. Metabol.* 58: 553–561.

45. Crilly, R.G. and Cox, L. (2013). A comparison of bone density and bone morphology between patients presenting with hip fractures, spinal fractures or a combination of the two. *BMC Musculoskelet. Disord.* 14: 68.

46. Langdahl, B., Ferrari, S., and Dempster, D.W. (2016). Bone modeling and remodeling: potential as therapeutic targets for the treatment of osteoporosis. *Ther Adv Musculoskelet Dis* 8: 225–235.

47. Ott, S.M. (2018). Cortical or trabecular bone: what's the difference? *Am. J. Nephrol.* 47: 373–375.

48. Subramanya, A.R. and Ellison, D.H. (2014). Distal convoluted tubule. *CJASN* 9: 2147–2163.

49. Loupy, A., Ramakrishnan, S.K., Wootla, B. et al. (2012). PTH-independent regulation of blood calcium concentration by the calcium-sensing receptor. *J. Clin. Invest.* 122: 3355–3367.

50. Blaine, J., Chonchol, M., and Levi, M. (2015). Renal control of calcium, phosphate, and magnesium homeostasis. *CJASN* 10: 1257–1272.

51. Alexander, R.T. and Dimke, H. (2017). Effect of diuretics on renal tubular transport of calcium and magnesium. *American Journal of Physiology-Renal Physiology* 312: F998–F1015.

52. Edwards, A. and Bonny, O. (2018). A model of calcium transport and regulation in the proximal tubule. *Am. J. Physiol. Renal Physiol.* 315: F942–F953.

53. Moor, M.B. and Bonny, O. (2016). Ways of calcium reabsorption in the kidney. *American Journal of Physiology-Renal Physiology* 310: F1337–F1350.

54. Bilezikian, J.P. (2020). Hypoparathyroidism. *J. Clin. Endocrinol. Metabol.* 105: 1722–1736.

55. Brandi, M.L., Bilezikian, J.P., Shoback, D. et al. (2016). Management of hypoparathyroidism: summary statement and guidelines. *J. Clin. Endocrinol. Metabol.* 101: 2273–2283.

56. Shoback, D. (2008). Clinical practice. Hypoparathyroidism. *N. Engl. J. Med.* 359: 391–403.

57. Lee, C.-T., Chen, H.-C., Lai, L.-W. et al. (2007). Effects of furosemide on renal calcium handling. *American Journal of Physiology-Renal Physiology* 293: F1231–F1237.

58. Lieben, L., Carmeliet, G., and Masuyama, R. (2011). Calcemic actions of vitamin D: effects on the intestine, kidney and bone. *Best Pract. Res. Clin. Endocrinol. Metab.* 25: 561–572.

59. Haussler, M.R., Livingston, S., Sabir, Z.L. et al. (2020). Vitamin D receptor mediates a myriad of biological actions dependent on its 1,25-dihydroxyvitamin D ligand: distinct regulatory themes revealed by induction of klotho and fibroblast growth factor-23. *JBMR Plus* 5: e10432.

60. Diaz de Barboza, G., Guizzardi, S., and Tolosa de Talamoni, N. (2015). Molecular aspects of intestinal calcium absorption. *World J. Gastroenterol.* 21: 7142–7154.

61. Buckley, A. and Turner, J.R. (2018). Cell biology of tight junction barrier regulation and mucosal disease. *Cold Spring Harb. Perspect. Biol.* 10: a029314.

62. Peng, J.-B., Suzuki, Y., Gyimesi, G., and Hediger, M.A. (2018). Chapter 13 – TRPV5 and TRPV6 calcium-selective channels. In: *Calcium Entry Channels in Non-Excitable Cells* (ed. J.A. Kozak and J.W. Putney Jr.). Boca Raton (FL): CRC Press/Taylor & Francis. https://www.ncbi.nlm.nih.gov/books/NBK531440/. 10.1201/9781315152592-13.

63. Choi, K.-C. and Jeung, E.-B. (2008). Molecular mechanism of regulation of the calcium-binding protein calbindin-D9k,and its physiological role(s) in mammals: a review of current research. *J. Cell. Mol. Med.* 12: 409–420.

64. Areco, V.A., Kohan, R., Talamoni, G. et al. (2020). Intestinal Ca2+ absorption revisited: a molecular and clinical approach. *World J. Gastroenterol.* 26: 3344–3364.

65. Areco, V., Rivoira, M.A., Rodriguez, V. et al. (2015). Dietary and pharmacological compounds altering intestinal calcium absorption in humans and animals. *Nutr. Res. Rev.* 28: 83–99.

66. Bilezikian, J.P., Brandi, M.L., Cusano, N.E. et al. (2016). Management of hypoparathyroidism: present and future. *J. Clin. Endocrinol. Metab.* 101: 2313–2324.

67. Streeten, E.A., Mohtasebi, Y., Konig, M. et al. (2017). Hypoparathyroidism: less severe hypocalcemia with treatment with vitamin D2 compared with calcitriol. *J. Clin. Endocrinol. Metabol.* 102: 1505–1510.

68. Saha, S., Vishnubhatla, S., and Goswami, R. (2021). Alfacalcidol versus calcitriol in the management of patient with hypoparathyroidism: a randomized control trial. *J. Clin. Endocrinol. Metab.* https://doi.org/10.1210/clinem/dgab114.

69. Ramirez, J.A., Goodman, W.G., Gornbein, J. et al. (1993). Direct in vivo comparison of calcium-regulated parathyroid hormone secretion in normal volunteers and patients with secondary hyperparathyroidism. *J. Clin. Endocrinol. Metabol.* 76: 1489–1494.

70. Malberti, F., Farina, M., and Imbasciati, E. (1999). The PTH-calcium curve and the set point of calcium in primary and secondary hyperparathyroidism. *Nephrol. Dial. Transplant.* 14: 2398–2406.

71. Akkan, T., Dagdeviren, M., Koca, A.O. et al. (2020). Alternate-day calcium dosing may be an effective treatment option for chronic hypoparathyroidism. *J. Endocrinol. Investig.* 43: 853–858.

72. Cusano, N.E., Rubin, M.R., and Bilezikian, J.P. (2015). PTH(1-84) replacement therapy for the treatment of hypoparathyroidism. *Expert. Rev. Endocrinol. Metab.* 10: 5–13.

73. Fasciotto, B.H., Denny, J.C., Greeley, G.H., and Cohn, D.V. (2000). Processing of chromogranin A in the parathyroid: generation of parastatin-related peptides. *Peptides* 21: 1389–1401.

74. D'Amour, P., Brossard, J.-H., Rousseau, L. et al. (2005). Structure of non-(1-84) PTH fragments secreted by parathyroid glands in primary and secondary hyperparathyroidism. *Kidney Int.* 68: 998–1007.

75. D'Amour, P. (2006). Circulating PTH molecular forms: what we know and what we don't. *Kidney Int. Suppl.* S29–S33.

76. Daugaard, H., Egfjord, M., Lewin, E., and Olgaard, K. (1994). Metabolism of N-terminal and C-terminal parathyroid hormone fragments by isolated perfused rat kidney and liver. *Endocrinology* 134: 1373–1381.

77. Rejnmark, L., Underbjerg, L., and Sikjaer, T. (2015). Hypoparathyroidism: replacement therapy with parathyroid hormone. *Endocrinol Metab (Seoul)* 30: 436–442.

78. Rubin, M.R., Cusano, N.E., Fan, W.-W. et al. (2016). Therapy of hypoparathyroidism with PTH(1–84): a prospective six year investigation of efficacy and safety. *J. Clin. Endocrinol. Metab.* 101: 2742–2750.

79. Mannstadt, M., Clarke, B.L., Vokes, T. et al. (2013). Efficacy and safety of recombinant human parathyroid hormone (1-84) in hypoparathyroidism (REPLACE): a double-blind, placebo-controlled, randomised, phase 3 study. *Lancet Diabetes Endocrinol.* 1: 275–283.

80. Linglart, A., Levine, M.A., and Jüppner, H. (2018). Pseudohypoparathyroidism. *Endocrinol. Metab. Clin. N. Am.* 47: 865–888.

81. Liu, J., Erlichman, B., and Weinstein, L.S. (2003). The stimulatory G protein alpha-subunit Gs alpha is imprinted in human thyroid glands: implications for thyroid function in pseudohypoparathyroidism types 1A and 1B. *J. Clin. Endocrinol. Metab.* 88: 4336–4341.

82. Bastepe, M. (2008). The GNAS locus and pseudohypoparathyroidism. *Adv. Exp. Med. Biol.* 626: 27–40.

83. Bastepe, M. (2018). GNAS mutations and heterotopic ossification. *Bone* 109: 80–85.

84. Turan, S. and Bastepe, M. (2015). GNAS spectrum of disorders. *Curr. Osteoporos. Rep.* 13: 146–158.

85. Thiele, S., Mantovani, G., Barlier, A. et al. (2016). From pseudohypoparathyroidism to inactivating PTH/PTHrP signalling disorder (iPPSD), a novel classification proposed by the EuroPHP network. *Eur. J. Endocrinol.* 175: P1–P17.

86. Mantovani, G. and Elli, F.M. (2019). Inactivating PTH/PTHrP signaling disorders. *Front. Horm. Res.* 51: 147–159.

87. Dixit, A., Chandler, K.E., Lever, M. et al. (2013). Pseudohypoparathyroidism type 1b due to paternal uniparental disomy of chromosome 20q. *J. Clin. Endocrinol. Metab.* 98: E103–E108.

88. Elli, F.M., deSanctis, L., Ceoloni, B. et al. (2013). Pseudohypoparathyroidism type Ia and pseudopseudohypoparathyroidism: the growing spectrum of GNAS inactivating mutations. *Hum. Mutat.* 34: 411–416.

89. Simpson, C., Grove, E., and Houston, B.A. (2015). Pseudopseudohypoparathyroidism. *Lancet* 385: 1123.

90. Mantovani, G., Bastepe, M., Monk, D. et al. (2018). Diagnosis and management of pseudohypoparathyroidism and related disorders: first international Consensus Statement. *Nat. Rev. Endocrinol.* 14: 476–500.

91. Rubin, M.R. (2019). Skeletal manifestations of hypoparathyroidism. *Bone* 120: 548–555.

92. Ralston, S.H., Langston, A.L., and Reid, I.R. (2008). Pathogenesis and management of Paget's disease of bone. *Lancet* 372: 155–163.

93. Hansen, M.F., Seton, M., and Merchant, A. (2006). Osteosarcoma in Paget's disease of bone. *J. Bone Miner. Res.* 21 (Suppl 2): P58–P63.

94. Shaker, J.L. (2009). Paget's disease of bone: a review of epidemiology, pathophysiology and management. *Ther Adv Musculoskelet Dis* 1: 107–125.

95. Singer, F.R., Bone, H.G., Hosking, D.J. et al. (2014). Paget's disease of bone: an endocrine society clinical practice guideline. *J. Clin. Endocrinol. Metab.* 99: 4408–4422.

96. Ralston, S.H., Corral-Gudino, L., Cooper, C. et al. (2019). Diagnosis and management of Paget's disease of bone in adults: a clinical guideline. *J. Bone Miner. Res.* 34: 579–604.

97. Corral-Gudino, L., Tan, A.J., Del Pino-Montes, J., and Ralston, S.H. (2017). Bisphosphonates for Paget's disease of bone in adults. *Cochrane Database Syst. Rev.* 12: CD004956–CD004956.

98. Naot, D., Musson, D.S., and Cornish, J. (2018). The activity of peptides of the calcitonin family in bone. *Physiol. Rev.* 99: 781–805.

99. Masi, L. and Brandi, M.L. (2007). Calcitonin and calcitonin receptors. *Clin. Cases Miner. Bone Metab.* 4: 117–122.

100. Kumar, A., Potts, J.D., and DiPette, D.J. (2019). Protective role of α-calcitonin gene-related peptide in cardiovascular diseases. *Front. Physiol.* 10.

101. Plosker, G.L. and McTavish, D. (1996). Intranasal salcatonin (salmon calcitonin). A review of its pharmacological properties and role in the management of postmenopausal osteoporosis. *Drugs Aging* 8: 378–400.

102. Singer, F.R. (1991). Clinical efficacy of salmon calcitonin in Paget's disease of bone. *Calcif. Tissue Int.* 49 (Suppl 2): S7–S8.

103. Reginster, J.Y. and Lecart, M.P. (1995). Efficacy and safety of drugs for Paget's disease of bone. *Bone* 17: 485S–488S.

104. Wootton, R., Reeve, J., Spellacy, E., and Tellez-Yudilevich, M. (1978). Skeletal blood flow in Paget's disease of bone and its response to calcitonin therapy. *Clin. Sci. Mol. Med.* 54: 69–74.

105. Hansen, M.F., Nellissery, M.J., and Bhatia, P. (1999). Common mechanisms of osteosarcoma and Paget's disease. *J. Bone Miner. Res.* 14 (Suppl 2): 39–44.

106. Gennari, L., Rendina, D., Falchetti, A., and Merlotti, D. (2019). Paget's disease of bone. *Calcif. Tissue Int.* 104: 483–500.

107. Shoaib, Z., Fan, T.M., and Irudayaraj, J.M.K. (2022). Osteosarcoma mechanobiology and therapeutic targets. *Br. J. Pharmacol.* 179: 201–217.

108. Gorlick, R. and Khanna, C. (2010). Osteosarcoma. *J. Bone Miner. Res.* 25: 683–691.

109. Ralston, S.H., Hoey, S.A., Gallacher, S.J. et al. (1994). Cytokine and growth factor expression in Paget's disease: analysis by reverse-transcriptton/polymerase chain reaction. *Rheumatology* 33: 620–625.

110. Corre, I., Verrecchia, F., Crenn, V. et al. (2020). The osteosarcoma microenvironment: a complex but targetable ecosystem. *Cell* 9: 976.

111. Carpenter TO, Imel, E.A., Holm, I.A. et al. (2011). A clinician's guide to X-linked hypophosphatemia. *J. Bone Miner. Res.* 26: 1381–1388.

112. Jacquillet, G. and Unwin, R.J. (2019). Physiological regulation of phosphate by vitamin D, parathyroid hormone (PTH) and phosphate (Pi). *Pflugers Arch.* 471: 83–98.

113. Prasad, N. and Bhadauria, D. (2013). Renal phosphate handling: physiology. *Indian J Endocrinol Metab* 17: 620–627.

114. Hernando, N. and Wagner, C.A. (2018). Mechanisms and regulation of intestinal phosphate absorption. *Compr. Physiol.* 8: 1065–1090.

115. Christov, M. and Jüppner, H. (2018). Phosphate homeostasis disorders. *Best Pract. Res. Clin. Endocrinol. Metab.* 32: 685–706.

116. Lecoq, A.-L., Brandi, M.L., Linglart, A., and Kamenický, P. (2020). Management of X-linked hypophosphatemia in adults. *Metabolism* 103S: 154049.

117. Haffner, D., Emma, F., Eastwood, D.M. et al. (2019). Clinical practice recommendations for the diagnosis and management of X-linked hypophosphataemia. *Nat. Rev. Nephrol.* 15: 435–455.

118. Verge, C.F., Lam, A., Simpson, J.M. et al. (1991). Effects of therapy in X-linked hypophosphatemic rickets. *N. Engl. J. Med.* 325: 1843–1848.

119. Rothenbuhler, A., Schnabel, D., Högler, W., and Linglart, A. (2020). Diagnosis, treatment-monitoring and follow-up of children and adolescents with X-linked hypophosphatemia (XLH). *Metabolism* 103S: 153892.

120. Prié, D. and Friedlander, G. (2010). Reciprocal control of 1,25-dihydroxyvitamin D and FGF23 formation involving the FGF23/klotho system. *CJASN* 5: 1717–1722.

121. Portale, A.A., Carpenter TO, Brandi, M.L. et al. (2019). Continued beneficial effects of burosumab in adults with X-linked hypophosphatemia: results from a 24-week treatment continuation period after a 24-week double-blind placebo-controlled period. *Calcif. Tissue Int.* 105: 271–284.

122. Imel, E.A., Glorieux, F.H., Whyte, M.P. et al. (2019). Burosumab versus conventional therapy in children with X-linked hypophosphataemia: a randomised, active-controlled, open-label, phase 3 trial. *Lancet* 393: 2416–2427.

123. Padidela, R., Cheung, M.S., Saraff, V., and Dharmaraj, P. (2020). Clinical guidelines for burosumab in the treatment of XLH in children and adolescents: British paediatric and adolescent bone group recommendations. *Endocr. Connect.* 9: 1051–1056.

124. Insogna, K.L., Briot, K., Imel, E.A. et al. (2018). A randomized, double-blind, placebo-controlled, phase 3 trial evaluating the efficacy of burosumab, an anti-FGF23 antibody, in adults with X-linked hypophosphatemia: week 24 primary analysis. *J. Bone Miner. Res.* 33: 1383–1393.

125. Bikle, D.D. (2014). Vitamin D metabolism, mechanism of action, and clinical applications. *Chem. Biol.* 21: 319–329.

126. Christakos, S., Ajibade, D.V., Dhawan, P. et al. (2010). Vitamin D: metabolism. *Endocrinol. Metab. Clin. N. Am.* 39: 243–253.

127. Saponaro, F., Saba, A., and Zucchi, R. (2020). An update on vitamin D metabolism. *Int. J. Mol. Sci.* 21: 6573.

128. Bikle, D. and Christakos, S. (2020). New aspects of vitamin D metabolism and action - addressing the skin as source and target. *Nat. Rev. Endocrinol.* 16: 234–252.

129. McKenna, M.J., Freaney, R., Casey, O.M. et al. (1983). Osteomalacia and osteoporosis: evaluation of a diagnostic index. *J. Clin. Pathol.* 36: 245–252.

130. Sayilekshmy, M., Hansen, R.B., Delaissé, J.-M. et al. (2019). Innervation is higher above bone remodeling surfaces and in cortical pores in human bone: lessons from patients with primary hyperparathyroidism. *Sci. Rep.* 9: 5361.

131. Choksi, P., Jepsen, K.J., and Clines, G.A. (2018). The challenges of diagnosing osteoporosis and the limitations of currently available tools. *Clinical Diabetes and Endocrinology* 4: 12.

132. Wang, J., Zhou, B., Liu, X.S. et al. (2015). Trabecular plates and rods determine elastic modulus and

yield strength of human trabecular bone. *Bone* 72: 71–80.

133. Florencio-Silva, R., Sasso, G.R.d.S., Sasso-Cerri, E. et al. (2015). Biology of bone tissue: structure, function, and factors that influence bone cells. *Biomed. Res. Int.* 2015: 421746.

134. Schaffler, M.B. and Kennedy, O.D. (2012). Osteocyte signaling in bone. *Curr. Osteoporos. Rep.* 10: 118–125.

135. Hu, L., Yin, C., Zhao, F. et al. (2018). Mesenchymal stem cells: cell fate decision to osteoblast or adipocyte and application in osteoporosis treatment. *Int. J. Mol. Sci.* 19: 360.

136. Almeida, M., Laurent, M.R., Dubois, V. et al. (2017). Estrogens and androgens in skeletal physiology and pathophysiology. *Physiol. Rev.* 97: 135–187.

137. Xu, F. and Teitelbaum, S.L. (2013). Osteoclasts: new insights. *Bone Res* 1: 11–26.

138. Bellido, T., Plotkin, L.I., and Bruzzaniti, A. (2019). Chapter 3 - Bone cells. In: *Basic and applied bone biology*, 2nde (ed. D.B. Burr and M.R. Allen), 37–55. Academic Press.

139. DiGirolamo, D.J., Clemens, T.L., and Kousteni, S. (2012). The skeleton as an endocrine organ. *Nat. Rev. Rheumatol.* 8: 674–683.

140. Allen, M.R. and Burr, D.B. (2014). Chapter 4 - Bone modeling and remodeling. In: *Basic and Applied Bone Biology* (ed. D.B. Burr and M.R. Allen), 75–90. San Diego: Academic Press.

141. Hadjidakis, D.J. and Androulakis, I.I. (2006). Bone remodeling. *Ann. N. Y. Acad. Sci.* 1092: 385–396.

142. Roelofs, A.J., Stewart, C.A., Sun, S. et al. (2012). Influence of bone affinity on the skeletal distribution of fluorescently labeled bisphosphonates in vivo. *J. Bone Miner. Res.* 27: 835–847.

143. Dempster, D.W., Chines, A., Bostrom, M.P. et al. (2020). Modeling-based bone formation in the human femoral neck in subjects treated with denosumab. *J. Bone Miner. Res.* 35: 1282–1288.

144. Damasiewicz, M.J. and Nickolas, T.L. (2020). Bisphosphonate therapy in CKD: the current state of affairs. *Curr. Opin. Nephrol. Hypertens.* 29: 221–226.

145. Pazianas, M., Abrahamsen, B., Ferrari, S., and Russell, R.G.G. (2013). Eliminating the need for fasting with oral administration of bisphosphonates. *Ther. Clin. Risk Manag.* 9: 395–402.

146. Olson, K. and Van Poznak, C. (2007). Significance and impact of bisphosphonate-induced acute phase responses. *J. Oncol. Pharm. Pract.* 13: 223–229.

147. Eastell, R., Rosen, C.J., Black, D.M. et al. (2019). Pharmacological management of osteoporosis in postmenopausal women: an endocrine society* clinical practice guideline. *J. Clin. Endocrinol. Metabol.* 104: 1595–1622.

148. Black, D.M., Delmas, P.D., Eastell, R. et al. (2007). Once-yearly zoledronic acid for treatment of postmenopausal osteoporosis. *N. Engl. J. Med.* 356: 1809–1822.

149. Black, D.M., Cummings, S.R., Karpf, D.B. et al. (1996). Randomised trial of effect of alendronate on risk of fracture in women with existing vertebral fractures. Fracture Intervention Trial Research Group. *Lancet* 348: 1535–1541.

150. Harris, S.T., Watts, N.B., Genant, H.K. et al. (1999). Effects of risedronate treatment on vertebral and nonvertebral fractures in women with postmenopausal osteoporosis – a randomized controlled trial. *JAMA* 282: 1344–1352.

151. Chesnut, C.H., Skag, A., Christiansen, C. et al. (2004). Effects of oral ibandronate administered daily or intermittently on fracture risk in postmenopausal osteoporosis. *J. Bone Miner. Res.* 19: 1241–1249.

152. Zaheer, S., LeBoff, M., and Lewiecki, E.M. (2015). Denosumab for the treatment of osteoporosis. *Expert Opin. Drug Metab. Toxicol.* 11: 461–470.

153. Cummings, S.R., San Martin, J., McClung, M.R. et al. (2009). Denosumab for prevention of fractures in postmenopausal women with osteoporosis. *N. Engl. J. Med.* 361: 756–765.

154. Saul, D. and Drake, M.T. (2021). Update on approved osteoporosis therapies including combination and sequential use of agents. *Endocrinol. Metab. Clin. N. Am.* 50: 179–191.

155. Tam, C.S., Heersche, J.N.M., Murray, T.M., and Parsons, J.A. (1982). Parathyroid hormone stimulates the bone apposition rate independently of its resorptive action: differential effects of intermittent and continuous administration. *Endocrinology* 110: 506–512.

156. Park, J.H., Lee, N.K., and Lee, S.Y. (2017). Current understanding of RANK signaling in osteoclast differentiation and maturation. *Mol. Cells* 40: 706–713.

157. Bonnet, N., Conway, S.J., and Ferrari, S.L. (2012). Regulation of beta catenin signaling and parathyroid hormone anabolic effects in bone by the matricellular protein periostin. *PNAS* 109: 15048–15053.

158. O'Brien, C.A., Plotkin, L.I., Galli, C. et al. (2008). Control of bone mass and remodeling by PTH receptor signaling in osteocytes. *PLoS ONE* 3: e2942.

159. Estell, E.G. and Rosen, C.J. (2021). Emerging insights into the comparative effectiveness of anabolic therapies for osteoporosis. *Nat. Rev. Endocrinol.* 17: 31–46.

160. Kramer, I., Halleux, C., Keller, H. et al. (2010). Osteocyte Wnt/β-catenin signaling is required for normal bone homeostasis. *Mol. Cell Biol.* 30: 3071–3085.

161. Padhi, D., Allison, M., Kivitz, A.J. et al. (2014). Multiple doses of sclerostin antibody romosozumab in healthy men and postmenopausal women with low bone mass: a randomized, double-blind, placebo-controlled study. *J. Clin. Pharmacol.* 54: 168–178.

162. Loots, G.G., Kneissel, M., Keller, H. et al. (2005). Genomic deletion of a long-range bone enhancer misregulates sclerostin in Van Buchem disease. *Genome Res.* 15: 928–935.

163. Balemans, W., Ebeling, M., Patel, N. et al. (2001). Increased bone density in sclerosteosis is due to the deficiency of a novel secreted protein (SOST). *Hum. Mol. Genet.* 10: 537–543.

164. Hodsman, A.B., Bauer, D.C., Dempster, D.W. et al. (2005). Parathyroid hormone and teriparatide for the treatment of osteoporosis: a review of the evidence and suggested guidelines for its use. *Endocr. Rev.* 26: 688–703.

165. Li, S.-S., He, S.-H., Xie, P.-Y. et al. (2021). Recent progresses in the treatment of osteoporosis. *Front. Pharmacol.* 12: 717065.

166. Wan, M., Yang, C., Li, J. et al. (2008). Parathyroid hormone signaling through low-density lipoprotein-related protein 6. *Genes Dev.* 22: 2968–2979.

167. Yang, D., Singh, R., Divieti, P. et al. (2007). Contributions of parathyroid hormone (PTH)/PTH-related peptide receptor signaling pathways to the anabolic effect of PTH on bone. *Bone* 40: 1453–1461.

168. Lombardi, G., Di Somma, C., Rubino, M. et al. (2011). The roles of parathyroid hormone in bone remodeling: prospects for novel therapeutics. *J. Endocrinol. Investig.* 34: 18–22.

169. Dempster, D.W., Zhou, H., Recker, R.R. et al. (2018). Remodeling- and modeling-based bone formation with teriparatide versus denosumab: a longitudinal analysis from baseline to 3 months in the AVA study. *J. Bone Miner. Res.* 33: 298–306.

170. Obermayer-Pietsch, B.M., Marin, F., McCloskey, E.V. et al. (2008). Effects of two years of daily teriparatide treatment on BMD in postmenopausal women with severe osteoporosis with and without prior antiresorptive treatment. *J. Bone Miner. Res.* 23: 1591–1600.

171. Neer, R.M., Arnaud, C.D., Zanchetta, J.R. et al. (2001). Effect of parathyroid hormone (1-34) on fractures and bone mineral density in postmenopausal women with osteoporosis. *N. Engl. J. Med.* 344: 1434–1441.

172. Sikon, A. and Batur, P. (2010). Profile of teriparatide in the management of postmenopausal osteoporosis. *Int. J. Women's Health* 2: 37–44.

173. van Maren, M.A., Wyers, C.E., Driessen, J.H.M. et al. (2019). Two-year persistence with teriparatide improved significantly after introduction of an educational and motivational support program. *Osteoporos. Int.* 30: 1837–1844.

174. Gilsenan, A., Harding, A., Kellier-Steele, N. et al. (2018). The Forteo Patient Registry linkage to multiple state cancer registries: study design and results from the first 8 years. *Osteoporos. Int.* 29: 2335–2343.

175. Rizzoli, R., Kraenzlin, M., and Lippuner, K. (2011). Indications to teriparatide treatment in patients with osteoporosis. *Swiss Med. Wkly.* https://doi.org/10.4414/smw.2011.13297.

176. Ferrari, S., Rizzoli, R., and Bonjour, J.-P. (1994). Effects of epidermal growth factor on parathyroid hormone-related protein production by mammary epithelial cells. *J. Bone Miner. Res.* 9: 639–644.

177. Winter, E.M. and Appelman-Dijkstra, N.M. (2017). Parathyroid hormone–related protein–induced hypercalcemia of pregnancy successfully reversed by a dopamine agonist. *J. Clin. Endocrinol. Metabol.* 102: 4417–4420.

178. Wysolmerski, J.J. (2012). Parathyroid hormone-related protein: an update. *J. Clin. Endocrinol. Metab.* 97: 2947–2956.

179. Mannstadt, M., Jüppner, H., and Gardella, T.J. (1999). Receptors for PTH and PTHrP: their biological importance and functional properties. *American Journal of Physiology-Renal Physiology* 277: F665–F675.

180. Rude, R.K., Haussler, M.R., and Singer, F.R. (1984). Postpartum resolution of hypocalcemia in a lactating hypoparathyroid patient. *Endocrinol. Jpn.* 31: 227–233.

181. Haas, A.V. and LeBoff, M.S. (2018). Osteoanabolic agents for osteoporosis. *J Endocr Soc* 2: 922–932.

182. Hattersley, G., Dean, T., Corbin, B.A. et al. (2016). Binding selectivity of abaloparatide for PTH-type-1-receptor conformations and effects on downstream signaling. *Endocrinology* 157: 141–149.

183. Miller, P.D., Hattersley, G., Lau, E. et al. (2019). Bone mineral density response rates are greater in patients treated with abaloparatide compared with those treated with placebo or teriparatide: results from the ACTIVE phase 3 trial. *Bone* 120: 137–140.

184. Sleeman, A. and Clements, J.N. (2019). Abaloparatide: a new pharmacological option for osteoporosis. *Am. J. Health Syst. Pharm.* 76: 130–135.

185. Cosman, F., Nieves, J.W., and Dempster, D.W. (2017). Treatment sequence matters: anabolic and antiresorptive therapy for osteoporosis. *J. Bone Miner. Res.* 32: 198–202.

186. Uluçkan, Ö., Segaliny, A., Botter, S. et al. (2015). Preclinical mouse models of osteosarcoma. *Bonekey Rep* 4: 670.

187. Miller, P.D., Hattersley, G., Riis, B.J. et al. (2016). Effect of abaloparatide vs placebo on new vertebral fractures in postmenopausal women with osteoporosis: a randomized clinical trial. *JAMA* 316: 722–733.

188. Greenblatt, M.B., Tsai, J.N., and Wein, M.N. (2017). Bone turnover markers in the diagnosis and monitoring of metabolic bone disease. *Clin. Chem.* 63: 464–474.

189. Jain, S. and Camacho, P. (2018). Use of bone turnover markers in the management of osteoporosis. *Curr. Opin. Endocrinol. Diabetes Obes.* 25: 366.

190. Christenson, R.H. (1997). Biochemical markers of bone metabolism: an overview. *Clin. Biochem.* 30: 573–593.

191. Naylor, K. and Eastell, R. (2012). Bone turnover markers: use in osteoporosis. *Nat. Rev. Rheumatol.* 8: 379–389.

192. Shetty, S., Kapoor, N., Bondu, J.D. et al. (2016). Bone turnover markers: emerging tool in the management of osteoporosis. *Indian J Endocrinol Metab* 20: 846–852.

193. Cloos, P.A.C., Lyubimova, N., Solberg, H. et al. (2004). An immunoassay for measuring fragments of newly synthesized collagen type I produced during metastatic invasion of bone. *Clin. Lab.* 50: 279–289.

194. Gillett, M.J., Vasikaran, S.D., and Inderjeeth, C.A. (2021). The role of PINP in diagnosis and management of metabolic bone disease. *Clin. Biochem. Rev.* 42: 3–10.

195. Brown, J.P., Don-Wauchope, A., Douville, P. et al. (2022). Current use of bone turnover markers in the management of osteoporosis. *Clin. Biochem.* 109–110: 1–10.

196. Practitioners TRAC of general Bone turnover markers. In: Australian Family Physician. https://www.racgp.org.au/afp/2013/may/bone-turnover-markers.

197. Thouverey, C. and Caverzasio, J. (2015). Sclerostin inhibits osteoblast differentiation without affecting BMP2/SMAD1/5 or Wnt3a/β-catenin signaling but through activation of platelet-derived growth factor receptor signaling in vitro. *Bonekey Rep* 4: 757.

198. Poole, K.E.S., Van Bezooijen, R.L., Loveridge, N. et al. (2005). Sclerostin is a delayed secreted product of osteocytes that inhibits bone formation. *FASEB J.* 19: 1842–1844.

199. Wijenayaka, A.R., Kogawa, M., Lim, H.P. et al. (2011). Sclerostin stimulates osteocyte support of osteoclast activity by a RANKL-dependent pathway. *PLoS ONE* 6: e25900.

200. Bandeira, L., Lewiecki, E.M., and Bilezikian, J.P. (2017). Romosozumab for the treatment of osteoporosis. *Expert. Opin. Biol. Ther.* 17: 255–263.

201. Costa, A.G., Bilezikian, J.P., and Lewiecki, E.M. (2014). Update on romosozumab: a humanized monoclonal antibody to sclerostin. *Expert. Opin. Biol. Ther.* 14: 697–707.

202. Shah, A.D., Shoback, D., and Lewiecki, E.M. (2015). Sclerostin inhibition: a novel therapeutic approach in the treatment of osteoporosis. *Int. J. Women's Health* 7: 565–580.

203. Kalervo Väänänen, H. and Härkönen, P.L. (1996). Estrogen and bone metabolism. *Maturitas* 23: S65–S69.

204. Khalid, A.B. and Krum, S.A. (2016). Estrogen Receptors Alpha and Beta in Bone. *Bone* 87: 130–135.

205. Lara-Castillo, N. (2021). Estrogen signaling in bone. *Appl. Sci.* 11: 4439.

206. Khosla, S. (2010). Update on estrogens and the skeleton. *J. Clin. Endocrinol. Metab.* 95: 3569–3577.

207. Krum, S.A. (2011). Direct transcriptional targets of sex steroid hormones in bone. *J. Cell. Biochem.* 112: 401–408.

208. Gennari, L., Merlotti, D., and Nuti, R. (2010). Selective estrogen receptor modulator (SERM)

for the treatment of osteoporosis in postmenopausal women: focus on lasofoxifene. *Clin. Interv. Aging* 5: 19–29.

209. Archer, D.F. (2011). The gynecologic effects of lasofoxifene, an estrogen agonist/antagonist, in postmenopausal women. *Menopause* 18: 6–7.

210. Silverman, S.L., Chines, A.A., Kendler, D.L. et al. (2012). Sustained efficacy and safety of bazedoxifene in preventing fractures in postmenopausal women with osteoporosis: results of a 5-year, randomized, placebo-controlled study. *Osteoporos. Int.* 23: 351–363.

211. Gennari, L. (2009). Lasofoxifene, a new selective estrogen receptor modulator for the treatment of osteoporosis and vaginal atrophy. *Expert. Opin. Pharmacother.* 10: 2209–2220.

212. An, K.-C. (2016). Selective estrogen receptor modulators. *Asian Spine J* 10: 787–791.

213. Love, R.R., Barden, H.S., Mazess, R.B. et al. (1994). Effect of tamoxifen on lumbar spine bone mineral density in postmenopausal women after 5 years. *Arch. Intern. Med.* 154: 2585–2588.

214. Delmas, P.D., Bjarnason, N.H., Mitlak, B.H. et al. (1997). Effects of raloxifene on bone mineral density, serum cholesterol concentrations, and uterine endometrium in postmenopausal women. *N. Engl. J. Med.* 337: 1641–1647.

215. Silverman, S.L., Christiansen, C., Genant, H.K. et al. (2008). Efficacy of bazedoxifene in reducing new vertebral fracture risk in postmenopausal women with osteoporosis: results from a 3-year, randomized, placebo-, and active-controlled clinical trial. *J. Bone Miner. Res.* 23: 1923–1934.

216. Castelo-Branco, C. (1998). Management of osteoporosis. An overview. *Drugs Aging* 12 (Suppl 1): 25–32.

217. Clarke, B.L. and Khosla, S. (2010). Female reproductive system and bone. *Arch. Biochem. Biophys.* 503: 118–128.

218. Ji, M.-X. and Yu, Q. (2015). Primary osteoporosis in postmenopausal women. *Chronic Dis Transl Med* 1: 9–13.

219. Pickar, J.H., Boucher, M., and Morgenstern, D. (2018). Tissue selective estrogen complex (TSEC): a review. *Menopause* 25: 1033–1045.

220. Lindsay, R. (2011). Preventing osteoporosis with a tissue selective estrogen complex (TSEC) containing bazedoxifene/conjugated estrogens (BZA/CE). *Osteoporos. Int.* 22: 447–451.

221. Kloosterboer, H.J. and Ederveen, A.G.H. (2002). Pros and cons of existing treatment modalities in osteoporosis: a comparison between tibolone, SERMs and estrogen (+/−progestogen) treatments. *J. Steroid Biochem. Mol. Biol.* 83: 157–165.

222. Kloosterboer, H.J. (2004). Tissue-selectivity: the mechanism of action of tibolone. *Maturitas* 48 (Suppl 1): S30–S40.

223. Reed, M.J. and Kloosterboer, H.J. (2004). Tibolone: a selective tissue estrogenic activity regulator (STEAR). *Maturitas* 48 (Suppl 1): S4–S6.

224. de Gooyer, M.E., Overklift Vaupel Kleyn, G.T., Smits, K.C. et al. (2001). Tibolone: a compound with tissue specific inhibitory effects on sulfatase. *Mol. Cell. Endocrinol.* 183: 55–62.

225. Chesnut, C.H., Silverman, S., Andriano, K. et al. (2000). A randomized trial of nasal spray salmon calcitonin in postmenopausal women with established osteoporosis: the prevent recurrence of osteoporotic fractures study. PROOF Study Group. *Am. J. Med.* 109: 267–276.

226. Wu, C.-H., Chang, Y.-F., Chen, C.-H. et al. (2021). Consensus statement on the use of bone turnover markers for short-term monitoring of osteoporosis treatment in the Asia-Pacific region. *J. Clin. Densitom.* 24: 3–13.

227. Fontalis, A. and Eastell, R. (2020). The challenge of long-term adherence: the role of bone turnover markers in monitoring bisphosphonate treatment of osteoporosis. *Bone* 136: 115336.

228. Gennari, C. (2001). Calcium and vitamin D nutrition and bone disease of the elderly. *Public Health Nutr.* 4: 547–559.

229. Reid, I.R. and Bolland, M.J. (2020). Calcium and/or vitamin D supplementation for the prevention of fragility fractures: who needs it? *Nutrients* 12: 1011.

230. Yao, P., Bennett, D., Mafham, M. et al. (2019). Vitamin D and calcium for the prevention of fracture: a systematic review and meta-analysis. *JAMA Netw. Open* 2: e1917789.

231. Black, D.M. and Schafer, A.L. (2013). The search for the optimal anabolic osteoporosis therapy. *J. Bone Miner. Res.* 28: 2263–2265.

232. Khosla, S. (2017). Romosozumab – on track or derailed? *Nat. Rev. Endocrinol.* 13: 697–698.

233. Tabacco, G. and Bilezikian, J.P. (2019). Osteoanabolic and dual action drugs. *Br. J. Clin. Pharmacol.* 85: 1084–1094.

234. General (US) O of the S. (2004). The basics of bone in health and disease. Bone Health and Osteoporosis: A Report of the Surgeon General.

235. Lassen, N.E., Andersen, T.L., Pløen, G.G. et al. (2017). Coupling of bone resorption and formation in real time: new knowledge gained from human haversian BMUs. *J. Bone Miner. Res.* 32: 1395–1405.

236. Caetano-Lopes, J., Canhão, H., and Fonseca, J.E. (2007). Osteoblasts and bone formation. *Acta Reumatol. Port.* 32: 103–110.

237. Kodama, J. and Kaito, T. (2020). Osteoclast multinucleation: review of current literature. *Int. J. Mol. Sci.* 21: 5685.

238. Wang, L., You, X., Zhang, L. et al. (2022). Mechanical regulation of bone remodeling. *Bone Res* 10: 1–15.

239. Föger-Samwald, U., Dovjak, P., Azizi-Semrad, U. et al. (2020). Osteoporosis: pathophysiology and therapeutic options. *EXCLI J.* 19: 1017–1037.

CHAPTER 6

Reproductive Organ Therapies

6.1 POLYCYSTIC OVARY SYNDROME

6.1.1 Biguanides (Metformin)

6.1.1.1 Physiology

Insulin-to-insulin-receptor interaction and post-receptor signaling was reviewed in Section 4.1.1. Insulin plays an essential role in various physiologic processes, including adrenal steroid synthesis, hepatic glucose output, peripheral glucose uptake, and ovarian androgen secretion. In addition, insulin impairs hepatic synthesis of sex hormone-binding globulin (SHBG), a function central to our understanding of some of the manifestations of polycystic ovary syndrome.

Adrenal Steroidogenesis

Insulin stimulates the synthesis of adrenal steroids, including androgens and cortisol [1]. Steroidogenic factor 1 (SF-1) is a ubiquitous transcription factor present in various tissues, including the adrenal glands and gonads. SF-1 promotes the transcription of critical adrenal steroidogenic genes, including CYP11A1, CYP17, and StAR (see Chapter 3) [2, 3]. More recently, it has been shown that insulin promotes the function of SF-1 by impairing the activity of a *canonical inhibitor* of SF-1 function [4].

Hepatic Glucose Output and Peripheral Glucose Uptake

The role of insulin in glucose metabolism is summarized in Figure 6.1.

Insulin inhibits glycogenolysis by binding to insulin receptors in the liver [5]. The direct suppression of glucagon secretion by insulin further reduces hepatic glucose output [6]. Additionally, peripheral uptake of glucose is regulated by insulin. Insulin reduces circulating glucose levels in the postprandial state by stimulating glucose uptake in insulin-sensitive tissues such as skeletal muscle [7].

Conversely, glucagon, an essential counter-regulatory hormone to insulin, promotes hepatic gluconeogenesis and lipolysis, contributing to increased peripheral glucose concentration.

Regulation of Sex Hormone-Binding Globulin by Insulin

SHBG is a glycoprotein that transports various sex steroids to their target tissues [8, 9]. There is an inverse relationship between SHBG and insulin [10, 11]. However, the mechanism underlying the regulation of SHBG by insulin is yet to be elucidated [12] (see Table 6.1).

Endocrinology: Pathophysiology to Therapy, First Edition. Akuffo Quarde.
© 2024 John Wiley & Sons Ltd. Published 2024 by John Wiley & Sons Ltd.

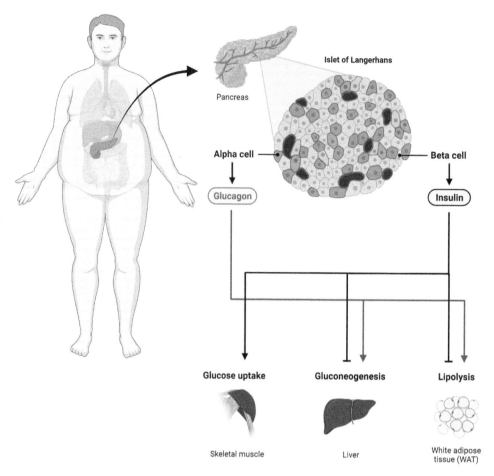

FIGURE 6.1   Role of insulin and glucagon in glucose metabolism.

TABLE 6.1   Regulators of SHBG production.

Promotes SHBG production	Inhibits SHBG production
Cortisol, estradiol, T3 and T4, dexamethasone, testosterone	Insulin, prolactin, IGF-1, epidermal growth factor

T3, Tri-iodothyronine; T4, Tetra-iodothyronine; IGF-1, Insulin-like growth factor 1.
Source: Adapted from [11].

 Pathophysiology Pearl

Role of insulin resistance in PCOS

Insulin resistance accounts for various manifestations of PCOS (see Figure 6.2).

1. Hyperinsulinemia stimulates androgen synthesis by promoting the effects of luteinizing hormone on theca cells of the ovaries [14]. Also, the trophic effects of ACTH on adrenocortical cells (androgen production by the zona reticularis) are further accentuated by hyperinsulinemia [15]. Consequently, hyperandrogenemia leads to the arrest of ovarian follicular growth, leading to anovulation and infertility [16].

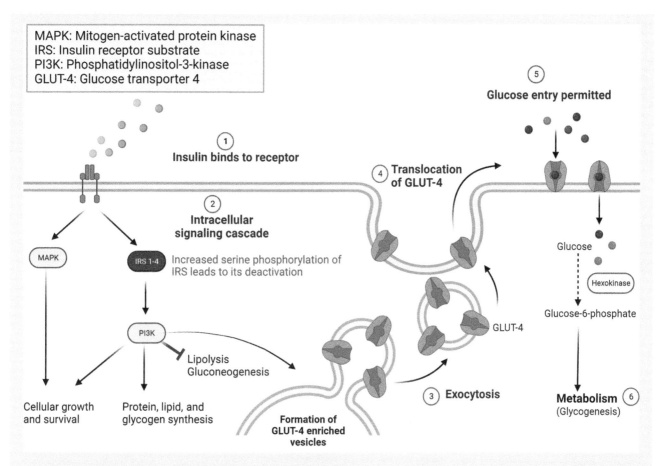

FIGURE 6.2   Molecular mechanisms of insulin resistance in PCOS. Defects in downstream signaling after insulin-to-insulin-receptor interaction account for hyperinsulinemia in PCOS. Increased serine phosphorylation of IRS-1 (deactivation) in skeletal muscle contrasts with reduced tyrosine phosphorylation of IRS-1 (activation) in patients with PCOS. This leads to a series of downstream effects, including impaired activation of PI3K, which leads to reduced expression of GLUT-4 receptors and, thus, low glucose uptake by peripheral tissues. Ultimately, hyperinsulinemia leads to some of the hormonal perturbations of PCOS. *Source*: Adapted from [20].

2. Hyperinsulinemia also inhibits the synthesis of SHBG, which exacerbates hyperandrogenemia by increasing the fraction of unbound (free) to bound androgens [17, 18].

3. Insulin resistance in the setting of PCOS impairs hepatic glycogenesis (conversion of glucose into glycogen) and peripheral glucose uptake [19]. Also, increased lipolysis in adipose tissue due to insulin resistance promotes the release of free fatty acids (which further exacerbates insulin resistance). Consequently, this sets up a vicious cycle of persistent insulin resistance [20].

6.1.1.2   Mechanism of Action

Metformin, a biguanide, is an insulin-sensitizing drug (ISD) that improves insulin resistance in PCOS. Although the mechanism of action of metformin has not been fully elucidated, it has been shown to activate the adenosine monophosphate-activated protein kinase (AMPK) pathway. A process that impairs hepatic glucose output, reduces fatty acid oxidation and increases glucose uptake by peripheral tissues. See Section 4.1.2 for additional information regarding the mechanism of action of metformin.

By improving insulin resistance, metformin helps mitigate some hormonal perturbations in PCOS.

Clinical Pearl

What is the history of polycystic ovary syndrome?

Polycystic ovary syndrome (PCOS) was eponymously named Stein-Leventhal syndrome based on a case series of seven women with clinical hyperandrogenism (hirsutism), oligomenorrhea, and enlarged ovaries, reported in 1935 [21]. Interestingly, this condition may have been first described by Antonio Vallisneri, an Italian physician, in 1721. He described a young, obese, and infertile woman with enlarged ovaries like those of a dove's eggs [22]. In recent times, the definition of PCOS has undergone various modifications based on recommendations from different groups of experts [23–26]. These definitions, in part, depend on specific clinical, biochemical, or ultrasonographic features (see Table 6.2). The pathophysiologic basis of PCOS is complex and is incompletely understood at this time [27].

The diagnostic criteria for PCOS vary across various practice guidelines (see Table 6.2).

TABLE 6.2   Diagnostic criteria for PCOS.

Diagnostic feature	NIH (1990) [23]	ESHRE/ASRM (2003) [24]	AE-PCOS (2006) [25]	NIH extension of ESHRE/ASRM (2012) [26]
Hyperandrogenism (HA)	+	+/–	+	A, B, C
Oligo/amenorrhea(OA)	+	+/–	+/–	A, B, D
Polycystic ovary morphology (PCOM)		+/–	+/–	A, C, D

+, refers to a required diagnostic feature; +/– refers to a diagnostic feature that may or may not be present.
NIH, National Institutes of Health (HA and OA required); ESHRE/ASRM, European Society for Human Reproduction and Embryology/American Society for Reproductive Medicine (also known as "Rotterdam Criteria") (Any 2 of 3 diagnostic features); AE-PCOS, Androgen Excess PCOS Society (HA with either OA or PCOM); OD, ovulatory dysfunction (includes OA or other ovulatory dysfunction such as infertility); A, Phenotype A (HA + OD + PCOM); B, Phenotype B (HA + OD); C, Phenotype C (HA + PCOM); D, Phenotype D (OD + PCOM).

Practice Pearl(s)

- Metformin should not be used as a first-line pharmacological option in anovulatory infertility (PCOS).
- Metformin does not reduce the risk of spontaneous abortions in women with PCOS.

- For patients undergoing assisted reproductive techniques, concomitant metformin reduces the risk of ovarian hyperstimulation syndrome [28].

Clinical Trial Evidence

(See Table 6.3)

TABLE 6.3   Clinical trials assessing the role of metformin in PCOS.

	Population	Intervention	Outcome
Hyperglycemia	Patients between 18 and 40 years of age with PCOS by the NIH criteria (n = 39).	Metformin ER 1500 mg/day for 12 weeks.	IVGTT at baseline and study conclusion was compared. Insulin response to glucose increased (P = 0.002), and basal glucose levels decreased (P = 0.001) compared to baseline [29].

TABLE 6.3 (Continued)

	Population	Intervention	Outcome
Hirsutism	Adult women with PCOS in 39 RCTs were analyzed in this Cochrane systematic review (n = 2047).	Metformin compared to OCP.	Metformin was less effective in improving hirsutism compared to OCP in patients with a BMI of 25–30 kg/m². (MD of 1.92, 95% CI 1.21–2.64) [30].
Menstrual regulation	Adult women with PCOS in 39 RCTs were analyzed in this Cochrane systematic review (n = 2047).	Metformin compared to OCP.	Metformin was less effective in improving menstrual patterns compared to OCP. (MD of 6.05, 95% CI 2.37–9.74) [30].
Infertility	This Cochrane systematic review analyzed adult women with PCOS in 6 RCTs.	ART in combination with metformin or placebo.	Compared to placebo, Metformin treatment did not improve various reproductive endpoints, including pregnancies or live births. There was, however, a statistically significant reduction in the risk of OHSS (pooled OR of 0.27, 95% CI 0.16–0.47) with metformin compared to placebo [31].

ER, extended-release; IVGTT, intravenous glucose tolerance test; OCP, oral contraceptive pill; BMI, Body Mass Index; MD, mean difference; ART, assisted reproductive techniques; OR, odds ratio; OHSS, ovarian hyperstimulation syndrome.

6.1.2 Combination Oral Contraceptive Pills

6.1.2.1 Physiology

The GnRH Pulse Generator and Normal Reproduction

The gonadotropin-releasing hormone (GnRH) pulse generator controls fertility by initiating the classic GnRH ultradian frequency, which regulates the synthesis of estradiol and progesterone by the ovaries [32]. More recently, the elusive GnRH pulse generator has been localized to the arcuate nucleus (ARN) of the hypothalamus. It is comprised of kisspeptin neurons with projections to distal dendrons of GnRH neurons (see Figure 6.3) [32–34].

The release of GnRH into the hypophyseal portal circulation promotes LH and FSH synthesis and secretion by pituitary gonadotrophs. The mode of release of GnRH, be it in a *pulsatile* or *surge-like fashion*, determines its downstream effects. Pulsatile GnRH release promotes ovarian follicle maturation. On the other hand, a surge-like increase in GnRH release accounts for the widely accepted *"LH surge"* required for ovulation [35].

In normal female reproductive physiology, progesterone reduces the GnRH pulse frequency (thus LH release) through its inhibitory effects on GnRH neurons (Table 6.4).

 Historical Pearl

Discovery of Kisspeptin

The gene encoding kisspeptins was designated as KiSS1 by investigators from the Penn State College of Medicine in Hershey, Pennsylvania. The gene's name is derived from the famous *"Hershey's Kisses"* chocolate brand [42].

The Two-Cell Two-Gonadotropin Hypothesis

In normal physiology, androgen synthesis by the theca interna cells of the ovary is induced by

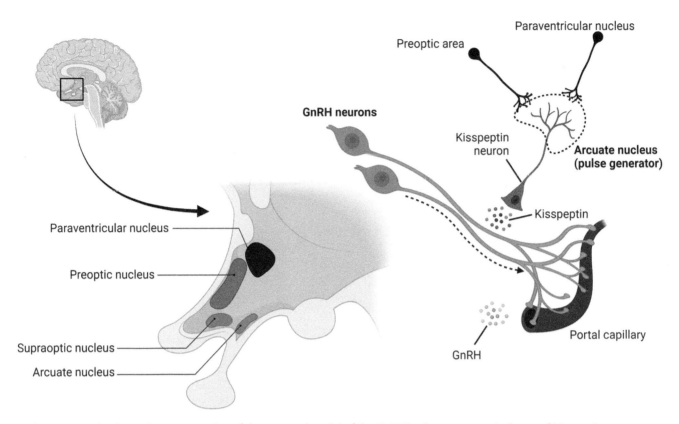

FIGURE 6.3 A schematic representation of the proposed model of the GnRH pulse generator. A cluster of kisspeptin neurons in the arcuate nucleus (ARN) of the hypothalamus possesses an intrinsic capacity to activate distal dendrons of the GnRH neuron. Additional modulators of GnRH release include the inputs from the preoptic area (POA), paraventricular nucleus (PVN), and yet-to-be-elucidated centers. *Source*: Adapted from [33].

TABLE 6.4 Regulation of the GnRH pulse generator.

Increases GnRH pulse frequency	Reduces GnRH pulse frequency
Estradiol [36]	Estradiol [36]
Leptin [37]	Progesterone [39]
Dihydrotestosterone [38]	Cortisol [40]
	Prolactin [41]

Source: Adapted from [36–41].

luteinizing hormone. Androgens are then transferred to the neighboring granulosa cells, where follicle-stimulating hormone stimulates aromatase activity, which mediates the conversion of androgens into estrogen. This is widely accepted as the *two-cell, two-gonadotropin theory of estrogen biosynthesis* [43] (Figure 6.4).

LH binds to the luteinizing hormone receptor (LHR), a G-protein coupled receptor, thus increasing intracytoplasmic cyclic adenosine monophosphate (cAMP) in the theca cell. cAMP derived from ATP then activates protein kinase A (PKA), which induces the expression of various steroidogenic enzymes involved in androgen synthesis (testosterone, andro-stenedione, and dehydroepiandrosterone). Likewise, FSH, by binding to its respective G-protein coupled receptor, also increases intracytoplasmic cAMP, which activates intracytoplasmic PKA. Androgens derived from the theca cell are ferried to the granu-losa cell, where aromatase (activated by PKA) pro-motes their conversion to estrogens (estradiol and estrone) [44, 45].

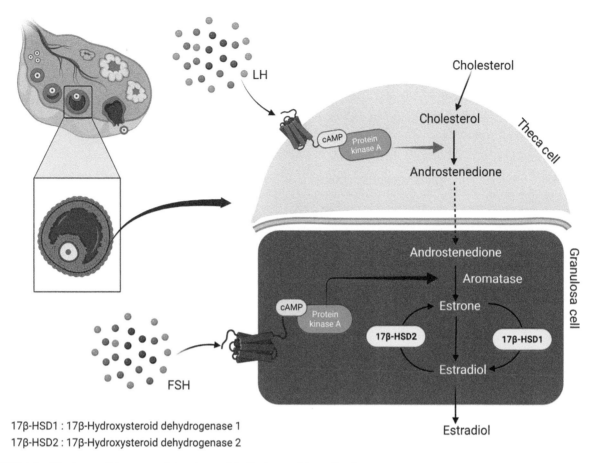

17β-HSD1 : 17β-Hydroxysteroid dehydrogenase 1
17β-HSD2 : 17β-Hydroxysteroid dehydrogenase 2

FIGURE 6.4   The two-cell two-gonadotropin model of estrogen biosynthesis.

6.1.2.2   Mechanism of Action

Estrogen and progestin-containing oral contraceptive pills (OCPs) are pivotal in improving various clinical manifestations of PCOS, including oligomenorrhea, hirsutism, and acne. The mechanism of action of OCPs is shown in Table 6.5.

Therapeutic benefits of OCPs include regulating menstrual cycles, mitigating the clinical effects of hyperandrogenemia (such as hirsutism and acne), prevention of endometrial hyperplasia, and contraception (for patients on anti-androgen medications) [46].

TABLE 6.5   Sites of action of OCPs in PCOS.

Site of action	Estrogen	Progestin
GnRH pulse generator	Suppresses FSH > LH	Suppresses LH release
Androgens	Increases SHBG → Decreases free androgen	Decreases ovarian androgen production (impairs LH-mediated production of androgens by theca cells). Androgen receptor blocking effects.[a]
Endometrium	Stabilizes the endometrium	Prevents endometrial hyperplasia.
Ovarian follicles	Suppresses recruitment and maturation of the dominant follicle	Inhibits the LH surge required for ovulation.

[a] Androgen receptor blocking effects are due to specific progestins, e.g. drospirenone.
Source: Adapted from [46].

Practice Pearl(s)

Oral contraceptive pills with low androgenic or anti-androgenic progestin activity are reasonable in PCOS (e.g. drospirenone) [47] (see Table 6.6). However, it should be noted that no specific OCP has been shown in clinical trials to be the best option in PCOS; as such current practice guidelines do not recommend the use of a specific OCP in PCOS [49, 50]. Although progestin-only therapies (depot injections or oral) offer some endometrial protective benefits, they are associated with breakthrough (or prolonged) uterine bleeding [51].

TABLE 6.6   Progestogenic and androgenic potencies of low-dose combined oral contraceptives.

Components of combined oral contraceptive			Activity of progestins	
Brand name(s)	Estrogen(dose)	Progestin(dose)	Progestogenic	Androgenic
Orthonovum 1/35	Ethinyl estradiol (35 mcg)	Norethindrone(1 mg)	+++	+++
Loestrin 1.5/30	Ethinyl estradiol (30 mcg)	Norethindrone(1.5 mg)		
Levlen, Nordette	Ethinyl estradiol (30 mcg)	Levonorgestrel (0.15 mg)	+++	+++
Levlite, Alesse	Ethinyl estradiol (20 mcg)	Levonorgestrel (0.1 mg)		
Ortho Tri-Cyclen	Ethinyl estradiol (35 mcg)	Norgestimate (0.18–0.25 mg)	++	+
Ortho Tri-Cyclen LO	Ethinyl estradiol (25 mcg)	Norgestimate (0.18–0.25 mg)		
Yasmin	Ethinyl estradiol (30 mcg)	Drospirenone (3 mg)	+	Antiandrogenic
Yaz	Ethinyl estradiol (20 mcg)	Drospirenone (3 mg)		
Natazia	Estradiol valerate (1–3 mg)	Dienogest(2–3 mg)	+	Antiandrogenic

Source: Adapted from [46, 48].

Clinical Trial Evidence

Also, see Table 6.3 (role of OCP in menstrual regulation and hirsutism).

6.1.3 Mineralocorticoid Antagonists

6.1.3.1 Physiology

Effects of androgen in the skin can be reviewed in greater detail in Sections 6.1.7 and 6.1.8.

6.1.3.2 Mechanism of Action

Spironolactone, a diuretic and aldosterone antagonist, also has antagonistic properties at the androgen receptor [52]. Additionally, spironolactone inhibits ovarian and adrenal steroidogenesis. Thus its utility in the management of acne and hirsutism in PCOS [53].

Additional antiandrogenic effects of spironolactone

- Inhibits the activity of 5 alpha-reductase (critical in converting testosterone to its active form, dihydrotestosterone).
- It increases the activity of aromatase (conversion of testosterone to estrogen).
- Increases SHBG [54].

Practice Pearl(s)

Spironolactone titrated to a dose of 200 mg/day (for 6–9 months), is effective in improving moderate-to-severe hirsutism in patients with polycystic ovary syndrome [53, 55] (Table 6.7). A starting dose of 25 mg twice daily and increasing to a maximum dose of 100 mg twice daily is reasonable.

Patients should be on oral contraceptive pills for at least 6 months before initiating spironolactone due to its effects on the development of male genitalia during intrauterine life. Furthermore, spironolactone can exacerbate menstrual irregularity if not used concomitantly with oral contraceptive therapy [52, 58].

Spironolactone can cause a myriad of side effects due to its diuretic and anti-mineralocorticoid action. These include postural hypotension, dizziness, and hyperkalemia. The side effects are tolerable as long as patients on long-term therapy are closely monitored [59].

TABLE 6.7   Clinical trials assessing the role of spironolactone in PCOS.

Study	Population	Intervention	Outcome
Spironolactone plus metformin in PCOS	56 overweight/obese patients with PCOS[a]	Randomized to metformin 1700 mg daily (n = 28) or metformin 1700 mg + spironolactone 25 mg daily (n = 28) for 6 months.	Modified Ferriman–Gallway score[b] was significantly lower in the spironolactone + metformin group compared to the metformin only group (P < 0.001) [56].
Spironolactone versus metformin in PCOS (Open-label study)	82 women with PCOS (NIH criteria)	Randomized to metformin 500 mg twice a day (n = 41) or spironolactone 25 mg twice a day (n = 41).	Hirsutism score was significantly lower in the spironolactone group compared to the metformin group, with a much tolerable side effect profile [57].

[a] Patients on oral contraceptives, anti-hypertensives, anti-diabetic, or weight loss medications were excluded.
[b] Hirsutism score.

Clinical Trial Evidence
See Table 6.7 for a summary of relevant trials evaluating the role of spironolactone in PCOS.

6.1.4 Gonadotropins

6.1.4.1 Physiology

Physiology of Follicular Development

The menstrual cycle and, in effect, ovarian follicular development are regulated by the hypothalamus, pituitary gland, and ovaries. The frequency of firing of the GnRH pulse generator at various stages of the menstrual cycle determines the extent of synthesis and secretion of follicle-stimulating hormone and luteinizing hormone. The term gonadotropins refers to follicle-stimulating hormone and luteinizing hormone. Follicle-stimulating hormone is critical in the recruitment and development of ovarian follicles while luteinizing hormone mediates the process of ovulation. Review regulation of the GnRH pulse generator in Section 6.1.2.

Ovarian follicular development can be categorized into two distinct but interrelated stages, often described as the *gonadotropin-independent* and *gonadotropin-dependent phases*. The independent gonadotropin phase is characterized by the growth of a primordial ovarian follicle into a pre-antral follicle (before the follicle develops a fluid-filled space or antrum). Gonadotropin-dependent phase promotes the development and release of the dominant follicle [60] (see Figure 6.5).

The gonadotropin-independent and -dependent phases of folliculogenesis show the transition from a primordial follicle to the corpus albicans (see Figure 6.5). Adapted and modified from Orisaka et al. [60]

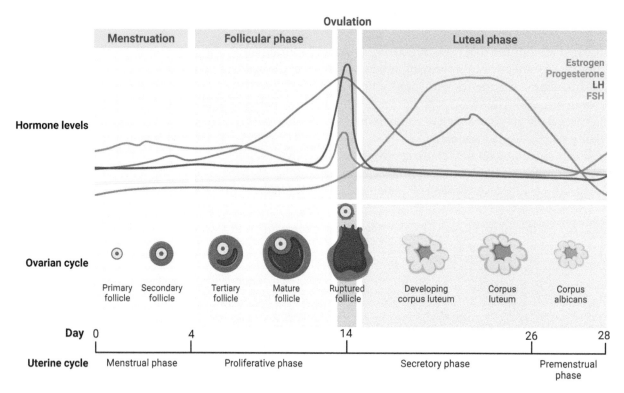

FIGURE 6.5   A schematic representation of folliculogenesis.

Gonadotropin-Independent Phase

The primordial follicle has a nucleus surrounded by a single layer of squamous granulosa cells. Recruited primordial follicles transform into primary follicles (transition of squamous to cuboidal granulosa cells). Subsequently, primary follicles develop into secondary follicles (transition from a cuboidal to stratified columnar epithelium). Additionally, the secondary follicle has an internal *theca interna* layer and an outer *theca externa* layer [61]. Next, the secondary follicle differentiates into a pre-antral follicle. Formation of the pre-antral follicle marks the transition point from gonadotropin-independent to gonadotropin-dependent folliculogenesis. Various intraovarian regulators control this follicular development phase, including growth factors and cytokines [62, 63].

Gonadotropin-Dependent Phase

Granulosa and theca interna cells of the pre-antral follicle express FSH and LH receptors, respectively. FSH binds to its cognate FSH receptor on the granulosa cells of the pre-antral follicle, leading to follicular growth and the development of a fluid-filled follicular space (antrum). Also, the binding of LH to LH receptors on theca interna cells results in the production of androgens [64]. Androgens paradoxically promote both follicular growth and regression, depending on the stage of follicular development [65]. Stimulation of androgen receptors on granulosa cells of follicles in the early gonadotropin-dependent phase augments FSH-mediated follicular development. Conversely, during the late preovulatory stage, elevated levels of androgens lead to arrested antral follicular development [65, 66].

In addition, some androgens will be converted into estrogen by granulosa cells (see the two-cell two gonadotropin model in Figure 6.4). Consequently, elevated levels of circulating estrogen inhibit the *GnRH pulse generator*, which blunts the release of FSH during the follicular (preovulatory) phase of the menstrual cycle. As a result, smaller follicles with a lower density of FSH receptors degenerate while the dominant (more prominent) follicle continues to develop. In contrast to most stages of the menstrual cycle, estrogen increases the GnRH pulse frequency during the midcycle, which increases the circulating levels of LH ("LH surge"). The LH surge leads to the release of a mature oocyte by the preovulatory follicle [67].

The empty follicle produced at the end of ovulation transforms into the *corpus luteum*, which secretes progesterone and estrogen critical in maintaining pregnancy. However, if implantation fails, the corpus luteum regresses into a bundle of connective tissue known as the *corpus albicans*.

6.1.4.2 Mechanism of Action

The principal reason for infertility in PCOS is anovulation, making gonadotropins a suitable option for patients desiring fertility (Table 6.8).

TABLE 6.8 Mechanism of action of gonadotropins in assisted reproduction.

Agent	Mechanism(s)
Recombinant FSH (rFSH)	1. FSH stimulates the recruitment and subsequent development of a cohort of pre-antral follicles [68, 69]. 2. FSH also rescues follicles destined for atresia [70].
Recombinant Luteinizing hormone (rLH), human chorionic gonadotropin (hCG)	1. Enhances final follicular maturation. 2. Promotes maturation of the follicular oocyte from its germinal vesicle stage (prophase I of the cell cycle) to metaphase II of meiosis. 3. Maintain luteal function prior to the establishment of placental steroidogenesis [71].

hCG binds to the LH receptor due to its structural homology to LH.

Practice Pearl(s)

Gonadotropin therapy is a suitable second-line option for patients with PCOS who are clomiphene or letrozole resistant.

Table 6.9 summarizes the dosing schedule of gonadotropins in ovulation induction.

TABLE 6.9 Dosing schedule of gonadotropins.

Treatment	Dose and timing
rFSH[a]	75 IU administered subcutaneously on a daily basis for to up 14 days until follicular maturity is achieved [72].
hCG[b]	5000–10,000 IU administered intramuscularly or subcutaneously.

[a] Dose of rFSH is increased on a weekly basis if there is a suboptimal response. Treatment is terminated after 35 days if there is a suboptimal response [72] – monitoring of response through transvaginal ultrasounds and serial serum estradiol levels. If more than four follicles have a diameter of 14 mm or greater, the cycle is canceled due to the risk of ovarian hyperstimulation syndrome [73].
[b] Progesterone concentration above 5 ng/mL confirms ovulation. Follicular rupture occurs within 48 hours of hCG administration [74]. (Progesterone levels assessed on day 7 and pregnancy test on day 14).

Clinical Trial Evidence

This systematic review measured various outcomes among women with PCOS treated with gonadotropins (urinary gonadotropins were compared to rFSH). All study participants had previously failed clomiphene citrate therapy. Those on co-treatment with metformin, letrozole, LH, or clomiphene citrate were excluded from the systematic review (see Table 6.10).

There was no statistically significant difference between comparisons of gonadotropins in terms of live birth rate, the incidence of multigestational pregnancies, or OHSS [75].

(continued)

(continued)

TABLE 6.10 Comparison of fertility outcomes of gonadotropin preparations.

Study endpoint	Urinary-derived gonadotropins	Recombinant FSH	OR (95% CI)
Live birth rate per woman	157 per 1000	191 per 1000	1.26 (0.80–1.99)
Incidence of OHSS	22 per 1000	33 per 1000	1.52 (0.81–2.84)
Incidence of multi-pregnancy rate per woman	30 per 1000	26 per 1000	0.86 (0.44–1.65)

OHSS, ovarian hyperstimulation syndrome; OR, odds ratio.
Urinary-derived gonadotropins included FSH, human menopausal gonadotropin (HMG), purified FSH, highly purified FSH, and highly purified HMG.

6.1.5 Clomiphene Citrate

6.1.5.1 Physiology

The role of estrogen in regulating the GnRH pulse generator was reviewed in Section 6.1.2.

6.1.5.2 Mechanism of Action

Clomiphene demonstrates its therapeutic effects in the setting of an intact hypothalamic–pituitary axis and optimal endogenous estrogen production (e.g. PCOS). Clomiphene is a selective estrogen receptor modular (SERM); as such, it can bind to estrogen receptors in various sensitive tissues, including the hypothalamus, ovaries, and endometrial lining [76]. Furthermore, it can exert both partial agonist and antagonist effects depending on the tissue in question.

For example, at the level of the hypothalamus, clomiphene acts as an antagonist, thus preventing negative feedback inhibition of the GnRH pulse generator by endogenous estrogen [77]. In patients with PCOS, clomiphene increases the pulse amplitude but not the pulse frequency of the GnRH pulse generator. As a result, the levels of LH and FSH increase, thereby enhancing the recruitment and maturation of ovarian follicles [78].

Practice Pearl(s)

Clomiphene citrate is traditionally initiated within 5 days of spontaneous menstruation or progestin-induced withdrawal bleeding. The starting dose of clomiphene citrate is 50 mg daily for 5 days. Ovulation is expected within 5–10 days after the last dose of clomiphene citrate; therefore, ovulation monitoring is required within this time window. If there is therapeutic failure, the dose of clomiphene citrate can be increased by 50 mg/day during the next cycle, up to a maximum daily dose of 250 mg [76].

Alternative Indications for Clomiphene Use

1. Male hypogonadism [79]
2. Gynecomastia (it is, however, not as effective as tamoxifen) [80]

Clinical Trial Evidence

In this meta-analysis of 3 trials and 133 participants with PCOS, clomiphene citrate resulted in a statistically significant increase in pregnancy and ovulation rates per woman, compared to placebo [81] (see Table 6.11).

TABLE 6.11 A meta-analysis of clomiphene citrate versus placebo in PCOS.

Study endpoint	Clomiphene Citrate	Placebo	OR (95% CI)
Pregnancy rate (per woman)	14	2	5.77 (1.55–21.48)
Ovulation rate (per woman)	45	14	7.47 (3.24–17.23)

OR, odds ratio.

6.1.6 Letrozole

6.1.6.1 Physiology

The role of estrogen in regulating the GnRH pulse generator was reviewed in Section 6.1.2.

6.1.6.2 Mechanism of Action

Letrozole is a competitive nonsteroidal *aromatase inhibitor* that exerts its therapeutic effects in PCOS by blocking the conversion of androgens to estrogens. Low circulating estrogen levels blunt its negative feedback effect on the GnRH pulse generator, which subsequently increases GnRH pulse frequency and gonadotropin release [82].

Practice Pearl(s)

Letrozole at a dose of 2.5 mg daily is initiated after three days of either spontaneous menstruation or progestin-induced bleed (medroxyprogesterone acetate, 5 mg daily for 10 days). Like clomiphene, letrozole is administered for 5 consecutive days. Furthermore, for patients who experience a poor ovulatory response, a gradual increase in dose to 7.5 mg daily during subsequent cycles is recommended for a total of 5 cycles [83].

Clinical Trial Evidence

In this meta-analysis of patients with PCOS, letrozole was compared to clomiphene citrate. Letrozole resulted in a statistically significant increase in clinical pregnancy rates and live birth rates compared to clomiphene. There was no statistically significant difference in ovarian hyperstimulation syndrome rates, miscarriage rates, or multigestational rates [84] (Table 6.12).

TABLE 6.12 A meta-analysis of clomiphene citrate versus letrozole in PCOS.

Study endpoint	Clomiphene citrate	Letrozole	OR (95% CI)
Live birth rate	214 per 1000	314 per 1000	1.68 (1.42–1.99)
Clinical pregnancy rate	264 per 1000	359 per 1000	1.56 (1.37–1.78)

OR, odds ratio.

6.1.7 Androgen Receptor Antagonist

6.1.7.1 Physiology

Structure of the Hair Follicle

Hair plays various biological and psychosocial functions. Hair is required for the dispersion of the secretions of sweat glands and, more importantly, protection from cold weather. The distribution of hair in humans contributes to some phenotypic differences between the sexes [85]. Consequently, conditions such as hirsutism, androgenetic alopecia (AGA), and hypertrichosis may have significant psychosexual consequences.

The hair follicle has two major components, the root (within the skin) and the shaft (visible above the skin) [86]. The triad of a sebaceous gland, arrector pili muscle, and the hair follicle is called a *pilosebaceous unit* [87].

The shaft comprises various filaments and proteins derived from matrix cells present in the hair bulb (part of the root). Melanocytes present in the matrix cells are responsible for the pigmentation of the shaft [88].

A group of specialized mesenchymal fibroblasts located at the base of the hair follicle forms the dermal papilla. Dermal papilla cells control the growth and differentiation of matrix cells. Other cells present in the hair follicle include melanocytes, Langerhans' cells (antigen-presenting cells), and Merkel cells (neural cells) [89].

Phases of Hair Growth

The anagen phase represents the initial growth of the hair follicle. Progressive elongation of filaments (derived from matrix cells) leads to the protrusion of the follicle from the skin. A subsequent catagen phase is characterized by regression of the hair follicle, leading to the formation of club hair (keratinized and dead hair). A final telogen phase (a period of quiescence) results in the shedding of club hair. This phase is not a terminal phase of hair growth since it lays the foundation for critical regulatory factors needed to restart the anagen phase [90].

Role of Androgens in Hair Formation

Androgens promote hair growth at various sites, including the scalp, beard, pubic, and axillary regions. Even so, androgens paradoxically result in AGA of the scalp [91].

Clinical Pearl

Androgenetic alopecia in men presents as frontal recession and loss of hair at the vertex of the scalp. Conversely, there is a loss of hair over the crown with relative sparing of frontal hair in women [89].

Although the exact mechanism of androgen-mediated regulation of hair growth is yet to be fully elucidated, dermal papilla cells appear to be the site of action of androgens [92, 93]. By binding to receptors on dermal papilla cells, androgens cause the release of regulatory factors critical in the growth of hair follicles [92]. Type 2 5 alpha-reductase enzyme in the hair follicle is critical in regulating the levels of dihydrotestosterone (DHT), a potent androgen. There is experimental evidence that this enzyme is present in a higher concentration in balding scalps compared to non-balding scalps [94].

See Table 6.13 for the mechanism of action of androgen receptor blockers.

Role of Androgens in Acne Formation

DHT regulates the production of sebum by sebaceous glands. The type 1 5 alpha-reductase isoenzyme is responsible for regulating tissue-specific concentrations of DHT in sebaceous glands [96].

6.1.7.2   Mechanism of Action

TABLE 6.13   Mechanism of action of androgen receptor blockers.

Drug	Mechanism of action	Clinical effects
Spironolactone	Aldosterone receptor blocker that inhibits the binding of testosterone and dihydrotestosterone to the androgen receptor. Increases SHBG and inhibits 5 alpha-reductase.	Treatment of acne and alopecia, hirsutism.
Flutamide	A selective non-steroidal androgen receptor blocker.	Treatment of acne, hirsutism, and alopecia.

Source: Adapted from [95].

Practice Pearl(s)

Refer to Table 6.14 for a summary of androgen receptor blockers used in treating PCOS.

TABLE 6.14   Androgen receptor blockers in clinical practice.

Drug	Dosage	Monitoring/Side effects
Spironolactone	100–200 mg/day in two divided doses.	Female patients should be on concomitant contraceptive therapy. It can cause gastrointestinal discomfort and menstrual irregularity [97].
Flutamide	62.5–250 mg/day.	Combination therapy with oral contraceptive therapy is recommended [98]. It is associated with hepatotoxicity (close monitoring of liver function tests is required) [99].

Source: Adapted from [97–99].

Clinical Trial Evidence

In this six-month randomized study, 48 patients with hirsutism were randomized to either 100 mg/day of cyproterone acetate or 100 mg/day of spironolactone. All subjects received additional therapy with estrogen therapy (contraception). Compared to the baseline, both cyproterone acetate and spironolactone led to a 16.8% (P-value < 0.001) and 17.1% (P-value < 0.001) decline in total hair diameter, respectively. More importantly, there was no between-group difference in their effect on total hair diameter [100].

6.1.8   5-Alpha Reductase Inhibitor (Finasteride)

6.1.8.1   Physiology

The role of androgens in hair growth was reviewed earlier in Section 6.1.7.

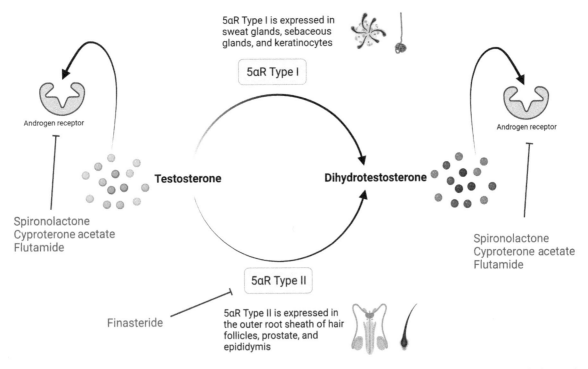

FIGURE 6.6 Schematic representation of the mechanism of action of various androgen-receptor modulators in hirsutism. The site of action of androgen receptor blockers (flutamide, spironolactone, and cyproterone acetate) and 5 alpha-reductase inhibitors (finasteride) is shown. The distribution of the subtypes of 5 alpha-reductase enzymes is tissue specific. *Source*: Adapted from [95].

6.1.8.2 Mechanism of Action

Finasteride impairs the conversion of testosterone to dihydrotestosterone (the active metabolite of testosterone) by inhibiting the type 2 isoenzyme of 5 alpha-reductase [101]. Also, see Figure 6.6.

Practice Pearl(s)

It is potentially teratogenic and is prescribed off-label for androgenetic alopecia and hirsutism. The recommended dose range of oral finasteride is 0.5–5 mg/day [102].

Finasteride gel 0.25%, applied twice daily, is efficacious in treating both hirsutism and acne, with very minimal side effects [103].

Clinical Trial Evidence

In this controlled clinical study by Tolino et al., 15 women with polycystic ovary syndrome were treated with oral finasteride 5 mg daily for a period of 6 months. The mean **Ferriman–Gallway score**

(clinical assessment of the degree of hirsutism) declined from 24.6 (with a standard deviation of 1.8) at baseline to 8.9 (standard deviation of 2.4) after 6 months of therapy (P-value of < 0.05) [104].

6.1.9 Weight loss interventions

6.1.9.1 Physiology

Essential concepts in obesity (see Section 7.2).

6.1.9.2 Mechanism of Action

The mechanism of action of various medical weight loss therapies (see Section 7.2).

Practice Pearl(s)

Weight loss therapy through medical nutrition therapy, medications, or bariatric surgery can lead to significant improvement in metabolic and reproductive perturbations in polycystic ovary syndrome [49].

Clinical Trial Evidence

The efficacy of weight loss interventions in the management of PCOS is shown in Table 6.15.

TABLE 6.15 Studies evaluating the role of weight-loss interventions in PCOS.

Study	Population	Intervention	Outcome(s)
Bariatric surgery	Premenopausal women with PCOS ($n = 17$)	A longitudinal nonrandomized study. Patients underwent bariatric surgery.	The mean weight loss after at least 6 months post-surgery was 41 kg (SD of 9, up to 61% of initial body weight). There was a statistically significant decline in hirsutism score, testosterone, androstenedione, DHEAs, and HOMA-IR scores [105].
Nutrition therapy	Premenopausal women with PCOS($n = 65$)	1200–1400 kcal/day diet for 6 months, subsequently placed on a mild calorie restrictive diet and physical activity.	Amelioration of clinical features of PCOS (oligomenorrhea, hyperandrogenism, and ovulatory dysfunction) occurred in 36.9% of participants [106].

SD, standard deviation; DHEAs, dehydroepiandrosterone sulfate; HOMA-IR, insulin resistance estimated by homeostasis model assessment.
Source: Adapted from [105, 106].

Concepts to Ponder Over

Differential diagnoses of oligomenorrhea.

- Pregnancy
- Non classic CAH
- Thyroid disease
- Hyperprolactinemia
- Hypothalamic amenorrhea
- Premature ovarian insufficiency
- Androgen-secreting tumor
- Acromegaly
- Cushing syndrome

6.2 MALE HYPOGONADISM

Historical Pearl

In a rather crude experiment carried out in 1889, Brown-Séquard injected testicular extracts from a dog and guinea pig into his subcutaneous tissue. In a letter published in *The Lancet* journal, he described various effects of his extract, including an increase in muscle strength, improved urinary flow, and improved cognition [107, 108]. The treatment of an ailing organ with a similar organ (mainly from animals) hails from antiquity – a treatment paradigm that was known as *similia similibus* [109]. This organotherapeutic "hormone replacement" approach is arguably the basis of modern endocrinology [108].

6.2.1 Testosterone Hormone Replacement

6.2.1.1 Physiology

Regulation of Testosterone Production

Hypothalamic neurons secrete GnRH, which gains access to anterior pituitary gonadotrophs via the *hypothalamic-hypophyseal venous portal system*. Pulsatile secretion of GnRH subsequently promotes the release of both LH and FSH by gonadotrophs. The stimulation of Leydig cells of the testes by LH results in the production of testosterone. Secretion of testosterone also occurs in a pulsatile and diurnal fashion, with peak concentrations around 8 a.m. and nadir around 8 p.m. [110]. Testosterone regulates its plasma concentration through negative feedback inhibition of both GnRH neurons in the hypothalamus and gonadotropins (LH and FSH) in the anterior pituitary gland [111]. The role of FSH in spermiogenesis (see Section 6.2.3).

Testosterone Production by Leydig Cells

LH stimulates the LH receptor (a G protein-coupled receptor), which subsequently results in the activation of adenylyl cyclase. Adenylyl cyclase mediates an increase in intracellular cyclic AMP formation, promoting protein kinase A activation and subsequent phosphorylation of various intracellular proteins required for steroidogenesis. Steroidogenic acute regulatory protein (StAR) and translocator proteins are essential intracellular proteins required to transport cholesterol into the mitochondria [112].

The mobilization of cholesterol from various sources, including plasma membrane, lipid droplets, and the *de novo* cholesterol synthesis pathway, initiates steroidogenesis. The transport of cholesterol into the mitochondria of Leydig cells is the rate-limiting step of testosterone synthesis [112]. 17 hydroxylase enzyme is central to the synthesis of androgens. The lack of 11 and 21 hydroxylase enzymes in Leydig cells prevents the production of glucocorticoids and mineralocorticoids [113].

Metabolism of Testosterone

Testosterone undergoes metabolism through various pathways, enhancing its biological function at the androgen receptor, converting it into estrogen to extend its effects in various tissues, or inactivating it (see Figure 6.7).

About 7 mg of testosterone is produced a day [114]. Approximately 90% of this undergoes metabolism in the liver, resulting in inactive metabolites – etiocholanolone and androsterone. 5–10% of endogenous testosterone is converted to dihydrotestosterone, further enhancing its effects on the androgen receptor. Also, dihydrotestosterone undergoes inactivation in the liver to produce androstanediol, androsterone, and androstenedione. The remaining 0.1% of endogenous testosterone gets converted into estradiol by aromatase present in the skeletal and central nervous systems [115].

Physiologic Effects of Testosterone in Men

Testosterone exerts its physiologic effects through various pathways:

- Conversion of testosterone into dihydrotestosterone by the 5 alpha-reductase enzyme.
- Conversion of testosterone into estradiol by the aromatase enzyme.
- Binding directly to the androgen receptor, which subsequently triggers various downstream processes. See Table 6.16.

Transportation of Testosterone

Testosterone is present in plasma, either bound to circulating proteins or an unbound free form. Approximately 53–55% of testosterone is bound to

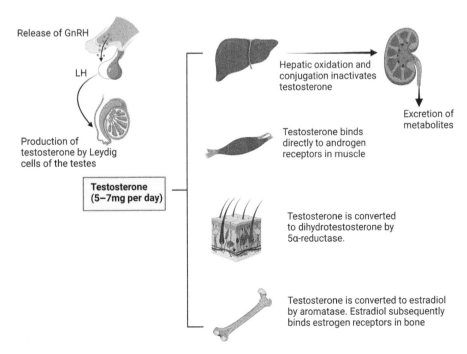

FIGURE 6.7   Metabolism of testosterone.

TABLE 6.16   Mechanism of the physiologic effects of testosterone.

Physiologic effect	Mechanism
Increase in bone mineral density	1. Promotes bone formation by binding to androgen receptors on osteoblasts. 2. Promotes insulin-like growth factor 1 mediated proliferation of chondrocytes and osteoblasts. 3. Estrogen (produced through the action of aromatase on testosterone) inhibits RANKL-mediated bone resorption [116].
Hair growth and sebum production	1. Growth of androgen-dependent hair by activating androgen receptors on dermal papilla cells. 2. Androgen receptors on sebaceous glands are activated by testosterone leading to an increased risk for acne [117].
Muscle growth	The mechanism underlying muscle protein synthesis and hypertrophy is unknown [118].
Reproductive roles	1. Descent of the testes, spermatogenesis, phallic and testicular enlargement. 2. Increase in libido [119].
Erythropoiesis (increase in hemoglobin and hematocrit)	1. Increased synthesis of erythropoietin. 2. Suppression of hepcidin (an inhibitor of intestinal iron absorption)... 3. Increase in iron mobilization [120].

RANKL, Receptor activator of nuclear factor kappa B ligand.
Source: Adapted from [116–120].

TABLE 6.17   Regulators of sex hormone-binding globulin.

Increase in SHBG	Decrease in SHBG
Hyperthyroidism	Hypothyroidism
Estrogens	Progestins, androgens, and glucocorticoids
Cirrhosis	Nephrosis
Aging	Acromegaly and diabetes mellitus
HIV infection	Obesity

HIV, Human immunodeficiency virus infection.
Source: Adapted from [122].

albumin, 43–45% is bound to SHBG with 1–2% in an active free form [121].

Regulation of Sex Hormone-Binding Globulin

SHBG is a glycoprotein with an affinity for various sex steroids, including testosterone, dihydrotestosterone, and estradiol [11]. Various pathophysiologic states that influence the concentration of serum SHBG are shown in Table 6.17.

6.2.1.2   Mechanism of Action

Testosterone exerts its physiologic effects by binding to the androgen receptor. Subsequent signaling after testosterone-to-androgen receptor interaction occurs via either a classical (gene expression) or a nonclassical (kinase activation) pathway [123] (Figure 6.8).

In the classical signaling pathway, testosterone diffuses through the plasma membrane and binds its cognate cytosolic receptor [124]. A conformational change in the cytosolic androgen receptor allows it to be separated from associated heat shock proteins (HSP 70 and HSP 90). The androgen receptor subsequently traverses the nuclear membrane and binds to androgen response elements (AREs) on DNA. Consequently, various transcription factors mediate the transcription and translation of specific androgen-inducible genes [123]. The nonclassical pathway (not shown) is initiated via the interaction of testosterone with the cytosolic androgen receptor. This leads to the activation of the mitogen-activated protein kinase (MAPK) cascade – sequential phosphorylation of various proteins, including RAF, MEK, and ERK. Finally, phosphorylation of CREB results in the activation of various CREB-regulated genes responsible for various physiological effects of testosterone [124].

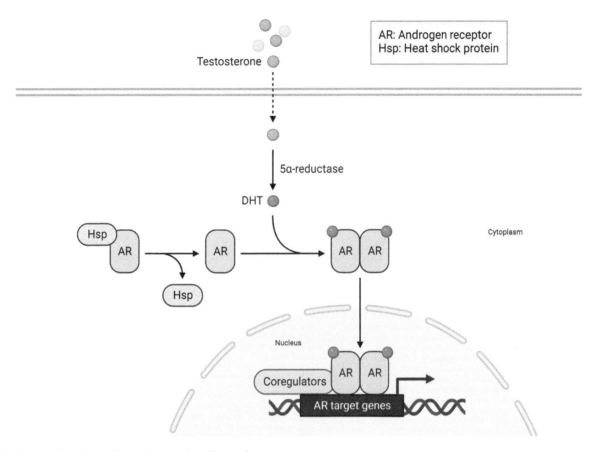

FIGURE 6.8   The classical testosterone signaling pathway.

Practice Pearl(s)

The typical dosing schedule of various testosterone preparations is shown in Table 6.18.

TABLE 6.18   Dosing schedule and practical guide to testosterone replacement.

Preparation	Dose (route, schedule)	Practical guide
Testosterone cypionate or enanthate	150–200 mg (IM, every two weeks)	Highly variable serum testosterone (significant fluctuation in hypogonadal symptoms). Risk of erythrocytosis.
Testosterone patch	2–4 mg (TD, every 24 hours)	Stable serum testosterone concentration. Less likely to cause erythrocytosis.
Testosterone gel	20.25–81 mg of 1.62% gel Or 50–100 mg of 1% gel (TD, every 24 hours)	Potential transfer to sexual partners or children.

Other preparations include long-acting intramuscular testosterone undecanoate, subcutaneous testosterone pellets, buccal tablets, and nasal gels.

IM, intramuscular; TD, transdermal.

Source: Adapted from Ref. [122].

Clinical Trial Evidence

A series of clinical trials, known as *The Testosterone Trials,* assessed the efficacy of testosterone therapy in men older than 65 years of age with hypogonadism (total serum testosterone <275 ng/dL and hypogonadal symptoms). Study participants were randomized to either testosterone gel (intervention) or placebo for a total of 12 months. For participants in the intervention arm of the study, the goal serum testosterone was in the mid-normal range for younger men (19–40 years of age). See Table 6.19.

TABLE 6.19   Summary of the testosterone trials.

Testosterone trial	Outcome
Sexual function trial	PDQ-Q4 score: The mean difference in the change from baseline between the intervention and placebo arms was 0.58 (95% CI 0.38–0.78, P-value < 0.0001).
Physical function trial	Increase in 6-minute walking distance by at least 50 m: Difference between the intervention and placebo arms, OR of 1.42 (95% CI 0.83–2.45, P-value = 0.20).
Vitality trial	Increase in FACIT score (a higher score implies less fatigue) of at least 4 points: The difference between the intervention and placebo arms, OR 1.23 (0.83–1.84, P-value = 0.03).

PDQ-Q4, psychosexual daily questionnaire; CI, confidence interval; OR, odds ratio; FACIT, Functional assessment of chronic illness therapy.
Source: Adapted from [125].

6.2.2   Human Chorionic Gonadotropin

6.2.2.1   Physiology

Human chorionic gonadotropin (hCG) regulates the production of progesterone and other factors critical in maintaining fetal viability during the first trimester of pregnancy [126]. hCG, a member of the glycoprotein hormone family, is comprised of α and β subunits, which are non-covalently linked. hCG, FSH, LH, and thyroid-stimulating hormone (TSH) share structural homology in their α-subunit [127]. Conversely, the amino acid sequence of the β-subunit is hormone-specific and distinguishes hCG from other members of the glycoprotein hormone family.

Spermatogenesis is dependent on intratesticular testosterone concentration (see Section 6.2.3). For patients on exogenous testosterone therapy, testosterone-mediated negative feedback inhibition of the hypothalamus and pituitary gland impairs the pulsatile release of GnRH and LH, respectively [128]. Consequently, Leydig cells of the testes cannot produce intratesticular testosterone critical in maintaining spermatogenesis and testicular volume [129–131].

6.2.2.2   Mechanism of Action

hCG is a placental-derived analog of LH and is extracted either from the urine of pregnant women or synthesized using recombinant DNA technology [132].

hCG has a half-life of 24 hours [133] compared to LH (half-life of 60 minutes), making the former a reasonable therapeutic option in managing male infertility [127]. Due to their similarity in the α-subunit amino acid sequence, hCG can occupy the LH receptor and activate downstream processes typically mediated by LH (see Section 6.2.1).

Practice Pearl(s)

Testosterone replacement therapy is associated with oligospermia, an undesirable clinical effect in younger hypogonadal men seeking to preserve their fertility [131]. This makes HCG a viable alternative to testosterone in this subset of hypogonadal men [128, 134, 135]. Furthermore, hCG is less likely to cause elevated hematocrit, hyperestrogenemia, or prostatic enlargement than conventional testosterone replacement therapy [128].

hCG requires functioning testicular tissue; as such, it can only be used in men with secondary causes of hypogonadism. Testosterone replacement therapy is recommended for men with primary hypogonadism [128].

Clinical Trial Evidence

Clinical trials evaluating the role of hCG in male hypogonadism are summarized in Table 6.20.

TABLE 6.20   The efficacy of hCG in male hypogonadism.

Study	Population	Intervention(s)	Outcome
CC or hCG in male hypogonadism	HH + Low serum testosterone (<300 ng/dL) with hypogonadal symptoms (n = 282)	Randomized to oral CC 50 mg daily, SC hCG 5000 IU twice a week or both for three months.	The mean baseline testosterone increased from 2.31 nmol/L to a final average of 5.17 nmol/L with no statistically significant difference between the treatment groups [136].
Concomitant Testosterone and hCG therapy in male hypogonadism	HH + Low serum testosterone (<300 ng/dL) with hypogonadal symptoms (n = 26)	Retrospective review of patients treated with TRT (IM or TD testosterone) and IM hCG 500 IU every other day. Mean follow-up of 6.2 months.	The mean serum testosterone level increased from a baseline of 207.2 ng/dL to 1055.5 ng/dL during treatment (P-value <0.0001). Semen indices, such as volume, density, and sperm motility, remained unchanged at the end of the study [137].

CC, clomiphene citrate; SC, subcutaneous; IU, international units; HH, hypogonadotropic hypogonadism; TRT, testosterone replacement therapy; IM, intramuscular; TD, transdermal.

6.2.3   Follicle-Stimulating Hormone

6.2.3.1   Physiology

Regulation of Sertoli Cell Function

Testosterone derived from Leydig cells of the testes diffuses into the seminiferous tubules to access Sertoli cells. Testosterone (a steroid hormone) subsequently diffuses through the plasma membrane and then binds directly to androgen receptors in the cytoplasm of Sertoli cells. Consequently, the synthesis of various androgen-inducible genes required for Sertoli cell function and spermatogenesis occurs (see Figure 6.8 for the classical pathway of testosterone signaling) [138].

FSH binds to the FSH receptor (a G protein-coupled receptor) on Sertoli cells, leading to downstream processes critical in Sertoli cell function [139]. Sertoli cells are responsible for the provision of nutrients required for germ cell function and optimal spermatogenesis [140]. Although FSH is needed for Sertoli cell function, in the absence of intratesticular androgens, the generation of spermatids is impaired [141] (Figure 6.9).

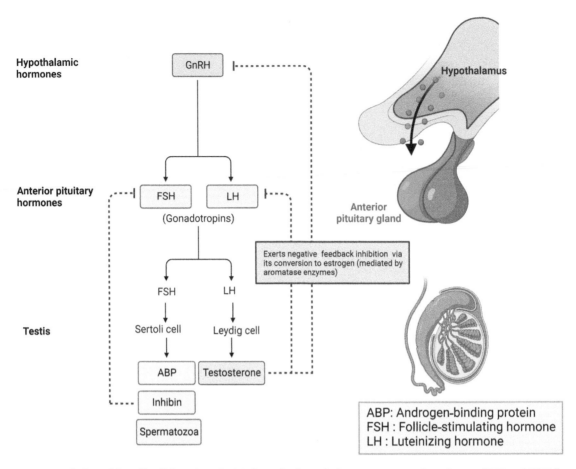

FIGURE 6.9   Regulation of Sertoli cell function. GnRH from the hypothalamus promotes the release of LH and FSH from the anterior pituitary gland. LH stimulates the biosynthesis and release of testosterone by Leydig cells of the testes, while FSH mediates the proliferation of Sertoli cells and the release of inhibin by seminiferous tubules. Inhibin and testosterone are involved in negative feedback inhibition of FSH and LH release, respectively. Also, testosterone exerts additional negative feedback regulation of GnRH release at the level of the hypothalamus. *Source*: Adapted from [142].

6.2.3.2   Mechanism of Action

Recombinant human FSH (rhFSH) binds to a complementary G protein-coupled receptor on Sertoli cells. Consequently, this leads to various complex intracellular processes which enhance the expression of genes required for gametogenesis [143].

Practice Pearl(s)

Idiopathic hypogonadotropic hypogonadism (congenital hypogonadotropic hypogonadism) and Kallmann syndrome are characterized by impaired synthesis or secretion of hypothalamic-derived GnRH. As a result of diminished stimulation of the anterior pituitary gland, there is impaired gonadal steroidogenesis and gametogenesis in males [144].

Concomitant administration of rhFSH and hCG is efficacious in initiating spermatogenesis in males with idiopathic hypogonadotropic hypogonadism [145]. It is worth noting that gonadotropin-deficient men can produce both testosterone and an adequate amount of sperm while on monotherapy with hCG. Nonetheless, the addition of rhFSH to therapy further enhances sperm production in these men [146].

Furthermore, men with inactivating mutations of the FSH continue to make sperm (all be it lower than normal males) despite having small testes. The direct activation of the FSH receptor is, therefore, not required for the maintenance of gametogenesis in men. In essence, FSH receptor activation is more relevant in female than male infertility [147].

Clinical Trial Evidence

The results of a clinical trial evaluating the efficacy of rhFSH in male hypogonadism are shown in Table 6.21.

TABLE 6.21 Efficacy of recombinant human FSH in male hypogonadism.

Study	Population	Intervention(s)	Outcome
rhFSH + hCG in IHH	Azoospermic men with IHH and a mean testicular volume ≤ 4 mL (n = 26)	rhFSH 150–225 IU three times a week, administered subcutaneously. Pretreatment with hCG for up to 6 months to maintain normal serum testosterone.	The primary efficacy endpoint, defined as attaining a sperm concentration of $\geq 1.5 \times 10^6$ per mL, occurred in 19 subjects (63.2%). The mean increase in sperm concentration compared to baseline was 2.8×10^6 per mL after 9 months of therapy (P-value = 0.027) [145].

IHH, idiopathic hypogonadotropic hypogonadism.
Testicular volume was assessed with a Prader orchidometer.

6.2.4 Clomiphene Citrate

6.2.4.1 Physiology

The hypothalamic–pituitary–gonadal axis and its negative feedback loops were discussed in Section 6.2.3.

6.2.4.2 Mechanism of Action

Clomiphene citrate (Clomid®) is a selective estrogen receptor modulator (SERM) that exerts estrogen antagonist properties in the hypothalamus and anterior pituitary, resulting in increased GnRH and gonadotropin release, respectively [132].

The hypothalamus, anterior pituitary gland, and testes work in concert to promote both spermatogenesis and testosterone in males. The sequential release of GnRH, LH, and FSH results in gonadal steroidogenesis and gametogenesis. Testosterone is subsequently converted to estrogen by the aromatase enzyme. Next, estrogen inhibits hypothalamic GnRH secretion, thus reducing testosterone and sperm production. Clomiphene citrate competes with endogenous estrogen for binding sites at the level of the hypothalamus. Consequently, estrogen cannot inhibit GnRH production, which increases LH and FSH, promoting eventual testosterone production and spermiogenesis [148].

Practice Pearl(s)

The initial recommended dose of clomiphene citrate is 25 mg/day or 50 mg every other day. The dose can then be gradually escalated to 50 mg/day [132].

Clomiphene citrate may be considered in men with functional hypogonadotropic hypogonadism, such as patients with sleep apnea initiating a weight loss program or nocturnal continuous positive airway pressure (CPAP) therapy. Hypogonadism in these patients is typically temporary; as such, a short course of clomiphene is a reasonable alternative in place of conventional testosterone replacement therapy [149].

> ## Clinical Trial Evidence
>
> The results of a clinical trial evaluating the efficacy of clomiphene citrate in male hypogonadism are shown in Table 6.22.
>
> **TABLE 6.22**   Efficacy of clomiphene citrate in male hypogonadism.
>
> | Study | Population | Intervention(s) | Outcome |
> |---|---|---|---|
> | CC monotherapy in hypogonadism | Men with hypogonadism, defined as serum testosterone <300 ng/dL on two consecutive early morning TT assessments (n = 86). | PO clomiphene citrate 25 mg every other day titrated to 50 mg every other day, to a target total testosterone of 550 ng/dL. Mean duration of treatment was 19 months. | There was a statistically significant increase in TT and gonadotropins (LH and FSH), comparing baseline to post-treatment levels (P-value of < 0.01) [150]. |
>
> TT, total testosterone; PO, per os (by mouth).

Concepts to Ponder Over

What is the expected trend in testosterone across the lifespan of men?

When evaluating hypogonadism in older men, it is worth noting that total testosterone decreases while sex-hormone-binding globulin increases with age [151].

Aromatase inhibitors in male hypogonadism

Aromatase inhibitors blunt the conversion of androgens into estrogens, thus blunting negative feedback control of GnRH production by estrogen. There is, however, no consistent evidence that aromatase inhibitors are efficacious in increasing serum testosterone or spermiogenesis [152].

What is the expected trend in testosterone across the lifespan of men?

Testosterone levels in men typically follow a pattern across the lifespan. Testosterone generally increase during adolescence, peaks in early adulthood, and then gradually decline as men age. This decline is commonly referred to as "andropause" or "late-onset hypogonadism" [153, 154].

6.3   MENOPAUSE

6.3.1   Menopausal Hormone Therapy

6.3.1.1   Physiology

Hot Flashes and Thermoregulation

Hot flashes, also known as vasomotor symptoms of menopause, are classically reported as sudden onset of diaphoresis and warmth involving the chest, neck, and face. Also, hot flashes last under 5 minutes but can sometimes persist for as long as an hour [155]. Heat-dissipating processes such as cutaneous vasodilation account for the typical vasomotor symptoms of menopause. Although the exact pathophysiologic basis of hot flashes is not entirely understood, there is evidence that estrogen-sensitive neuronal pathways regulate the classical thermoregulatory center [156].

Clinical Pearl

What is the definition of menopause?

Menopause is defined as the permanent cessation of menses. Traditionally, this condition is diagnosed after at least 12 months have elapsed without menstrual bleeding [157].

Laboratory tests may not be required if a comprehensive history and physical exam can identify other potential causes for amenorrhea or distressing symptoms.

Under certain conditions, measuring FSH and estradiol levels or antimullerian hormone levels in women may be necessary. Among them are:

- If they have undergone a hysterectomy without oophorectomy and are aged under 40 [158];
- If they use estrogen-containing contraceptives (which tend to suppress FSH and increase estradiol levels) [159];
- If they continue menstruating after reaching 55 (this could indicate postmenopausal status but with bleeding endometrial neoplasm or another uterine pathology) [160].

Estrogen plays a critical role in regulating the thermoregulatory center in the hypothalamus. Various estrogen-sensitive neurons, including 5-hydroxytryptamine (5HT, from the midbrain), norepinephrine (NE, from the brain stem), and KNDy (kisspeptin, neurokinin B, dynorphin from the ARN) neurons project onto the thermoregulatory center [156].

Although the exact mechanism is unclear, elevation in NE levels within the brain results in a narrowing of the inter-threshold zone of the thermoregulatory center. Consequently, slight elevations in core body temperature result in hot flashes. Interestingly, this is typically followed by minor shivers (at the end of a spell), further affirming the narrowing of the inter-threshold zone [161]. Conversely, elevated levels of 5HT in the brain result in the widening of the inter-threshold zone, thus relieving hot flashes [155, 162].

Role of Estrogen in Bone Health

The role of estrogen in bone health was discussed in Section 5.5.6.

6.3.1.2   Mechanism of Action

Estrogens With or Without Progestins

The effects of estrogen in the pathogenesis of hot flashes were described earlier.

 Clinical Pearl

Conditions masquerading as vasomotor symptoms of menopause [163].

- Autoimmune thyroid disease
- Insulinoma
- Carcinoid syndrome
- Recurrent hypoglycemia
- Anxiety disorder
- Leukemia/Lymphoma
- Mast cell disorders

Practice Pearl(s)

- Estrogen administered orally or transdermally has equal efficacy in ameliorating vasomotor symptoms of menopause. In patients with an intact uterus, concomitant progestins are required to reduce the risk of endometrial hyperplasia and cancer [164] (see Table 6.23).
- Menopausal hormone therapy (estrogen with or without progestin) primarily relieves vasomotor symptoms (hot flashes) of menopause. Postmenopausal women may notice improved sleep and emotional lability on menopausal hormone therapy.
- Local application of vaginal estrogen relieves dryness and dyspareunia (genitourinary syndrome of menopause).
- Contraindications to oral estrogens include a diagnosis of thrombophilia, venous thromboembolism, hypertriglyceridemia, active gall bladder disease, or migraine headaches with aura (Table 6.24).

(continued)

(continued)

TABLE 6.23 Estrogen-based therapies with efficacy in vasomotor symptoms.

Estrogen-based treatment (route)	Standard dose (Low dose)
Conjugated estrogen (oral)	0.625 mg/d (0.3–0.45 mg/d)
Micronized estradiol-17β (oral)	1 mg/d (0.5 mg/d)
Estradiol-17β (transdermal)	0.0375–0.05 mg/d (0.025 mg/d)
Conjugated estrogen + bazedoxifene[a] (oral)	0.45 mg/d + 20 mg/d

[a] Combined estrogen agonist/antagonist.
Source: Adapted from [165].

TABLE 6.24 Comparison of oral and transdermal estrogens.

Effect(s)	Oral estrogen	Transdermal estrogen
First metabolism in the liver	Yes	No
Low-density lipoprotein	↓↓	↓
High-density lipoprotein	↑↑	↑
Triglycerides	↑↑	→
Coagulation factors	↑↑	→

Coagulation factors include factor VII and prothrombin.
Source: Adapted from [166].

Clinical Trial Evidence

The efficacy of menopausal hormone therapy in mitigating vasomotor symptoms and osteoporotic-related fractures is shown in Table 6.25.

TABLE 6.25 Clinical studies evaluating the safety and efficacy of hormone therapy in mitigating hot flashes and osteoporosis.

Clinical feature	Population	Intervention	Outcome
Hot flashes	Menopausal women (spontaneous menopause or bilateral oophorectomy) with hot flashes (n = 1104) were assessed in a meta-analysis.	Oral hormone therapy[a] versus placebo.	Reduction in weekly hot flashes comparing hormone therapy to placebo (WMD −17.92, 95% CI −22.86 to −12.99) [167].
Osteoporosis	Postmenopausal women were assessed in a meta-analysis.	Hormone therapy versus placebo (or calcium/vitamin D).	Incidence of vertebral fractures comparing hormone therapy to placebo (RR 0.66, 95% CI 0.41–1.07). Incidence of nonvertebral fractures (RR 0.87, 95% CI 0.71–1.08) [168].

[a] Hormone therapy – estrogens alone or combined with progestins in either a cyclic or continuous regimen.
WMD, weighted mean difference.
Source: Adapted from [167, 168].

Clinical Pearl

Historical understanding of the menopause

There was a time in our shameful past as medical professionals when women were coerced into undergoing **bilateral oophorectomy** (removal of the ovaries) for hysteria, anorexia nervosa, anxiety disorder, and a myriad of other neuropsychiatric ailments. The central dogma of that day was that the nervous system controlled all parts of the human body. Quite disconcertingly, the belief was that the ovaries were essential nerve centers governing women's behavior. This fueled the practice of ovarian removal and its unintended consequence of premature menopause. Unfortunately, over 100 000 young women underwent this procedure in Europe and subsequently developed severe vasomotor symptoms of menopause.

In his seminal work on the internal secretions of the ovaries, Josef von Halban (1870–1937), a pioneer in hormone science, disproved the long-held belief that the ovaries were in direct communication with the nervous system. Halban showed that the ovaries exerted systemic effects by directly releasing a special chemical (estrogen) into the bloodstream. He removed bits of the ovaries and uterus and transplanted these into the skin of guinea pigs. He was able to show that despite being anatomically displaced, the ovaries allowed an immature spayed guinea pig to attain normal puberty, confirming the role of a yet-to-be-characterized hormone we now know as **estrogen.**

6.3.2   SSRI/SNRI

6.3.2.1   Physiology

5-Hydroxytryptamine (serotonin) plays a critical role in regulating the thermoregulatory center.

6.3.2.2   Mechanism of Action

In the postmenopausal state, the loss of estrogen results in reduced activation and production of 5HT by central serotonergic neurons. As a result of reduced serum serotonin levels, the sensitivity of serotonergic neurons increases, which causes hot flushes. Selective serotonergic reuptake inhibitors relieve hot flushes by increasing serotonin levels

leading to widening of the inter-threshold zone of the thermoregulatory center [169].

Practice Pearl(s)

Paroxetine is the only selective serotonin receptor inhibitor approved for the treatment of hot flashes in the United States. Low-dose paroxetine between 10 and 20 mg is efficacious in reducing hot flashes [170].

Clinical Trial Evidence

In a meta-analysis of 11 randomized control trials, 2069 menopausal women aged between 36 and 76 years were followed up for 1–9 months. The mean duration since menopause was 2.3–6.6 years. SSRIs compared to placebo resulted in a statistically significant reduction in vasomotor symptom frequency, with a reported difference in means of -0.93 (95% CI -1.46 to -0.37, $I^2 = 21\%$) [171].

Concepts to Ponder Over

A woman with breast cancer developed vasomotor symptoms after starting tamoxifen. Is SSRI therapy a reasonable option for this patient who cannot be on conventional menopausal hormone therapy?

Cytochrome-P450 isoenzyme 2D6 (CYP2D6) is responsible for the conversion of tamoxifen (a prodrug) into its active metabolite (endoxifen). Some SSRIs (paroxetine and fluoxetine) are potent inhibitors of CYP2D6, potentially reducing the clinical efficacy of tamoxifen in the management of breast cancer [172].

Outline possible mitigating strategies in the above scenario

1. Switching from tamoxifen to anastrozole [173].
2. Opt for SSRIs that do not inhibit CYP2D6, such as citalopram, sertraline, and escitalopram [172].

6.4   TURNER'S SYNDROME

 Historical Pearl

This syndrome is traditionally attributed to Henry Turner due to his description of the triad of infantilism, webbed neck, and cubitus valgus in 1938 [174].

6.4.1   Hormone Replacement Therapy

6.4.1.1   Physiology

The Effects of Estrogen on Metabolism

Estrogen exerts its effects by binding to its cognate nuclear receptors, Estrogen Receptor alpha (ERα) and Estrogen Receptor beta (ERβ). In normal physiology, estrogen receptors are attached to Heat Shock Protein 90 (HSP90) present in the cytosol. The binding of estrogen to estrogen receptors promotes the dissociation of the latter from HSP90. Consequently, estrogen receptors bind estrogen response elements (sequences on DNA) responsible for either promoting or inhibiting gene transcription [175].

6.4.1.2   Mechanism of Action

See Table 6.26.

Practice Pearl(s)

Hormone replacement therapy is required for pubertal induction and long-term bone health [178]. Transdermal estrogen is the preferred route of administration in pubescent girls. Progestin therapy is conventionally initiated after two years of estrogen therapy (or breakthrough bleeding) to provide endometrial protection in these patients with an intact uterus [179, 180].

For adult women, transdermal estrogen (25–150 mcg/day) or oral estrogen (1–4 mg) promotes skeletal and metabolic health [178, 181]. Progestins can be administered in a sequential fashion ten days out of the month or as a continuous estrogen–progestin regimen. A progestin-containing intrauterine device combined with either oral or transdermal estradiol is recommended for patients with irregular uterine bleeds or in whom uterine bleeds are undesirable [178]. Hormone replacement therapy should be continued throughout adult life until the average age of menopause.

TABLE 6.26   Physiologic effects of estrogen.

Physiologic role	Mechanism
Mammary gland	Estrogen promotes the proliferation of mammary tissue during puberty. Also responsible for cyclical proliferation and involution during the menstrual cycle (reproductive years) [176].
Bone	It promotes initial pubertal growth spurt and paradoxically limits final skeletal height by inducing ossification (closure) of the epiphyseal growth plate [176]. The effects of estrogen on bone resorption (Section 5.5.6).
Lipid metabolism	Estrogen lowers triacylglycerols by increasing the expression of apolipoproteins required for lipid transport [177].
Glucose metabolism	Estrogen exerts a myriad of effects on lipid metabolism by, Increasing peripheral tissue sensitivity by increasing the expression of glucose transporter 4 (GLUT4) – required for glucose uptake by skeletal muscle and adipose tissue. Reducing inflammation in adipose tissue (thus, insulin resistance) [177].

Source: Adapted from [176, 177].

Clinical Trial Evidence

(Table 6.27)

TABLE 6.27   A meta-analysis of the efficacy of transdermal versus oral estrogen in Turner syndrome.

Parameter	Outcome
Bone Mineral Density	Compared to OE, TDE caused a greater increase in whole-body BMD Z-score. A mean difference of −0.071 (95% CI, −0.125 to −0.017).
Lipids	OE, compared to TDE led to a statistically significant decrease in LDL-C levels. Mean difference 5.87 (95% CI, 2.18–9.55).[a]
Insulin	There was no statistically significant difference in fasting insulin levels.

OE, oral estrogen; TDE, transdermal estrogen; BMD, bone mineral density.
[a] There was no significant difference in serum triglycerides, comparing OE and TDE.
Source: Adapted from [182].

6.4.2   Therapies for Metabolic Disorders

6.4.2.1   Physiology

See Section 6.4.1.

6.4.2.2   Mechanism of Action

See Section 6.4.1.

Practice Pearl(s)

Patients with Turner's syndrome are at risk for various metabolic conditions, including diabetes mellitus, hyperlipidemia, and hypothyroidism (see Table 6.28).

TABLE 6.28   Metabolic monitoring guidelines for patients with Turner's syndrome.

Metabolic feature	Screening
Hyperglycemia	Annual hemoglobin A1c and fasting glucose
Hyperlipidemia	Annual lipid panel
Hypothyroidism	Annual thyroid function tests

Source: Adapted from [179].

Clinical Trial Evidence

See Table 6.27.

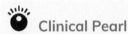 **Clinical Pearl**

What is Short Stature

Short stature is a general term that applies to children whose height is two standard deviations (SD) or more below the mean for children of that sex, age, and population. Statistics show that 23 per 1000 individuals have this diagnosis [183]. Short stature may be idiopathic, secondary to organ disease, or arise from an endocrine disorder. Endocrine causes include childhood-onset growth hormone deficiency (GHD), primary insulin-like growth factor 1 deficiency, and defects in their pathways [184].

Genetic variations in growth must first be considered when searching for a pathological cause of short stature. In other words, children often have similar growth patterns and the onset of puberty as their parents. Therefore, a history of pubertal development and evidence of the heights of their family members should be obtained. Moreover, families in which short stature is frequent can show different patterns of growth that are considered normal. One pattern is the constitutional delay of growth and development, where children are known as "late bloomers."

For pathological short stature, disproportionate short stature means the trunk is longer or shorter in comparison with the limbs. This type is seen in skeletal dysplasias, SHOX gene mutations, or after spine radiation. Proportional short stature refers to an expected trunk length compared to the limbs. This pattern is seen in inherited limitations on bone growth, babies small for gestational age, genetic and chromosomal abnormalities, or in cases where the mother received radiation during pregnancy.

6.4.3   Therapies for Linear Growth

6.4.3.1   Physiology

The etiology of short stature is multifactorial, including estrogen deficiency, perturbations in GH/IGF-1 signaling, and short stature homeobox-containing (SHOX) gene deficiency [185]. Haploinsufficiency of the SHOX gene might be the etiology of short stature in Turner syndrome through loss of normal chondrocyte function at the epiphyseal growth plate [186].

6.4.3.2   Mechanism of Action

Growth hormone promotes longitudinal growth.

Practice Pearl(s)

Early initiation of growth hormone therapy in girls with Turner syndrome has various demonstrable benefits, including skeletal growth, increased bone mineral density, and optimal metabolic parameters (improvement in glucose and lipid panel) [180].

(continued)

(continued)

Even if short stature may be a sign of underlying pathology, it is not a disease. However, it is considered a problem because it is socially perceived to be a disability [187]. One option is growth hormone therapy which comes with its risks – short term such as insulin resistance (with increased incidence of type 2 diabetes mellitus in children with other risk factors), pseudotumor cerebri, and slipped capital femoral epiphyses [188].

Growth hormone treatment should be initiated around 4–6 years of age, especially if the affected child grows at a height velocity less than the 50% percentile for age and gender. At a dose of 45–50 mcg/kg/day, growth hormone can be further titrated to a maximum dose of 68 mcg/kg/day. Serum insulin-like growth factor 1 should be evaluated at least annually during treatment [181].

Clinical Trial Evidence

In a meta-analysis of 11 studies comparing recombinant human growth hormone(rhGH) to placebo, rhGH resulted in a statistically significant increase in the final height of subjects with Turner syndrome (mean difference of 7.22 cm, 95% CI 5.27–9.18, $P < 0.001$). The reported height velocity comparing rhGH to placebo was also statistically significant (mean difference of 2.68 cm/year, 95% CI 2.34–3.02, $P < 0.001$) [189].

 Concepts to Ponder Over

What is the underlying pathophysiology of short stature in Turner syndrome?

Alterations in the SHOX gene (Short stature homeobox-containing gene) located on the short arm of the X chromosome have been implicated as the causal factor for the diminished height characteristic of Turner syndrome (TS) patients. In females with normal genotypes, two copies of the SHOX gene are inherited, one on the active and the other on the inactive X chromosome, thereby ensuring the gene's evasion of Lyonization effects.

Interestingly, the SHOX gene is also present on the Y chromosome in genetic males. Hence, the eventual height outcome is dose-dependent on the SHOX gene [190]. The SHOX gene is expressed in mesenchymal tissue and plays a pivotal role in the formation of chondroblasts in the long bones of both the upper and lower limbs. When only a single copy of the SHOX gene is available, a condition termed haploinsufficiency, as is the case with TS, it proves insufficient to fully support the growth of long bones. This mechanism explains the resultant short stature observed in individuals with Turner syndrome [191, 192].

PRACTICE-BASED QUESTIONS

1. Which of the following best describes the role of insulin in adrenal steroidogenesis?

   a. Insulin stimulates the breakdown of adrenal steroids
   b. Insulin inhibits the synthesis of adrenal steroids
   c. Insulin has no effect on adrenal steroidogenesis
   d. Insulin promotes the synthesis of adrenal steroids

   Answer: d) Insulin promotes the synthesis of adrenal steroids. Insulin stimulates the synthesis of adrenal steroids, including androgens and cortisol, by promoting the function of steroidogenic factor 1 (SF-1). SF-1 is a transcription factor that enhances the transcription of critical adrenal steroidogenic genes. Insulin impairs the activity of a canonical inhibitor of SF-1 function, increasing adrenal steroid synthesis.

2. What is the mechanism underlying the regulation of sex hormone-binding globulin (SHBG) by insulin?

   a. It promotes SHBG production
   b. It inhibits SHBG production
   c. It has no effect on SHBG production
   d. The mechanism is not yet known

   Answer: b) It inhibits SHBG production. There is an inverse relationship between SHBG and insulin. Insulin inhibits the synthesis of SHBG, exacerbating hyperandrogenemia by increasing the fraction of unbound (free) to bound androgens. The mechanism underlying this regulation is not yet fully elucidated.

3. What is the mechanism of action of metformin in PCOS?

   a. It promotes the synthesis of adrenal steroids
   b. It inhibits the synthesis of androgens
   c. It improves insulin resistance
   d. It reduces SHBG production

Answer: c) It improves insulin resistance. Metformin is an insulin-sensitizing drug that improves insulin resistance in PCOS by activating the adenosine monophosphate-activated protein kinase (AMPK) pathway. This process impairs hepatic glucose output, reduces fatty acid oxidation, and increases glucose uptake by peripheral tissues. By improving insulin resistance, metformin helps mitigate some hormonal perturbations in PCOS.

4. What is the mode of release of GnRH that promotes ovarian follicle maturation?

   a. Pulsatile
   b. Surge-like
   c. Continuous
   d. Sporadic

Answer: a) Pulsatile. Pulsatile GnRH release promotes ovarian follicle maturation. On the other hand, a surge-like increase in GnRH release accounts for the widely accepted "LH surge" required for ovulation. The GnRH pulse generator, localized to the arcuate nucleus of the hypothalamus, controls fertility by initiating the classic GnRH ultradian frequency, which regulates the synthesis of estradiol and progesterone by the ovaries.

5. Which hormone reduces the GnRH pulse frequency, ultimately leading to decreased LH and FSH secretion in normal female physiology?

   a. Estradiol
   b. Progesterone
   c. Leptin
   d. Cortisol

Answer: b) Progesterone. Progesterone inhibits GnRH neurons, leading to a decrease in the GnRH pulse frequency and, ultimately, a decrease in LH and FSH secretion.

6. What is the mechanism of action of estrogen and progestin-containing oral contraceptive pills (OCPs) in PCOS?

   a. Suppress LH release
   b. Increases free androgen levels
   c. Inhibits LH surge required for ovulation
   d. Decreases ovarian androgen production

Answer: d) Decreases ovarian androgen production. Estrogen and progestin-containing OCPs decrease ovarian androgen production in patients with PCOS. Estrogen increases sex hormone-binding globulin, which decreases free androgen levels, and progestin suppresses LH release. Progestin also has androgen receptor-blocking effects. The inhibition of ovarian androgen production is essential in mitigating the clinical effects of hyperandrogenemia, such as hirsutism and acne, and prevention of endometrial hyperplasia.

7. What is the mechanism of action of spironolactone in managing acne and hirsutism in PCOS?

   a. Inhibits 5 alpha-reductase activity
   b. Increases ovarian and adrenal steroidogenesis
   c. Inhibits the activity of aromatase
   d. Increases sex hormone-binding globulin

Answer: a) Inhibits 5 alpha-reductase activity. Spironolactone is a diuretic and aldosterone antagonist with antagonistic properties at the androgen receptor. It inhibits the activity of 5 alpha-reductase, which is critical in converting testosterone to its active form, dihydrotestosterone. Spironolactone also increases the activity of aromatase, which converts testosterone to estrogen and increases sex hormone-binding globulin. Patients with moderate-to-severe hirsutism in PCOS can benefit from spironolactone therapy, but it should be initiated only after at least six months of oral contraceptive pill use. Spironolactone can exacerbate menstrual irregularity if not used concomitantly with oral contraceptive therapy and can cause postural hypotension, dizziness, and hyperkalemia as side effects.

8. Which phase of ovarian follicular development is controlled by growth factors and cytokines?

   a. Gonadotropin-independent phase
   b. Gonadotropin-dependent phase
   c. Antral follicular phase
   d. Luteal phase

Answer: a) Gonadotropin-independent phase. The transition from a primordial follicle to a pre-antral follicle is controlled by various intra-ovarian regulators, including growth factors and cytokines.

9. What is the mechanism of action of clomiphene citrate?

    a. It stimulates the growth and development of a cohort of pre-antral follicles

    b. It enhances final follicular maturation

    c. It increases the pulse amplitude of the GnRH pulse generator

    d. It blocks the conversion of androgens to estrogens

Answer: c) It increases the pulse amplitude of the GnRH pulse generator. Clomiphene citrate is a selective estrogen receptor modular (SERM) that acts as an antagonist at the level of the hypothalamus, preventing negative feedback inhibition of the GnRH pulse generator by endogenous estrogen. As a result, the levels of LH and FSH increase, enhancing the recruitment and maturation of ovarian follicles.

10. What is the dosing schedule of letrozole for patients with PCOS?

    a. 50 mg daily for 5 days

    b. 2.5 mg daily for 5 days

    c. 75 IU administered subcutaneously on a daily basis for up to 14 days

    d. 5000–10,000 IU administered intramuscularly or subcutaneously

Answer: b) 2.5 mg daily for 5 days. Letrozole is a competitive nonsteroidal aromatase inhibitor that blocks the conversion of androgens to estrogens, which subsequently increases GnRH pulse frequency and gonadotropin release. For patients who experience a poor ovulatory response, a gradual increase in dose to 7.5 mg daily during subsequent cycles is recommended for a total of 5 cycles.

11. What is the role of androgens in hair formation?

    a. Androgens promote hair growth at various sites

    b. Androgens result in androgenetic alopecia (AGA) of the scalp

    c. Androgens have no effect on hair formation

    d. Androgens result in excessive hair growth (hypertrichosis)

Answer: a) Androgens promote hair growth at various sites. Androgens promote hair growth at various sites, including the scalp, beard, pubic and axillary regions. However, androgens paradoxically result in androgenetic alopecia (AGA) of the scalp.

12. What is the primary hormone responsible for regulating testosterone production in the testes?

    a. FSH

    b. LH

    c. GnRH

    d. Estrogen

Answer: b) LH. The secretion of testosterone is primarily regulated by luteinizing hormone (LH), which is secreted by the anterior pituitary gland in response to gonadotropin-releasing hormone (GnRH) from the hypothalamus. FSH (follicle-stimulating hormone) also plays a role in testosterone production, but it is mainly responsible for spermatogenesis.

13. Which factor is essential for transporting cholesterol into the mitochondria of Leydig cells for testosterone synthesis?

    a. 17 hydroxylase

    b. 11 hydroxylase

    c. 21 hydroxylase

    d. Steroidogenic acute regulatory protein (StAR)

Answer: d) Steroidogenic acute regulatory protein (StAR). The transportation of cholesterol into the mitochondria of Leydig cells is the rate-limiting step of testosterone synthesis. The steroidogenic acute regulatory protein (StAR) is an essential intracellular protein required to transport cholesterol into the mitochondria.

14. What is the primary mechanism by which testosterone promotes bone formation?

    a. Activation of osteoclasts

    b. Inhibition of RANKL-mediated bone resorption

    c. Promotion of insulin-like growth factor 1-mediated proliferation of chondrocytes and osteoblasts

    d. Conversion to estrogen.

Answer: c) Promotion of insulin-like growth factor 1-mediated proliferation of chondrocytes and osteoblasts. Testosterone promotes bone formation by binding to androgen receptors on osteoblasts, which subsequently promotes insulin-like growth factor 1-mediated proliferation of chondrocytes and osteoblasts. Additionally, estrogen (produced through the action of aromatase on testosterone) inhibits RANKL-mediated bone resorption.

15. What is the most stable form of testosterone replacement therapy?

    a. Testosterone cypionate or enanthate
    b. Testosterone patch
    c. Testosterone gel
    d. Long-acting intramuscular testosterone undecanoate

    Answer: b) Testosterone patch. Testosterone replacement therapy can be administered via various methods, including injections, patches, gels, pellets, tablets, and nasal gels. The testosterone patch is the most stable form of testosterone replacement therapy, with a stable serum testosterone concentration and less likelihood of causing erythrocytosis. Testosterone cypionate or enanthate, while commonly used, can lead to highly variable serum testosterone levels and significant fluctuations in hypogonadal symptoms.

16. What is the role of human chorionic gonadotropin (hCG) in male infertility?

    a. Inhibition of sperm production
    b. Enhancement of testosterone production
    c. Activation of the follicle-stimulating hormone (FSH) receptor
    d. Inhibition of the luteinizing hormone (LH) receptor

    Answer: b) Enhancement of testosterone production. hCG, a placental-derived analog of LH, can occupy the LH receptor and activate downstream processes typically mediated by LH. It is extracted either from the urine of pregnant women or synthesized using recombinant DNA technology. In males, hCG enhances testosterone production, which is critical in maintaining spermatogenesis and testicular volume, making it a viable alternative to testosterone in younger hypogonadal men seeking to preserve their fertility.

17. What is the mechanism of action of clomiphene citrate (Clomid) in male hypogonadism?

    a. Activation of the FSH receptor
    b. Inhibition of the GnRH receptor
    c. Inhibition of estrogen production
    d. Inhibition of testosterone production

    Answer: c) Inhibition of estrogen production. Clomiphene citrate is a selective estrogen receptor modulator (SERM) that exerts estrogen antagonist properties in the hypothalamus and anterior pituitary, resulting in increased GnRH and gonadotropin release, respectively. It competes with endogenous estrogen for binding sites at the level of the hypothalamus, which inhibits estrogen's negative feedback control of GnRH production, leading to increased LH and FSH and eventual testosterone production and spermiogenesis.

18. What is the pathophysiologic basis of hot flashes in menopause?

    a. Increased cutaneous vasodilation
    b. Narrowing of the inter-threshold zone of the thermoregulatory center
    c. Widening of the inter-threshold zone of the thermoregulatory center
    d. Decreased norepinephrine levels in the brain

    Answer: b) Narrowing of the inter-threshold zone of the thermoregulatory center. The exact pathophysiologic basis of hot flashes is not entirely understood, but there is evidence that estrogen-sensitive neuronal pathways regulate the classical thermoregulatory center. Elevated levels of norepinephrine within the brain result in the narrowing of the inter-threshold zone of the thermoregulatory center. Consequently, slight elevations in core body temperature result in hot flashes. This is typically followed by minor shivers (at the end of a spell), further affirming the narrowing of the inter-threshold zone. Conversely, elevated levels of 5HT in the brain result in the widening of the inter-threshold zone, thus relieving hot flashes.

19. Which selective serotonergic reuptake inhibitor is approved for the treatment of hot flashes in the United States?

    a. Fluoxetine
    b. Citalopram
    c. Sertraline
    d. Paroxetine

    Answer: d) Paroxetine. Paroxetine is the only selective serotonin receptor inhibitor approved for the treatment of hot flashes in the United States.

20. What is the preferred route of administration of estrogen in pubescent girls with Turner syndrome?

    a. Oral
    b. Transdermal
    c. Intramuscular
    d. Intranasal

    Answer: b) Transdermal. Transdermal estrogen is the preferred route of administration in pubescent girls with Turner syndrome. Progestin therapy is conventionally initiated after two years of estrogen therapy (or breakthrough bleeding) to provide endometrial protection in these patients with an intact uterus.

REFERENCES

1. Martikainen, H., Salmela, P., Nuojua-Huttunen, S. et al. (1996). Adrenal steroidogenesis is related to insulin in hyperandrogenic women. *Fertil. Steril.* 66: 564–570.

2. Schimmer, B.P. and White, P.C. (2010). Minireview: steroidogenic factor 1: its roles in differentiation, development, and disease. *Mol. Endocrinol.* 24: 1322–1337.

3. Lin, L. and Achermann, J.C. (2008). Steroidogenic factor-1 (SF-1, Ad4BP, NR5A1) and disorders of testis development. *SXD* 2: 200–209.

4. Kinyua, A.W., Doan, K.V., Yang, D.J. et al. (2018). Insulin regulates adrenal steroidogenesis by stabilizing sf-1 activity. *Sci. Rep.* 8: 5025.

5. Ramnanan, C.J., Edgerton, D.S., Rivera, N. et al. (2010). Molecular characterization of insulin-mediated suppression of hepatic glucose production in vivo. *Diabetes* 59: 1302–1311.

6. Pedersen, C., Kraft, G., Edgerton, D.S. et al. (2020). The kinetics of glucagon action on the liver during insulin-induced hypoglycemia. *Am. J. Physiol. Endocrinol. Metabolism* 318: E779–E790.

7. Handberg, A., Vaag, A., Beck-Nielsen, H., and Vinten, J. (1992). Peripheral glucose uptake and skeletal muscle GLUT4 content in man: effect of insulin and free fatty acids. *Diabet. Med.* 9: 605–610.

8. Wallace, I.R., McKinley, M.C., Bell, P.M., and Hunter, S.J. (2013). Sex hormone binding globulin and insulin resistance. *Clin. Endocrinol.* 78: 321–329.

9. Akin, F., Bastemir, M., and Kaptanoglu, B. (2007). Relationship between insulin and sex hormone-binding globulin levels during weight loss in obese women. *Ann. Nutr. Metab.* 51: 557–562.

10. Strain, G., Zumoff, B., Rosner, W., and Pi-Sunyer, X. (1994). The relationship between serum levels of insulin and sex hormone-binding globulin in men: the effect of weight loss. *J. Clin. Endocrinol. Metab.* 79: 1173–1176.

11. Hautanen, A. (2000). Synthesis and regulation of sex hormone-binding globulin in obesity. *Int. J. Obes. Relat. Metab. Disord.* 24 (Suppl 2): S64–S70.

12. Simó, R., Sáez-López, C., Barbosa-Desongles, A. et al. (2015). Novel insights in SHBG regulation and clinical implications. *Trends Endocrinol. Metab.* 26: 376–383.

13. Zeng, X., Xie, Y., Liu, Y. et al. (2020). Polycystic ovarian syndrome: correlation between hyperandrogenism, insulin resistance and obesity. *Clin. Chim. Acta* 502: 214–221.

14. Nestler, J.E. (1997). Role of hyperinsulinemia in the pathogenesis of the polycystic ovary syndrome, and its clinical implications. *Semin. Reprod. Endocrinol.* 15: 111–122.

15. Unluhizarci, K., Karaca, Z., and Kelestimur, F. (2021). Role of insulin and insulin resistance in androgen excess disorders. *World J. Diabetes* 12: 616–629.

16. Witchel, S.F., Oberfield, S.E., and Peña, A.S. (2019). Polycystic ovary syndrome: pathophysiology, presentation, and treatment with emphasis on adolescent girls. *J. Endocr. Soc.* 3: 1545–1573.

17. Rosenfield, R.L. and Ehrmann, D.A. (2016). The pathogenesis of polycystic ovary syndrome (PCOS): the hypothesis of PCOS as functional ovarian hyperandrogenism revisited. *Endocr. Rev.* 37: 467–520.

18. Diamanti-Kandarakis, E. and Dunaif, A. (2012). Insulin resistance and the polycystic ovary syndrome revisited: an update on mechanisms and implications. *Endocr. Rev.* 33: 981–1030.

19. Rice, S., Christoforidis, N., Gadd, C. et al. (2005). Impaired insulin-dependent glucose metabolism in

granulosa-lutein cells from anovulatory women with polycystic ovaries. *Hum. Reprod.* 20: 373–381.

20. Sam, S. (2015). Adiposity and metabolic dysfunction in polycystic ovary syndrome. *Horm. Mol. Biol. Clin. Invest.* 21: 107–116.

21. Stein, I.F. and Leventhal, M.L. (1935). Amenorrhea associated with bilateral polycystic ovaries. *Am. J. Obstet. Gynecol.* 29: 181–191.

22. Battaglia, C. (2003). The role of ultrasound and Doppler analysis in the diagnosis of polycystic ovary syndrome. *Ultrasound Obstet. Gynecol.* 22: 225–232.

23. Zawadzki, J.K. and Dunaif, A. (1992). Diagnostic criteria for polycystic ovary syndrome: towards a rational approach. In: *Polycystic Ovary Syndrome* (ed. A.G.J. Dunaif and F. Haseltine), 377–384. Boston: Blackwell Scientific.

24. The Rotterdam ESHRE/ASRM-sponsored PCOS consensus workshop group (2004). Revised 2003 consensus on diagnostic criteria and long-term health risks related to polycystic ovary syndrome (PCOS). *Hum. Reprod.* 19: 41–47.

25. Azziz, R., Carmina, E., Dewailly, D. et al. (2006). Criteria for defining polycystic ovary syndrome as a predominantly hyperandrogenic syndrome: an androgen excess society guideline. *J. Clin. Endocrinol. Metabol.* 91: 4237–4245.

26. Johnson T., Kaplan L., Ouyang P., and Rizza P. (2019). *National Institutes of Health Evidence-Based Methodology Workshop on Polycystic Ovary Syndrome.* NIH EbMW Reports. Bethesda, MD: National Institutes of Health, 2012; 1: 1–14. Executive summary Available at: https://prevention.nih.gov/docs/programs/pcos/FinalReport pdf.

27. Ibáñez, L., Oberfield, S.E., Witchel, S. et al. (2017). An International consortium update: pathophysiology, diagnosis, and treatment of polycystic ovarian syndrome in adolescence. *HRP* 88: 371–395.

28. Hashim, H.A. (2016). Twenty years of ovulation induction with metformin for PCOS; what is the best available evidence? *Reprod. Biomed. Online* 32: 44–53.

29. Pau, C.T., Keefe, C., Duran, J., and Welt, C.K. (2014). Metformin improves glucose effectiveness, not insulin sensitivity: predicting treatment response in women with polycystic ovary syndrome in an open-label, interventional study. *J. Clin. Endocrinol. Metab.* 99: 1870–1878.

30. Fraison, E., Kostova, E., Moran, L.J. et al. (2020). Metformin versus the combined oral contraceptive pill for hirsutism, acne, and menstrual pattern in polycystic ovary syndrome. *Cochrane Database Syst. Rev.* 2020: CD005552.

31. Tso L.O., Costello M.F., Albuquerque L.E., et al. (2009). Metformin treatment before and during IVF or ICSI in women with polycystic ovary syndrome. *Cochrane Database Syst. Rev.* (2):CD006105. https://doi.org/10.1002/14651858.CD006105.pub2s.

32. Voliotis, M., Li, X.F., De Burgh, R. et al. (2019). The origin of GnRH pulse generation: an integrative mathematical-experimental approach. *J. Neurosci.* 39: 9738–9747.

33. Herbison, A.E. (2018). The gonadotropin-releasing hormone pulse generator. *Endocrinology* 159: 3723–3736.

34. Plant T.M. (2020). The neurobiological mechanism underlying hypothalamic GnRH pulse generation: the role of kisspeptin neurons in the arcuate nucleus. https://doi.org/10.12688/f1000research.18356.2

35. Maeda, K.-I., Ohkura, S., Uenoyama, Y. et al. (2010). Neurobiological mechanisms underlying GnRH pulse generation by the hypothalamus. *Brain Res.* 1364: 103–115.

36. Knobil, E., Plant, T.M., Wildt, L. et al. (1980). Control of the rhesus monkey menstrual cycle: permissive role of hypothalamic gonadotropin-releasing hormone. *Science* 207: 1371–1373.

37. Welt, C.K., Chan, J.L., Bullen, J. et al. (2004). Recombinant human leptin in women with hypothalamic amenorrhea. *N. Engl. J. Med.* 351: 987–997.

38. Pielecka, J., Quaynor, S.D., and Moenter, S.M. (2006). Androgens increase gonadotropin-releasing hormone neuron firing activity in females and interfere with progesterone negative feedback. *Endocrinology* 147: 1474–1479.

39. Skinner, D.C., Evans, N.P., Delaleu, B. et al. (1998). The negative feedback actions of progesterone on gonadotropin-releasing hormone secretion are transduced by the classical progesterone receptor. *Proc. Natl. Acad. Sci. U. S. A.* 95: 10978–10983.

40. Saketos, M., Sharma, N., and Santoro, N.F. (1993). Suppression of the hypothalamic-pituitary-ovarian axis in normal women by glucocorticoids. *Biol. Reprod.* 49: 1270–1276.

41. Lecomte, P., Lecomte, C., Lansac, J. et al. (1997). Pregnancy after intravenous pulsatile gonadotropin-releasing hormone in a hyperprolactinaemic woman resistant to treatment with dopamine agonists. *Eur. J. Obstet. Gynecol. Reprod. Biol.* 74: 219–221.

42. Lee, J.H., Miele, M.E., Hicks, D.J. et al. (1996). KiSS-1, a novel human malignant melanoma metastasis-suppressor gene. *J. Natl. Cancer Inst.* 88: 1731–1737.

43. Liu, Y.-X. and Hsueh, A.J.W. (1986). Synergism between granulosa and theca-interstitial cells in estrogen biosynthesis by gonadotropin-treated rat ovaries: studies on the two-cell, two-gonadotropin hypothesis using steroid antisera1. *Biol. Reprod.* 35: 27–36.

44. McNatty, K.P., Makris, A., DeGrazia, C. et al. (1979). The production of progesterone, androgens, and estrogens by granulosa cells, thecal tissue, and stromal tissue from human ovaries in vitro. *J. Clin. Endocrinol. Metab.* 49: 687–699.

45. Knecht, M., Amsterdam, A., and Catt, K. (1981). The regulatory role of cyclic AMP in hormone-induced of granulosa cell differentiation. *J. Biol. Chem.* 256: 10628–10633.

46. Nader, S. and Diamanti-Kandarakis, E. (2007). Polycystic ovary syndrome, oral contraceptives and metabolic issues: new perspectives and a unifying hypothesis. *Hum. Reprod.* 22: 317–322.

47. Mathur, R., Levin, O., and Azziz, R. (2008). Use of ethinylestradiol/drospirenone combination in patients with the polycystic ovary syndrome. *Ther. Clin. Risk Manag.* 4: 487–492.

48. Shah, D. and Patil, M. (2018). Consensus statement on the use of oral contraceptive pills in polycystic ovarian syndrome women in India. *J. Hum. Reprod. Sci.* 11: 96–118.

49. Legro, R.S., Arslanian, S.A., Ehrmann, D.A. et al. (2013). Diagnosis and treatment of polycystic ovary syndrome: an endocrine society clinical practice guideline. *J. Clin. Endocrinol. Metab.* 98: 4565–4592.

50. American College of Obstetricians and Gynecologists' Committee on Practice Bulletins—Gynecology (2018). ACOG Practice Bulletin No. 194: polycystic ovary syndrome. *Obstet. Gynecol.* 131: e157–e171.

51. Kovacs, G. (1996). Progestogen-only pills and bleeding disturbances. *Hum. Reprod.* 11 (Suppl 2): 20–23.

52. Martin, K.A., Anderson, R.R., Chang, R.J. et al. (2018). Evaluation and treatment of hirsutism in premenopausal women: an endocrine society clinical practice guideline. *J. Clin. Endocrinol. Metab.* 103: 1233–1257.

53. Armanini, D., Andrisani, A., Bordin, L., and Sabbadin, C. (2016). Spironolactone in the treatment of polycystic ovary syndrome. *Expert. Opin. Pharmacother.* 17: 1713–1715.

54. Corvol, P., Michaud, A., Menard, J. et al. (1975). Antiandrogenic effect of spirolactones: mechanism of action. *Endocrinology* 97: 52–58.

55. Cumming, D.C., Yang, J.C., Rebar, R.W., and Yen, S.S. (1982). Treatment of hirsutism with spironolactone. *JAMA* 247: 1295–1298.

56. Mazza, A., Fruci, B., Guzzi, P. et al. (2014). In PCOS patients the addition of low-dose spironolactone induces a more marked reduction of clinical and biochemical hyperandrogenism than metformin alone. *Nutr. Metab. Cardiovasc. Dis.* 24: 132–139.

57. Ganie, M.A., Khurana, M.L., Eunice, M. et al. (2004). Comparison of efficacy of spironolactone with metformin in the management of polycystic ovary syndrome: an open-labeled study. *J. Clin. Endocrinol. Metabol.* 89: 2756–2762.

58. Spritzer, P.M., Lisboa, K.O., Mattiello, S., and Lhullier, F. (2000). Spironolactone as a single agent for long-term therapy of hirsute patients. *Clin. Endocrinol.* 52: 587–594.

59. Williams, E.M., Katholi, R.E., and Karambelas, M.R. (2006). Use and side-effect profile of spironolactone in a private cardiologist's practice. *Clin. Cardiol.* 29: 149–153.

60. Orisaka, M., Miyazaki, Y., Shirafuji, A. et al. (2021). The role of pituitary gonadotropins and intraovarian regulators in follicle development: a mini-review. *Reprod. Med. Biol.* 20: 169–175.

61. Rimon-Dahari, N., Yerushalmi-Heinemann, L., Alyagor, L., and Dekel, N. (2016). Ovarian folliculogenesis. *Results Probl. Cell Differ.* 58: 167–190.

62. Orisaka, M., Tajima, K., Tsang, B.K., and Kotsuji, F. (2009). Oocyte-granulosa-theca cell interactions during preantral follicular development. *J. Ovarian Res.* 2: 9.

63. Knight, P.G. and Glister, C. (2006). TGF-beta superfamily members and ovarian follicle development. *Reproduction* 132: 191–206.

64. Macklon, N.S. and Fauser, B.C. (1998). Follicle development during the normal menstrual cycle. *Maturitas* 30: 181–188.

65. Hillier, S.G. and Tetsuka, M. (1997). Role of androgens in follicle maturation and atresia. *Baillieres Clin. Obstet. Gynaecol.* 11: 249–260.

66. Walters, K.A., Paris, V.R., Aflatounian, A., and Handelsman, D.J. (2019). Androgens and ovarian function: translation from basic discovery research to clinical impact. *J. Endocrinol.* 242: R23–R50.

67. Dunlop, C.E. and Anderson, R.A. (2014). The regulation and assessment of follicular growth. *Scand. J. Clin. Lab. Invest.* 74: 13–17.

68. Macklon, N.S. and Fauser, B.C. (2001). Follicle-stimulating hormone and advanced follicle development in the human. *Arch. Med. Res.* 32: 595–600.

69. Kovacs, P., Sajgo, A., Kaali, S.G., and Pal, L. (2012). Detrimental effects of high-dose gonadotropin on outcome of IVF: making a case for gentle ovarian stimulation strategies. *Reprod. Sci.* 19: 718–724.

70. Hsueh, A.J.W., Kawamura, K., Cheng, Y., and Fauser, B.C.J.M. (2015). Intraovarian control of early folliculogenesis. *Endocr. Rev.* 36: 1–24.

71. Leão R. de B.F. and Esteves S.C. (2014). Gonadotropin therapy in assisted reproduction: an evolutionary perspective from biologics to biotech. *Clinics (Sao Paulo)* 69:279–293

72. Homburg, R. and Howles, C.M. (1999). Low-dose FSH therapy for anovulatory infertility associated with polycystic ovary syndrome: rationale, results, reflections and refinements. *Hum. Reprod. Update* 5: 493–499.

73. Streda, R., Mardesic, T., Sobotka, V. et al. (2012). Comparison of different starting gonadotropin doses (50, 75 and 100 IU daily) for ovulation induction combined with intrauterine insemination. *Arch. Gynecol. Obstet.* 286: 1055–1059.

74. Fischer, R.A., Nakajima, S.T., Gibson, M., and Brumsted, J.R. (1993). Ovulation after intravenous and intramuscular human chorionic gonadotropin. *Fertil. Steril.* 60: 418–422.

75. Weiss, N.S., Kostova, E., Nahuis, M. et al. (2019). Gonadotrophins for ovulation induction in women with polycystic ovarian syndrome. *Cochrane Database Syst. Rev.* 1 (1): CD010290.

76. Von Hofe, J. and Bates, G.W. (2015). Ovulation induction. *Obstet. Gynecol. Clin. N. Am.* 42: 27–37.

77. Adashi, E.Y. (1984). Clomiphene citrate: mechanism(s) and site(s) of action--a hypothesis revisited. *Fertil. Steril.* 42: 331–344.

78. Kettel, L.M., Roseff, S.J., Berga, S.L. et al. (1993). Hypothalamic-pituitary-ovarian response to clomiphene citrate in women with polycystic ovary syndrome. *Fertil. Steril.* 59: 532–538.

79. Bach, P.V., Najari, B.B., and Kashanian, J.A. (2016). Adjunct management of male hypogonadism. *Curr. Sex. Health Rep.* 8: 231–239.

80. Agrawal, S., Ganie, M.A., and Nisar, S. (2017). Gynaecomastia. In: *Basics of Human Andrology: A Textbook* (ed. A. Kumar and M. Sharma), 451–458. Singapore: Springer.

81. Brown, J., Farquhar, C., Beck, J. et al. (2009). Clomiphene and anti-oestrogens for ovulation induction in PCOS. *Cochrane Database Sysst. Rev.* (4): CD002249.

82. Casper, R.F. and Mitwally, M.F.M. (2011). Use of the aromatase inhibitor letrozole for ovulation induction in women with polycystic ovarian syndrome. *Clin. Obstet. Gynecol.* 54: 685–695.

83. Legro, R.S., Brzyski, R.G., Diamond, M.P. et al. (2014). Letrozole versus clomiphene for infertility in the polycystic ovary syndrome. *N. Engl. J. Med.* 371: 119–129.

84. Franik, S., Eltrop, S.M., Kremer, J.A. et al. (2018). Aromatase inhibitors (letrozole) for subfertile women with polycystic ovary syndrome. *Cochrane Database Syst. Rev.* 5: CD010287.

85. Buffoli, B., Rinaldi, F., Labanca, M. et al. (2014). The human hair: from anatomy to physiology. *Int. J. Dermatol.* 53: 331–341.

86. Schlake, T. (2007). Determination of hair structure and shape. *Semin. Cell Dev. Biol.* 18: 267–273.

87. Agarwal, R., Katare, O.P., and Vyas, S.P. (2000). The pilosebaceous unit: a pivotal route for topical drug delivery. *Methods Find. Exp. Clin. Pharmacol.* 22: 129–133.

88. Ranson, M., Posen, S., and Mason, R.S. (1988). Extracellular matrix modulates the function of human melanocytes but not melanoma cells. *J. Cell. Physiol.* 136: 281–288.

89. Paus, R. and Cotsarelis, G. (1999). The biology of hair follicles. *N. Engl. J. Med.* 341: 491–497.

90. Schneider, M.R., Schmidt-Ullrich, R., and Paus, R. (2009). The hair follicle as a dynamic miniorgan. *Curr. Biol.* 19: R132–R142.

91. Chen, X., Liu, B., Li, Y. et al. (2020). Dihydrotestosterone regulates hair growth through the Wnt/β-catenin pathway in C57BL/6 mice and in vitro organ culture. *Front. Pharmacol.* 10: 1528.

92. Randall, V.A., Thornton, M.J., Hamada, K., and Messenger, A.G. (1994). Androgen action in cultured dermal papilla cells from human hair follicles. *Skin Pharmacol.* 7: 20–26.

93. Hibberts, N.A., Howell, A.E., and Randall, V.A. (1998). Balding hair follicle dermal papilla cells contain higher levels of androgen receptors than those from non-balding scalp. *J. Endocrinol.* 156: 59–65.

94. Thornton, M.J., Hamada, K., Randall, V.A., and Messenger, A.G. (1998). Androgen-dependent beard dermal papilla cells secrete autocrine growth factor(s) in response to testosterone unlike scalp cells. *J. Investig. Dermatol.* 111: 727–732.

95. Ju, Q., Tao, T., Hu, T. et al. (2017). Sex hormones and acne. *Clin. Dermatol.* 35: 130–137.

96. Leyden, J., Bergfeld, W., Drake, L. et al. (2004). A systemic type I 5 alpha-reductase inhibitor is ineffective in the treatment of acne vulgaris. *J. Am. Acad. Dermatol.* 50: 443–447.

97. Cumming, D.C. (1990). Use of spironolactone in treatment of hirsutism. *Cleve. Clin. J. Med.* 57: 285–287.

98. Generali, J.A. and Cada, D.J. (2014). Flutamide: hirsutism in women. *Hosp. Pharm.* 49: 517.

99. Iguchi, T., Tamada, S., Kato, M. et al. (2019). Enzalutamide versus flutamide for castration-resistant prostate cancer after combined androgen blockade therapy with bicalutamide: a retrospective study. *Int. J. Clin. Oncol.* 24: 848–856.

100. O'Brien, R.C., Cooper, M.E., Murray, R.M. et al. (1991). Comparison of sequential cyproterone acetate/estrogen versus spironolactone/oral contraceptive in the treatment of hirsutism. *J. Clin. Endocrinol. Metab.* 72: 1008–1013.

101. Moghetti, P., Tosi, F., Tosti, A. et al. (2000). Comparison of spironolactone, flutamide, and finasteride efficacy in the treatment of hirsutism: a randomized, double blind, placebo-controlled trial1. *J. Clin. Endocrinol. Metabol.* 85: 89–94.

102. Hu, A.C., Chapman, L.W., and Mesinkovska, N.A. (2019). The efficacy and use of finasteride in women: a systematic review. *Int. J. Dermatol.* 58: 759–776.

103. Tahvilian, R., Ebrahimi, A., Beiki, O. et al. (2015). Preparation and clinical evaluation of Finastride gel in the treatment of idiopathic Hirsutism. *J. Drug Assessment* 4: 12.

104. Tolino, A., Petrone, A., Sarnacchiaro, F. et al. (1996). Finasteride in the treatment of hirsutism: new therapeutic perspectives. *Fertil. Steril.* 66: 61–65.

105. Escobar-Morreale, H.F., Botella-Carretero, J.I., Alvarez-Blasco, F. et al. (2005). The polycystic ovary syndrome associated with morbid obesity may resolve after weight loss induced by bariatric surgery. *J. Clin. Endocrinol. Metab.* 90: 6364–6369.

106. Pasquali, R., Gambineri, A., Cavazza, C. et al. (2011). Heterogeneity in the responsiveness to long-term lifestyle intervention and predictability in obese women with polycystic ovary syndrome. *Eur. J. Endocrinol.* 164: 53–60.

107. Brown-Séquard (1889). Note on the effects produced on man by subcutaneous injections of a liquid obtained from the testicles of animals. *Lancet* 134:105–107

108. Hoberman, J.M. and Yesalis, C.E. (1995). The history of synthetic testosterone. *Sci. Am.* 272: 76–81.

109. Schmidt, J.M. (2021). Similia similibus curentur: theory, history, and status of the constitutive principle of homeopathy. *Homeopathy* 110: 212–221.

110. Crawford, E.D., Poage, W., Nyhuis, A. et al. (2015). Measurement of testosterone: how important is a morning blood draw? *Curr. Med. Res. Opin.* 31: 1911–1914.

111. Vingren, J.L., Kraemer, W.J., Ratamess, N.A. et al. (2010). Testosterone physiology in resistance exercise and training: the up-stream regulatory elements. *Sports Med.* 40: 1037–1053.

112. Wang, Y., Chen, F., Ye, L. et al. (2017). Steroidogenesis in Leydig cells: effects of aging and environmental factors. *Reproduction* 154: R111–R122.

113. Zirkin, B.R. and Papadopoulos, V. (2018). Leydig cells: formation, function, and regulation. *Biol. Reprod.* 99: 101.

114. Piper, T., Putz, M., Schänzer, W. et al. (2017). Epiandrosterone sulfate prolongs the detectability of testosterone, 4-androstenedione, and dihydrotestosterone misuse by means of carbon isotope ratio mass spectrometry. *Drug Test. Anal.* 9: 1695–1703.

115. Čeponis, J., Wang, C., Swerdloff, R.S., and Liu, P.Y. (2017). Anabolic and metabolic effects of testosterone and other androgens: direct effects and role of testosterone metabolic products. In: *Endocrinology of the Testis and Male Reproduction* (ed. M. Simoni and I.T. Huhtaniemi), 373–394. Cham: Springer International Publishing.

116. Shigehara, K., Izumi, K., Kadono, Y., and Mizokami, A. (2021). Testosterone and bone health in men: a narrative review. *J. Clin. Med.* 10: 530.

117. Zouboulis, C.C. and Degitz, K. (2004). Androgen action on human skin – from basic research to clinical significance. *Exp. Dermatol.* 13: 5–10.

118. Sheffield-Moore, M. (2000). Androgens and the control of skeletal muscle protein synthesis. *null* 32: 181–186.

119. Kalfa, N., Gaspari, L., Ollivier, M. et al. (2019). Molecular genetics of hypospadias and cryptorchidism recent developments. *Clin. Genet.* 95: 122–131.

120. Bachman, E., Travison, T.G., Basaria, S. et al. (2014). Testosterone induces erythrocytosis via increased erythropoietin and suppressed hepcidin: evidence for a new erythropoietin/hemoglobin set point. *J. Gerontol. Ser. A Biol. Med. Sci.* 69: 725.

121. Czub, M.P., Venkataramany, B.S., Majorek, K.A. et al. (2019). Testosterone meets albumin – the molecular mechanism of sex hormone transport by serum albumins. *Chem. Sci.* 10: 1607.

122. Bhasin, S., Brito, J.P., Cunningham, G.R. et al. (2018). Testosterone therapy in men with hypogonadism: an endocrine society* clinical practice guideline. *J. Clin. Endocrinol. Metabol.* 103: 1715–1744.

123. Walker, W.H. (2011). Testosterone signaling and the regulation of spermatogenesis. *Spermatogenesis* 1: 116.

124. Shihan, M., Bulldan, A., and Scheiner-Bobis, G. (2014). Non-classical testosterone signaling is mediated by a G-protein-coupled receptor interacting with Gnα11. *Biochim. Biophys. Acta* 1843: 1172–1181.

125. Snyder, P.J., Bhasin, S., Cunningham, G.R. et al. (2016). Effects of testosterone treatment in older men. *N. Engl. J. Med.* 374: 611–624.

126. Järvelä, I.Y., Ruokonen, A., and Tekay, A. (2008). Effect of rising hCG levels on the human corpus luteum during early pregnancy. *Hum. Reprod.* 23: 2775–2781.

127. le Cotonnec, J.Y., Porchet, H.C., Beltrami, V., and Munafo, A. (1998). Clinical pharmacology of recombinant human luteinizing hormone: Part I. Pharmacokinetics after intravenous administration to healthy female volunteers and comparison with urinary human luteinizing hormone. *Fertil. Steril.* 69: 189–194.

128. Fink, J., Schoenfeld, B.J., Hackney, A.C. et al. (2021). Human chorionic gonadotropin treatment: a viable option for management of secondary hypogonadism and male infertility. *Expert. Rev. Endocrinol. Metab.* 16: 1–8.

129. Jan, Z., Pfeifer, M., and Zorn, B. (2012). Reversible testosterone-induced azoospermia in a 45-year-old man attending an infertility outpatient clinic. *Andrologia* 44 (Suppl 1): 823–825.

130. Najari, B. (2018). Azoospermia With Testosterone Therapy Despite Concomitant Intramuscular Human Chorionic Gonadotropin. *Rev. Urol.* 20: 137–139.

131. Vicari, E., Mongioì, A., Calogero, A.E. et al. (1992). Therapy with human chorionic gonadotrophin alone induces spermatogenesis in men with isolated hypogonadotrophic hypogonadism-long-term follow-up. *Int. J. Androl.* 15: 320–329.

132. Lo, E.M., Rodriguez, K.M., Pastuszak, A.W., and Khera, M. (2018). Alternatives to testosterone therapy: a review. *Sex Med. Rev.* 6: 106–113.

133. Damewood, M.D., Shen, W., Zacur, H.A. et al. (1989). Disappearance of exogenously administered human chorionic gonadotropin. *Fertil. Steril.* 52: 398–400.

134. Lee, J.A. and Ramasamy, R. (2018). Indications for the use of human chorionic gonadotropic hormone for the management of infertility in hypogonadal men. *Trans.l Androl. Urol.* 7: S348–S352.

135. Trinh, T.S., Hung, N.B., Hien, L.T.T. et al. (2021). Evaluating the combination of human chorionic gonadotropin and clomiphene citrate in treatment of male hypogonadotropic hypogonadism: a prospective study. *Res. Rep. Urol.* 13: 357–366.

136. Habous, M., Giona, S., Tealab, A. et al. (2018). Clomiphene citrate and human chorionic gonadotropin are both effective in restoring testosterone in hypogonadism: a short-course randomized study. *BJU Int.* 122: 889–897.

137. Hsieh, T.-C., Pastuszak, A.W., Hwang, K., and Lipshultz, L.I. (2013). Concomitant intramuscular human chorionic gonadotropin preserves spermatogenesis in men undergoing testosterone replacement therapy. *J. Urol.* 189: 647–650.

138. Walker, W.H. and Cheng, J. (2005). FSH and testosterone signaling in Sertoli cells. *Reproduction* 130: 15–28.

139. Oduwole, O.O., Peltoketo, H., and Huhtaniemi, I.T. (2018). Role of follicle-stimulating hormone in spermatogenesis. *Front. Endocrinol. (Lausanne)* 9: 763.

140. Ni, F.-D., Hao, S.-L., and Yang, W.-X. (2019). Multiple signaling pathways in Sertoli cells: recent findings in spermatogenesis. *Cell Death Dis.* 10: 1–15.

141. Khanehzad, M., Abbaszadeh, R., Holakuyee, M. et al. (2021). FSH regulates RA signaling to commit spermatogonia into differentiation pathway and meiosis. *Reprod. Biol. Endocrinol.* 19: 4.

142. Shah, W., Khan, R., Shah, B. et al. (2021). The molecular mechanism of sex hormones on sertoli cell development and proliferation. *Front. Endocrinol.* 12.

143. Casarini, L. and Crépieux, P. (2019). Molecular mechanisms of action of FSH. *Front. Endocrinol. (Lausanne)* 10: 305–305.

144. Behre, H.M. (2019). Clinical use of FSH in male infertility. *Front. Endocrinol. (Lausanne)* 10: 322–322.

145. Bouloux, P., Warne, D.W., Loumaye, E., and FSH Study Group in Men's Infertility (2002). Efficacy and safety of recombinant human follicle-stimulating hormone in men with isolated hypogonadotropic hypogonadism. *Fertil. Steril.* 77: 270–273.

146. Zacharin, M., Sabin, M.A., Nair, V.V., and Dagabdhao, P. (2012). Addition of recombinant follicle-stimulating hormone to human chorionic gonadotropin treatment in adolescents and young adults with hypogonadotropic hypogonadism promotes normal testicular growth and may promote early spermatogenesis. *Fertil. Steril.* 98: 836–842.

147. Tapanainen, J.S., Aittomäki, K., Min, J. et al. (1997). Men homozygous for an inactivating mutation of the follicle-stimulating hormone (FSH) receptor gene present variable suppression of spermatogenesis and fertility. *Nat. Genet.* 15: 205–206.

148. Herzog, B.J., Nguyen, H.M.T., Soubra, A., and Hellstrom, W.J.G. (2020). Clomiphene citrate for male hypogonadism and infertility: an updated review. *Androgens: Clinical Res. Therap.* 1: 62–69.

149. Guay, A.T., Jacobson, J., Perez, J.B. et al. (2003). Clomiphene increases free testosterone levels in men with both secondary hypogonadism and erectile dysfunction: who does and does not benefit? *Int. J. Impot. Res.* 15: 156–165.

150. Katz, D.J., Nabulsi, O., Tal, R., and Mulhall, J.P. (2012). Outcomes of clomiphene citrate treatment in young hypogonadal men. *BJU Int.* 110: 573–578.

151. McBride, J.A., Carson, C.C. III, and Coward, R.M. (2016). Testosterone deficiency in the aging male. *Ther. Adv. Urol.* 8: 47.

152. Ronde W. de and Jong F.H. de (2011). Aromatase inhibitors in men: effects and therapeutic options. *Reprod. Biol. Endocrinol.* 9:93

153. Harman, S.M., Metter, E.J., Tobin, J.D. et al. (2001). Longitudinal effects of aging on serum total and free testosterone levels in healthy men. *J. Clin. Endocrinol. Metab.* 86: 724–731.

154. Feldman, H.A., Longcope, C., Derby, C.A. et al. (2002). Age trends in the level of serum testosterone and other hormones in middle-aged men: longitudinal results from the massachusetts male aging study. *J. Clin. Endocrinol. Metabol.* 87: 589–598.

155. Freedman, R.R. (2014). Menopausal hot flashes: mechanisms, endocrinology, treatment. *J. Steroid Biochem. Mol. Biol.* 142: 115–120.

156. Rance, N.E., Dacks, P.A., Mittelman-Smith, M.A. et al. (2013). Modulation of body temperature and LH secretion by hypothalamic KNDy (kisspeptin, neurokinin B and dynorphin) neurons: a novel hypothesis on the mechanism of hot flushes. *Front. Neuroendocrinol.* 34: 211–227.

157. Takahashi, T.A. and Johnson, K.M. (2015). Menopause. *Med. Clin. North Am.* 99: 521–534.

158. Moorman, P.G., Myers, E.R., Schildkraut, J.M. et al. (2011). Effect of hysterectomy with ovarian preservation on ovarian function. *Obstet. Gynecol.* 118: 1271–1279.

159. Quinn, M., Cedars, M.I., Huddleston, H.G., and Santoro, N. (2022). Antimüllerian hormone use and misuse in current reproductive medicine practice: a clinically oriented review. *F&S Rev.* 3: 1–10.

160. Freeman, E.W., Sammel, M.D., Lin, H., and Gracia, C.R. (2012). Anti-Mullerian hormone as a predictor of time to menopause in late reproductive age women. *J. Clin. Endocrinol. Metab.* 97: 1673–1680.

161. Freedman, R.R. and Krell, W. (1999). Reduced thermoregulatory null zone in postmenopausal women with hot flashes. *Am. J. Obstet. Gynecol.* 181: 66–70.

162. Freedman, R.R. (2005). Pathophysiology and treatment of menopausal hot flashes. *Semin. Reprod. Med.* 23: 117–125.

163. North American Menopause Society (2014). *Menopause Practice: A Clinician's Guide.* Mayfield Heights, OH: North American Menopause Society.

164. Kaunitz, A.M. and Manson, J.E. (2015). Management of Menopausal Symptoms. *Obstet. Gynecol.* 126: 859–876.

165. (2014). ACOG Practice Bulletin No. 141: management of menopausal symptoms. *Obstet. Gynecol.* 123: 202–216.

166. Black, D. (2020). The safety of oral versus transdermal estrogen. *Menopause* 27: 1328–1329.

167. MacLennan A.H., Broadbent J.L., Lester S., and Moore V. (2004). Oral oestrogen and combined oestrogen/progestogen therapy versus placebo for hot flushes. *Cochrane Database Syst. Rev.* https://doi.org/10.1002/14651858.CD002978.pub2

168. Wells, G., Tugwell, P., Shea, B. et al. (2002). Meta-analyses of therapies for postmenopausal osteoporosis. V. Meta-analysis of the efficacy of hormone replacement therapy in treating and preventing osteoporosis in postmenopausal women. *Endocr. Rev.* 23: 529–539.

169. Uchida, M. and Kobayashi, O. (2018). Novel effect of α-lactalbumin on the yohimbine-induced hot flush increase of the tail skin temperature in ovariectomized rats. *Biosci. Biotechnol. Biochem.* 82: 862–868.

170. Stearns, V., Slack, R., Greep, N. et al. (2005). Paroxetine is an effective treatment for hot flashes: results from a prospective randomized clinical trial. *J. Clin. Oncol.* 23: 6919–6930.

171. Shams, T., Firwana, B., Habib, F. et al. (2014). SSRIs for hot flashes: a systematic review and meta-analysis of randomized trials. *J. Gen. Intern. Med.* 29: 204–213.

172. Juurlink, D. (2016). Revisiting the drug interaction between tamoxifen and SSRI antidepressants. *BMJ* 354: i5309.

173. (2011). Tamoxifen and CYP 2D6 inhibitors: caution. *Prescrire Int.* 20: 182–184.

174. Turner, H.H. (1938). A syndrome of infantilism, congenital webbed neck, and cubitus valgus. *Endocrinology* 23: 566–574.

175. Osborne, C.K. and Schiff, R. (2005). Estrogen-receptor biology: continuing progress and therapeutic implications. *J. Clin. Oncol.* 23: 1616–1622.

176. Nilsson, S., Mäkelä, S., Treuter, E. et al. (2001). Mechanisms of estrogen action. *Physiol. Rev.* 81: 1535–1565.

177. Alemany, M. (2021). Estrogens and the regulation of glucose metabolism. *World J. Diabetes* 12: 1622–1654.

178. Klein, K.O., Rosenfield, R.L., Santen, R.J. et al. (2018). Estrogen replacement in turner syndrome: literature review and practical considerations. *J. Clin. Endocrinol. Metab.* 103: 1790–1803.

179. Shankar, R.K. and Backeljauw, P.F. (2018). Current best practice in the management of Turner syndrome. *Ther. Adv. Endocrinol. Metab.* 9: 33–40.

180. Clemente E.G., Maravol P.V., and Tanager C.L. (2019). Gonadal dysgenesis: a clinical overview of Turner syndrome. *Pediatr. Med.* 2:31. https://doi.org/10.21037/pm.2019.06.10.

181. Gravholt, C.H., Andersen, N.H., Conway, G.S. et al. (2017). Clinical practice guidelines for the care of girls and women with Turner syndrome: proceedings from the 2016 Cincinnati International Turner Syndrome Meeting. *Eur. J. Endocrinol.* 177: G1–G70.

182. Zaiem, F., Alahdab, F., Nofal, A.A. et al. (2017). Oral versus transdermal estrogen in turner syndrome: a systematic review and meta-analysis. *Endocr. Pract.* 23: 408–421.

183. Tanner, J.M. and Davies, P.S. (1985). Clinical longitudinal standards for height and height velocity for North American children. *J. Pediatr.* 107: 317–329.

184. Rosenfeld, R.G. (2006). Molecular mechanisms of IGF-I deficiency. *Horm. Res.* 65 (Suppl 1): 15–20.

185. van der Eerden, B.C.J., Karperien, M., and Wit, J.M. (2003). Systemic and local regulation of the growth plate. *Endocr. Rev.* 24: 782–801.

186. Binder, G. (2011). Short stature due to SHOX deficiency: genotype, phenotype, and therapy. *Horm. Res. Paediatr.* 75: 81–89.

187. Allen, D.B. (2006). Growth hormone therapy for short stature: is the benefit worth the burden? *Pediatrics* 118: 343–348.

188. Carel, J.-C. and Butler, G. (2010). Safety of recombinant human growth hormone. *Endocr. Dev.* 18: 40–54.

189. Li, P., Cheng, F., and Xiu, L. (2018). Height outcome of the recombinant human growth hormone treatment in Turner syndrome: a meta-analysis. *Endocr. Connect.* 7: 573–583.

190. Seo, G.H., Kang, E., Cho, J.H. et al. (2015). Turner syndrome presented with tall stature due to overdosage of the SHOX gene. *Ann. Pediatr. Endocrinol. Metab.* 20: 110–113.

191. Oliveira, C.S. and Alves, C. (2011). The role of the SHOX gene in the pathophysiology of Turner syndrome. *Endocrinol. Nutr.* 58: 433–442.

192. Ross, J.L., Kowal, K., Quigley, C.A. et al. (2005). The phenotype of short stature homeobox gene (SHOX) deficiency in childhood: contrasting children with Leri-Weill Dyschondrosteosis and Turner Syndrome. *J. Pediatr.* 147: 499–507.

CHAPTER 7

Therapies in Disorders of Lipid Metabolism and Obesity

7.1 HYPERLIPOPROTEINEMIA SYNDROMES

7.1.1 Ezetimibe

7.1.1.1 Physiology

What Are Lipoproteins?

Lipoproteins are complex molecules composed of cholesterol esters (CEs) and triacylglycerols, surrounded by a layer of free cholesterol, apolipoproteins, and phospholipids. This unique structure enables lipoproteins to transport water-insoluble cholesterol and triacylglycerols through the bloodstream to their intended destinations (Figure 7.1). The different types of lipoproteins, including high-density lipoproteins (HDL), low-density lipoproteins (LDL), very low-density lipoproteins (VLDL), and intermediate-density lipoproteins (IDL), vary in their composition and function [1, 2].

The classification of lipoproteins is based on their size, lipid composition, and the specific apolipoprotein subtype they contain. There are several types of lipoproteins, including LDL, HDL, VLDL, IDL, and chylomicrons [3].

HDL, or high-density lipoproteins, contain roughly equal parts of protein and lipid. They differ in their content of various components like triglycerides (TAGs), apolipoproteins, lipid transfer enzymes, and proteins. HDL also carries liposoluble vitamins and antioxidants. Its protective benefits are mainly due to its role in reverse cholesterol transport. Factors such as HDL metabolism, the concentration of various HDL subclasses, and genetic factors can all impact HDL's anti-atherogenic properties. Thus, standard plasma measurements may not fully reflect the range of HDL's effects. Recent studies suggest that the function of HDL may be more crucial than its plasma concentration, as there are populations with low HDL levels yet without an increased risk of coronary heart disease [4].

VLDLs are also triglyceride-rich and contain both Apo C-II and Apo E; however, unlike their chylomicron counterparts, they contain less TAGs, are smaller, and now contain Apo B-100 instead of Apo B-48. This change is important because Apo B-100 acts as a physiological ligand for LDL receptors (LDL-R) [5].

Chylomicrons are a type of lipoprotein responsible for carrying dietary fats, cholesterol, and fat-soluble nutrients through the digestive tract. Their surface consists of phospholipids (ApoB48), as well as approximately 90% triglyceride by weight (chylomicron's core being less dense than plasma) [3].

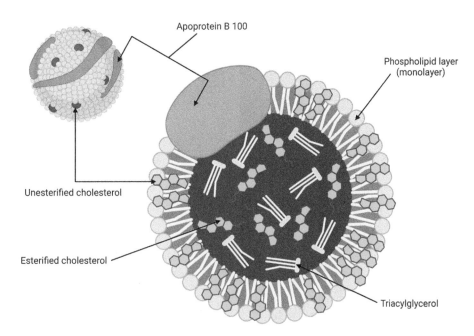

Apoprotein B 100

Phospholipid layer
(monolayer)

Unesterified cholesterol

Esterified cholesterol

Triacylglycerol

FIGURE 7.1 Structure of LDL cholesterol. Esterified cholesterol and triacylglycerol in a lipid core, surrounded by a phospholipid monolayer containing apolipoproteins and unesterified cholesterol.

What Are Apolipoproteins?

Apolipoproteins are complex proteins found on the surface of lipoproteins that serve an integral function in lipoprotein physiology. Apolipoproteins provide structural integrity to lipoproteins while modulating related enzymatic activity as well as acting as ligands for various receptors in specific target tissues [6].

Apolipoproteins can be divided into several distinct classes depending on where they exist within lipoproteins. Some of the key apolipoproteins include Apolipoprotein B (apoB), Apolipoprotein A1 (apoA1), ApoE, and ApoC. ApoB can be found primarily on LDL and VLDL particles, where it helps manage cholesterol metabolism. ApoA1 plays an integral part in HDL transport processes that remove extra cholesterol from peripheral tissues and carries them to the liver for further processing [3].

ApoE can be found on several lipoproteins, including VLDL, IDL, and chylomicrons; its presence facilitates their removal from circulation [7]. ApoC is present in VLDLs and HDLs and plays an essential part in the metabolism of TAGs [8].

What Is the Significance of Lipoprotein Metabolism?

The main purpose of lipoprotein metabolism is to transfer dietary sources of TAGs for energy metabolism or storage in muscles or fat tissue, respectively. Lipoprotein produced by the liver includes VLDLs and chylomicrons which are responsible for carrying TAGs from intestines to peripheral tissues [9].

Lipoprotein metabolism enables the cycling of cholesterol between the liver and peripheral tissues, an essential process in producing steroid hormones, cell membranes, and bile acids. HDL plays an essential role in this cycle by collecting excess cholesterol from peripheral tissues and returning it for processing and excretion by the liver. LDL delivers cholesterol directly into peripheral tissues, which could contribute to plaque formation in arteries.

Endogenous and Exogenous Lipoprotein Pathway

The endogenous and exogenous lipoprotein pathways are two distinct mechanisms by which lipids, including cholesterol and TAGs, are transported through the body (see Figure 7.2).

The **endogenous pathway** is responsible for the production and transport of lipids that are synthesized by the liver. This pathway begins with the synthesis of VLDL, which is then secreted into the bloodstream. VLDL particles are then metabolized by lipoprotein lipase (LPL) in peripheral tissues, releasing fatty acids and producing IDL particles. IDL particles can either be taken up by the liver or further metabolized into LDL particles, which deliver cholesterol to peripheral tissues.

The **exogenous pathway**, on the other hand, is responsible for the transport of lipids that are derived

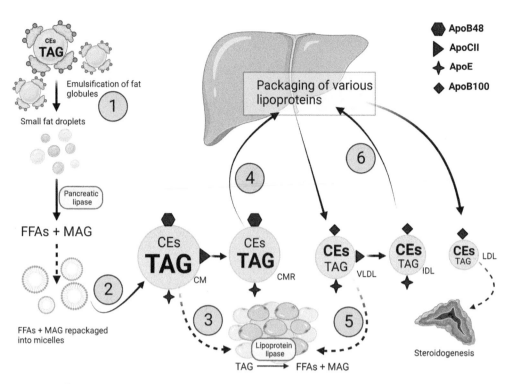

FIGURE 7.2   Summary of the exogenous and endogenous pathways of lipoprotein metabolism.

from dietary sources. This pathway begins with the ingestion of dietary fats, which are packaged into chylomicrons in the intestines. Chylomicrons are then transported through the lymphatic system and into the bloodstream, where they are metabolized by LPL in peripheral tissues, releasing fatty acids and producing chylomicron remnants that are taken up by the liver for further processing.

Bile acids are responsible for the emulsification of fat globules into small fatty droplets (step 1). This step facilitates the hydrolysis of triacylglycerides (TAG) into free fatty acids (FFAs) and monoacylglycerol (MAG) by pancreatic lipase (PL) in the intestinal lumen. Chylomicrons (CMs), formed from packaging TAG, cholesterol ester (CE) and various apoproteins into packages (step 2). They are then transported to target tissues where lipoprotein lipase (LPL hydrolyzes TAGs (step 3). Chylomicron remnants (CMR) formed after this hydrolysis are then transported to the liver for further processing (step 4). VLDL is produced in the liver and then transported to target tissues where TAG stores are released for hydrolysis by LPL (step 5). IDL, formed after processing VLDL in target tissues, is transported back to the liver (step 6). LDL, which is rich in cholesterol esters (CE), plays a critical role in steroidogenesis in various tissues and is also integral in atherogenesis (step 7) [5].

Bile salts emulsify fat globules into smaller fatty droplets that contain TAGs and CEs. Dietary triglycerides are then hydrolyzed into free fatty acids (FFAs) and monoacylglycerol (MAG) in the intestinal lumen by pancreatic lipases. This initial step enables the eventual transfer of TAGs from the intestinal lumen into the circulatory system. Following the hydrolysis of TAGs into FFAs and MAG, these products are repackaged into micelles, which can diffuse into the cytosol of the enterocyte [9, 10]. After entering the enterocyte, FFAs and MAG are resynthesized into TAGs to prepare for transport into the circulatory system. Chylomicrons are then formed within the enterocyte by packaging the newly formed TAGs, along with CEs, cholesterol, and apolipoprotein B-48 (Apo B-48) [11]. This marks the completion of the formation of the initial lipoprotein in the exogenous lipoprotein pathway [12].

Chylomicrons circumvent the portal circulation and enter the systemic circulation through the thoracic duct [11, 13]. Once in the systemic circulation, HDL transfers apolipoprotein CII (Apo-CII) and apolipoprotein E (Apo-E) to the chylomicrons. Apo-E facilitates the binding of lipoproteins to specific LDL-R or LDL-like receptors found in various tissues such as the liver and adrenal cortex. Apo-CII plays a crucial role in activating LPL, which is present in the capillary endothelium [14].

Once they reach adipose tissue and muscle, chylomicrons encounter LPL (which is produced by adipocytes and muscle cells) on the endothelial lining of capillaries. LPL hydrolyzes TAGs into FFAs and MAG, which can then be taken up by adipocytes and muscle cells for energy metabolism [9]. Chylomicron remnants, which are produced after this step, release the previously acquired apo-CII back to HDL, as it is no longer needed for LPL activity [14]. This marks the end of the exogenous lipoprotein pathway, which enables the transfer of dietary sources of fatty acids from the intestine to muscle and adipose tissue for both storage and metabolism [15].

Chylomicron remnants, which primarily consist of cholesterol and CEs, attach to the hepatic LDL-R and are conveyed into the liver [16]. Upon entering the liver, TAGs, CEs, and Apo-B100 are repackaged into VLDL. Similar to chylomicrons, VLDL in circulation acquires Apo-E and Apo-CII from HDL. VLDL is conveyed to adipose tissue and muscle, where LPL enables the hydrolysis of TAGs into FFAs and MAG. FFAs can be stored in fatty tissue or utilized for energy metabolism by muscle. The depletion of TAGs from VLDL results in the formation of IDL or VLDL remnants. Following the formation of IDL, Apo-CII is once again released back to HDL [14, 17].

IDL found in the bloodstream, with Apo-E bound to its surface, demonstrates an affinity for binding to tissues that possess LDL or LDL-like receptors. It attaches to the hepatic LDL-R and is conveyed to the liver for further processing. Apo-B100 and CEs are then consolidated to create a new lipoprotein, which is referred to as LDL [14].

LDL can attach to LDL-like receptors in the gonads for gonadal steroidogenesis [18] and the adrenal cortex for adrenal steroidogenesis [19, 20]. Additionally, it can bind to LDL-R found in muscle and adipose tissue, where it is conveyed for additional processing. Ultimately, LDL returns to the liver to conclude the endogenous lipoprotein pathway, which primarily aims to convey cholesterol and TAGs from the liver to peripheral tissues [21].

To understand how cholesterol is absorbed in the small intestine, it is vital to know the basic steps involved in both dietary and biliary cholesterol handling [22]. Cholesterol absorption occurs through several processes in the small intestine. Regardless of its origin, free cholesterol first binds to the Niemann-Pick C1-like 1 (NPC1L1) protein located on the luminal side of the enterocyte plasma membrane [23]. The NPC1L1-cholesterol complex then binds to clathrin/AP2, which enables vesicular endocytosis of the NPC1L1–cholesterol complex into the enterocyte. Indeed, without the activity of clathrin/AP2, the endocytosis of NPC1L1 and cholesterol would not occur. [24, 25].

Once the NPC1L1–cholesterol complex is endocytosed, cholesterol is released, and NPC1L1 is returned to the plasma membrane for additional cholesterol binding/absorption. The cholesterol released into the cytosol is then esterified by *acyl-coenzyme A: cholesterol acyltransferase (ACAT)* to form CEs. These newly formed CEs combine with triacylglycerol particles (from absorbed FFAs) and ApoB-48 to form chylomicrons. The newly formed ApoB-48 containing chylomicrons are then taken up into the portal or lymphatic circulation for use by the rest of the body [26] (Figure 7.3).

7.1.1.2 Mechanism of Action

Ezetimibe and its main metabolite, ezetimibe glucuronide, inhibit the absorption of cholesterol in the small intestine [27]. They accomplish this by directly binding to a transmembrane loop of the NPC1L1 protein, which is responsible for transporting cholesterol into enterocytes (cells in the small intestine lining) [28].

Binding to NPC1L1, ezetimibe, and ezetimibe glucuronide prevents the protein from interacting with clathrin and AP2, which are required for its internalization into the cell [29]. This means that the enterocyte cannot take up the cholesterol/NPC1L1 complex, resulting in decreased absorption of cholesterol from the diet.

The net effect of this inhibition of cholesterol absorption is a reduction in LDL-C levels in the bloodstream and modest reductions in total cholesterol and TAGs. Clinical studies have shown that treatment with ezetimibe can lead to LDL-C reductions of 18–20%, making it a useful medication for managing hypercholesterolemia [30].

Practice Pearl(s)

- It lowers LDL-C levels by 13–20%, can be used either alone or in combination with other drugs, and is indicated for various types of hyperlipidemia [31].
- Ezetimibe can be combined with statins and has been shown to improve cardiovascular outcomes in post-acute coronary syndrome patients. The American College of Cardiology recommends considering ezetimibe therapy in addition to statin therapy for patients who have not achieved target LDL reduction [32].

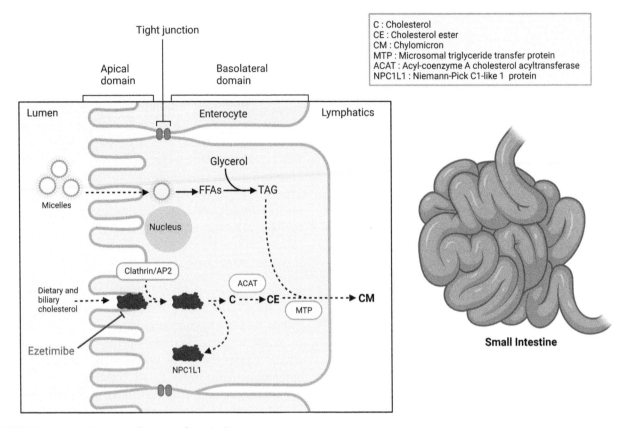

FIGURE 7.3 Mechanism of action of ezetimibe.

Clinical Trial Evidence

The IMPROVE-IT (Improved Reduction of Outcomes: Vytorin Efficacy International Trial) study, involving over 18,000 patients, was designed to evaluate whether adding ezetimibe to simvastatin would further reduce cardiovascular events compared to simvastatin alone in patients who had experienced an acute coronary syndrome (ACS) event like a heart attack or unstable angina. This was particularly interesting since patients enrolled in the study had LDL cholesterol levels already at or below current guideline targets. The trial aimed to see if further lowering would yield additional benefits (see Table 7.1 for a summary of the trial results).

TABLE 7.1 Efficacy of ezetimibe in patients with acute coronary syndrome (IMPROVE-IT study).

Study	Population	Intervention	Outcome
IMPROVE-IT	Patients hospitalized for acute coronary syndrome within the last 10 days, with LDL cholesterol levels between 50–100 mg/dL if receiving lipid-lowering therapy, or 50–125 mg/dL if not receiving lipid-lowering therapy.	Double-blind, randomized trial comparing the combination of simvastatin (40 mg) and ezetimibe (10 mg) against simvastatin (40 mg) and placebo (n = 18,144).	The event rate for the primary end point at 7 years was 32.7% in the simvastatin–ezetimibe group, compared to 34.7% in the simvastatin-monotherapy group. The addition of ezetimibe to statin therapy resulted in further lowering of LDL cholesterol levels and improved cardiovascular outcomes [33].

7.1.2 Statins

7.1.2.1 Physiology

HMG CoA reductase (3-hydroxy-3-methylglutaryl coenzyme A reductase) is a key enzyme in the biosynthesis of cholesterol. This enzyme catalyzes the rate-limiting step in the mevalonate pathway, ultimately producing cholesterol and other isoprenoids such as ubiquinone, heme, and farnesyl groups attached to cellular proteins. The HMG CoA reductase-catalyzed reaction is the rate-limiting step in the mevalonate pathway, meaning it determines the overall rate of cholesterol synthesis. Because of its crucial role, the enzyme serves as a key target for regulating cholesterol levels in the body [34].

7.1.2.2 Mechanism of Action

Statins function as competitive inhibitors of HMG CoA reductase, the enzyme responsible for the rate-limiting step in cholesterol biosynthesis (see Figure 7.4). These agents bind to a part of the HMG CoA binding site on the enzyme, HMG CoA reductase, effectively blocking the access of the substrate (HMG CoA) to the active site of the enzyme [35, 36].

As a result of statin-induced inhibition of HMG CoA reductase, intrahepatic cholesterol levels decrease. This reduction in liver cholesterol prompts an increase in the turnover of LDL receptors due to an accelerated rate of hepatic LDL-R cycling [37]. This process leads to enhanced clearance of LDL cholesterol from the bloodstream, thereby reducing blood cholesterol levels.

In addition to their effect on LDL cholesterol, statins also reduce the production of VLDL by influencing the hepatic secretion of apoB. apoB is a crucial component of VLDL particles, and its altered secretion impacts VLDL production [38].

By targeting HMG CoA reductase, statins play a vital role in controlling cholesterol levels and preventing cardiovascular diseases. The dual action of these drugs, both on LDL and VLDL cholesterol, highlights their therapeutic significance in managing hypercholesterolemia and reducing the risk of atherosclerosis and other related complications.

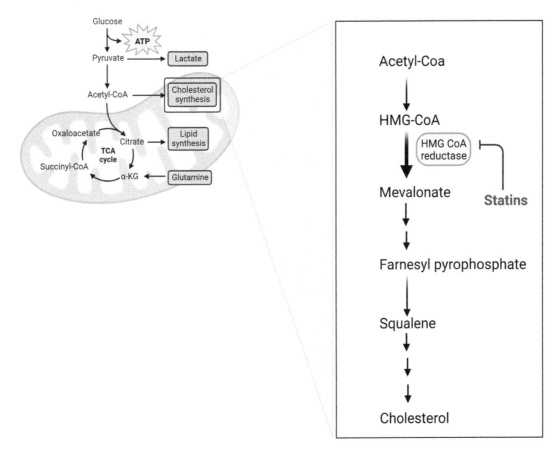

FIGURE 7.4 Schematic representation of the cholesterol synthesis pathway.

Practice Pearl(s)

- Cholesterol synthesis mostly occurs at night, influenced by the fasting state. Indeed statins with shorter half-lives are best administered in the evening or at bedtime [39].
- Routine monitoring of serum creatine kinase (CK) levels and liver enzymes is not recommended. It is, however, reasonable to obtain baseline levels prior to initiating treatment with statins [40].

 Pathophysiology Pearl

Diurnal rhythm of cholesterol synthesis

Cholesterol production predominantly occurs in the liver, and its synthesis is controlled by the enzyme HMG-CoA reductase (3-hydroxy-3-methyl-glutaryl-CoA reductase). The activity of this enzyme is influenced by the circadian rhythm, with cholesterol synthesis generally peaking during the night [41].

Although all statins undergo metabolism in the liver, there is considerable variation in their elimination half-lives. For example, *simvastatin, fluvastatin, and lovastatin* have *shorter elimination half-lives* compared to other statins in the class. These agents with shorter half-lives need to be administered at bedtime to optimize their efficacy, ensuring the highest statin concentration coincides with peak endogenous cholesterol synthesis, which occurs during the night. [42].

In contrast, *rosuvastatin, atorvastatin, pitavastatin, and pravastatin* have *longer elimination half-lives*. This extended duration allows these statins to maintain therapeutic drug concentrations throughout a 24-hour period, offering more flexibility in dosing schedules [42]. Consequently, these agents can be administered at different times of the day without compromising their effectiveness.

It is important to note that the circadian rhythm of cholesterol production plays a key role in determining the optimal dosing time for statins by aligning the peak statin concentration with the time when cholesterol synthesis is the highest.

Statin therapy is a widely used treatment approach for managing dyslipidemia, particularly high levels of low-density lipoprotein cholesterol (LDL-C), which is a significant risk factor for cardiovascular disease. The intensity of statin therapy is categorized based on

the degree of LDL-C reduction achieved by various statins at their respective doses.

There are three main levels of statin therapy intensity:

1. *High-intensity statin therapy*: High-intensity statins aim to reduce LDL-C levels by at least 50%. They are generally prescribed for individuals at high risk of atherosclerotic cardiovascular disease (ASCVD) or those with extremely high LDL-C levels. Common high-intensity statin regimens include:
   - Atorvastatin: 40–80 mg/day
   - Rosuvastatin: 20–40 mg/day [43]

2. *Moderate-intensity statin therapy*: Moderate-intensity statins are intended to reduce LDL-C levels by 30–49%. They are often prescribed for individuals with moderate ASCVD risk or those who cannot tolerate high-intensity statin therapy due to side effects. Examples of moderate-intensity statin regimens include:
   - Atorvastatin: 10–20 mg/day
   - Rosuvastatin: 5–10 mg/day
   - Simvastatin: 20–40 mg/day
   - Pravastatin: 40–80 mg/day
   - Lovastatin: 40 mg/day
   - Fluvastatin XL: 80 mg/day
   - Pitavastatin: 2–4 mg/day [44]

3. *Low-intensity statin therapy*: Low-intensity statins aim to reduce LDL-C levels by less than 30%. They are typically prescribed for individuals with a lower ASCVD risk, older adults, or those who have contraindications or intolerance to higher-intensity statins. Some low-intensity statin regimens are:
   - Simvastatin: 10 mg/day
   - Pravastatin: 10–20 mg/day
   - Lovastatin: 20 mg/day
   - Fluvastatin: 20–40 mg/day
   - Pitavastatin: 1 mg/day [45]

The choice of statin intensity depends on the individual's risk factors, baseline LDL-C levels, comorbidities, and potential side effects. It is crucial to monitor the patient's lipid levels, liver function, and any side effects throughout the course of therapy to make necessary adjustments to the treatment plan. In some cases, non-statin lipid-lowering medications may be added or used as alternatives if statin therapy is not well tolerated or if the desired LDL-C reduction is not achieved.

Clinical Trial Evidence

A summary of landmark trials that evaluated the efficacy of statin therapy in reducing cardiovascular events is shown in Table 7.2.

TABLE 7.2   Landmark trials of statins in patients with cardiovascular disease.

Study	Population	Intervention	Outcome
PROVE IT–TIMI 22	Patients hospitalized for an acute coronary syndrome within the last 10 days (n = 4162)	Comparison of daily 40 mg pravastatin (standard therapy) versus 80 mg atorvastatin (intensive therapy)	The rates of the primary end point at two years were 26.3% in the pravastatin group and 22.4% in the atorvastatin group, indicating a 16% reduction in the hazard ratio in favor of atorvastatin. Intensive lipid-lowering statin regimen provides greater protection against death or major cardiovascular events than standard therapy [46].
MIRACL	Adults aged 18 years or older with unstable angina or non–Q-wave acute myocardial infarction	A randomized, double-blind trial with atorvastatin (80 mg/d) or placebo treatment initiated between 24 and 96 h after hospital admission (n = 3086)	There were no significant differences in risk of death, nonfatal myocardial infarction, or cardiac arrest between the groups, but the atorvastatin group had a lower risk of symptomatic ischemia requiring emergency rehospitalization. There were fewer strokes in the atorvastatin group than in the placebo group [47].
4S	Patients with angina pectoris or previous myocardial infarction and serum cholesterol 5·5–8·0 mmol/L on a lipid-lowering diet	Double-blind treatment with simvastatin or placebo (n = 4444)	The simvastatin group had lower death rates (8%) compared to the placebo group (12%). The 6-year survival probabilities in the placebo and simvastatin groups were 87.6% and 91.3%, respectively. There were fewer coronary deaths and major coronary events in the simvastatin group compared to the placebo group. Additionally, the risk of undergoing myocardial revascularisation procedures was reduced by 37% in the simvastatin group [48].

PROVE IT–TIMI 22, Pravastatin or Atorvastatin Evaluation and Infection Therapy–Thrombolysis in Myocardial Infarction 22; MIRACL, The Myocardial Ischemia Reduction with Aggressive Cholesterol Lowering; 4S, Scandinavian Simvastatin Survival Study.

7.1.3   PCSK9-Inhibitors

7.1.3.1   Physiology

Proprotein convertase subtilisin/kexin type 9 (PCSK9) is a serine protease enzyme encoded by the PCSK9 gene, which is primarily expressed in the liver. This enzyme plays a pivotal role in modulating cholesterol homeostasis by regulating the low-density lipoprotein receptor (LDL-R) lifecycle [49].

Under physiological conditions, LDL-Rs situated on the surface of hepatocytes bind circulating LDL-C particles and internalize them. Subsequently, the intracellular LDL-C particles undergo degradation, with cholesterol being utilized or excreted. This mechanism is crucial for maintaining optimal cholesterol levels in the bloodstream.

However, PCSK9 interferes with this process by binding to LDL-R on hepatocytes. Upon PCSK9–LDL-R interaction, the receptor is internalized and directed toward lysosomal degradation rather than recycling to the cell surface. Consequently, the availability of LDL-Rs on the hepatocyte surface decreases, leading to reduced LDL-C clearance from the blood. This, in turn, results in elevated plasma LDL-C levels, thereby increasing the risk of ASCVD [50].

7.1.3.2   Mechanism of Action

PCSK9 inhibitors disrupt the interaction between PCSK9 and LDL-R, increasing hepatic LDL-R expression and decreasing plasma LDL-C levels. Alirocumab and evolocumab are fully humanized monoclonal antibodies that target and bind free plasma PCSK9, facilitating its degradation. Consequently, less free PCSK9 is available in plasma to interact with LDL-R. This increased LDL-R recycling to the hepatocyte surface allows the liver to remove more LDL-C from circulation, leading to reduced plasma LDL-C levels [51, 52].

Importantly, these antibodies are specific for PCSK9 and do not bind to other members of the PCSK enzyme superfamily.

An alternative approach to inhibiting PCSK9 is by blocking its synthesis, which relies on messenger RNA (mRNA) [14]. Inclisiran, an antisense oligonucleotide, silences mRNA and serves as an example of this mechanism. By inhibiting the synthesis of PCSK9, inclisiran reduces the availability of PCSK9 in the plasma, ultimately enhancing LDL-R recycling and lowering plasma LDL-C levels (see Section 7.1.9).

Practice Pearl(s)

- The recommended dosage of evolocumab is 140 mg subcutaneously every two weeks or 420 mg once monthly (secondary prevention of ASCVD).
- The recommended starting dose of evolocumab is 420 mg subcutaneously once monthly, which can be increased to 420 mg every 2 weeks (homozygous familial hypercholesterolemia).
- The starting dose of alirocumab is 150 mg every two weeks or 300 mg every month.

Clinical Trial Evidence

The FOURIER (Further Cardiovascular Outcomes Research with PCSK9 Inhibition in Subjects with Elevated Risk) and ODYSSEY OUTCOMES (Evaluation of Cardiovascular Outcomes After an Acute Coronary Syndrome During Treatment With Alirocumab) trials were landmark studies that evaluated the cardiovascular benefits of PCSK9 inhibitors, a class of drugs that emerged as a novel therapeutic approach to lowering LDL cholesterol beyond what had been achievable with statins alone. Refer to Table 7.3 for a summary of both trials.

TABLE 7.3   Trials of PCSK9 inhibitors.

Study	Population	Intervention	Outcome
Evolocumab (FOURIER)	Patients with atherosclerotic cardiovascular disease and LDL cholesterol levels of 70 mg/dL (1.8 mmol/L) or higher who were receiving statin therapy.	Random assignment to receive evolocumab (either 140 mg every 2 wk or 420 mg monthly) or matching placebo as subcutaneous injections (n = 27,564).	The reduction in LDL cholesterol levels with evolocumab, as compared with placebo, was 59%, from a median baseline value of 92 mg/dL (2.4 mmol/L) to 30 mg/dL (0.78 mmol/L) ($P < 0.001$). Evolocumab treatment significantly reduced the risk of the primary end point (cardiovascular death, myocardial infarction, stroke, hospitalization for unstable angina, or coronary revascularization) [50].

TABLE 7.3 (Continued)

Study	Population	Intervention	Outcome
Alirocumab (ODYSSEY OUTCOMES)	Patients who had an acute coronary syndrome 1–12 months prior, on high-intensity or maximum tolerated dose statin therapy.	Alirocumab subcutaneously at a dose of 75 mg every 2 weeks, with dose adjustments to target specific LDL cholesterol levels.	Alirocumab group had a reduced risk of recurrent ischemic cardiovascular events compared to the placebo group. Adverse events were similar between groups, except for more local injection-site reactions in the alirocumab group [53].

7.1.4 Omega-3 Fatty Acids

7.1.4.1 Physiology

See Section 7.1.1.

7.1.4.2 Mechanism of Action

Sources of fatty acids include diet, adipose tissue, and de novo synthesis in the liver.

Omega-3 fatty acids exert their lipid-lowering effects primarily through the reduction of hepatic production of triglyceride-rich, VLDLs. Several potential cellular mechanisms contribute to this process.

1. Omega 3 fatty acids accumulate in both plasma and bile after oral administration, subsequently inhibiting triglyceride hydrolysis and absorption at the intestinal brush border. This ultimately results in a reduction in hepatic VLDL production [54].
2. Omega 3 fatty acids inhibit the production of acyl-CoA, which plays a crucial role in triglyceride synthesis. Additionally, omega-3 fatty acids enhance hepatic mitochondrial and peroxisomal beta oxidation, promoting the breakdown of fatty acids [55].

Practice Pearl(s)

The suggested prescription omega fatty acid formulations are distinct from numerous over-the-counter fish oil supplements, which typically comprise 30–50% omega-3 fatty acids and are administered at lower doses. Conversely, the commercial product Vascepa comprises over 95% icosapent ethyl [56], highlighting a key difference in composition and concentration between prescription preparations and common fish oil supplements.

The suggested dose of icosapent ethyl (vascepa) is 2 g twice daily with meals. This formulation of omega-3 fatty acids contains mainly EPA.

The suggested dose of generic omega-3 fatty acids or the commercial brand Lovaza is either 2 g twice a day or 4 g once daily with food. These formulations contain both EPA and docosahexaenoic acid DHA [57].

Clinical Trial Evidence

The REDUCE-IT (Reduction of Cardiovascular Events with Icosapent Ethyl–Intervention Trial) study is a landmark cardiovascular outcomes study that assessed the efficacy of icosapent ethyl, a highly purified eicosapentaenoic acid (EPA) derived from fish oil, in reducing major adverse cardiovascular events. Initiated against growing interest in the cardioprotective effects of omega-3 fatty acids, the trial aimed to determine whether icosapent ethyl could provide additional cardiovascular benefits beyond standard statin therapy (see Table 7.4).

(continued)

(continued)

TABLE 7.4   Cardiovascular efficacy of icosapent ethyl therapy.

Study	Population	Intervention	Outcome
REDUCE-IT	Patients with cardiovascular disease or diabetes and other risk factors, high triglyceride levels, and receiving statin therapy.	Administration of 2 g of icosapent ethyl twice daily (total daily dose, 4 g) or placebo.	Significant decrease in the risk of ischemic events, including cardiovascular death. However, higher rates of hospitalization for atrial fibrillation or flutter and a slight increase in serious bleeding events were observed compared to the placebo group [58].

7.1.5   Fibrates

7.1.5.1   Physiology

Metabolism of HDL Cholesterol

HDL cholesterol metabolism is primarily associated with reverse cholesterol transport RCT, a crucial process that removes excess cholesterol from peripheral tissues and returns it to the liver for excretion. The RCT process helps maintain cholesterol homeostasis and protect against atherosclerosis development (see Figure 7.5).

Nascent HDL formation: Apolipoprotein A-1 (ApoA-1) interacts with the ATP-binding cassette transporter A1 (ABCA1) present on the cell membranes of peripheral tissues, such as muscles and adipose tissue. This interaction facilitates the transfer of free cholesterol and phospholipids from these tissues to ApoA-1, forming nascent discoidal HDL particles. *Maturation of HDL:* The enzyme lecithin cholesterol acyltransferase (LCAT) converts free cholesterol in nascent HDL particles into cholesterol esters. This process results in the formation of mature,

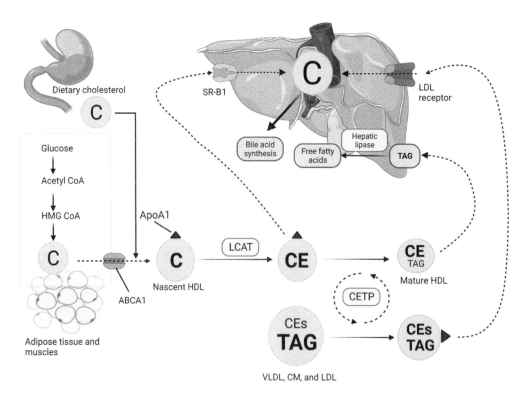

FIGURE 7.5   Schematic representation of HDL metabolism.

spherical HDL particles that contain a hydrophobic core of cholesterol esters surrounded by phospholipids and ApoA-1 [14].

Cholesterol ester exchange: Cholesterol ester transfer protein (CETP) mediates the exchange of cholesterol esters and triglycerides between HDL and other circulating lipoproteins, such as chylomicrons, very low-density lipoproteins (VLDL), and low-density lipoproteins (LDL). CETP transfers cholesterol esters from HDL to these lipoproteins and takes up triglycerides in return [59]. *Hepatic uptake and excretion:* HDL particles bind to the hepatic scavenger receptor class B type 1 (SR-B1), which facilitates the selective uptake of cholesterol esters from HDL into the liver. The liver then converts cholesterol into bile acids, which are secreted into the bile and ultimately excreted via the gastrointestinal tract. The remaining smaller HDL particles can be recycled to participate in further cholesterol uptake from peripheral tissues [60, 61].

Role of Hepatic Lipase in HDL Metabolism

Hepatic lipase (HL) plays a significant role in HDL metabolism within the liver. It is a lipolytic enzyme synthesized by hepatocytes and anchored to the liver endothelial cell surface. HL influences HDL metabolism by catalyzing the hydrolysis of lipids in lipoproteins, particularly HDL. Its primary actions on HDL metabolism include:

1. HL hydrolyzes the phospholipids and TAGs present in HDL particles. This action leads to the release of FFAs and results in the formation of smaller, denser HDL particles, which are often referred to as HDL3. This remodeling process enables the HDL particles to continue participating in RCT [62].

2. As a consequence of the HDL remodeling by HL, the apolipoprotein A-1 (ApoA-1) component of the HDL particle may dissociate. The dissociated ApoA-1 can then return to peripheral tissues to interact with the ATP-binding cassette transporter A1 (ABCA1) and initiate the formation of new nascent HDL particles.

3. HL activity may influence the clearance of HDL particles from circulation. The smaller, denser HDL particles generated after HL-mediated remodeling can be more readily cleared from the bloodstream, either through the hepatic scavenger receptor class B type 1 (SR-B1) or the LDL-R. The interaction with these receptors facilitates the delivery of cholesterol to the liver for bile acid synthesis and excretion [63].

7.1.5.2 Mechanism of Action

Fibrates are a class of lipid-lowering drugs that primarily target the ability of peroxisome proliferator-activated receptor-alpha (PPARα) to modulate lipid metabolism. They are particularly effective in reducing elevated triglyceride levels and are often prescribed for patients with hypertriglyceridemia. The mechanism of action of fibrates involves several processes that influence lipid metabolism, as detailed below [64]:

1. Fibrates act as agonists for PPARα, a nuclear hormone receptor predominantly expressed in tissues with high oxidative capacity, such as the liver, heart, and skeletal muscle. By binding to and activating PPARα, fibrates regulate the transcription of target genes involved in various aspects of lipid metabolism.

2. Fibrates upregulate the expression of genes involved in fatty acid uptake and transport and enzymes responsible for mitochondrial and peroxisomal beta oxidation [65]. This increase in fatty acid oxidation reduces the availability of fatty acids for triglyceride synthesis in the liver, ultimately leading to lower plasma triglyceride levels.

3. Fibrates also decrease the production and secretion of VLDL particles by the liver. This reduction is partly due to the enhanced fatty acid oxidation, which lowers the availability of TAGs for VLDL assembly and secretion [66].

4. They also increase the expression of LPL, an enzyme that hydrolyzes TAGs in lipoproteins, thereby promoting the clearance of circulating triglyceride-rich lipoproteins such as VLDL and chylomicrons [67].

5. Fibrates upregulate the expression of ApoA-1 and apolipoprotein A-II (ApoA-II), which are major components of HDL particles [68]. This upregulation can contribute to an increase in HDL cholesterol levels, which is generally considered cardioprotective.

7.1.6　Inclisiran

7.1.6.1　Physiology

Small interfering RNA (siRNA) technology is a novel tool for silencing (or inhibiting) specific genes in cells, providing a way to study gene function, regulate gene expression, and develop therapies for various diseases [73]. The pathophysiological basis of siRNA technology relies on the naturally occurring RNA interference (RNAi) pathway; a post-transcriptional gene silencing mechanism conserved among eukaryotes [74].

The RNAi pathway is initiated by the presence of double-stranded RNA (dsRNA) molecules in the cell. These dsRNA molecules can be exogenously introduced or generated endogenously. Dicer, an RNase III endonuclease, cleaves these long dsRNAs into short 20–30 nucleotide fragments called siRNAs [75]. Each siRNA molecule consists of the guide strand and the passenger strand.

The guide strand, also known as the antisense strand, is the key component in the RNAi pathway. The guide strand is complementary to the target mRNA sequence that needs to be silenced. After the formation of siRNA, the guide strand is incorporated into the RNA-induced silencing complex (RISC). The RISC then uses the guide strand as a template to recognize and bind to the target mRNA. Once bound, the Argonaute protein within the RISC cleaves the target mRNA, effectively silencing the gene expression [76].

The passenger strand (sense strand) complements the guide strand. After the formation of siRNA, the passenger strand is typically degraded or ejected from the RISC complex [77]. The role of PCSK9 in LDL cholesterol metabolism was discussed in Section 7.1.3.

7.1.6.2　Mechanism of Action

siRNA inhibitors of PCSK9 synthesis, such as inclisiran, are a novel class of lipid-lowering agents that utilize RNA interference (RNAi) technology to target and degrade PCSK9 mRNA [78, 79]. This mechanism of action results in reduced PCSK9 protein synthesis, ultimately leading to lower LDL cholesterol (LDL-C) levels [79] (Figure 7.6).

The mechanism of action of siRNA inhibitors of PCSK9 synthesis involves the following steps:

1. The siRNA molecule, which is complementary to a specific region of the PCSK9 mRNA, is introduced into the target cells, typically hepatocytes.

2. Once inside the cell, the siRNA associates with a group of proteins to form the RISC.

3. The RISC complex, guided by the siRNA, binds to the complementary PCSK9 mRNA. This binding leads to the cleavage and degradation of the target mRNA.

4. As a result of mRNA degradation, the translation of PCSK9 protein is inhibited, leading to reduced PCSK9 synthesis.

5. With lower levels of PCSK9, there is less degradation of LDL-R on hepatocyte surfaces. This results in increased LDL-R expression and activity, allowing for enhanced clearance of circulating LDL-C [80].

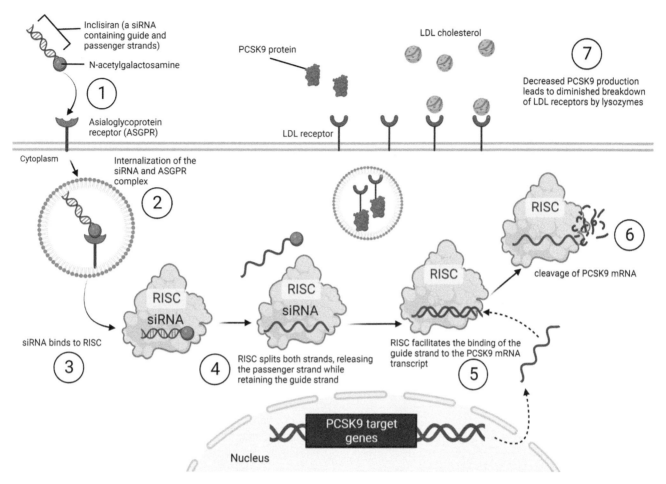

FIGURE 7.6   Mechanism of action of inclisiran.

Practice Pearl(s)

SC inclisiran 284 mg initially, followed by a repeat injection at 3 months and then every 6 months.

Clinical Trial Evidence

The study, comprising two trials (ORION-10 and ORION-11), assessed the effectiveness of inclisiran, an inhibitor of hepatic synthesis of proprotein convertase subtilisin–kexin type 9, in reducing low-density lipoprotein (LDL) cholesterol levels. Participants were patients with atherosclerotic cardiovascular disease or an equivalent risk who had high LDL cholesterol levels despite receiving the maximum tolerated dose of statin therapy.

In both trials, patients were given inclisiran or a placebo via subcutaneous injection initially, on day 90, and every 6 months thereafter for a period of 540 days. The key outcomes measured were the change in LDL cholesterol level from baseline to day 510 and the time-adjusted change in LDL cholesterol level from baseline after day 90 up to day 540.

Results showed that inclisiran led to significant reductions in LDL cholesterol levels by approximately 50% in both ORION-10 and ORION-11 trials. The adverse events were generally similar for both inclisiran and placebo groups, although there were more injection-site adverse reactions reported with inclisiran. These reactions were generally mild, and none were severe or persistent. Thus, the study concluded that inclisiran, administered every 6 months, effectively reduced LDL cholesterol levels by around 50%, despite a higher occurrence of injection-site adverse events compared to placebo [81].

7.1.7   Niacin

7.1.7.1   Physiology

See Section 7.1.5.

7.1.7.2   Mechanism of Action

Niacin, also known as nicotinic acid or vitamin B3, is a water-soluble vitamin that is used for the treatment of lipid disorders due to its ability to favorably modify the lipid profile.

Firstly, niacin inhibits hormone-sensitive lipase in adipose tissue, resulting in decreased lipolysis, hence decreasing the substrate availability of hepatic triglyceride for VLDL synthesis.

As a consequence of reduced VLDL availability, even less LDL cholesterol is packaged and released by the liver.

Furthermore, niacin promotes the synthesis of apolipoprotein A-I (apoA-I), a key component of HDL cholesterol [82]. These actions collectively lead to an increase in plasma HDL cholesterol levels (also see Section 7.1.5).

Also, niacin has been shown to lower lipoprotein A levels, a highly atherogenic lipoprotein, by mechanisms that are not yet fully understood [83].

Practice Pearl(s)

The recommended initial dose is 250 mg once daily (with food), which can be increased to a maximum of 1.5–2 g daily in 2–3 divided doses.

Niacin is associated with an increased risk of flushing. To mitigate this, high-dose aspirin may be taken prophylactically within 30 minutes of niacin administration.

Clinical Trial Evidence

The AIM-HIGH (Atherothrombosis Intervention in Metabolic Syndrome with Low HDL/High Triglycerides: Impact on Global Health Outcomes) trial evaluated the cardiovascular benefits of adding niacin to statin therapy in patients with established vascular disease. While statins effectively lower LDL cholesterol, the trial focused on patients with residual risk manifested by low HDL cholesterol levels and elevated triglycerides, a lipid profile niacin might optimally address.

Building on the backdrop of the AIM-HIGH trial, HPS2-THRIVE (Heart Protection Study 2–Treatment of HDL to Reduce the Incidence of Vascular Events) further investigated niacin's role in cardiovascular

protection but in a much larger and diverse cohort. The study combined niacin with laropiprant, a drug meant to reduce the facial flushing commonly associated with niacin, aiming to improve patient adherence.

Together, the results from AIM-HIGH and HPS2-THRIVE dampened enthusiasm for using niacin as adjunctive therapy for cardiovascular prevention in the era of effective statin therapy. These trials emphasized the importance of rigorous, large-scale randomized trials to validate the cardiovascular benefits of lipid-modifying therapies, even for those with a long history of use, like niacin. See Table 7.5 for a summary of the results of the AIM-HIGH and HPS2-THRIVE trials.

TABLE 7.5   Trials assessing the efficacy of niacin.

Study	Population	Intervention	Outcome
AIM-HIGH	Patients with established cardiovascular disease and LDL cholesterol levels of less than 70 mg/dL.	Patients were randomly assigned to receive either extended-release niacin (1500–2000 mg/day) or a placebo. All patients also received simvastatin (40–80 mg/day) plus ezetimibe (10 mg/day) if needed.	Despite significant improvements in HDL cholesterol and triglyceride levels with niacin addition, there was no incremental clinical benefit observed during a 36-month follow-up period. Primary endpoint events occurred in 16.4% of patients in the niacin group and 16.2% in the placebo group [84].

TABLE 7.5   (Continued)

Study	Population	Intervention	Outcome
HPS2-THRIVE [85]	Adults with vascular disease.	Participants were randomly assigned to receive 2 g of extended-release niacin and 40 mg of laropiprant or a matching placebo daily(n = 25,673).	Despite a decrease in LDL cholesterol and an increase in HDL cholesterol with the addition of niacin-laropiprant, there was no significant reduction in major vascular events [85].

 Concepts to Ponder

Summary of the effects of lipid-lowering therapies on lipid levels

Lipid-lowering therapies primarily aim to decrease the risk of atherosclerotic cardiovascular disease (ASCVD). Different classes of these agents target various aspects of the lipid profile, and thus, their effects on lipids can be diverse (see Table 7.6).

What is advanced lipid testing?

Advanced lipid testing represents a more comprehensive evaluation of blood lipids beyond the conventional lipid profile test. The standard lipid profile typically measures total cholesterol, low-density lipoprotein (LDL) cholesterol, high-density lipoprotein (HDL) cholesterol, and triglycerides. Advanced lipid testing is an invaluable screening test [86].

TABLE 7.6   The effects of various lipid-lowering therapies on lipid levels.

Lipid therapy	LDL	HDL	TAGS
Ezetimibe	↓↓	↑	↓
Fibrate	↓↓	↑↑	↓↓↓
Statins	↓↓↓	↑	↓↓
Omega 3FA	Variable effects	↑	↓↓
PCSK9i	↓↓↓	↑	↓↓
Niacin	↓	↑↑	↓↓
Bile acid sequestrants	↓↓	→↑	→↑

- To assess the residual risk for cardiovascular disease in patients already on lipid-lowering therapy [87].
- Patients with borderline risk for Atherosclerotic Cardiovascular Disease (ASCVD) based on traditional risk calculators [88].
- A strong family history of ASCVD [86].

Examples of advanced lipid tests

- Lipoprotein a
- LDL particle size (small dense LDL is artherogenic)
- Apolipoprotein B

7.2   OBESITY

7.2.1   Phentermine-Topiramate

7.2.1.1   Physiology

The anorexigenic (satiety-promoting) and orexigenic (hunger-stimulating) pathways consist of an intricate network of hormones, neurotransmitters, and neural circuits, all intricately interwoven to maintain our body's energy balance [89].

The anorexigenic pathway is a complex signaling system that regulates food intake and energy balance. It involves communication between peripheral tissues, such as adipose tissue, and central nervous system (CNS)structures, including the hypothalamus and higher cortical centers [90, 91]. The role of other mediators of the anorexigenic pathway is shown in Figure 7.7.

Adipose tissue produces and releases the hormone leptin in proportion to the amount of stored fat [92]. As fat stores increase, leptin levels rise, signaling the

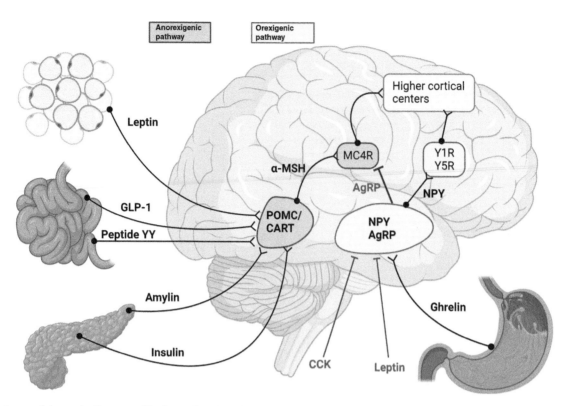

FIGURE 7.7   Schematic diagram of both orexigenic and anorexigenic pathways. There are connections between peripheral organs and relay centers in the hypothalamus en route to higher cortical centers.

body to decrease food intake and increase energy expenditure [91].

Leptin circulates in the bloodstream, crosses the blood–brain barrier via specific transporters, and finally reaches the arcuate nucleus of the hypothalamus in order to exert its anorexigenic pathway [93].

The arcuate nucleus contains two distinct populations of neurons: one that produces neuropeptide Y (NPY) and agouti-related peptide (AgRP) and another that produces pro-opiomelanocortin (POMC) and cocaine- and amphetamine-regulated transcript (CART) [94]. Leptin binds to its receptors on these neurons, inhibiting NPY/AgRP neurons and stimulating POMC/CART neurons [95].

NPY is an orexigenic peptide, while AgRP acts as an antagonist of the melanocortin receptors [96]. Leptin suppresses the orexigenic effects of NPY while promoting the anorexigenic pathway via POMC/CART activation, decreasing food intake and promoting weight loss [97].

POMC is processed into alpha-melanocyte-stimulating hormone (α-MSH), which binds to melanocortin receptors and exerts anorexigenic effects [98]. CART also has anorexigenic

properties [99]. Activation of POMC/CART neurons by leptin contributes to reduced food intake and increased energy expenditure [100].

Signals from the arcuate nucleus are transmitted to higher cortical centers involved in the regulation of appetite, satiety, and energy balance [101]. These centers integrate information from various sources, including hormonal and neural signals, to modulate feeding behavior [102].

7.2.1.2   Mechanism of Action

Phentermine is a sympathomimetic amine that acts as an appetite suppressant and is used for the short-term management of obesity in conjunction with a reduced-calorie diet and exercise. The precise mechanism of action of phentermine is not entirely understood, but it is believed to exert its effects primarily through the CNS by stimulating the release of certain neurotransmitters.

Phentermine stimulates the release of catecholamines, primarily norepinephrine (NE), and to a lesser extent, dopamine (DA) and serotonin (5-HT), in the hypothalamus and other regions of the brain.

The increased levels of NE, DA, and 5-HT in the hypothalamus, specifically in the arcuate nucleus, lead to the activation of neurons that express POMC and CART. Activation of POMC/CART neurons promotes the release of α-MSH, which in turn binds to melanocortin receptors (MC4R) in the brain. This ultimately suppresses appetite and reduces food intake [103].

Practice Pearl(s)

The starting dosage for phentermine-topiramate consists of 3.75/23 mg administered for a 14-day period, followed by a dose of 7.5/46 mg. If a 3% reduction in baseline body weight is not observed after 12 weeks, the dosage can be escalated to 11.25/69 mg for an additional 14 days and subsequently increased to 15/92 mg daily [104].

Clinical Trial Evidence

Among the numerous clinical trials undertaken to assess potential weight loss therapies, two noteworthy studies are the CONQUER and EQUIP trials.

The Comprehensive Assessment of Long-term Effects of Reducing Intake of Energy (CONQUER) trial aimed to evaluate the efficacy and safety of phentermine–topiramate extended-release combination as a weight-loss therapy. Efficacy and safety of Qsymia (phentermine and topiramate extended-release) Indicated for Weight Loss in Patients with Obesity and Patients who are Overweight with at least one Weight-related Comorbidity: a Randomized, Placebo-controlled, Phase 3 Study (EQUIP) was another pivotal trial. This study primarily evaluated a higher dosage of phentermine–topiramate extended-release for weight loss in obese participants without diabetes. The EQUIP trial reinforced the findings of the CONQUER trial, presenting substantial weight reduction in participants treated with the drug combination relative to the placebo group. Refer to Table 7.7 for a summary of the results of the CONQUER and EQUIP trials.

TABLE 7.7 Trials evaluating the efficacy of phentermine and topiramate in obesity.

Study	Population	Intervention	Outcome
CONQUER	Overweight or obese adults (aged 18–70 years), with a body-mass index of 27–45 kg/m(2) and two or more comorbidities (hypertension, dyslipidemia, diabetes or prediabetes, or abdominal obesity).	Random assignment to one of the following groups: Placebo, once-daily Phentermine 7.5 mg plus Topiramate 46.0 mg, once-daily Phentermine 15.0 mg plus Topiramate 92.0 mg (n = 2487).	Patients on Phentermine 7.5 mg plus Topiramate 46.0 mg and Phentermine 15.0 mg plus Topiramate 92.0 mg showed significant weight reduction compared to placebo. [105].
EQUIP	Men and women with class II and III obesity (BMI ≥ 35 kg/m(2)).	Random assignment to one of the following groups: Placebo, Phentermine/Topiramate 3.75/23 mg, or Phentermine/Topiramate 15/92 mg, added to a reduced-energy diet.	Patients on Phentermine/Topiramate 3.75/23 mg and Phentermine/Topiramate 15/92 mg showed significant weight reduction compared to placebo [106].

7.2.2 Liraglutide

7.2.2.1 Physiology

The Brain–Gut Axis

The brain–gut axis is a complex bidirectional communication system that connects the CNS with peripheral signals, mainly from the gastrointestinal (GI) tract. This intricate system regulates appetite, energy balance, and metabolism. Gut hormones and peptides, including glucagon-like peptide-1 (GLP-1), cholecystokinin (CCK), polypeptide Y, and ghrelin, play various roles in the brain–gut axis.

CCK is secreted by I-cells in the small intestine in response to the presence of nutrients in the proximal small intestine [107]. It acts locally to stimulate gallbladder contraction and pancreatic enzyme secretion while also acting centrally to promote satiety and reduce food intake [108]. CCK promotes satiety by inhibiting NPY/AgRP neurons in the arcuate nucleus (orexigenic pathway) [109].

NPY is a potent orexigenic peptide produced by the small intestine and acts primarily in the arcuate nucleus of the hypothalamus. It stimulates food intake and is involved in the regulation of energy balance [110].

Ghrelin (the "hunger hormone") is a potent peripheral orexigenic peptide. It is secreted by the gastric fundus about 1–2 hours before meal ingestion. It stimulates appetite and food intake by acting on NPY/AgRP neurons in the arcuate nucleus of the hypothalamus (orexigenic pathway) [111]. See Figure 7.7.

GLP-1 is an incretin hormone released by the L-cells in the intestine in response to nutrient ingestion (see Chapter 4). It slows gastric emptying, stimulates insulin secretion, and inhibits glucagon secretion. Even more importantly, GLP-1 acts as an anorexigenic factor, decreasing food intake and promoting satiety [112]. It exerts these effects through the stimulation of POMC and CART neurons in the arcuate nucleus [113].

7.2.2.2　Mechanism of Action

GLP-1 agonists stimulate the anorexigenic pathway by binding to GLP-1 receptors (GLP-1R) present on POMC/CART neurons in the arcuate nucleus of the hypothalamus. Upon activation by GLP-1, POMC/CART neurons stimulate the synthesis and release of α-MSH. Next, α-MSH binds to melanocortin-4 receptors (MC4R) found on second-order neurons in the hypothalamus, which relays signals to higher cortical centers that ultimately lead to early satiety [114,115].

Pathophysiology Pearl

Tirzepatide is a novel dual glucose-dependent insulinotropic polypeptide (GIP) and glucagon-like peptide-1 (GLP-1) receptor agonist, which has shown promise in treating obesity. Tirzepatide's site of action in the arcuate nucleus involves binding to GLP-1 receptors on POMC/CART neurons (anorexigenic pathway) [116].

Practice Pearl(s)

For weight loss, liraglutide (Saxenda®) should be started at a dose of 0.6 mg subcutaneously once daily for one week. After the initial week, the dose should be increased by 0.6 mg increments each week until the maintenance dose of 3.0 mg once daily is reached. The dose should not exceed 3.0 mg daily, and liraglutide can be administered at any time of day, with or without meals [117].

For patients on semaglutide (Wegovy™), the initial dose should be 0.25 mg subcutaneously once weekly for four weeks. Following this period, the dose should be increased to 0.5 mg once weekly for the next four weeks. If further dose escalation is needed, the dose can be increased to 1.0 mg once weekly for 4 weeks. The dose can be increased to 2.0 mg for a further month and then a maximum of 2.4 mg weekly [118].

Clinical Trial Evidence

The growing prevalence of obesity has intensified the search for effective therapeutic agents. Among the promising candidates are the glucagon-like peptide-1 (GLP-1) agonists, traditionally used in diabetes management but now recognized for their potential in weight loss. The Satiety and Clinical Adiposity–Liraglutide Evidence (SCALE) trial investigated the efficacy of liraglutide, a GLP-1 receptor agonist, in weight management. The study showed that liraglutide, when used at higher doses than typically prescribed for diabetes, led to significant weight loss compared to placebo, alongside improvements in several health parameters.

The Semaglutide Treatment Effect in People with Obesity (STEP 1) trial assessed the weight loss potential of semaglutide, another GLP-1 receptor agonist. Participants receiving semaglutide experienced a substantial reduction in body weight relative to those on placebo, underscoring the potential of this agent as a powerful tool in obesity management (see Table 7.8).

TABLE 7.8   Trials evaluating the efficacy of GLP-1 agonists in obesity.

Study	Population	Intervention	Outcome
SCALE	Patients without type 2 diabetes, with a BMI of at least 30 or a BMI of at least 27 if they had treated or untreated dyslipidemia or hypertension.	Study participants were randomly assigned in a 2:1 ratio to receive once-daily subcutaneous injections of liraglutide at a dose of 3.0 mg or placebo; all participants also received lifestyle modification counseling ($n = 3731$).	The liraglutide group lost a mean of 8.4 ± 7.3 kg of body weight, while the placebo group lost a mean of 2.8 ± 6.5 kg (difference of -5.6 kg; 95% confidence interval, -6.0–-5.1; $P < 0.001$) [119].
STEP 1	Adults with a BMI of 30 or greater (≥ 27 in persons with ≥ 1 weight-related coexisting condition), who did not have diabetes.	Participants were randomly assigned in a 2:1 ratio to receive once-weekly subcutaneous injections of semaglutide at a dose of 2.4 mg or placebo ($n = 1961$).	The mean change in body weight from baseline to week 68 was -14.9% in the semaglutide group and -2.4% with placebo, treatment difference of -12.4% (95% confidence interval, -13.4–-11.5; $P < 0.001$) [118].

7.2.3   Bupropion–Naltrexone

7.2.3.1   Physiology

Also, see Section 7.2.1.

7.2.3.2   Mechanism of Action

The combination of sustained-release (SR) bupropion and naltrexone has been shown to be effective in the treatment of obesity through their synergistic effects on appetite regulation and energy expenditure.

Bupropion, an atypical antidepressant, and a DA/NE reuptake inhibitor, is believed to promote weight loss through its stimulatory effect on POMC neurons in the arcuate nucleus of the hypothalamus. Activation of POMC neurons leads to the release of α-MSH, which binds to MC4R in downstream brain regions. This binding results in a decrease in food intake and an increase in energy expenditure [120].

Naltrexone, an opioid receptor antagonist, primarily blocks the mu-opioid receptor. Its role in weight loss is thought to be related to its ability to counteract the inhibitory effect of beta-endorphins on POMC neurons. Under normal circumstances, beta-endorphins, which are opioid peptides, suppress POMC neuronal activity. By antagonizing the mu-opioid receptor, naltrexone prevents beta-endorphins from inhibiting POMC neurons, thus promoting the release of α-MSH and enhancing the anorexigenic pathway (see Figure 7.7) [121].

Practice Pearl(s)

Initially, administer a single tablet containing a combination of 8 mg naltrexone and 90 mg bupropion once daily in the morning for a duration of 1 week. Subsequently, based on patient tolerability, escalate the dosage in weekly intervals as follows: during the second week, administer one tablet twice daily; during the third week, administer two tablets in the morning and one tablet in the evening; and thereafter, administer two tablets twice daily. The maximum recommended dosage is four tablets per day, equivalent to 32 mg naltrexone and 360 mg bupropion [122].

Clinical Trial Evidence

The Contrave Obesity Research (COR-1) trial was designed to evaluate the safety and efficacy of Contrave (Naltrexone/Bupropion) in overweight and obese participants. This pivotal trial demonstrated that individuals treated with Contrave experienced significantly greater weight loss compared to those

(continued)

(continued)

on placebo. Additionally, several health-related quality-of-life measures were improved in the Contrave group. The results from the COR-1 trial played a foundational role in substantiating the benefits of Contrave as a novel approach to obesity management (see Table 7.9).

TABLE 7.9 Clinical trial evaluating the efficacy of naltrexone and bupropion in obesity.

Study	Population	Intervention	Outcome
Contrave obesity research (COR)-1	Men and women aged 18–65 y with a BMI of 30–45 kg/m² and uncomplicated obesity or BMI 27–45 kg/m² with dyslipidemia or hypertension.	Participants were randomly assigned in a 1 : 1 : 1 ratio to receive: 1) NB32: naltrexone 32 mg/day + bupropion 360 mg/day, 2) NB16: naltrexone 16 mg/day + bupropion 360 mg/day, or 3) matching placebo.	The proportion of participants achieving a decrease in body weight of 5% or more: 16% (placebo), 48% (NB32; $p < 0.0001$ vs. placebo), and 39% (NB16; $p < 0.0001$ vs. placebo) [123].

7.2.4 Intestinal Lipase Inhibitor

7.2.4.1 Physiology

The role of pancreatic lipases in the hydrolysis of dietary triglycerides in the intestine was reviewed in Section 7.1.1.

7.2.4.2 Mechanism of Action

Orlistat is a gastrointestinal (GI) lipase inhibitor that is used to treat obesity. Its mechanism of action involves the reversible inhibition of pancreatic lipases, which are essential enzymes responsible for the hydrolysis of dietary triglycerides into absorbable FFAs and monoglycerides. By inhibiting these lipases, orlistat prevents the breakdown and subsequent absorption of dietary fat in the GI tract. Consequently, a portion of the consumed fat is excreted in the feces, reducing overall caloric intake and promoting weight loss. It is important to note that orlistat does not act centrally; its effects are confined to the GI tract.

> **Practice Pearl(s)**
>
> The recommended dose of orlistat is 120 mg three times a day with fat-based meals.

Clinical Trial Evidence

The Xenical in the Prevention of Diabetes in Obese Subjects (XENDOS) trial was a landmark study that evaluated the long-term efficacy of orlistat in weight management and its potential role in diabetes prevention. Spanning over four years, this trial included obese subjects. It assessed weight loss outcomes and the incidence of type 2 diabetes in participants treated with orlistat versus those on placebo. The results indicated that orlistat users experienced sustained weight loss over the trial period and had a reduced risk of developing type 2 diabetes compared to the placebo group (see Table 7.10).

The XENDOS trial provided valuable insights into the dual benefits of orlistat: as a weight management tool and as a preventive measure against type 2 diabetes in obese individuals.

TABLE 7.10 Clinical trial evaluating the efficacy of orlistat in obesity.

Study	Population	Intervention	Outcome
XENDOS	Patients with a BMI >/=30 kg/m², having either normal (79%) or impaired glucose tolerance (IGT) (21%).	Participants were randomized to receive lifestyle changes plus either orlistat 120 mg or placebo, three times daily, in a 4-y, double-blind, prospective study.	Mean weight loss was significantly greater with orlistat (5.8 vs. 3.0 kg with placebo; $P < 0.001$) [124].

7.2.5   Bariatric Surgery

7.2.5.1   Physiology

Hormonal regulation of appetite has been reviewed in previous sections of this chapter.

7.2.5.2   Mechanism of Action

Metabolic surgery, also known as bariatric surgery, is a surgical intervention aimed at promoting weight loss and improving obesity-related comorbidities. The mechanisms of action of metabolic surgery are complex and multifactorial. Some of the key mechanisms include:

1. Bariatric surgeries, such as gastric banding and sleeve gastrectomy, physically limit the stomach's capacity, reducing food intake and promoting satiety [125, 126].
2. Procedures like Roux-en-Y gastric bypass (RYGB) lead to reduced absorption of nutrients by bypassing a portion of the small intestine [126].
3. Metabolic surgery alters the gut hormone profile, including increased GLP-1 and reduced ghrelin levels, resulting in appetite suppression and enhanced insulin sensitivity [127].
4. Metabolic surgeries can induce changes in the gut microbiota composition, leading to enhanced energy expenditure, altered short-chain fatty acid production, and improved glucose metabolism [128].

Practice Pearl(s)

Refer to Figure 7.8 for a summary of various forms of bariatric surgery.

Laparoscopic Roux-en-Y Gastric Bypass (LRYGB)

Laparoscopic Roux-en-Y gastric bypass (LRYGB) is a widely performed bariatric surgery that promotes significant weight loss and improves obesity-related comorbidities. This procedure combines both restrictive and malabsorptive mechanisms to achieve its metabolic effects.

In LRYGB, the surgeon creates a small gastric pouch (roughly 30 ml in volume) by dividing the stomach. This restrictive step limits the amount of food that can be consumed at a time, promoting early satiety. Next, the small intestine is divided approximately 30–50 cm distal to the ligament of Treitz. The distal part of the divided small intestine (the Roux limb) is then connected to the newly formed gastric pouch, effectively bypassing a significant portion of the stomach and the proximal small intestine (duodenum and part of the jejunum). This malabsorptive step reduces the absorption of nutrients, particularly fats and fat-soluble vitamins.

The remaining proximal part of the divided small intestine, known as the biliopancreatic limb, is connected to the Roux limb 75–150 cm distal to the gastrojejunostomy, forming the Y-shaped configuration. This connection, called the jejunojejunostomy, allows digestive enzymes and bile to mix with the food, enabling digestion and absorption in the distal small intestine [129].

Sleeve Gastrectomy

Sleeve gastrectomy, or laparoscopic sleeve gastrectomy (LSG), is a widely adopted bariatric surgical intervention that promotes substantial weight loss by primarily employing restrictive mechanisms. The procedure entails the resection of approximately 75–80% of the stomach, resulting in a tubular gastric remnant, often likened to a "sleeve" or "banana" shape, with a markedly reduced volume capacity for food.

The residual tubular portion of the stomach is secured with surgical staples and sealed, culminating in the formation of the gastric sleeve. This newly fashioned, smaller stomach significantly curtails food intake by facilitating early satiety, thus restricting caloric consumption and promoting weight loss.

A notable advantage of LSG over other bariatric procedures, such as Roux-en-Y gastric bypass, is the absence of intestinal rerouting or a malabsorptive component. As a result, LSG is associated with a lower risk of nutritional deficiencies [130].

Laparoscopic Adjustable Gastric Banding (LAGB)

Laparoscopic adjustable gastric banding (LAGB) is a minimally invasive bariatric surgery intended to induce weight loss primarily through restrictive

(continued)

(continued)

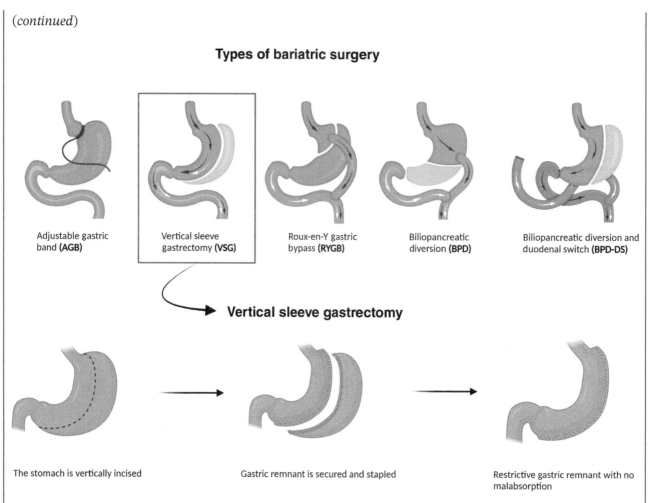

FIGURE 7.8   Types of bariatric surgery.

mechanisms. This procedure involves the placement of an adjustable, inflatable silicone band around the upper portion of the stomach, creating a small gastric pouch and a narrow outlet leading to the rest of the stomach. The restricted stomach capacity facilitates early satiety, limiting caloric intake and promoting weight loss.

The adjustability of the gastric band is a key feature, as it enables the band's diameter to be modified based on the patient's weight loss progress and tolerability. By injecting or removing saline through the access port, the band's constriction can be controlled, thereby regulating the size of the stomach pouch and the rate at which food passes through the outlet.

LAGB has the advantage of being a reversible procedure with a relatively low risk of complications and nutritional deficiencies compared to other bariatric surgeries. However, it often results in slower and less substantial weight loss than more invasive procedures, such as Roux-en-Y gastric bypass or sleeve gastrectomy [131].

Biliopancreatic Diversion with Duodenal Switch (BPD-DS)

Biliopancreatic diversion with duodenal switch (BPD-DS) is a complex bariatric surgery combining restrictive and malabsorptive mechanisms to achieve significant weight loss. This procedure is typically reserved for patients with severe obesity or those without adequate weight loss with other bariatric surgeries. BPD-DS consists of two main components: a vertical sleeve gastrectomy (VSG) and an intestinal bypass.

In the first step, a vertical sleeve gastrectomy is performed, which involves the removal of a large portion of the stomach, leaving a tubular gastric pouch.

The second step involves the creation of the intestinal bypass. The duodenum is divided just past the pylorus, and the distal portion of the small intestine (the ileum) is connected to the duodenal stump. This rerouting of the intestinal tract creates the "duodenal switch." The remaining portion of the small intestine, carrying bile and pancreatic enzymes, is then connected to the ileum approximately 100 cm proximal to the ileocecal valve. This configuration results in a short "common channel" where digestion and absorption occur, thereby limiting the absorption of nutrients and calories, leading to the malabsorptive component of the surgery [132].

Clinical Trial Evidence

The Surgical Therapy And Medications Potentially Eradicate Diabetes Efficiently (STAMPEDE) trial was a seminal study that compared the efficacy of intensive medical therapy alone with that of medical therapy combined with Roux-en-Y gastric bypass (RYGB) or sleeve gastrectomy in patients with uncontrolled type 2 diabetes. The results showed that patients undergoing RYGB and medical therapy experienced superior glycemic control and needed fewer medications than those receiving medical therapy alone (see Table 7.11).

TABLE 7.11   Clinical trial evaluating the efficacy of metabolic surgery in obesity.

Study	Population	Intervention	Outcome
STAMPEDE	Obese patients with uncontrolled type 2 diabetes.	1. Intensive medical therapy alone. 2. Medical therapy plus Roux-en-Y gastric bypass. 3. Medical therapy plus sleeve gastrectomy.	Weight loss was greater in the gastric-bypass group (−29.4 ± 9.0 kg) and sleeve-gastrectomy group (−25.1 ± 8.5 kg) than in the medical-therapy group (−5.4 ± 8.0 kg). The use of drugs to lower glucose, lipid, and blood-pressure levels decreased significantly after both surgical procedures but increased in patients receiving medical therapy only [133].

 Concepts to Ponder

How do corticosteroids promote weight gain?

As you may recall, alpha MSH is the ligand for the hypothalamic MC4 receptor (MC4R) in the anorexigenic pathway. Pro-opiomelanocortin in the hypothalamus is converted to ACTH, beta-lipoprotein, and gamma melanocyte-stimulating hormone (γMSH) [134]. Next, γMSH is processed into alpha MSH (αMSH) and corticotropin-like intermediate peptide (CLIP). Cortisol exerts negative feedback control POMC processing at the level of the hypothalamus under physiological conditions. For patients on exogenous glucocorticoid therapy, there is profound suppression of POMC synthesis and hence, αMSH production [135]. This reduces signaling of the anorexigenic pathway in favor of the orexigenic pathway (neuropeptide Y/agouti-related peptide). Review both the anorexigenic and orexigenic pathways. See Figure 7.7.

Why do patients with Addison's disease have significant anorexia?

Hypocortisolemia in Addison's disease lifts the normal negative feedback inhibition of POMC by cortisol. Significant overproduction of POMC, ACTH, and αMSH promotes the anorexigenic pathway, resulting in poor oral intake [136] (see Figure 7.9).

(continued)

(continued)

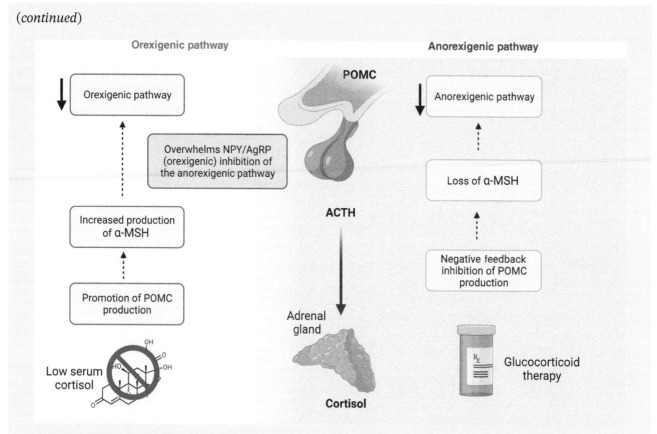

FIGURE 7.9   Comparison of the effects of exogenous steroids and Addison's disease on the anorexigenic and orexigenic pathways, respectively.

7.3   LIPODYSTROPHY SYNDROMES

7.3.1   Insulin Sensitizers

7.3.1.1   Physiology

Location and Types of Adipose Tissues

Adipose tissue is a specialized connective tissue that primarily functions in energy storage, insulation, metabolism, immune response, and hormone secretion [137]. There are two main types of adipose tissue, *white adipose tissue (WAT)* and *brown adipose tissue (BAT)* [138].

WAT is the most abundant type of adipose tissue and is primarily involved in energy storage and the secretion of adipokines and cytokines that regulate metabolism, inflammation, and insulin sensitivity [139].

WAT can be further subdivided into two subtypes based on its anatomical location and function:

a. *Subcutaneous adipose tissue (SAT):* SAT is located beneath the skin and accounts for approximately 80% of human body fat [140].

It is mainly found in the buttocks, thighs, and abdomen and plays a role in insulation and energy storage [141].

b. *Visceral adipose tissue (VAT):* VAT is found within the abdominal cavity, surrounding internal organs such as the liver, intestines, and pancreas [142]. It accounts for approximately 20% of total body fat. It is associated with a higher risk of metabolic disorders, as it secretes pro-inflammatory adipokines and releases FFAs into the portal circulation, which can contribute to insulin resistance and dyslipidemia [143].

BAT promotes thermogenesis [144] through a process mediated by uncoupling protein 1 (UCP1), uniquely expressed in brown adipocytes [145]. BAT is predominantly found in infants and decreases in abundance with age, but it can still be found in adults in small amounts [146]. In adults, BAT is primarily located in the cervical, supraclavicular, and paravertebral regions and around the heart, kidneys, and major blood vessels [147]. See Figure 7.10.

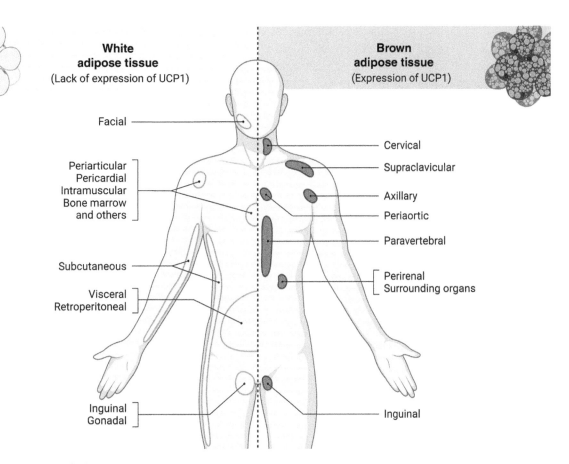

FIGURE 7.10   Location of adipose tissue.

Adipocyte Physiology

Adipocytes are specialized cells primarily responsible for storing energy as TAGs and releasing fatty acids during periods of increased energy demand [148]. Besides their energy storage function, adipocytes serve as endocrine cells, secreting numerous hormones and cytokines that modulate systemic metabolism, inflammation, and insulin sensitivity [149].

Adiponectin possesses anti-inflammatory, anti-atherogenic, and insulin-sensitizing properties. Secreted primarily by adipocytes, adiponectin enhances insulin sensitivity by promoting glucose uptake in skeletal muscle and suppressing hepatic gluconeogenesis [150]. Also, the levels of adiponectin have an inverse relationship with the degree of adiposity, highlighting its protective role against insulin resistance and type 2 diabetes development [150].

Furthermore, adiponectin exerts a host of anti-inflammatory effects, the most essential being its ability to inhibit the production of pro-inflammatory cytokines such as TNF-alpha and interleukin-6 (IL-6) [150].

As a pro-inflammatory cytokine, TNF-alpha is secreted by various cell types, including adipocytes [151]. It has been implicated in the pathogenesis of insulin resistance and the chronic low-grade inflammatory state characteristic of obesity. TNF-alpha contributes to insulin resistance by impairing insulin signaling pathways and promoting the production of other inflammatory mediators [151]. Moreover, it enhances lipolysis and free fatty acid release, further exacerbating insulin resistance [151].

Resistin is another adipokine central to the pathogenesis of insulin resistance. While predominantly secreted by adipocytes in rodents, human resistin production mainly occurs in macrophages present in adipose tissue [152]. Resistin has been shown to impair insulin signaling and glucose uptake in skeletal muscle, contributing to insulin resistance. Furthermore, resistin promotes the production of pro-inflammatory cytokines such as TNF-alpha and IL-6, further exacerbating inflammation and insulin resistance [152].

Peroxisome proliferator-activated receptor gamma is a nuclear transcription factor that plays a crucial role in adipogenesis, lipid metabolism, and insulin sensitivity [153]. PPAR-gamma activation in adipocytes promotes lipid storage and insulin sensitivity by regulating the expression of genes involved in lipid and glucose metabolism, respectively [6].

7.3.1.2 Mechanism of Action

Insulin sensitizers, such as thiazolidinediones (TZDs) and metformin, have been used as treatment options for lipodystrophy syndromes due to their ability to improve insulin sensitivity and ameliorate metabolic complications associated with these disorders [154].

TZDs, such as pioglitazone, are peroxisome proliferator-activated receptor-gamma (PPAR-gamma) agonists. TZDs activate PPAR-gamma in adipose tissue and other insulin-responsive tissues in lipodystrophy syndromes, promoting adipocyte differentiation and enhancing insulin-stimulated glucose uptake [155]. This results in improved insulin sensitivity. Additionally, TZDs may exert anti-inflammatory effects, which can contribute to improved insulin action in lipodystrophy syndromes [156].

Practice Pearl(s)

See Section 4.1.6 for the mechanism of action of pioglitazone in insulin resistance.

Clinical Trial Evidence

There is limited randomized clinical trial data on using insulin sensitizers in lipodystrophy syndromes. They have been shown in case reports to improve some metabolic parameters such as hyperglycemia and hypertriglyceridemia [157–159].

 Pathophysiology Pearl

Compare the various types of adipose tissue distribution in lipodystrophy syndromes

The distribution of adipose tissue atrophy is variable in patients with lipodystrophy syndromes and is largely dependent on the underlying cause [160, 161] (see Table 7.12).

TABLE 7.12 Distribution of fat loss in lipodystrophy syndromes.

Type of lipodystrophy	Distribution of adipose atrophy
Familial partial lipodystrophy (Dunnigan variety)	Loss of subcutaneous tissue fat in the extremities and trunk. Increased fat deposition in the supraclavicular region [162].
Acquired generalized lipodystrophy	A generalized progressive loss of subcutaneous tissue fat [116].
Acquired partial lipodystrophy (APL, Barraquer–Simons syndrome)	Selective loss of subcutaneous tissue fat involving the trunk, upper limbs, and head [117, 118].
Localized lipodystrophy	Medication-induced loss of subcutaneous tissue. It tends to involve sites of injection, e.g. insulin-mediated lipodystrophy [119].

7.3.2 Leptin

7.3.2.1 Physiology

Leptin and Adipocyte Physiology

Leptin (also known as the "satiety hormone") is a crucial hormone in adipocyte physiology, playing a central role in regulating energy balance, appetite, and metabolism [91]. Primarily secreted by WAT, leptin signals the body's energy stores, conveying information about adipose tissue mass to the CNS, specifically the hypothalamus [92].

Leptin plays an essential role in energy homeostasis by modulating food intake and expenditure [91]. Leptin exerts its anorexigenic effects by binding to its receptor, the leptin receptor (LEPR), expressed in the arcuate nucleus of the hypothalamus. Here, leptin inhibits the expression of orexigenic neuropeptides, such as NPY and agouti-related protein (AgRP), while stimulating the expression of anorexigenic neuropeptides, including POMC and CART [95]. The net effect is a reduction in appetite and hence food intake (see Figure 7.7).

Additionally, leptin influences energy expenditure by modulating the activity of the sympathetic nervous system and increasing thermogenesis in BAT [91]. It also contributes to glucose homeostasis by enhancing insulin sensitivity in peripheral tissues, such as skeletal muscle and liver [163].

In obesity, a state of hyperleptinemia and leptin resistance often arises, in which the elevated leptin levels fail to suppress appetite and promote energy expenditure effectively, thereby contributing to the maintenance of obesity and the development of related metabolic complications, such as insulin resistance and type 2 diabetes [164].

Lipodystrophy Syndrome and Leptin

Leptin is a crucial hormone in adipocyte physiology, and its role is particularly important in the context of lipodystrophy syndromes, a group of rare disorders characterized by partial or total loss of adipose tissue [165]. These syndromes result in a deficiency of leptin, which in turn leads to alterations in energy balance, appetite, and metabolism [166].

In lipodystrophy syndromes, the reduction or absence of adipose tissue impairs the production and secretion of leptin [167]. Consequently, leptin deficiency disrupts normal signaling to the CNS, specifically the hypothalamus, which regulates energy homeostasis by modulating both food intake and energy expenditure [168]. Leptin deficiency in lipodystrophy leads to increased appetite, and reduced energy expenditure, contributing to the development of metabolic complications often associated with these syndromes [169].

Additionally, leptin's role in enhancing insulin sensitivity in peripheral tissues, such as skeletal muscle and liver, is compromised in lipodystrophy syndromes due to its deficiency [170]. This results in the development of insulin resistance and hyperinsulinemia, which are commonly observed in patients with lipodystrophy [171].

Furthermore, the absence of leptin's regulatory effect on the immune system in lipodystrophy may lead to abnormal immune and inflammatory responses, exacerbating the risk of developing other complications [172].

7.3.2.2 Mechanism of Action

One therapeutic approach for treating leptin deficiency in lipodystrophy syndromes is the administration of recombinant human leptin, known as metreleptin [166]. Metreleptin therapy has been shown to improve metabolic parameters, such as glycemic control and lipid profiles, reduce food intake and increase energy expenditure in patients with lipodystrophy [173]. However, the long-term efficacy and safety of metreleptin treatment for lipodystrophy syndrgVomes require further investigation [174].

Practice Pearl(s)

For patients with a baseline weight of 40 kg or less, the initial subcutaneous dosage of metreleptin is 0.06 mg/kg once daily. The dose can be adjusted by 0.02 mg/kg daily, based on the patient's response and tolerability, with a maximum dose of 0.13 mg/kg once daily [175].

For patients with a baseline weight above 40 kg, the initial subcutaneous dosage is 2.5 mg for males and 5 mg for females, administered once daily. Depending on the patient's response and tolerability, the dose can be steadily adjusted by 1.25–2.5 mg daily, with a maximum dose of 10 mg once daily [175].

Clinical Trial Evidence

Refer to Table 7.13 for the summary of a trial evaluating the efficacy of leptin in lipodystrophy syndromes.

TABLE 7.13 Results of a study evaluating the safety and efficacy of recombinant human leptin therapy in patients with lipodystrophy syndromes.

Study	Population	Intervention	Outcome
Leptin replacement for severe lipodystrophy	Patients with severe lipodystrophy not related to HIV infection.	Administration of recombinant human methionyl leptin (metreleptin). Typical daily replacement doses were 0.06–0.08 mg/kg for female patients and 0.04 mg/kg for male patients, delivered via subcutaneous injection twice daily.	Improvement in glycemic control, insulin sensitivity, plasma triglycerides, caloric intake, liver volume and lipid content, intramyocellular lipid content, and neuroendocrine and immunologic endpoints. The treatment with metreleptin was well tolerated [176].

Concepts to Ponder

What is congenital leptin deficiency?

Congenital leptin deficiency occurs as a result of a genetic mutation in the leptin gene, which results in the transcription of a defective protein (leptin) [177].

Patients with congenital leptin deficiency present with significant early-onset obesity [178] due to food-seeking behavior, which starts at a very young age [177]. Leptin, a hormone secreted by *white adipose tissue*, is involved in triggering satiety through the central anorexigenic pathway [178]. Indeed, leptin binds to leptin receptors present on pro-opiomelanocortin (POMC) processing neurons in the arcuate nucleus of the hypothalamus to cause satiety (this was reviewed in earlier in Section 7.2.1) [179]. Congenital leptin deficiency, therefore, causes hyperphagia and promotes excess weight gain due to the absence of normal leptin signaling [178].

Also, leptin increases energy expenditure by potentiating sympathetic nerve activity in *brown adipose tissue*, a process which results in increased thermogenesis. Consequently, reduced energy expenditure in the setting of leptin deficiency contributes to obesity [180].

What are the other endocrine effects of leptin?

1. *Hypothalamic–pituitary–thyroidal axis:* Leptin regulates the release of thyroid-stimulating hormone (TSH) [181]. Central hypothyroidism occurs due to leptin-mediated signaling defects in the hypothalamic–pituitary–thyroid axis. It is worth noting that optimal leptin replacement therapy completely corrects hypothyroidism [182].
2. *Hypogonadotropic–pituitary–gonadal axis:* Leptin regulates the release of gonadotropin-releasing hormone (GnRH) [180]. Patients with congenital leptin deficiency are hypogonadal due to defective GnRH signaling [181].

PRACTICE-BASED QUESTIONS

1. A 68-year-old woman with a history of hyperlipidemia and coronary artery disease is currently taking atorvastatin. Despite adhering to her medication regimen, her LDL cholesterol levels remain above the target range (recent LDL cholesterol was 114 mg/dL). Her physician decides to add another medication to her current therapy.
   Which medication is most likely to be added?

   a. Rosuvastatin
   b. Ezetimibe
   c. Fenofibrate
   d. Alirocumab

   Answer: b. Ezetimibe. **Explanation:** Ezetimibe inhibits the absorption of cholesterol in the small intestine, leading to a decrease in the total amount of cholesterol available to the liver. This causes the liver to take more cholesterol out of the bloodstream, lowering the overall cholesterol levels. It is especially effective when used in combination with a statin, like atorvastatin.

2. A 72-year-old male with a history of hyperlipidemia and coronary artery disease presents to his primary care provider for a routine follow-up. His current medications include rosuvastatin and ezetimibe. He has been compliant with his medications, and his LDL cholesterol levels are on target.
   What is the likely mechanism of action of ezetimibe in this patient?

   a. Inhibition of HMG-CoA reductase
   b. Inhibition of cholesterol absorption in the small intestine
   c. Increase in the production of bile acids
   d. Activation of peroxisome proliferator-activated receptor-alpha (PPAR-α)

   Answer: b. Inhibition of cholesterol absorption in the small intestine. **Explanation:** Ezetimibe acts by inhibiting a protein called Niemann-Pick C1-Like 1 (NPC1L1) on the intestinal cells. NPC1L1 is responsible for the uptake of cholesterol into these cells. Therefore, inhibition of this protein by ezetimibe decreases cholesterol absorption, reducing the delivery of cholesterol to the liver and lowering cholesterol levels in the blood.

3. A 68-year-old man with a history of hypertension, type 2 diabetes mellitus, and coronary artery disease (CAD) presents for a routine follow-up visit. His current medications include metformin, lisinopril, and aspirin. His LDL-C level is 140 mg/dL. Given the patient's risk factors and medical history, what would be the most appropriate statin therapy?

a. High-intensity statin therapy
b. Moderate-intensity statin therapy
c. Low-intensity statin therapy
d. No statin therapy

Answer: a) High-intensity statin therapy. **Explanation:** The patient has multiple risk factors for atherosclerotic cardiovascular disease (ASCVD), including hypertension, diabetes, and CAD. Furthermore, his LDL-C level is high. As per the guidelines, high-intensity statin therapy, which aims to reduce LDL-C levels by at least 50%, is recommended for patients at high risk for ASCVD and those with extremely high LDL-C levels. Examples of high-intensity statin therapy include atorvastatin (40–80 mg/day) and rosuvastatin (20–40 mg/day).

4. A 50-year-old woman with a history of hypothyroidism and a recent diagnosis of hyperlipidemia with an LDL-C level of 160 mg/dL is started on atorvastatin 80 mg daily. What is the expected reduction in her LDL-C level following high-intensity statin therapy?

a. 10–29%
b. 30–49%
c. At least 50%
d. No significant reduction

Answer: c) At least 50%. **Explanation:** High-intensity statin therapy, such as atorvastatin 80 mg daily, is expected to reduce LDL-C levels by at least 50%.

5. A 62-year-old man with a history of ischemic stroke is started on simvastatin for secondary prevention. What would be the optimal time of day to administer simvastatin to this patient?

a. Morning
b. Afternoon
c. Evening
d. No specific timing necessary

Answer: c) Evening. **Explanation:** Simvastatin has a shorter half-life, and given that cholesterol synthesis is highest during the night, it is most effective when administered in the evening or at bedtime.

6. A 75-year-old woman with a history of rheumatoid arthritis and mild hyperlipidemia is started on statin therapy. Her LDL-C level is 110 mg/dL. What would be the most appropriate statin therapy?

a. High-intensity statin therapy
b. Moderate-intensity statin therapy
c. Low-intensity statin therapy
d. No statin therapy

Answer: c) Low-intensity statin therapy. **Explanation:** Given the patient's age and relatively mild hyperlipidemia, low-intensity statin therapy would be appropriate. This regimen aims to reduce LDL-C levels by less than 30%. It is typically prescribed for older adults, individuals with lower ASCVD risk, or those with contraindications or intolerance to higher-intensity statins. Some low-intensity statin regimens include simvastatin 10 mg daily, pravastatin 10–20 mg daily, and lovastatin 20 mg daily.

7. A 55-year-old female patient with elevated triglyceride levels is being prescribed Vascepa. What is the suggested dose of this medication?

a. 2 g once daily with meals
b. 2 g twice daily with meals
c. 4 g once daily with meals
d. 4 g twice daily with meals

Answer: B. The suggested dose of icosapent ethyl (Vascepa) is 2 g twice daily with meals. Options A, C, and D are incorrect as they do not match the recommended dosage of this medication.

8. In the metabolism of HDL cholesterol, which protein mediates the exchange of cholesterol esters and triglycerides between HDL and other circulating lipoproteins?

a. Apolipoprotein A-1 (ApoA-1)
b. ATP-binding cassette transporter A1 (ABCA1)
c. Cholesterol ester transfer protein (CETP)
d. Hepatic scavenger receptor class B type 1 (SR-B1)

Answer: c. CETP mediates the exchange of cholesterol esters and triglycerides between HDL and other circulating lipoproteins. Options A, B, and D are proteins that play significant roles in the metabolism of HDL cholesterol, but they do not mediate this particular process.

9. A 70-year-old man with hypertriglyceridemia is being started on fenofibrate. It is important to monitor which of the following in this patient?

a. Creatinine levels
b. Liver enzymes

c. Serum potassium levels

d. Hemoglobin A1C

Answer: b. It is crucial to monitor liver enzymes in patients taking fenofibrate due to the risk of drug-induced liver injury. Options A, C, and D are important to monitor in certain patient populations or those taking certain medications, but they are not the primary concern when starting a patient on fenofibrate.

10. A 55-year-old man with a history of familial hypercholesterolemia is under your care. Despite maximal statin therapy, his LDL cholesterol remains high. You decide to add Inclisiran to his regimen. What mechanism does Inclisiran use to lower LDL cholesterol?

a. Inhibits HMG-CoA reductase

b. Upregulates ApoB100 synthesis

c. Inhibits PCSK9 mRNA

d. Increases LDL receptor degradation

Answer: c. Inclisiran, a small interfering RNA (siRNA), inhibits the synthesis of PCSK9 by targeting and degrading PCSK9 mRNA. This results in a decrease in PCSK9 protein synthesis, which in turn leads to less degradation of LDL receptors on hepatocyte surfaces. More LDL receptors lead to enhanced clearance of circulating LDL cholesterol, thereby lowering LDL cholesterol levels.

11. A 40-year-old woman with mixed dyslipidemia has been prescribed Niacin to improve her lipid profile. How does Niacin primarily function to manage her condition?

a. Increases synthesis of Apolipoprotein B

b. Inhibits hormone-sensitive lipase in adipose tissue

c. Increases LDL receptor degradation

d. Stimulates PCSK9 production

Answer: b. Niacin primarily inhibits hormone-sensitive lipase in adipose tissue, which results in decreased lipolysis. This reduction decreases the substrate availability for hepatic triglyceride and very-low-density lipoprotein (VLDL) synthesis. Consequently, less LDL

cholesterol is packaged and released by the liver, improving the patient's lipid profile.

12. Which hormone, produced and released by adipose tissue, plays a significant role in regulating food intake and energy balance as part of the anorexigenic pathway?

a. Ghrelin

b. Insulin

c. Leptin

d. Glucagon

Answer: c. Leptin, produced and released by adipose tissue, plays a significant role in the anorexigenic pathway. As fat stores increase, leptin levels rise, signaling the body to decrease food intake and increase energy expenditure. Leptin exerts its effects by reaching the arcuate nucleus of the hypothalamus, where it inhibits Neuropeptide Y/agouti-related peptide neurons and stimulates pro-opiomelanocortin/ cocaine- and amphetamine-regulated transcript neurons.

13. A 45-year-old man with obesity has been started on Phentermine for short-term management of his weight. The primary mode of action of this drug involves which neurotransmitter?

a. Dopamine

b. GABA

c. Acetylcholine

d. Norepinephrine

Answer: d. Phentermine primarily stimulates the release of catecholamines, particularly norepinephrine, in the hypothalamus and other regions of the brain. The increased levels of norepinephrine lead to activation of neurons that express pro-opiomelanocortin (POMC) and cocaine- and amphetamine-regulated transcript (CART). This results in the release of alpha-melanocyte-stimulating hormone (α-MSH), which binds to melanocortin receptors in the brain, suppressing appetite and reducing food intake.

14. A 55-year-old man with a history of type 2 diabetes and obesity is currently taking metformin and atorvastatin. He has been struggling with weight loss and asks about medication options.

How does the medication tirzepatide aid in weight loss?

a. It stimulates the release of ghrelin.
b. It binds to GLP-1 receptors on POMC/CART neurons.
c. It inhibits the absorption of dietary fat.
d. It inhibits pancreatic lipase.

Answer: b. It binds to GLP-1 receptors on POMC/CART neurons. **Explanation:** Tirzepatide is a dual glucose-dependent insulinotropic polypeptide (GIP) and GLP-1 receptor agonist. It aids in weight loss by binding to GLP-1 receptors on POMC/CART neurons in the arcuate nucleus of the hypothalamus, thus promoting the anorexigenic pathway. This decreases food intake and promotes satiety.

15. A 38-year-old woman presents to the endocrinology clinic complaining of recent significant weight gain, despite no changes in diet or physical activity. Her past medical history is significant for rheumatoid arthritis and she takes prednisone 10 mg daily. She also complains of excessive hunger, which she finds difficult to control.
Which of the following mechanisms is most likely responsible for the patient's weight gain and increased appetite?

a. Increased production of pro-opiomelanocortin (POMC)
b. Suppression of POMC production
c. Overexpression of the MC4 receptor
d. Activation of the hypothalamic–pituitary–thyroid axis

Answer: b) Suppression of POMC production. **Explanation:** Patients on exogenous glucocorticoids like prednisone experience profound suppression of pro-opiomelanocortin (POMC) production in the hypothalamus, which in turn reduces the production of alpha melanocyte-stimulating hormone (αMSH). αMSH is involved in signaling the anorexigenic pathway, which promotes satiety. When this pathway is suppressed due to lower αMSH, the orexigenic pathway, which promotes hunger, dominates. Therefore, patients on long-term glucocorticoid therapy often experience weight gain and increased appetite.

16. A 55-year-old man presents with weight loss, anorexia, and fatigue. He has a history of Addison's disease, which is poorly controlled. Which of the following is most likely responsible for his symptoms?

a. Increased production of pro-opiomelanocortin (POMC)
b. Suppression of POMC production
c. Overexpression of the MC4 receptor
d. Activation of the hypothalamic–pituitary–thyroid axis

Answer: a) Increased production of pro-opiomelanocortin (POMC). **Explanation:** In Addison's disease, there is hypocortisolemia, which lifts the normal negative feedback inhibition of POMC by cortisol. This leads to an overproduction of POMC, ACTH, and αMSH. The overproduction of αMSH promotes the anorexigenic pathway, which suppresses hunger, and can result in poor oral intake and weight loss.

17. Which of the following hormones primarily secreted by adipocytes is anti-inflammatory, anti-atherogenic, and insulin-sensitizing?

a. Leptin
b. Resistin
c. Adiponectin
d. TNF-alpha

Answer: c) Adiponectin. **Explanation:** Adiponectin, secreted by adipocytes, enhances insulin sensitivity by promoting glucose uptake in skeletal muscle and suppressing hepatic gluconeogenesis. Additionally, it has anti-inflammatory effects, including the ability to inhibit the production of pro-inflammatory cytokines such as TNF-alpha and interleukin-6 (IL-6).

REFERENCES

1. Ginsberg, H.N. (1990). Lipoprotein physiology and its relationship to atherogenesis. *Endocrinol. Metab. Clin. N. Am.* 19: 211–228.
2. Pullinger, C.R. and Kane, J.P. (2006). Lipid and Lipoprotein Metabolism. *Reviews in Cell Biology and Molecular Medicine.* https://doi.org/10.1002/3527600906.mcb.200400101.

3. Ginsberg, H.N. (1998). Lipoprotein physiology. *Endocrinol. Metab. Clin. N. Am.* 27: 503–519.

4. Link, J.J., Rohatgi, A., and de Lemos, J.A. (2007). HDL cholesterol: physiology, pathophysiology, and management. *Curr. Probl. Cardiol.* 32: 268–314.

5. Tulenko, T.N. and Sumner, A.E. (2002). The physiology of lipoproteins. *J. Nucl. Cardiol.* 9: 638–649.

6. Alaupovic, P. (2003). The concept of apolipoprotein-defined lipoprotein families and its clinical significance. *Curr. Atheroscler. Rep.* 5: 459–467.

7. Marais, A.D. (2019). Apolipoprotein E in lipoprotein metabolism, health and cardiovascular disease. *Pathology* 51: 165–176.

8. Yamazaki, A., Ohkawa, R., Yamagata, Y. et al. (2021). Apolipoprotein C-II and C-III preferably transfer to both high-density lipoprotein (HDL)2 and the larger HDL3 from very low-density lipoprotein (VLDL). *Biol. Chem.* 402: 439–449.

9. Ramasamy, I. (2014). Recent advances in physiological lipoprotein metabolism. *Clin. Chem. Lab. Med.* 52: 1695–1727.

10. Hussain, M.M. (2014). Intestinal lipid absorption and lipoprotein formation. *Curr. Opin. Lipidol.* 25: 200–206.

11. Iqbal, J. and Hussain, M.M. (2009). Intestinal lipid absorption. *Am. J. Physiol. Endocrinol. Metab.* 296: E1183–E1194.

12. Wolska, A., Dunbar, R.L., Freeman, L.A. et al. (2017). Apolipoprotein C-II: New findings related to genetics, biochemistry, and role in triglyceride metabolism. *Atherosclerosis* 267: 49–60.

13. Kindel, T., Lee, D.M., and Tso, P. (2010). The mechanism of the formation and secretion of chylomicrons. *Atheroscler. Suppl.* 11: 11–16.

14. Cohen, D.E. and Fisher, E.A. (2013). Lipoprotein metabolism, dyslipidemia and nonalcoholic fatty liver disease. *Semin. Liver Dis.* 33: 380–388.

15. Daniels, T.F., Killinger, K.M., Michal, J.J. et al. (2009). Lipoproteins, cholesterol homeostasis and cardiac health. *Int. J. Biol. Sci.* 5: 474–488.

16. Willnow, T.E. (1997). Mechanisms of hepatic chylomicron remnant clearance. *Diabet. Med.* 14 (Suppl 3): S75–S80.

17. Beisiegel, U. (1998). Lipoprotein metabolism. *Eur. Heart J.* 19 (Suppl A): A20–A23.

18. Hu, J., Zhang, Z., Shen, W.-J., and Azhar, S. (2010). Cellular cholesterol delivery, intracellular processing and utilization for biosynthesis of steroid hormones. *Nutr. Metab. (Lond.)* 7: 47.

19. Miller, W.L. and Bose, H.S. (2011). Early steps in steroidogenesis: intracellular cholesterol trafficking. *J. Lipid Res.* 52: 2111–2135.

20. Bochem, A.E., Holleboom, A.G., Romijn, J.A. et al. (2013). High density lipoprotein as a source of cholesterol for adrenal steroidogenesis: a study in individuals with low plasma HDL-C. *J. Lipid Res.* 54: 1698–1704.

21. Geldenhuys, W.J., Lin, L., Darvesh, A.S., and Sadana, P. (2017). Emerging strategies of targeting lipoprotein lipase for metabolic and cardiovascular diseases. *Drug Discov. Today* 22: 352–365.

22. Davies, J.P., Scott, C., Oishi, K. et al. (2005). Inactivation of NPC1L1 causes multiple lipid transport defects and protects against diet-induced hypercholesterolemia. *J. Biol. Chem.* 280: 12710–12720.

23. Altmann, S.W., Davis, H.R., Zhu, L.-J. et al. (2004). Niemann-Pick C1 Like 1 protein is critical for intestinal cholesterol absorption. *Science* 303: 1201–1204.

24. Chang, T.-Y. and Chang, C. (2008). Ezetimibe blocks internalization of the NPC1L1/cholesterol complex. *Cell Metab.* 7: 469–471.

25. Wang, J., Chu, B.-B., Ge, L. et al. (2009). Membrane topology of human NPC1L1, a key protein in enterohepatic cholesterol absorption. *J. Lipid Res.* 50: 1653–1662.

26. Phan, B.A.P., Dayspring, T.D., and Toth, P.P. (2012). Ezetimibe therapy: mechanism of action and clinical update. *Vasc. Health Risk Manag.* 8: 415–427.

27. Kosoglou, T., Statkevich, P., Johnson-Levonas, A.O. et al. (2005). Ezetimibe: a review of its metabolism, pharmacokinetics and drug interactions. *Clin. Pharmacokinet.* 44: 467–494.

28. Weinglass, A.B., Kohler, M., Schulte, U. et al. (2008). Extracellular loop C of NPC1L1 is important for binding to ezetimibe. *Proc. Natl. Acad. Sci. U. S. A.* 105: 11140–11145.

29. Huang, C.-S., Yu, X., Fordstrom, P. et al. (2020). Cryo-EM structures of NPC1L1 reveal mechanisms of cholesterol transport and ezetimibe inhibition. Science. *Advances* 6: eabb1989.

30. Ge, L., Wang, J., Qi, W. et al. (2008). The cholesterol absorption inhibitor ezetimibe acts by blocking the sterol-induced internalization of NPC1L1. *Cell Metab.* 7: 508–519.

31. Grundy, S.M., Stone, N.J., Bailey, A.L. et al. (2019). 2018 AHA/ACC/AACVPR/AAPA/ABC/ACPM/ADA/AGS/APhA/ASPC/NLA/PCNA

Guideline on the management of blood cholesterol: executive summary: A report of the American College of Cardiology/American Heart Association Task Force on clinical practice guidelines. *J. Am. Coll. Cardiol.* 73: 3168–3209.

32. Gencer, B., Marston, N.A., Im, K. et al. (2020). Efficacy and safety of lowering LDL cholesterol in older patients: a systematic review and meta-analysis of randomised controlled trials. *Lancet* 396: 1637–1643.

33. Cannon, C.P., Blazing, M.A., Giugliano, R.P. et al. (2015). Ezetimibe added to statin therapy after acute coronary syndromes. *N. Engl. J. Med.* 372: 2387–2397.

34. DeBose-Boyd, R.A. (2008). Feedback regulation of cholesterol synthesis: sterol-accelerated ubiquitination and degradation of HMG CoA reductase. *Cell Res.* 18: 609–621.

35. Istvan, E. (2003). Statin inhibition of HMG-CoA reductase: a 3-dimensional view. *Atheroscler. Suppl.* 4: 3–8.

36. Carbonell, T. and Freire, E. (2005). Binding thermodynamics of statins to HMG-CoA reductase. *Biochemistry* 44: 11741–11748.

37. Young, S.G. and Fong, L.G. (2012). Lowering plasma cholesterol by raising LDL receptors—revisited. *N. Engl. J. Med.* 366: 1154.

38. Ness, G.C., Chambers, C.M., and Lopez, D. (1998). Atorvastatin action involves diminished recovery of hepatic HMG-CoA reductase activity. *J. Lipid Res.* 39: 75–84.

39. Schroor, M.M., Sennels, H.P., Fahrenkrug, J. et al. (2019). Diurnal variation of markers for cholesterol synthesis, cholesterol absorption, and bile acid synthesis: a systematic review and the bispebjerg study of diurnal variations. *Nutrients* 11: 1439.

40. Wiklund, O., Pirazzi, C., and Romeo, S. (2013). Monitoring of lipids, enzymes, and creatine kinase in patients on lipid-lowering drug therapy. *Curr. Cardiol. Rep.* 15: 397.

41. Plakogiannis, R. and Cohen, H. (2007). Optimal low-density lipoprotein cholesterol lowering-morning versus evening statin administration. *Ann. Pharmacother.* 41: 106–110.

42. Marcum, Z.A., Huang, H.-C., and Romanelli, R.J. (2019). Statin dosing instructions, medication adherence, and low-density lipoprotein cholesterol: a cohort study of incident statin users. *J. Gen. Intern. Med.* 34: 2559–2566.

43. Grundy, S.M., Stone, N.J., Blumenthal, R.S. et al. (2021). High-intensity statins benefit high-risk patients: why and how to do better. *Mayo Clin. Proc.* 96: 2660–2670.

44. Kim, S., Choi, H., and Won, C.W. (2022). Moderate-intensity statin use for primary prevention for more than 5 years is associated with decreased all-cause mortality in 75 years and older. *Arch. Gerontol. Geriatr.* 100: 104644.

45. Kim, J.Y., Choi, J., Kim, S.G., and Kim, N.H. (2022). Relative contributions of statin intensity, achieved low-density lipoprotein cholesterol level, and statin therapy duration to cardiovascular risk reduction in patients with type 2 diabetes: population based cohort study. *Cardiovasc. Diabetol.* 21: 28.

46. Cannon, C.P., Braunwald, E., McCabe, C.H. et al. (2004). Intensive versus moderate lipid lowering with statins after acute coronary syndromes. *N. Engl. J. Med.* 350: 1495–1504.

47. Schwartz, G.G., Olsson, A.G., Ezekowitz, M.D. et al. (2001). Effects of atorvastatin on early recurrent ischemic events in acute coronary syndromes The MIRACL Study: a randomized controlled trial. *JAMA* 285: 1711–1718.

48. Group SSSS (1994). Randomised trial of cholesterol lowering in 4444 patients with coronary heart disease: the Scandinavian Simvastatin Survival Study (4S). *Lancet* 344: 1383–1389.

49. Reiss, A.B., Shah, N., Muhieddine, D. et al. (2018). PCSK9 in cholesterol metabolism: from bench to bedside. *Clin. Sci. (Lond.)* 132: 1135–1153.

50. Lin, X.-L., Xiao, L.-L., Tang, Z.-H. et al. (2018). Role of PCSK9 in lipid metabolism and atherosclerosis. *Biomed. Pharmacother.* 104: 36–44.

51. Roth, E.M. and Davidson, M.H. (2018). PCSK9 inhibitors: mechanism of action, efficacy, and safety. *Rev. Cardiovasc. Med.* 19: S31–S46.

52. Sabatine, M.S. (2019). PCSK9 inhibitors: clinical evidence and implementation. *Nat. Rev. Cardiol.* 16: 155–165.

53. Steg, P.G., Szarek, M., Bhatt, D.L. et al. (2019). Effect of alirocumab on mortality after acute coronary syndromes. *Circulation* 140: 103–112.

54. Bornfeldt KE (2021) Triglyceride lowering by omega-3 fatty acids: a mechanism mediated by *N*-acyl taurines. *J. Clin. Invest.* https://doi.org/10.1172/JCI147558

55. Alves-Bezerra, M. and Cohen, D.E. (2017). Triglyceride metabolism in the liver. *Compr. Physiol.* 8: 1.

56. Ballantyne, C.M., Bays, H.E., Kastelein, J.J. et al. (2012). Efficacy and safety of eicosapentaenoic acid ethyl ester (AMR101) therapy in statin-treated patients with persistent high triglycerides (from the ANCHOR study). *Am. J. Cardiol.* 110: 984–992.

57. Skulas-Ray, A.C., Wilson, P.W.F., Harris, W.S. et al. (2019). Omega-3 fatty acids for the management of hypertriglyceridemia: a science advisory from the American Heart Association. *Circulation* 140: e673–e691.

58. Bhatt, D.L., Steg, P.G., Miller, M. et al. (2019). Cardiovascular risk reduction with icosapent ethyl for hypertriglyceridemia. *N. Engl. J. Med.* 380: 11–22.

59. Tall, A.R. (2010). Functions of cholesterol ester transfer protein and relationship to coronary artery disease risk. *J. Clin. Lipidol.* 4: 389–393.

60. Zhou, L., Li, C., Gao, L., and Wang, A. (2015). High-density lipoprotein synthesis and metabolism (Review). *Mol. Med. Rep.* 12: 4015–4021.

61. Afonso, M.S., Machado, R.M., Lavrador, M.S. et al. (2018). Molecular pathways underlying cholesterol homeostasis. *Nutrients* 10: 760.

62. Trajkovska, K.T. and Topuzovska, S. (2017). High-density lipoprotein metabolism and reverse cholesterol transport: strategies for raising HDL cholesterol. *Anatol. J. Cardiol.* 18: 149–154.

63. Staels, B. and Fonseca, V.A. (2009). Bile acids and metabolic regulation. *Diabetes Care* 32: S237–S245.

64. Staels, B., Dallongeville, J., Auwerx, J. et al. (1998). Mechanism of action of fibrates on lipid and lipoprotein metabolism. *Circulation* 98: 2088–2093.

65. Oosterveer, M.H., Grefhorst, A., van Dijk, T.H. et al. (2009). Fenofibrate simultaneously induces hepatic fatty acid oxidation, synthesis, and elongation in mice. *J. Biol. Chem.* 284: 34036–34044.

66. Fabbrini, E., Mohammed, B.S., Korenblat, K.M. et al. (2010). Effect of fenofibrate and niacin on intrahepatic triglyceride content, very low-density lipoprotein kinetics, and insulin action in obese subjects with nonalcoholic fatty liver disease. *J. Clin. Endocrinol. Metab.* 95: 2727–2735.

67. Schwandt, P. (1991). Fibrates and triglyceride metabolism. *Eur. J. Clin. Pharmacol.* 40: S41–S43.

68. Fruchart, J.-C. and Duriez, P. (2006). Mode of action of fibrates in the regulation of triglyceride and HDL-cholesterol metabolism. *Drugs Today (Barc)* 42: 39–64.

69. Ma, S., Liu, S., Wang, Q. et al. (2020). Fenofibrate-induced hepatotoxicity: a case with a special feature that is different from those in the LiverTox database. *J. Clin. Pharm. Ther.* 45: 204–207.

70. He, Y., Qin, M., and Chen, Y. (2021). Liver injury caused by fenofibrate within 48 h after first administration: a case report. *BMC Gastroenterol.* 21: 298.

71. Wiggins, B.S., Saseen, J.J., and Morris, P.B. (2016). Gemfibrozil in combination with statins-is it really contraindicated? *Curr. Atheroscler. Rep.* 18: 18.

72. Jun, M., Foote, C., Lv, J. et al. (2010). Effects of fibrates on cardiovascular outcomes: a systematic review and meta-analysis. *Lancet* 375: 1875–1884.

73. Hu, B., Zhong, L., Weng, Y. et al. (2020). Therapeutic siRNA: state of the art. *Sig. Transduct Target Ther.* 5: 1–25.

74. Svoboda, P. (2020). Key mechanistic principles and considerations concerning RNA interference. *Front. Plant Sci.* 11.

75. Song, M.-S. and Rossi, J.J. (2017). Molecular mechanisms of Dicer: endonuclease and enzymatic activity. *Biochem. J.* 474: 1603–1618.

76. Martinez, J., Patkaniowska, A., Urlaub, H. et al. (2002). Single-stranded antisense siRNAs guide target RNA cleavage in RNAi. *Cell* 110: 563–574.

77. Leuschner, P.J.F., Ameres, S.L., Kueng, S., and Martinez, J. (2006). Cleavage of the siRNA passenger strand during RISC assembly in human cells. *EMBO Rep.* 7: 314–320.

78. Frampton, J.E. (2023). Inclisiran: a review in hypercholesterolemia. *Am. J. Cardiovasc. Drugs* 23: 219–230.

79. Fitzgerald, K., White, S., Borodovsky, A. et al. (2017). A highly durable RNAi therapeutic inhibitor of PCSK9. *N. Engl. J. Med.* 376: 41–51.

80. Henney, N.C., Banach, M., and Penson, P.E. (2021). RNA silencing in the management of dyslipidemias. *Curr. Atheroscler. Rep.* 23: 69.

81. Ray, K.K., Wright, R.S., Kallend, D. et al. (2020). Two phase 3 trials of inclisiran in patients with elevated LDL cholesterol. *N. Engl. J. Med.* 382: 1507–1519.

82. Kamanna, V.S. and Kashyap, M.L. (2008). Mechanism of action of niacin. *Am. J. Cardiol.* 101: 20B–26B.

83. Stein, E.A. and Raal, F. (2016). Future directions to establish lipoprotein(a) as a treatment for atherosclerotic cardiovascular disease. *Cardiovasc. Drugs Ther.* 30: 101–108.

84. AIM-HIGH Investigators, Boden, W.E., Probstfield, J.L. et al. (2011). Niacin in patients with low HDL cholesterol levels receiving intensive statin therapy. *N. Engl. J. Med.* 365: 2255–2267.

85. HPS2-THRIVE Collaborative Group, Landray, M.J., Haynes, R. et al. (2014). Effects of extended-release niacin with laropiprant in high-risk patients. *N. Engl. J. Med.* 371: 203–212.

86. Chandra, A. and Rohatgi, A. (2014). The role of advanced lipid testing in the prediction of cardiovascular disease. *Curr. Atheroscler. Rep.* 16: 394.

87. German, C.A. and Shapiro, M.D. (2020). Assessing atherosclerotic cardiovascular disease risk with advanced lipid testing: state of the science. *Eur. Cardiol.* 15: e56.

88. Sykes, A.V., Patel, N., Lee, D., and Taub, P.R. (2022). Integrating advanced lipid testing and biomarkers in assessment and treatment. *Curr. Cardiol. Rep.* 24: 1647–1655.

89. Smitka, K., Papezova, H., Vondra, K. et al. (2013). The role of "mixed" orexigenic and anorexigenic signals and autoantibodies reacting with appetite-regulating neuropeptides and peptides of the adipose tissue-gut-brain axis: relevance to food intake and nutritional status in patients with anorexia nervosa and bulimia nervosa. *Int. J. Endocrinol.* 2013: 483145.

90. Morton, G.J., Cummings, D.E., Baskin, D.G. et al. (2006). Central nervous system control of food intake and body weight. *Nature* 443: 289–295.

91. Friedman, J.M. and Halaas, J.L. (1998). Leptin and the regulation of body weight in mammals. *Nature* 395: 763–770.

92. Zhang, Y., Proenca, R., Maffei, M. et al. (1994). Positional cloning of the mouse obese gene and its human homologue. *Nature* 372: 425–432.

93. Banks, W.A., Kastin, A.J., Huang, W. et al. (1996). Leptin enters the brain by a saturable system independent of insulin. *Peptides* 17: 305–311.

94. Schwartz, M.W., Woods, S.C., Porte, D. et al. (2000). Central nervous system control of food intake. *Nature* 404: 661–671.

95. Elmquist, J.K., Bjørbaek, C., Ahima, R.S. et al. (1998). Distributions of leptin receptor mRNA isoforms in the rat brain. *J. Comp. Neurol.* 395: 535–547.

96. Ollmann, M.M., Wilson, B.D., Yang, Y.K. et al. (1997). Antagonism of central melanocortin receptors in vitro and in vivo by agouti-related protein. *Science* 278: 135–138.

97. Cowley, M.A., Smart, J.L., Rubinstein, M. et al. (2001). Leptin activates anorexigenic POMC neurons through a neural network in the arcuate nucleus. *Nature* 411: 480–484.

98. Cone, R.D. (2005). Anatomy and regulation of the central melanocortin system. *Nat. Neurosci.* 8: 571–578.

99. Kristensen, P., Judge, M.E., Thim, L. et al. (1998). Hypothalamic CART is a new anorectic peptide regulated by leptin. *Nature* 393: 72–76.

100. Belgardt, B.F. and Brüning, J.C. (2010). CNS leptin and insulin action in the control of energy homeostasis. *Ann. N. Y. Acad. Sci.* 1212: 97–113.

101. Berthoud, H.-R. (2002). Multiple neural systems controlling food intake and body weight. *Neurosci. Biobehav. Rev.* 26: 393–428.

102. Morton, G.J., Meek, T.H., and Schwartz, M.W. (2014). Neurobiology of food intake in health and disease. *Nat. Rev. Neurosci.* 15: 367–378.

103. Son, J.W. and Kim, S. (2020). Comprehensive review of current and upcoming anti-obesity drugs. *Diabetes Metab. J.* 44: 802–818.

104. Lonneman DJ, Rey JA, McKee BD (2013) Phentermine/topiramate extended-release capsules (qsymia) for weight loss. P T 38:446–452

105. Gadde, K.M., Allison, D.B., Ryan, D.H. et al. (2011). Effects of low-dose, controlled-release, phentermine plus topiramate combination on weight and associated comorbidities in overweight and obese adults (CONQUER): a randomised, placebo-controlled, phase 3 trial. *Lancet* 377: 1341–1352.

106. Allison, D.B., Gadde, K.M., Garvey, W.T. et al. (2012). Controlled-release phentermine/topiramate in severely obese adults: a randomized controlled trial (EQUIP). *Obesity (Silver Spring)* 20: 330–342.

107. Desai, A.J., Dong, M., Harikumar, K.G., and Miller, L.J. (2016). Cholecystokinin-induced satiety, a key gut servomechanism that is affected by the membrane microenvironment of this receptor. *Int. J. Obes. Suppl.* 6: S22–S27.

108. Schjoldager, B.T. (1994). Role of CCK in gallbladder function. *Ann. N. Y. Acad. Sci.* 713: 207–218.

109. Chen, J., Scott, K.A., Zhao, Z. et al. (2008). Characterization of the feeding inhibition and neural activation produced by dorsomedial hypothalamic cholecystokinin administration. *Neuroscience* 152: 178–188.

110. Huang, Y., Lin, X., and Lin, S. (2021). Neuropeptide Y and metabolism syndrome: an update on perspectives of clinical therapeutic intervention strategies. *Front. Cell Dev. Biol.* 9: 695623. https://doi.org/10.3389/fcell.2021.695623.

111. Yamada, C. (2021). Relationship between orexigenic peptide ghrelin signal, gender difference and disease. *Int. J. Mol. Sci.* 22: 3763.

112. Drucker, D.J. (2018). Mechanisms of action and therapeutic application of glucagon-like peptide-1. *Cell Metab.* 27: 740–756.

113. Secher, A., Jelsing, J., Baquero, A.F. et al. (2014). The arcuate nucleus mediates GLP-1 receptor agonist liraglutide-dependent weight loss. *J. Clin. Invest.* 124: 4473–4488.

114. Welling, M.S., de Groot, C.J., Kleinendorst, L. et al. (2021). Effects of glucagon-like peptide-1 analogue treatment in genetic obesity: A case series. *Clinical Obesity* 11: e12481.

115. Wen, X., Zhang, B., Wu, B. et al. (2022). Signaling pathways in obesity: mechanisms and therapeutic interventions. *Sig. Transduct Target Ther.* 7: 1–31.

116. Mukherjee, S., Diéguez, C., Fernø, J., and López, M. (2023). Obesity wars: hypothalamic sEVs a new hope. *Trends Mol. Med.* https://doi.org/10.1016/j.molmed.2023.04.006.

117. Mehta, A., Marso, S.P., and Neeland, I.J. (2016). Liraglutide for weight management: a critical review of the evidence. *Obes. Sci. Pract.* 3: 3–14.

118. Wilding, J.P.H., Batterham, R.L., Calanna, S. et al. (2021). Once-weekly semaglutide in adults with overweight or obesity. *N. Engl. J. Med.* 384: 989–1002.

119. Pi-Sunyer, X., Astrup, A., Fujioka, K. et al. (2015). A randomized, controlled trial of 3.0 mg of liraglutide in weight management. *N. Engl. J. Med.* 373: 11–22.

120. Kim, K.K. (2019). Understanding the mechanism of action and clinical implications of anti-obesity drugs recently approved in Korea. *Korean J. Fam. Med.* 40: 63–71.

121. Billes, S.K., Sinnayah, P., and Cowley, M.A. (2014). Naltrexone/bupropion for obesity: An investigational combination pharmacotherapy for weight loss. *Pharmacol. Res.* 84: 1–11.

122. Early, J. and Whitten, J.S. (2015). Naltrexone/bupropion (contrave) for weight loss. *AFP* 91: 554–556.

123. Greenway, F.L., Fujioka, K., Plodkowski, R.A. et al. (2010). Effect of naltrexone plus bupropion on weight loss in overweight and obese adults (COR-I): a multicentre, randomised, double-blind, placebo-controlled, phase 3 trial. *Lancet* 376: 595–605.

124. Torgerson, J.S., Hauptman, J., Boldrin, M.N., and Sjöström, L. (2004). XENical in the prevention of diabetes in obese subjects (XENDOS) study: a randomized study of orlistat as an adjunct to lifestyle changes for the prevention of type 2 diabetes in obese patients. *Diabetes Care* 27: 155–161.

125. Brethauer, S.A., Aminian, A., Romero-Talamás, H. et al. (2013). Can diabetes be surgically cured? Long-term metabolic effects of bariatric surgery in obese patients with type 2 diabetes mellitus. *Ann. Surg.* 258: 628–636. discussion 636-637.

126. Cummings, D.E., Overduin, J., and Foster-Schubert, K.E. (2004). Gastric bypass for obesity: mechanisms of weight loss and diabetes resolution. *J. Clin. Endocrinol. Metabol.* 89: 2608–2615.

127. Holst, J.J., Madsbad, S., Bojsen-Møller, K.N. et al. (2018). Mechanisms in bariatric surgery: Gut hormones, diabetes resolution, and weight loss. *Surg. Obes. Relat. Dis.* 14: 708–714.

128. Ulker, İ. and Yildiran, H. (2019). The effects of bariatric surgery on gut microbiota in patients with obesity: a review of the literature. *Biosci. Microbiota. Food Health* 38: 3–9.

129. Mitchell, B.G. and Gupta, N. (2023). *Roux-en-Y Gastric Bypass*. StatPearls.

130. Karmali, S., Schauer, P., Birch, D. et al. (2010). Laparoscopic sleeve gastrectomy: an innovative new tool in the battle against the obesity epidemic in Canada. *Can. J. Surg.* 53: 126–132.

131. Furbetta, N., Cervelli, R., and Furbetta, F. (2020). Laparoscopic adjustable gastric banding, the past, the present and the future. *Ann. Transl. Med.* 8: S4.

132. Conner, J. and Nottingham, J.M. (2023). *Biliopancreatic Diversion With Duodenal Switch*. StatPearls.

133. Schauer, P.R., Kashyap, S.R., Wolski, K. et al. (2012). Bariatric surgery versus intensive medical therapy in obese patients with diabetes. *N. Engl. J. Med.* 366: 1567–1576.

134. D'Agostino, G. and Diano, S. (2010). Alpha-melanocyte stimulating hormone: production and degradation. *J. Mol. Med. (Berl)* 88: 1195–1201.

135. Wardlaw, S.L., McCarthy, K.C., and Conwell, I.M. (1998). Glucocorticoid regulation of hypothalamic proopiomelanocortin. *Neuroendocrinology* 67: 51–57.

136. Jada, K., Djossi, S.K., Khedr, A. et al. (2021). The pathophysiology of anorexia nervosa in hypothalamic endocrine function and bone metabolism. *Cureus.* https://doi.org/10.7759/cureus.20548.

137. Coelho, M., Oliveira, T., and Fernandes, R. (2013). Biochemistry of adipose tissue: an endocrine organ. *Arch. Med. Sci.* 9: 191–200.

138. Cannon, B. and Nedergaard, J. (2004). Brown adipose tissue: function and physiological significance. *Physiol. Rev.* 84: 277–359.

139. Lafontan, M. (2014). Adipose tissue and adipocyte dysregulation. *Diabetes Metab.* 40: 16–28.

140. Ibrahim, M.M. (2010). Subcutaneous and visceral adipose tissue: structural and functional differences. *Obes. Rev.* 11: 11–18.

141. Porter, S.A., Massaro, J.M., Hoffmann, U. et al. (2009). Abdominal subcutaneous adipose tissue: a protective fat depot? *Diabetes Care* 32: 1068–1075.

142. Tchernof, A. and Després, J.-P. (2013). Pathophysiology of human visceral obesity: an update. *Physiol. Rev.* 93: 359–404.

143. Neeland, I.J., Poirier, P., and Després, J.-P. (2018). Cardiovascular and metabolic heterogeneity of obesity: clinical challenges and implications for management. *Circulation* 137: 1391–1406.

144. Harms, M. and Seale, P. (2013). Brown and beige fat: development, function and therapeutic potential. *Nat. Med.* 19: 1252–1263.

145. Fedorenko, A., Lishko, P.V., and Kirichok, Y. (2012). Mechanism of fatty-acid-dependent UCP1 uncoupling in brown fat mitochondria. *Cell* 151: 400–413.

146. Cypess, A.M., Lehman, S., Williams, G. et al. (2009). Identification and importance of brown adipose tissue in adult humans. *N. Engl. J. Med.* 360: 1509–1517.

147. Nedergaard, J., Bengtsson, T., and Cannon, B. (2007). Unexpected evidence for active brown adipose tissue in adult humans. *Am. J. Physiol. Endocrinol. Metab.* 293: E444–E452.

148. Rosen, E.D. and Spiegelman, B.M. (2006). Adipocytes as regulators of energy balance and glucose homeostasis. *Nature* 444: 847–853.

149. Trayhurn, P. and Wood, I.S. (2004). Adipokines: inflammation and the pleiotropic role of white adipose tissue. *Br. J. Nutr.* 92: 347–355.

150. Yamauchi, T., Kamon, J., Waki, H. et al. (2001). The fat-derived hormone adiponectin reverses insulin resistance associated with both lipoatrophy and obesity. *Nat. Med.* 7: 941–946.

151. Hotamisligil, G.S., Shargill, N.S., and Spiegelman, B.M. (1993). Adipose expression of tumor necrosis factor-alpha: direct role in obesity-linked insulin resistance. *Science* 259: 87–91.

152. Steppan, C.M., Bailey, S.T., Bhat, S. et al. (2001). The hormone resistin links obesity to diabetes. *Nature* 409: 307–312.

153. Rosen, E.D., Sarraf, P., Troy, A.E. et al. (1999). PPAR gamma is required for the differentiation of adipose tissue in vivo and in vitro. *Mol. Cell* 4: 611–617.

154. Garg, A. (2011). Clinical review: Lipodystrophies: genetic and acquired body fat disorders. *J. Clin. Endocrinol. Metab.* 96: 3313–3325.

155. Lehmann, J.M., Moore, L.B., Smith-Oliver, T.A. et al. (1995). An antidiabetic thiazolidinedione is a high affinity ligand for peroxisome proliferator-activated receptor gamma (PPAR gamma). *J. Biol. Chem.* 270: 12953–12956.

156. Olefsky, J.M. and Saltiel, A.R. (2000). PPAR gamma and the treatment of insulin resistance. *Trends Endocrinol. Metab.* 11: 362–368.

157. Moreau, F., Boullu-Sanchis, S., Vigouroux, C. et al. (2007). Efficacy of pioglitazone in familial partial lipodystrophy of the Dunnigan type: a case report. *Diabetes Metab.* 33: 385–389.

158. Sleilati, G.G., Leff, T., Bonnett, J.W., and Hegele, R.A. (2007). Efficacy and safety of pioglitazone in treatment of a patient with an atypical partial lipodystrophy syndrome. *Endocr. Pract.* 13: 656–661.

159. Prasithsirikul, W. and Bunnag, P. (2004). Improvement of fat redistribution, insulin resistance and hepatic fatty infiltration in HIV-associated lipodystrophy syndrome by pioglitazone: a case report. *J. Med. Assoc. Thail.* 87: 166–172.

160. Corvillo, F. and Akinci, B. (2019). An overview of lipodystrophy and the role of the complement system. *Mol. Immunol.* 112: 223–232.

161. Giralt, M., Villarroya, F., and Araújo-Vilar, D. (2019). Lipodystrophy. In: *Encyclopedia of Endocrine Diseases*, 2nde (ed. I. Huhtaniemi and L. Martini), 482–495. Oxford: Academic Press.

162. Belo, S.P.M., Magalhães, Â.C., Freitas, P., and Carvalho, D.M. (2015). Familial partial lipodystrophy, Dunnigan variety - challenges for patient care during pregnancy: a case report. *BMC. Res. Notes* 8: 140.

163. Minokoshi, Y., Haque, M.S., and Shimazu, T. (1999). Microinjection of leptin into the ventromedial hypothalamus increases glucose uptake in peripheral tissues in rats. *Diabetes* 48: 287–291.

164. Myers, M.G., Leibel, R.L., Seeley, R.J., and Schwartz, M.W. (2010). Obesity and leptin resistance: distinguishing cause from effect. *Trends Endocrinol. Metab.* 21: 643–651.

165. Garg, A. (2004). Acquired and inherited lipodystrophies. *N. Engl. J. Med.* 350: 1220–1234.

166. Oral, E.A., Simha, V., Ruiz, E. et al. (2002). Leptin-replacement therapy for lipodystrophy. *N. Engl. J. Med.* 346: 570–578.

167. Petersen, K.F., Oral, E.A., Dufour, S. et al. (2002). Leptin reverses insulin resistance and hepatic steatosis in patients with severe lipodystrophy. *J. Clin. Invest.* 109: 1345–1350.

168. Friedman, J. (2014). 20 years of leptin: leptin at 20: an overview. *J. Endocrinol.* 223: T1–T8.

169. Capeau, J., Magré, J., Caron-Debarle, M. et al. (2010). Human lipodystrophies: genetic and acquired diseases of adipose tissue. *Endocr. Dev.* 19: 1–20.

170. Minokoshi, Y., Kim, Y.-B., Peroni, O.D. et al. (2002). Leptin stimulates fatty-acid oxidation by activating AMP-activated protein kinase. *Nature* 415: 339–343.

171. Chong, A.Y., Lupsa, B.C., Cochran, E.K., and Gorden, P. (2010). Efficacy of leptin therapy in the different forms of human lipodystrophy. *Diabetologia* 53: 27–35.

172. Matarese, G. and La Cava, A. (2004). The intricate interface between immune system and metabolism. *Trends Immunol.* 25: 193–200.

173. Chan, J.L., Lutz, K., Cochran, E. et al. (2011). Clinical effects of long-term metreleptin treatment in patients with lipodystrophy. *Endocr. Pract.* 17: 922–932.

174. Brown, R.J., Araujo-Vilar, D., Cheung, P.T. et al. (2016). The diagnosis and management of lipodystrophy syndromes: a multi-society practice guideline. *J. Clin. Endocrinol. Metab.* 101: 4500–4511.

175. Chou, K. and Perry, C.M. (2013). Metreleptin: first global approval. *Drugs* 73: 989–997.

176. Oral, E.A. and Chan, J.L. (2010). Rationale for leptin-replacement therapy for severe lipodystrophy. *Endocr. Pract.* 16: 324–333.

177. Wabitsch, M., Funcke, J.-B., Lennerz, B. et al. (2015). Biologically inactive leptin and early-onset extreme obesity. *N. Engl. J. Med.* 372: 48–54.

178. Wasim, M., Awan, F.R., Najam, S.S. et al. (2016). Role of leptin deficiency, inefficiency, and leptin receptors in obesity. *Biochem. Genet.* 54: 565–572.

179. Dodd, G., Descherf, S., Loh, K. et al. (2015). Leptin and insulin act on POMC neurons to promote the browning of white fat. *Cell* 160: 88–104.

180. Kelesidis, T., Kelesidis, I., Chou, S., and Mantzoros, C.S. (2010). Narrative review: the role of leptin in human physiology: emerging clinical applications. *Ann. Intern. Med.* 152: 93–100.

181. Paz-Filho, G., Mastronardi, C.A., and Licinio, J. (2015). Leptin treatment: facts and expectations. *Metabolism* 64: 146–156.

182. Paz-Filho, G., Delibasi, T., Erol, H.K. et al. (2009). Congenital leptin deficiency and thyroid function. *Thyroid. Res.* 2: 11.

CHAPTER 8

Miscellaneous Topics in Disorders of Endocrine Glands

8.1 RECENT TECHNOLOGICAL ADVANCES IN DIABETES CARE

8.1.1 Insulin Pumps

Insulin pumps are small computerized medical devices used by those living with type 1 diabetes to continuously administer insulin throughout their day, replicating the pancreas' normal physiological role of regulating blood glucose levels. A conventional insulin pump comprises a disposable reservoir for insulin storage and a thin, flexible tube (cannulae) that serves as a conduit for delivering insulin from the reservoir to the subcutaneous tissue [1].

Insulin pumps, also known as continuous subcutaneous insulin infusion (CSII) devices, deliver a steady and continuous stream of basal insulin at an adjustable basal rate to meet user needs and additional doses during mealtimes or to correct hyperglycemia. Physicians can program specific amounts to be delivered automatically by the insulin pump [2]. The typical programmed rates on an insulin pump include basal rates, insulin sensitivity factors, and insulin-to-carbohydrate ratios. A comparison of available insulin pumps in the United States of America is shown in Table 8.1.

8.1.2 Continuous Glucose Monitors

8.1.2.1 A Brief History of Glucose Monitoring

Blood glucose monitoring, essential in diabetes management, has evolved significantly over the past century. Major developments include Benedict's urine glucose testing reagent in 1908, the introduction of Clinitest in 1945, and Ames' Dextrostix, the first blood glucose test strip in 1965. By the mid-1970s, the idea of home-based glucose monitoring emerged, leading to the development of the Dextrometer in 1980. Throughout the 1980s, more affordable, less-invasive blood glucose meters and strips were introduced, making self-monitoring of blood glucose a standard of care. The advent of continuous glucose monitoring (CGM) revolutionized glucose monitoring, starting with the FDA-approved professional CGM in 1999 [3].

Types of CGMs

- Dexcom G6 and Dexcom G7
- Freestyle libre, Freestyle libre 2, and Freestyle Libre 3
- Eversense senseonics
- Medtronic guardian sensor 3, and guardian sensor 4 (see Table 8.2)

Endocrinology: Pathophysiology to Therapy, First Edition. Akuffo Quarde.
© 2024 John Wiley & Sons Ltd. Published 2024 by John Wiley & Sons Ltd.

TABLE 8.1   The types of insulin pumps.

Manufacturer	Medtronic	Insulet	Tandem diabetes care
Legacy models	MiniMed 508, Minimed Paradigm (511, 512, 712, 515, 715), MiniMed Paradigm REAL-time (522, 722), MiniMed Paradigm REAL-Time Revel, MiniMed (530G, 630G, 670G, 770G).	Omnipod DASH, Insulet Omnipod UST400, Omnipod Eros	Tandem T:Slim G4, Tandem T:Flex
Current model (Flagship)	Minimed 770G system	Omnipod 5	Tandem T:Slim X2
Features	Links to a CGM (Guardian Sensor 3, Guardian Link 3 transmitter, Accu-Check Guide Link meter, and Test strips). Integrated insulin pump and display screen. Smartphone app (displays your blood sugar trends over time).	Links to Dexcom G6. PDM (An android phone displays blood sugars and pump settings). Can link to personal smartphone.	Links to Dexcom G6. Integrated insulin pump and display screen.
Dimensions	3.78 length × 2.11 width × 0.96 depth (inches)	2.05 length × 1.53 width × 0.57 depth (inches)	3.13 length × 2.0 width × 0.6 depth (inches)
Compatible insulin	U-100 insulins: Novolog, Humalog, fiasp	U-100 insulins: Novolog, Humalog, admelog, fiasp	U-100 insulins: Novolog, Humalog
Basal increment	Variable 0.025, 0.05 and 0.1 units	0.05 units	0.1 units
Maximum basal rate	35 units per hour	30 units per hour	15 units per hour
Maximum bolus	25 units	30 units	25 units
The capacity of the reservoir	300 units	200 units	300 units
Battery life	AA battery replaceable	Rechargeable lithium battery (android phone as PDM)	The rechargeable lithium battery of the pump can last for up to 7 days (depending on settings).
Basal programming	Three basal patterns	12 basal patterns	6 patterns
Insulin on board	Yes. SmartGuard Auto Mode can only be used for patients requiring 8–250 units/24 h	Yes. SmartAdjust Technology	Yes. Control IQ and Basal IQ Technology
CGM integration	Yes (Compatible with Guardian System, change sensor every 7 days)	Yes (Compatible with Dexcom G6 CGM)	Yes (Compatible with Dexcom G6 CGM)
Calibration of CGM	Yes. At least twice a day using the accu-check Guide link	No	No
Future model	MiniMed 780G	N/A	Tandem Mobi (tubeless pump), Tandem TSlim X3
Major limitation	At least two capillary glucose checks are needed daily. Patients are tethered to a tubing.	Restricted to 200 units of insulin per day	Patients are tethered to a tubing.
Major advantage	Hybrid-closed loop system	Hybrid-closed loop system. Tubeless pump	Hybrid-closed loop system

TABLE 8.2   Comparison of popular continuous glucose monitors.

Feature	Dexcom G7	Guardian sensor 4	Freestyle libre 3	Eversense E3
Manufacturer	Dexcom	Medtronic	Abott	Senseonics
Mean absolute relative difference	8.20%	9.60%	7.90%	8.50%
Approved sites	Back of upper arms or upper buttocks	Back of upper arms or upper buttocks	Back of upper arms	Back of upper arms
Warm up	30 min	2 h	60 min warm up	24 h
Duration of wear	10 d	7 d	14 d	180 d
Insulin pump integration	Tandem T Slim X2 (pending as of March 2023)	Minimed 780G	Not yet	Not yet
Smartphone app	Yes	Yes	Yes (not compatible with all models)	Yes
Sharing of data	Yes (Dexcom follow)	Yes (Carelink Connect)	Yes (libre link app)	Yes
Water resistance	Yes	Yes	Yes	Yes

Source: Table is adapted from Refs. [4–7].

8.1.3   Pumps and CGMs in Practice

In clinical practice, the integration of insulin pumps and CGM systems offers a sophisticated approach to managing diabetes, facilitating improved glycemic control, and reducing the risk of diabetes-related complications. These advanced devices are crucial components of modern diabetes management, enabling patients to achieve better regulation of their blood glucose levels.

Insulin pumps are programmable devices designed to administer a continuous basal insulin infusion, with the capacity to deliver additional bolus doses as needed. This precise and adjustable method of insulin delivery supports patients in maintaining their blood glucose levels within the desired range.

CGM systems measure glucose concentrations in interstitial fluid throughout the day and night. Comprised of a subcutaneous sensor, a transmitter affixed to the sensor, and a display device or smartphone application that displays real-time glucose data, CGMs provide patients with continuous insights into their blood glucose levels, informing decisions regarding insulin dosing, nutrition, and physical activity. The sites of application of CGMs are shown in Figure 8.1.

The combination of insulin pumps and CGMs in clinical practice offers several advantages:

1. By continuously monitoring glucose levels and adjusting insulin delivery in response, patients can maintain their blood glucose levels within their target range more consistently.

2. CGM enables patients to rapidly identify and address impending hypoglycemic spells, which helps in mitigating the risk of severe hypoglycemia.

3. CGMs facilitate the tracking of glucose trends and patterns over time, assisting patients and physicians in making informed decisions regarding adjustments in diabetes treatment.

4. The integration of insulin pumps and CGMs (hybrid-closed loop insulin pump systems) empowers patients to effectively manage their diabetes under various circumstances, such as during exercise, travel, or changes in daily routines.

5. CGM and insulin pump therapy can alleviate the burden of diabetes management, leading to an enhanced quality of life for patients [8].

Clinical Pearl

Time in range (TIR): Time in range refers to the percentage of time an individual with diabetes spends within a specified target blood glucose range, typically between 70 mg/dL (3.9 mmol/L) and 180 mg/dL (10 mmol/L). TIR is an essential metric in diabetes management, as it provides insights into overall glycemic control and is associated with a reduced risk of both short-term and long-term complications. Continuous glucose monitoring (CGM) systems enable patients and healthcare providers to monitor TIR and make informed decisions regarding treatment adjustments [9].

Hybrid-closed loop insulin pump: A hybrid-closed loop insulin pump, also known as an artificial pancreas or an advanced insulin pump system, is a device that combines an insulin pump with continuous glucose monitoring (CGM) technology [10]. This system automatically adjusts basal insulin delivery in response to real-time glucose levels, providing a semiautomated approach to diabetes management. While the hybrid-closed loop system manages basal insulin adjustments, users are still required to administer bolus insulin doses for meals and correct high blood glucose levels manually [11].

Mean absolute relative difference (MARD): MARD is a statistical measurement used to assess the accuracy of continuous glucose monitoring (CGM) systems. It calculates the average difference between CGM glucose values and blood glucose values obtained through capillary blood testing or a laboratory method [12]. The MARD is expressed as a percentage, with lower values indicating higher accuracy. A lower MARD value signifies that the CGM system provides more reliable and precise glucose measurements, contributing to improved diabetes management and decision-making [13].

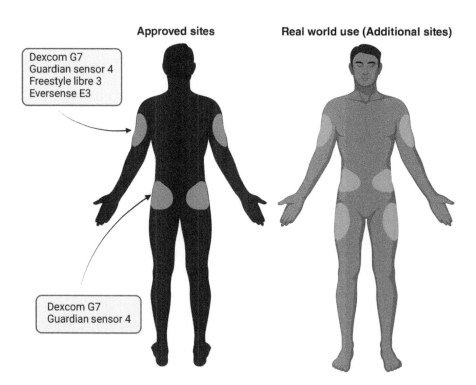

FIGURE 8.1   Locations for continuous glucose monitor placement. A comparison of approved and real-world use sites for CGM placement.

8.2   IMMUNE CHECKPOINT INHIBITOR-RELATED ENDOCRINOPATHIES

8.2.1   Hypophysitis

 Clinical Pearl

Immune checkpoint inhibitors enhance the immune system's ability to recognize and attack cancer cells. They target specific proteins on immune cells, called immune checkpoints, which play a critical role in modulating the immune response [14].

Under normal conditions, immune checkpoints help maintain self-tolerance and prevent the immune system from causing damage to healthy cells [15]. However, cancer cells can exploit these checkpoints to evade immune surveillance and destruction by expressing inhibitory proteins that bind to checkpoint receptors on immune cells, such as T cells. This binding effectively "switches off" the immune response against the cancer cells [16].

Immune checkpoint inhibitors work by blocking the interaction between checkpoint proteins and their ligands, thereby releasing the "brakes" on the immune system and allowing T cells to recognize and attack cancer cells more effectively. Some examples of targeted immune checkpoints include cytotoxic T-lymphocyte-associated protein 4 (CTLA-4), programmed cell death protein 1 (PD-1), and programmed death-ligand 1 (PD-L1) [17, 18].

Immune checkpoint inhibitors have shown promising results in treating various cancers, including melanoma, non-small cell lung cancer, and renal cell carcinoma, among others [19]. However, they can also cause immune-related adverse events due to increased immune activation, potentially leading to inflammation and damage to healthy tissues. The endocrine system is susceptible to these immune-related adverse events [20].

8.2.1.1   Checkpoints in Immune Regulation

CTLA-4 is expressed on the surface of T cells and competes with the co-stimulatory receptor CD28 for binding to both CD80 and CD86, present on antigen-presenting cells (APCs) [21]. While CD28 binding enhances T cell activation, CTLA-4 binding inhibits T cell activation. In cancer, overexpression of CTLA-4 can dampen the immune response against tumor cells by inhibiting T-cell activation, thus promoting tumor progression [22].

PD-1 is also expressed on the surface of T cells and binds to its ligands [23], programmed death ligand 1 (PD-L1), and programmed death ligand 2 (PD-L2), which can be found on tumor cells and some immune cells [24]. The binding of PD-1 to its ligands leads to the suppression of T cell activation and proliferation, promoting immune tolerance and allowing tumor cells to effectively evade immune detection [25].

Immune checkpoint inhibitors (ICIs) represent a new class of anticancer medications that have been developed to target these immune checkpoints and counteract the immunosuppressive effects of CTLA-4 and PD-1 activation pathways (Table 8.3).

Anti-CTLA-4 inhibitors, such as ipilimumab, disrupt the binding of CTLA-4 to CD80/CD86, preventing the inhibition of T cell activation and promoting an antitumor immune response [28].

Also, anti-PD-1 inhibitors, like nivolumab and pembrolizumab, block the interaction between PD-1 and its ligands, allowing T cells to maintain their activation and attack tumor cells [29] (see Figure 8.2).

TABLE 8.3   Sites of action of immune checkpoint inhibitors.

Immune checkpoint inhibitors	Site of action
Atezolizumab, avelumab, durvalumab [26]	PD-L1
Nivolumab, pembrolizumab, cemiplimab, dostarlimab	PD-1
Ipilimumab, tremelimumab [27]	CTLA-4

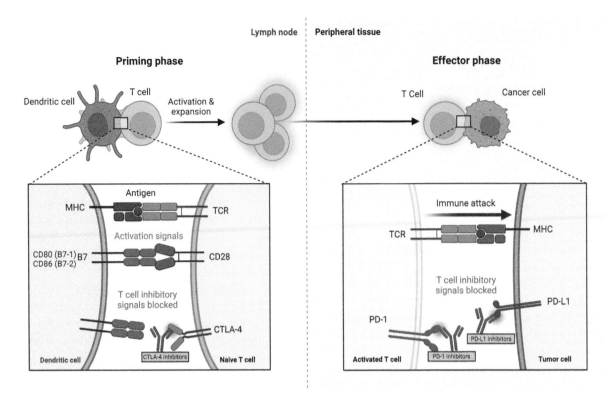

FIGURE 8.2 Mechanism of action of various immune check inhibitors. The phases of immune checkpoint processes, showing the role of the dendritic cell, T cell, and cancer cell during the priming and effector phases. The site of action of immune checkpoint inhibitors (CTLA-4 inhibitors, PD-1 inhibitors, and PD-L1 inhibitors) is shown.

 Pathophysiology Pearl

The proposed mechanisms of toxicity (irAEs) associated with ICIs

Immune-related adverse events in the setting of ICIs can affect any organ or tissue, with the endocrine system being no exception. See Figure 8.3.

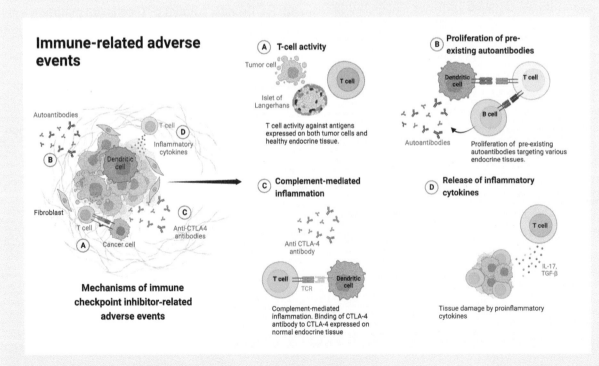

FIGURE 8.3 Mechanisms of immune checkpoint inhibitor-related adverse events. The proposed mechanisms include T cell activity against antigens on normal endocrine cells, proliferation of pre-existing antibodies, complement activation, and the release of proinflammatory cytokines. *Source*: Adapted from Ref. [30].

8.2.1.2 Hypophysitis – An Immune-Related Adverse Reaction

ICIs have been associated with various immune-related adverse events (irAEs), one of which is hypophysitis. Hypophysitis can result in the disruption of normal hormone production and regulation [31].

The association between ICIs and hypophysitis is thought to be due to the enhanced immune activation caused by these drugs. By blocking inhibitory immune checkpoints, such as CTLA-4 and PD-1/PD-L1, ICIs enable a more potent immune response against cancer cells. However, this heightened immune activation can also lead to the immune system mistakenly targeting and attacking healthy tissues, such as the pituitary gland, causing inflammation and subsequent dysfunction [32, 33].

Hypophysitis is more commonly observed with CTLA-4 inhibitors, such as ipilimumab, compared to PD-1 and PD-L1 inhibitors, like nivolumab and pembrolizumab. Nonetheless, the risk of hypophysitis should be considered when using any ICIs, and patients should be closely monitored for signs and symptoms [34, 35].

Hypophysitis is more common with CTLA-4 inhibitors than PD-1/PD-L1 inhibitors [36].

8.2.2 Thyroid Dysfunction

ICIs can cause thyroid dysfunction, which can manifest as hypothyroidism or overt hyperthyroidism [37]. This immune response can result in the destruction of thyroid tissue and the development of hypothyroidism or, initially, transient hyperthyroidism due to the release of preformed thyroid hormones through a process of destructive thyroiditis [38, 39].

Also, some tumor antigens might share structural similarities with thyroid antigens, leading to the activation of T cells that cross-react with both tumor and thyroid tissue (molecular mimicry). This cross-reactivity could result in an autoimmune attack on the thyroid gland, causing thyroid dysfunction [39, 40].

8.2.3 Autoimmune Diabetes

ICIs have been reported to cause autoimmune diabetes, also known as insulin-dependent diabetes or type 1 diabetes mellitus, as a rare immune-related adverse event (irAE) [41]. This occurs when the immune system mistakenly attacks and destroys insulin-producing beta cells in the pancreas, leading to insulin deficiency and hyperglycemia.

The precise mechanism by which ICIs induce autoimmune diabetes is not yet fully understood [42].

8.2.4 Hypoparathyroidism

The development of hypoparathyroidism due to ICIs is a irAE.

Early detection and management of hypoparathyroidism in patients receiving ICIs are essential to prevent complications, such as hypocalcemia and associated symptoms like muscle cramps, tetany, and seizures. Patients should be monitored for symptoms of hypoparathyroidism. Appropriate treatment, such as calcium and vitamin D supplementation, should be initiated if necessary.

8.3 PSEUDOENDOCRINE CONDITIONS

8.3.1 Adrenal Fatigue

Adrenal Fatigue (AF) has recently gained immense traction within alternative medicine circles. Proponents of AF suggest that chronic stress causes adrenal gland dysfunction, leading to nonspecific symptoms, including fatigue, body aches, and sleep disruption; however, mainstream medical authorities – The Endocrine Society specifically – do not recognize AF as an official endocrine disorder.

The theory underlying AF rests on the idea that chronic stress places an excessive strain on adrenal glands, which are responsible for producing stress hormones like cortisol. Over time, this pressure may cause them to fatigue out, leaving patients vulnerable to AF symptoms.

Evidence supporting AF remains scarce and often anecdotal. No research studies have conclusively established a connection between chronic stress and reduced adrenal function and AF, and there are no established diagnostic criteria or laboratory tests that reliably detect it. The Endocrine Society issued a statement emphasizing that AF is not a legitimate medical condition and no scientific studies supports its diagnosis or treatment. Furthermore, adrenal insufficiency – an endocrine disorder – should never be confused with AF as the former can pose life-threatening dangers necessitating proper diagnosis and therapy [43]. Although scientific evidence has not proven AF, numerous over-the-counter adrenal supplements are being sold as treatments. These supplements typically consist of vitamins, minerals, and herbs which could potentially have unintended negative side effects.

- Dietary supplements do not face the same stringent testing and regulations as prescription medicines, thus affecting their quality, safety, and efficacy to varying degrees.
- Some adrenal supplements contain ingredients that interfere with normal adrenal function, leading to reduced hormone production. Prolonged use may even result in real adrenal insufficiency, which requires urgent medical intervention. The US Food and Drug Administration recently warned the public of the risks posed by over-the-counter supplements like "Artri King", which contains high concentrations of dexamethasone [44].
- Individuals who diagnose and self-treat their AF could be overlooking other medical conditions that are potentially responsible for their symptoms, like anemia. By solely treating AF, they might miss an opportunity for proper medical intervention to address a real medical diagnosis.

Clinical Pearl

Pseudoendocrine syndromes are a group of conditions that may mimic the signs and symptoms of true endocrine disorders but are not caused by hormonal deficiency or excess states.

8.3.2   Relative Adrenal Insufficiency

Relative adrenal insufficiency (RAI) is a controversial phenomenon that has been increasingly recognized in critically ill patients, particularly in those with severe septic shock. It is described as a state where the adrenal glands produce an insufficient amount of cortisol relative to the body's needs during periods of extreme stress, such as severe sepsis [45]. In severe septic shock, the overwhelming systemic infection and inflammation can lead to profound alterations in the hypothalamic–pituitary–adrenal (HPA) axis, resulting in an inadequate cortisol production required to meet the body's stress response [46, 47]. Several factors may contribute to the development of RAI in septic shock, including:

1. *Impaired cortisol synthesis:* Inflammation can inhibit the enzymes responsible for cortisol synthesis, reducing the overall production of the hormone.
2. *Altered cortisol metabolism:* Inflammation can also affect the metabolism of cortisol, increasing its clearance from the body.
3. *Reduced cortisol availability:* High levels of circulating inflammatory mediators can lead to increased cortisol binding to its carrier protein, reducing the availability of free, biologically active cortisol.

Diagnosing RAI in septic shock is challenging due to the lack of a universally accepted diagnostic criteria. A commonly used diagnostic test is the adrenocorticotropic hormone (ACTH) stimulation test, which measures the adrenal glands' ability to produce cortisol in response to ACTH administration. However, the interpretation of the test results is subject to debate, and there is no consensus on the cortisol cutoff levels that indicate RAI [45, 48].

Some experts propose the use of dynamic tests, such as the delta cortisol or the cortisol-to-ACTH ratio, to assess adrenal function more accurately. These tests take into account the baseline cortisol levels and the individual patient's physiological response to stress [49].

The optimal dosing, duration, and tapering of glucocorticoids in RAI are not well established, and the management strategies may vary depending on the severity of the septic shock and the individual patient's response to treatment [50].

8.3.3   Low T3 Syndrome

Low T3 syndrome, also known as Wilson's syndrome, is a controversial pseudoendocrine condition characterized by low levels of triiodothyronine (T3) and normal levels of thyroxine (T4) and thyroid-stimulating hormone (TSH). Although some alternative health practitioners argue that this condition is a legitimate and underdiagnosed cause of fatigue, weight gain, and other nonspecific symptoms, current consensus guidelines do not recognize Wilson's syndrome as a legitimate endocrine disorder [51].

Dr. Denis Wilson first proposed Wilson's syndrome as a possible explanation for a subset of hypothyroid patients presenting with nonspecific symptoms such as fatigue, weight gain, brain fog, and cold intolerance, but with normal TSH and T4 levels. He hypothesized that these patients might have a deficiency in the conversion of T4 to the more biologically active T3 hormone, leading to a state of "functional hypothyroidism" that goes undetected by conventional thyroid function tests. It is worth noting that this is not the same condition as the previously described deiodinase deficiency state (Thr92Ala) mentioned in Section 2.1.3.

The proposed pathophysiology of Wilson's syndrome involves a decreased conversion of T4 to T3 in peripheral tissues, leading to low serum T3 levels. This decrease may be due to various factors such as stress, inflammation, or illness. However, no clear causative mechanism has been established, and the relationship between low T3 levels and the reported symptoms remains speculative at best.

Diagnosing Wilson's syndrome is beset with various challenges, as no universally accepted diagnostic criteria exist. Low T3 levels, normal T4 and TSH levels, and a constellation of nonspecific symptoms primarily define the condition. However, these symptoms are common and can be caused by numerous other medical conditions, making it difficult to determine whether a true association exists between low T3 levels and the reported symptoms.

Moreover, transient fluctuations in thyroid hormone levels can occur in healthy individuals and in response to various stressors, such as illness, surgery, or fasting. These fluctuations typically resolve without intervention and do not warrant treatment.

The treatment for Wilson's syndrome, as proposed by Dr. Wilson, involves the administration of time-released T3 hormone, often using a protocol called the "Wilson's Temperature Syndrome Protocol." However, there is no scientific evidence supporting the efficacy or safety of this treatment approach. Moreover, using T3 hormone supplementation in patients with normal TSH levels can lead to overtreatment and potential harm, such as the development of hyperthyroidism or cardiac complications [52].

8.3.4　Hashimoto Encephalopathy

Hashimoto encephalopathy (HE), also referred to as Steroid Responsive Encephalopathy Associated with Autoimmune Thyroiditis (SREAT), is a rare but potentially reversible neurological disorder associated with autoimmune thyroiditis that manifests with cognitive dysfunction, psychiatric symptoms, seizures, and focal neurological deficits [53]. The condition may be immune-mediated; early recognition and prompt treatment with corticosteroids could result in significant improvement or even complete resolution of symptoms.

HE can typically be diagnosed on clinical suspicion and the presence of elevated thyroid peroxidase (TPO) antibodies – commonly seen among those suffering from autoimmune thyroiditis; however, elevated TPO antibodies alone do not confirm a diagnosis, as they may also exist among people without neurological symptoms [54].

Lumbar puncture and cerebrospinal fluid (CSF) analysis can aid in diagnosing and ruling out other potential causes of encephalopathy, such as infections or inflammation conditions [55]. CSF analysis may show signs of HE, such as mild-to-moderate lymphocytic pleocytosis, elevated protein levels, or the presence of oligoclonal bands; however, these results are nonspecific and could occur as part of any number of other inflammatory or autoimmune conditions [56].

Other diagnostic tests, including brain imaging (MRI) and electroencephalography (EEG), may reveal nonspecific abnormalities that support the diagnosis of HE, but they cannot stand alone as conclusive tests [57, 58].

Prompt therapy with corticosteroids such as prednisone or intravenous methylprednisolone is the cornerstone of treatment for HE. Steroids appear to exert their therapeutic effect by reducing inflammation and modulating immune response; most patients respond quickly with either significant improvement or complete resolution of symptoms as soon as starting on steroids; however, some may require long-term immunosuppressive therapy.

8.4　DRUGS OF ABUSE WITH ENDOCRINE SIDE EFFECTS

8.4.1　Cannabis

Cannabis sativa contains many cannabinoids that exert their psychoactive properties by binding to cannabinoid receptors known as CB1 and CB2, found throughout the central nervous system and peripheral tissues, such as glandular tissues [36, 37]. Tetrahydrocannabinol (THC) acts as the principal psychoactive constituent. THC exerts its effects by binding to receptors on cannabinoid receptors throughout both organ systems: CNS, for instance, and peripheral tissues, including glandular ones [59, 60].

The Endocannabinoid System (ECS) plays an integral part in maintaining homeostasis and regulating numerous physiological processes, such as those overseen by the Endocrine System. As THC interacts with ECS receptors, it could significantly impact hormonal regulation and related physiological functions [61].

8.4.1.1 Effects of THC on the Hypothalamic–Pituitary–Gonadal (HPG) Axis

THC has been shown to alter the hypothalamic–pituitary–gonadal (HPG) axis by interfering with gonadotropin-releasing hormone (GnRH) production; as a result, this decreases the secretion of LH and FSH from the anterior pituitary, which ultimately results in reduced fertility for both genders [62]. These hormonal shifts could manifest themselves with menstrual cycle irregularities for women and decreased sperm count for males, compromising fertility in both sexes [63].

8.4.1.2 Effects of THC on Energy Homeostasis and Metabolic Regulation

THC has been shown to influence appetite regulation by acting on CB1 receptors in the hypothalamus and other brain regions. Acute administration typically increases appetite, while chronic use may alter body weight or lead to altered adiposity distribution [64]. Furthermore, THC has been shown to improve fasting insulin levels and the insulin resistance score, homeostasis model assessment of insulin resistance (HOMA-IR) [65].

8.4.2 Opioids

Opioids are a class of potent analgesic drugs that exert their effects through interactions with opioid receptors in the central and peripheral nervous systems. Opioids, including morphine, heroin, and prescription painkillers, are widely used for their potent analgesic properties [66]. They exert their effects by binding to and activating mu (μ), delta (δ), and kappa (κ) opioid receptors, which are widely distributed throughout both the central and peripheral nervous systems [67].

While the analgesic effects of opioids have been extensively studied, their impact on the endocrine system is an area of growing interest.

8.4.2.1 Effects of Opioids on the Hypothalamic–Pituitary–Adrenal (HPA) Axis

Studies in healthy volunteers have shown that naloxone, an opioid antagonist which acts on mu receptors, promotes increased corticotropin-releasing hormone and cortisol release. By inference, it has been postulated that opioids exert significant inhibition of the HPA axis at the level of the hypothalamus [68]. Chronic exposure to opioid analgesics can result in opioid-induced adrenal insufficiency (OIAI), with patients presenting with postural instability, fatigue, nausea, and weight loss [69].

 Practice Pearl

Opioid-induced adrenal insufficiency occurs in up to a third of patients on long-term treatment with opiates. As such, all patients on these agents who develop clinical symptoms concerning for adrenal insufficiency should be screened for this condition [68]. It is worth noting that glucocorticoid replacement therapy results in prompt resolution of symptoms in up to 70% of patients. Furthermore, discontinuation or dose reduction in opiates leads to the resolution of OIAI [70].

8.4.2.2 Effects of Opioids on the Hypothalamic–Pituitary–Gonadal (HPG) Axis

Opioids have been shown to disrupt the HPG axis by inhibiting the release of GnRH from the hypothalamus. This results in decreased secretion of luteinizing hormone (LH) and follicle-stimulating hormone (FSH) from the anterior pituitary, ultimately reducing testosterone and estradiol production [71]. Furthermore, opioids increase the release of prolactin which subsequently promotes hypogonadotropic hypogonadism. Opioid-induced hypogonadism can manifest as sexual dysfunction and infertility in both men and women [72].

8.4.3 Amphetamines

Amphetamines are stimulant drugs known for their potent effects on the central nervous system. While their impact on neurotransmitter release and neuronal function has been extensively studied, their influence on the endocrine system has received comparatively less attention.

8.4.3.1 Effects on the Hypothalamic–Pituitary–Adrenal Axis

Methamphetamine abuse (MA) can harm the HPA axis – an essential system involved with stress response – leading to functional and morphological alterations within this axis. Some of the deleterious effects of MA abuse include altered stress hormone release as well as changes to genes or proteins such as corticotropin-releasing factor (CRF), arginine vasopressin (AVP) receptor, and glucocorticoid receptor (GR) [73].

MA activates the HPA axis by stimulating secretagogues of ACTH, such as CRF and AVP, in hypothalamic paraventricular neurons (PVN). This action activates cells within the anterior pituitary gland that produce ACTH, which in turn triggers the adrenal cortex to release cortisol, which then circulates throughout the body to exert its physiological effects [74].

Although activation of the HPA axis can serve a protective function during times of threat or stress, prolonged activation may become harmful, leading to excessive levels of corticosteroids being released into the bloodstream and having adverse impacts on the brain tissue by way of increasing cell death, altering proliferation patterns or dendritic remodeling. Furthermore, prolonged exposure may influence gene and protein expression associated with HPA activation within our bodies [73].

These changes cause lasting disruption in HPA axis function, including altered levels of stress hormone release; this disruption is characteristic of depressive and anxiety spectrum disorders and its negative mood states, including anxiety and depression [75].

8.4.3.2 Effects on the Thyroid

Amphetamines and other amphetamine-like medications are known to have significant effects on the hypothalamic–pituitary–thyroid axis [76, 77]. Indeed, some studies have suggested that amphetamines could lead to alterations in TSH, T3, and T4 levels, although these results have not been consistent across all research [78].

8.4.4 Anabolic Androgenic Steroids

Anabolic androgenic steroids (AAS) are synthetic derivatives of testosterone that have gained popularity over time in both medical and nonmedical settings. Their use may be legal or illegal; regardless, its popularity continues to increase [79]. There are two distinct classes of anabolic steroids: 17 alpha alkyl derivatives such as oxandrolone, fluoxymesterone, and oxymetholone; and 17 beta ester derivatives like testosterone cypionate, testosterone enanthate, and testosterone propionate [80]. Nandrolone phenpropionate, classified as a C18 androgenic anabolic steroid, was one of the earliest anabolic steroids used as performance-enhancing medications by professional athletes during the 1960s and was banned from Olympic competition by the International Olympic Committee in 1974. All anabolic steroids are classified by U.S. Drug Enforcement Administration as Schedule III drugs [81–83].

The HPG axis is responsible for regulating reproductive function. AAS misuse can disrupt the HPG axis by accentuating a negative feedback loop that suppresses the release of GnRH from the hypothalamus [84]. This results in decreased secretion of LH and FSH from the anterior pituitary, ultimately leading to reduced endogenous testosterone production. The consequences of AAS-induced HPG axis disruption in men include testicular atrophy, decreased sperm count, and infertility [85]. In comparison, AAS misuse in women results in a deepening of the female voice and clitoromegaly [86].

Androgenic anabolic steroids acting via the androgen receptor primarily its physiologic effects at the level of skeletal muscle. Elevated testosterone levels promote an increase in muscle fiber size, ultimately promoting their strength and resistance to injury [87]. Abusers of androgenic steroids utilize these agents in hopes of improving their muscle strength and endurance.

8.4.5 SERMs

Selective estrogen receptor modulators (SERMs) is an umbrella term encompassing an assortment of compounds with tissue-selective activity when they bind with estrogen receptors (ERs). Depending on the tissue context, SERMs can act either as estrogen agonists or antagonists, leading to various pharmacological outcomes. Although predominantly used to treat various medical conditions like breast cancer, osteoporosis, and infertility, SERMs have recently come under scrutiny as potential drugs of abuse among athletes and bodybuilders alike [88]. Indeed, some athletes and bodybuilders abuse SERMs illegally as performance enhancers or to combat estrogenic side effects from anabolic steroids use, or to gain performance advantages over their fellow competitors [89].

Examples of SERMs abused by athletes include tamoxifen and clomiphene citrate. Tamoxifen is typically used along with aromatase inhibitors to limit the estrogenic side effects of being on supraphysiologic doses of androgens. Clomiphene citrate, on the other hand, helps in the recovery of the hypothalamic–pituitary–testicular axis after a prolonged period of androgen abuse.

In normal physiology, testosterone is converted to estradiol through the activity of the aromatase enzyme. Estradiol has various effects, including negative feedback inhibition of the HPG axis through its direct effects on endogenous gonadotropin (LH and FSH) production. Consequently, estradiol promotes the development of glandular breast tissue (gynecomastia), which is undesirable in male bodybuilders [90]. Aromatase inhibitors are used by male bodybuilders to offset this side effect. Also, negative feedback inhibition of gonadotrophs by elevated levels of estradiol promotes both infertility and reduction in the size of the testes. SERMs have antiestrogenic effects at the level of the anterior pituitary gland, which helps in mitigating the side effects of hyperestrogenemia on gonadotropin production [91].

Testosterone is also converted into the more active dihydrotestosterone (DHT) by the 5α-reductase enzyme in mainly the prostate gland, liver, and skin. The increased local activity of this enzyme in the scalp promotes male pattern hair loss, a potentially undesirable side effect of testosterone abuse [92].

 Practice Pearl

List important side effects of aromatase inhibitors and SERMs [93]

Aromatase inhibitors

Loss of bone mineral density
Sexual dysfunction (loss of libido)
Fat maldistribution (central adiposity)

SERMs

Headaches
Vasomotor symptoms
Vision changes

PRACTICE-BASED QUESTIONS

1. A 45-year-old woman presents to the clinic with a 3-month history of fatigue, body aches, and sleep disturbances. She has no significant medical history and takes no medications. She has read about adrenal fatigue and believes she may have it. What should be the appropriate response?

   a. Prescribe adrenal supplements
   b. Diagnose her with adrenal fatigue and start treatment
   c. Order an ACTH stimulation test
   d. Explain that adrenal fatigue is not recognized by mainstream medicine and investigate other potential causes of her symptoms

   Correct answer: d. Despite the patient's belief that she may have adrenal fatigue, mainstream medical authorities do not recognize it as an official endocrine disorder. Therefore, it is important to investigate other potential causes of her symptoms.

2. A 55-year-old man is admitted to the ICU with severe septic shock. The medical team is considering the possibility of relative adrenal insufficiency (RAI). Which of the following best describes the suspected mechanism of RAI in this patient?

   a. Overactivity of the adrenal glands leading to excess cortisol production
   b. Underactivity of the adrenal glands leading to insufficient cortisol production
   c. Impaired conversion of T4–T3
   d. Overactivity of the HPA axis leading to excessive cortisol release

   Correct answer: b. RAI is described as a state where the adrenal glands produce an insufficient amount of cortisol relative to the body's needs during periods of extreme stress, such as severe sepsis.

3. A 35-year-old woman presents with fatigue, weight gain, brain fog, and cold intolerance. Her TSH and T4 levels are normal, but T3 levels are low. She is concerned she might have Wilson's syndrome. What is the best next step in management?

   a. Start her on T3 hormone supplementation
   b. Reassure her that Wilson's syndrome is not recognized by mainstream endocrinology

c. Start her on a high dose of corticosteroids

d. Advise her to take over-the-counter adrenal supplements

Correct answer: b. While some practitioners argue that Wilson's syndrome is a legitimate cause of nonspecific symptoms, mainstream endocrinology practitioners do not recognize it as a legitimate endocrine disorder.

4. A 48-year-old woman presents to the neurology clinic with cognitive impairment, memory loss, confusion, and occasional hallucinations. She has a history of autoimmune thyroiditis. Thyroid peroxidase (TPO) antibodies are elevated. What is the most likely diagnosis?

a. Alzheimer's disease

b. Wilson's syndrome

c. Hashimoto encephalopathy

d. Adrenal fatigue

Correct answer: c. Hashimoto encephalopathy is a rare neurological disorder associated with autoimmune thyroiditis that presents with cognitive dysfunction, psychiatric symptoms, and elevated TPO antibodies.

5. A 60-year-old woman is diagnosed with Hashimoto encephalopathy and is started on treatment. Which of the following medications would be the cornerstone of her treatment?

a. Levothyroxine

b. Intravenous methylprednisolone

c. Naloxone

d. Adrenal supplements

Correct answer: b. Hashimoto encephalopathy is typically treated with corticosteroids such as prednisone or intravenous methylprednisolone to reduce inflammation and modulate immune response.

6. A 30-year-old male with a history of chronic cannabis use presents to the clinic complaining of sexual dysfunction and low libido. What mechanism best describes the potential impact of chronic cannabis use on his symptoms?

a. THC stimulates the production of gonadotropin-releasing hormone (GnRH).

b. THC increases the secretion of LH and FSH from the anterior pituitary.

c. THC decreases the secretion of LH and FSH from the anterior pituitary.

d. THC has no effect on the hypothalamic–pituitary–gonadal (HPG) axis.

Correct answer: c) THC decreases the secretion of LH and FSH from the anterior pituitary. Explanation: Chronic cannabis use is known to alter the hypothalamic–pituitary–gonadal (HPG) axis by interfering with gonadotropin-releasing hormone (GnRH) production, which leads to decreased secretion of LH and FSH from the anterior pituitary. This can result in reduced fertility in both males and females and sexual dysfunction in males, including low libido.

7. A 45-year-old woman with chronic low back pain managed with long-term opioid therapy presents with fatigue, nausea, and weight loss. She denies any changes in diet, exercise, or stress levels. What should be suspected in this case?

a. Opioid-induced adrenal insufficiency

b. Opioid-induced liver damage

c. Opioid-induced renal failure

d. Opioid-induced thyroid dysfunction

Correct answer: a) Opioid-induced adrenal insufficiency. **Explanation:** Chronic exposure to opioid analgesics can result in opioid-induced adrenal insufficiency (OIAI). Symptoms suggestive of OIAI include postural instability, fatigue, nausea, and weight loss.

8. A 28-year-old male with a history of methamphetamine abuse presents with symptoms of depression and anxiety. These symptoms are most likely due to changes in which system?

a. The hypothalamic–pituitary–thyroid (HPT) axis

b. The hypothalamic–pituitary–adrenal (HPA) axis

c. The hypothalamic–pituitary–gonadal (HPG) axis

d. The hypothalamic–pituitary–somatotropic (HPS) axis

Correct answer: b) The hypothalamic–pituitary–adrenal (HPA) axis. **Explanation**: Methamphetamine abuse can cause lasting disruptions in the hypothalamic–pituitary–adrenal (HPA) axis, including altered levels of stress hormone release. This disruption is characteristic of depressive and anxiety spectrum disorders.

9. A 35-year-old male bodybuilder is found to have gynecomastia and reduced testes size. He admits to the use of anabolic steroids. What could be a potential treatment strategy to mitigate these side effects?

   a. The use of aromatase inhibitors and SERMs
   b. Discontinuing the use of anabolic steroids
   c. Increasing the dose of anabolic steroids
   d. Supplementing with testosterone

   Answer: a) The use of aromatase inhibitors and SERMs. **Explanation**: Anabolic androgenic steroid (AAS) misuse can disrupt the HPG axis and promote the development of glandular breast tissue (gynecomastia) in males, which is undesirable for male bodybuilders. The use of aromatase inhibitors and selective estrogen receptor modulators (SERMs) can mitigate these side effects.

10. A 52-year-old woman with a 10-year history of type 1 diabetes comes to the clinic for her regular check-up. She has been managing her blood glucose levels using multiple daily injections and self-monitoring of blood glucose. Despite her best efforts, she struggles with frequent hypoglycemic episodes and wide fluctuations in her blood glucose levels. The clinician recommends considering an insulin pump and continuous glucose monitoring (CGM) system. Which of the following is NOT a benefit of using an insulin pump and CGM?

    a. Enhanced glycemic control
    b. Increased risk of hypoglycemia
    c. Trend analysis and pattern recognition
    d. Improved quality of life

    Correct answer: b. The use of an insulin pump and CGM actually reduces the risk of hypoglycemia. These systems enable patients to maintain tighter control of their blood glucose levels, identify low blood glucose levels more quickly, and adjust insulin doses accordingly, thereby decreasing the risk of hypoglycemic episodes.

11. A 30-year-old man with type 1 diabetes is currently using a hybrid-closed loop insulin pump system. What is the primary function of this type of insulin pump?

    a. It completely automates insulin delivery, requiring no input from the user.

    b. It administers bolus insulin doses for meals and corrects high blood glucose levels automatically.
    c. It automatically adjusts basal insulin delivery in response to real-time glucose levels.
    d. It eliminates the need for continuous glucose monitoring.

    Correct answer: c. A hybrid-closed loop insulin pump system, also known as an artificial pancreas, automatically adjusts basal insulin delivery based on real-time glucose levels. However, users are still required to manually administer bolus insulin doses for meals and to correct high blood glucose levels.

12. A 45-year-old woman with type 1 diabetes has started using a continuous glucose monitoring (CGM) system. Her endocrinologist is discussing the concept of "Time in Range" (TIR). What does this term refer to?

    a. The percentage of time the patient spends exercising each day
    b. The time it takes for insulin to start working
    c. The percentage of time the patient's blood glucose levels are within a specific target range
    d. The time it takes for the CGM system to adjust to changes in blood glucose levels

    Correct answer: c. Time in Range refers to the percentage of time an individual's blood glucose levels remain within a specified target range, typically between 70 mg/dL (3.9 mmol/L) and 180 mg/dL (10 mmol/L). It is an important metric in diabetes management and is closely associated with overall glycemic control.

13. A 55-year-old man with type 2 diabetes is considering the use of a CGM system. His doctor is explaining the importance of the Mean Absolute Relative Difference (MARD) in selecting a CGM system. What does a lower MARD value signify?

    a. The CGM system provides less reliable and less precise glucose measurements.
    b. The CGM system provides more reliable and precise glucose measurements.
    c. The CGM system has a higher risk of device malfunction.
    d. The CGM system has a lower rate of user satisfaction.

Correct answer: b. The Mean Absolute Relative Difference (MARD) is a statistical measurement used to assess the accuracy of continuous glucose monitoring (CGM) systems. A lower MARD value indicates that the CGM system provides more reliable and precise glucose measurements, which contributes to improved diabetes management and decision making.

REFERENCES

1. Nimri, R., Nir, J., and Phillip, M. (2020). Insulin pump therapy. *Am. J. Ther.* 27: e30–e41.

2. Sora, N.D., Shashpal, F., Bond, E.A., and Jenkins, A.J. (2019). Insulin pumps: review of technological advancement in diabetes management. *Am. J. Med. Sci.* 358: 326–331.

3. Moore, S.W. and Zaahl, M. (2010). Familial associations in medullary thyroid carcinoma with Hirschsprung disease: the role of the RET-C620 "Janus" genetic variation. *J. Pediatr. Surg.* 45: 393–396.

4. Dexcom G7 CGM - Powerfully simple diabetes management. Dexcom. https://www.dexcom.com/en-us/g7-cgm-system (accessed 14 May 2023).

5. Priyan, V. (2021). *Medtronic obtains CE mark for Guardian 4 Sensor and smart insulin pen.* Medical Device Network.

6. FreeStyle Libre 3 System | Our Smallest CGM Sensor. https://www.freestyle.abbott/us-en/products/freestyle-libre-3.html (accessed 14 May 2023).

7. Introducing the Eversense® E3 CGM System | Ascensia Diabetes Care. https://www.ascensiadiabetes.com/eversense/ (accessed 14 May 2023).

8. Martens, T., Beck, R.W., Bailey, R. et al. (2021). Effect of continuous glucose monitoring on glycemic control in patients with type 2 diabetes treated with basal insulin: a randomized clinical trial. *JAMA* 325: 2262–2272.

9. Gabbay, M.A.L., Rodacki, M., Calliari, L.E. et al. (2020). Time in range: a new parameter to evaluate blood glucose control in patients with diabetes. *Diabetol. Metab. Syndr.* 12: 22.

10. Boughton, C.K., Hartnell, S., Allen, J.M. et al. (2022). Training and support for hybrid closed-loop therapy. *J. Diabetes Sci. Technol.* 16: 218–223.

11. Usoh, C.O., Johnson, C.P., Speiser, J.L. et al. (2022). Real-world efficacy of the hybrid closed-loop system. *J. Diabetes Sci. Technol.* 16: 659–662.

12. Pleus, S., Stuhr, A., Link, M. et al. (2022). Variation of mean absolute relative differences of continuous glucose monitoring systems throughout the day. *J. Diabetes Sci. Technol.* 16: 649–658.

13. Reiterer, F., Polterauer, P., Schoemaker, M. et al. (2017). Significance and reliability of MARD for the accuracy of CGM systems. *J. Diabetes Sci. Technol.* 11: 59–67.

14. Darvin, P., Toor, S.M., Sasidharan Nair, V., and Elkord, E. (2018). Immune checkpoint inhibitors: recent progress and potential biomarkers. *Exp. Mol. Med.* 50: 1–11.

15. Lee, L., Gupta, M., and Sahasranaman, S. (2016). Immune checkpoint inhibitors: an introduction to the next-generation cancer immunotherapy. *J. Clin. Pharmacol.* 56: 157–169.

16. Hargadon, K.M., Johnson, C.E., and Williams, C.J. (2018). Immune checkpoint blockade therapy for cancer: an overview of FDA-approved immune checkpoint inhibitors. *Int. Immunopharmacol.* 62: 29–39.

17. Shiravand, Y., Khodadadi, F., Kashani, S.M.A. et al. (2022). Immune checkpoint inhibitors in cancer therapy. *Curr. Oncol.* 29: 3044–3060.

18. Marin-Acevedo, J.A., Kimbrough, E.O., and Lou, Y. (2021). Next generation of immune checkpoint inhibitors and beyond. *J. Hematol. Oncol.* 14: 45.

19. Atkins, M.B., Clark, J.I., and Quinn, D.I. (2017). Immune checkpoint inhibitors in advanced renal cell carcinoma: experience to date and future directions. *Ann. Oncol.* 28: 1484–1494.

20. Cappelli, L.C. and Bingham, C.O. (2021). Spectrum and impact of checkpoint inhibitor-induced irAEs. *Nat. Rev. Rheumatol.* 17: 69–70.

21. Sansom, D.M. (2000). CD28, CTLA-4 and their ligands: who does what and to whom? *Immunology* 101: 169–177.

22. Esensten, J.H., Helou, Y.A., Chopra, G. et al. (2016). CD28 costimulation: from mechanism to therapy. *Immunity* 44: 973–988.

23. Simon, S. and Labarriere, N. (2017). PD-1 expression on tumor-specific T cells: friend or foe for immunotherapy? *Onco. Targets. Ther.* 7: e1364828.

24. Philips, E.A., Garcia-España, A., Tocheva, A.S. et al. (2020). The structural features that distinguish PD-L2 from PD-L1 emerged in placental mammals. *J. Biol. Chem.* 295: 4372–4380.

25. Dong, Y., Sun, Q., and Zhang, X. (2016). PD-1 and its ligands are important immune checkpoints in cancer. *Oncotarget* 8: 2171–2186.

26. Rotte, A. (2019). Combination of CTLA-4 and PD-1 blockers for treatment of cancer. *J. Exp. Clin. Cancer Res.* 38: 255.

27. Seidel, J.A., Otsuka, A., and Kabashima, K. (2018). Anti-PD-1 and anti-CTLA-4 therapies in cancer: mechanisms of action, efficacy, and limitations. *Front. Oncol.* 8: 86.

28. Vandenborre, K., Van Gool, S.W., Kasran, A. et al. (1999). Interaction of CTLA-4 (CD152) with CD80 or CD86 inhibits human T-cell activation. *Immunology* 98: 413–421.

29. Fessas, P., Lee, H., Ikemizu, S., and Janowitz, T. (2017). A molecular and preclinical comparison of the PD-1–targeted T-cell checkpoint inhibitors nivolumab and pembrolizumab. *Semin. Oncol.* 44: 136–140.

30. Postow, M.A., Sidlow, R., and Hellmann, M.D. (2018). Immune-related adverse events associated with immune checkpoint blockade. *N. Engl. J. Med.* 378: 158–168.

31. Mahzari, M., Liu, D., Arnaout, A., and Lochnan, H. (2015). Immune checkpoint inhibitor therapy associated hypophysitis. *Clin. Med. Insights Endocrinol. Diabetes* 8: 21–28.

32. Mortensen MJ, Oatman O, Azadi A, Fonkem E, Yuen KCJ (2020). An update on immune checkpoint inhibitor-related hypophysitis.

33. Albarel, F., Gaudy, C., Castinetti, F. et al. (2015). Long-term follow-up of ipilimumab-induced hypophysitis, a common adverse event of the anti-CTLA-4 antibody in melanoma. *Eur. J. Endocrinol.* 172: 195–204.

34. Nguyen, H., Shah, K., Waguespack, S.G. et al. (2021). Immune checkpoint inhibitor related hypophysitis: diagnostic criteria and recovery patterns. *Endocr. Relat. Cancer* 28: 419–431.

35. Kotwal, A., Rouleau, S.G., Dasari, S. et al. (2022). Immune checkpoint inhibitor-induced hypophysitis: lessons learnt from a large cancer cohort. *J. Investig. Med.* 70: 939–946.

36. Di Dalmazi, G., Ippolito, S., Lupi, I., and Caturegli, P. (2019). Hypophysitis induced by immune checkpoint inhibitors: a 10-year assessment. *Expert. Rev. Endocrinol. Metab.* 14: 381–398.

37. Iwama, S., Kobayashi, T., Yasuda, Y., and Arima, H. (2022). Immune checkpoint inhibitor-related thyroid dysfunction. *Best Pract. Res. Clin. Endocrinol. Metab.* 36: 101660.

38. Muir, C.A., Wood, C.C.G., Clifton-Bligh, R.J. et al. (2022). Association of antithyroid antibodies in checkpoint inhibitor-associated thyroid immune-related adverse events. *J. Clin. Endocrinol. Metab.* 107: e1843–e1849.

39. Chera, A., Stancu, A.L., and Bucur, O. (2022). Thyroid-related adverse events induced by immune checkpoint inhibitors. *Front. Endocrinol.* 13: 1010279. https://doi.org/10.3389/fendo.2022.1010279.

40. Zhan, L., Feng, H., Liu, H. et al. (2021). Immune checkpoint inhibitors-related thyroid dysfunction: epidemiology, clinical presentation, possible pathogenesis, and management. *Front. Endocrinol. (Lausanne)* 12: 649863. https://doi.org/10.3389/fendo.2021.649863.

41. Kyriacou, A., Melson, E., Chen, W., and Kempegowda, P. (2020). Is immune checkpoint inhibitor-associated diabetes the same as fulminant type 1 diabetes mellitus? *Clin. Med. (Lond.)* 20: 417–423.

42. Chen, X., Affinati, A.H., Lee, Y. et al. (2022). Immune checkpoint inhibitors and risk of type 1 diabetes. *Diabetes Care* 45: 1170–1176.

43. Newman, M. (2017). Treating the symptoms that are believed to be adrenal fatigue. *Endocrine News.* https://endocrinenews.endocrine.org/myth-adrenal-fatigue/ (accessed 16 May 2023).

44. Research C for DE and (2022). *Public Notification: Artri King Contains Hidden Drug Ingredients.* FDA https://www.fda.gov/drugs/medication-health-fraud/public-notification-artri-ajo-king-contains-hidden-drug-ingredient.

45. Loriaux, D.L. and Fleseriu, M. (2009). Relative adrenal insufficiency. *Curr. Opin. Endocrinol. Diabetes Obes.* 16: 392–400.

46. Fleseriu, M. and Loriaux, D.L. (2009). "Relative" adrenal insufficiency in critical illness. *Endocr. Pract.* 15: 632–640.

47. de Jong, M.F.C., Beishuizen, A., Spijkstra, J.-J., and Groeneveld, A.B.J. (2007). Relative adrenal insufficiency as a predictor of disease severity, mortality, and beneficial effects of corticosteroid treatment in septic shock. *Crit. Care Med.* 35: 1896–1903.

48. Dickstein, G. (2005). On the term "relative adrenal insufficiency" – or what do we really measure with adrenal stimulation tests? *J. Clin. Endocrinol. Metabol.* 90: 4973–4974.

49. Meyer, N.J. and Hall, J.B. (2006). Relative adrenal insufficiency in the ICU: can we at least make the diagnosis? *Am. J. Respir. Crit. Care Med.* 174: 1282–1284.

50. Aucott, S.W. (2012). The challenge of defining relative adrenal insufficiency. *J. Perinatol.* 32: 397–398.

51. American Thyroid Association (2005). *American Thyroid Association Statement on "Wilson's Syndrome"*. https://www.thyroid.org/american-thyroid-association-statement-on-wilsons-syndrome/.

52. WTS Overview (2022). Wilson's Syndrome. https://www.wilsonssyndrome.com/identify/wts-overview/

53. Liyanage, C.K., Munasinghe, T.M.J., and Paramanantham, A. (2017). Steroid-responsive encephalopathy associated with autoimmune thyroiditis presenting with fever and confusion. *Case Rep. Neurol. Med.* 2017: 3790741.

54. Nagano, M., Kobayashi, K., Yamada-Otani, M. et al. (2019). Hashimoto's encephalopathy presenting with smoldering limbic encephalitis. *Intern. Med.* 58: 1167–1172.

55. Castillo, P., Woodruff, B., Caselli, R. et al. (2006). Steroid-responsive encephalopathy associated with autoimmune thyroiditis. *Arch. Neurol.* 63: 197–202.

56. Sharma, P.M.S., Javali, M., Mahale, R. et al. (2015). Hashimoto encephalopathy: a study of the clinical profile, radiological and electrophysiological correlation in a Tertiary Care Center in South India. *J. Neurosci. Rural Pract.* 6: 309–314.

57. Sharma, B., Bhavi, V.K., Nehra, H.R. et al. (2018). Steroid-responsive encephalopathy in autoimmune thyroiditis: a diagnostic enigma? *Thyroid Res. Pract.* 15: 52.

58. Jegatheeswaran, V., Chan, M., Chen, Y.A. et al. (2021). MRI findings of two patients with hashimoto encephalopathy. *Cureus* https://doi.org/10.7759/cureus.15697.

59. Brown, T.T. and Dobs, A.S. (2002). Endocrine effects of marijuana. *J. Clin. Pharmacol.* 42: 90S–96S.

60. Micale, V. and Drago, F. (2018). Endocannabinoid system, stress and HPA axis. *Eur. J. Pharmacol.* 834: 230–239.

61. Ranganathan, M., Braley, G., Pittman, B. et al. (2009). The effects of cannabinoids on serum cortisol and prolactin in humans. *Psychopharmacology* 203: 737–744.

62. Belladelli, F., Boeri, L., Capogrosso, P. et al. (2021). Substances of abuse consumption among patients seeking medical help for uro-andrological purposes: a sociobehavioral survey in the real-life scenario. *Asian J. Androl.* 23: 456.

63. Ilnitsky, S. and Van Uum, S. (2019). Marijuana and fertility. *CMAJ* 191: E638.

64. Sansone, R.A. and Sansone, L.A. (2014). Marijuana and body weight. *Innov. Clin. Neurosci.* 11: 50–54.

65. Penner, E.A., Buettner, H., and Mittleman, M.A. (2013). The impact of marijuana use on glucose, insulin, and insulin resistance among US adults. *Am. J. Med.* 126: 583–589.

66. Stein, C. (2018). New concepts in opioid analgesia. *Expert Opin. Investig. Drugs* 27: 765–775.

67. Pasternak, G.W. (1993). Pharmacological mechanisms of opioid analgesics. *Clin. Neuropharmacol.* 16: 1–18.

68. Donegan, D. and Bancos, I. (2018). Opioid-induced adrenal insufficiency. *Mayo Clin. Proc.* 93: 937–944.

69. Gordin, Y., Le, M., Quarde, A. et al. (2019). Recognizing adrenal insufficiency in substance use disorder: a case study of opioid-related suppression of hypothalamo-pituitary-adrenal axis. *Pain Med.* 20: 607–609.

70. Li, T., Donegan, D., Hooten, W.M., and Bancos, I. (2020). Clinical presentation and outcomes of opioid-induced adrenal insufficiency. *Endocr. Pract.* 26: 1291–1297.

71. Reddy, R.G., Aung, T., Karavitaki, N., and Wass, J.A.H. (2010). Opioid induced hypogonadism. *BMJ* 341: c4462.

72. Vuong, C., Van Uum, S.H.M., O'Dell, L.E. et al. (2010). The effects of opioids and opioid analogs on animal and human endocrine systems. *Endocr. Rev.* 31: 98–132.

73. Zuloaga, D., Jacobskind, J., and Raber, J. (2015). Methamphetamine and the hypothalamic-pituitary-adrenal axis. *Front. Neurosci.* 9.

74. Strajhar, P., Vizeli, P., Patt, M. et al. (2019). Effects of lisdexamfetamine on plasma steroid concentrations compared with d-amphetamine in healthy subjects: a randomized, double-blind, placebo-controlled study. *J. Steroid Biochem. Mol. Biol.* 186: 212–225.

75. Barr, A.M., Hofmann, C.E., Weinberg, J., and Phillips, A.G. (2002). Exposure to repeated, intermittent d-amphetamine induces sensitization of HPA axis to a subsequent stressor. *Neuropsychopharmacology* 26: 286–294.

76. Morley, J.E., Shafer, R.B., Elson, M.K. et al. (1980). Amphetamine-induced hyperthyroxinemia. *Ann. Intern. Med.* 93: 707–709.

77. Viswanath, O., Menapace, D.C., and Headley, D.B. (2017). Methamphetamine use with subsequent thyrotoxicosis/thyroid storm, agranulocytosis, and modified total thyroidectomy: a case report. *Clin. Med. Insights Ear Nose Throat* 10: 1179550617741293.

78. Little, K.Y., Garbutt, J.C., Mayo, J.P., and Mason, G. (2008). Lack of acute d-amphetamine effects on thyrotropin release. *Neuroendocrinology* 48: 304–307.

79. Ganesan, K., Rahman, S., and Zito, P. (2023). *Anabolic Steroids*. StatPearls.

80. Attarzadeh Hosseini, S.R., Rashid Lamir, A., and Dehbashi, M. (2016). Comparison of the effects of 17-alpha-alkyl steroids and 17-beta-hydroxy esters on the levels of liver enzymes and hematologicalfactors in male bodybuilders. *Internal Medicine Today* 22: 21–26.

81. Lusetti, M., Licata, M., Silingardi, E. et al. (2018). Appearance/image- and performance-enhancing drug users: a forensic approach. *Am J Forensic Med Pathol* 39: 325–329.

82. Jones, I.A., Togashi, R., Hatch, G.F.R. et al. (2018). Anabolic steroids and tendons: a review of their mechanical, structural, and biologic effects. *J. Orthop. Res.* 36: 2830–2841.

83. Armstrong, J.M., Avant, R.A., Charchenko, C.M. et al. (2018). Impact of anabolic androgenic steroids on sexual function. *Transl Androl Urol* 7: 483–489.

84. Vilar Neto, J.O., da Silva, C.A., Lima, A.B. et al. (2018). Disorder of hypothalamic-pituitary-gonadal axis induced by abusing of anabolic-androgenic steroids for short time: a case report. *Andrologia* 50: e13107.

85. El Osta, R., Almont, T., Diligent, C. et al. (2016). Anabolic steroids abuse and male infertility. *Basic Clin Androl* 26: 2.

86. Börjesson, A., Ekebergh, M., Dahl, M.-L. et al. (2021). Women's experiences of using anabolic androgenic steroids. frontiers in sports and active. *Living* 3.

87. Kam, P.C.A. and Yarrow, M. (2005). Anabolic steroid abuse: physiological and anaesthetic considerations. *Anaesthesia* 60: 685–692.

88. Kwok, K.Y., Chan, G.H.M., Kwok, W.H. et al. (2017). In vitro phase I metabolism of selective estrogen receptor modulators in horse using ultra-high performance liquid chromatography-high resolution mass spectrometry. *Drug Test. Anal.* 9: 1349–1362.

89. Vassallo, S.U. (2015). *Athletic Performance Enhancers*. Goldfrank's Toxicologic Emergencies.

90. Basaria, S. (2010). Androgen abuse in athletes: detection and consequences. *J. Clin. Endocrinol. Metabol.* 95: 1533–1543.

91. Rochoy, M., Danel, A., Chazard, E. et al. (2022). Doping with aromatase inhibitors and oestrogen receptor modulators in steroid users: analysis of a forum to identify dosages, durations and adverse drug reactions. *Therapies* 77: 683–691.

92. Swerdloff, R.S., Dudley, R.E., Page, S.T. et al. (2017). Dihydrotestosterone: biochemistry, physiology, and clinical implications of elevated blood levels. *Endocr. Rev.* 38: 220–254.

93. Bonnecaze, A.K., O'Connor, T., and Burns, C.A. (2021). Harm reduction in male patients actively using anabolic androgenic steroids (AAS) and performance-enhancing drugs (PEDs): a review. *J. Gen. Intern. Med.* 36: 2055–2064.

CHAPTER 9

Dynamic Tests in Clinical Endocrinology

9.1 PITUITARY GLAND

9.1.1 ACTH Stimulation Test (Adrenal Insufficiency)

9.1.1.1 Physiology

The ACTH stimulation test (adrenocorticotropic hormone, ACTH) is a diagnostic test used to evaluate adrenal gland function and diagnose conditions such as adrenal insufficiency and congenital adrenal hyperplasia [1, 2].

The hypothalamic–pituitary–adrenal axis (HPA) is a complex network of hormonal interactions that regulate the body's response to stress, immune function, and energy metabolism [3]. The HPA axis involves three key components: the hypothalamus, the pituitary gland, and the adrenal glands.

In response to stress or other stimuli, the hypothalamus releases CRH, which travels to the anterior pituitary gland [4]. In the anterior pituitary gland, CRH stimulates the release of ACTH. ACTH then enters the bloodstream and travels to the adrenal gland, located on the top of the kidneys [1].

The adrenal cortex is the outer layer of the adrenal gland, responsible for producing cortisol and other steroid hormones. ACTH stimulates the adrenal cortex to produce and release cortisol, which is a glucocorticoid hormone involved in the regulation of metabolism, immune function, and the stress response [2].

A negative feedback loop regulates cortisol levels in the bloodstream. For example, high levels of cortisol suppress the release of CRH and ACTH, leading to decreased cortisol production. On the contrary, low cortisol levels stimulate the release of CRH and ACTH, increasing cortisol production [3].

9.1.1.2 Mechanism of Action

The ACTH (cortrosyn or cosyntropin) stimulation test is performed to determine whether adrenal glands can produce cortisol appropriately in response to stimulation by exogenous ACTH [1].

A typical response to the cosyntropin stimulation test is characterized by a maximum cortisol level exceeding 18 mcg/dL at the 30- or 60-minute mark ([1]. In primary adrenal failure cases, cortisol concentration remains unchanged from the baseline level (usually <5 µg/dL), with an increase of less than 9 µg/dL after cosyntropin administration. More importantly, the maximum value of cortisol is typically below 18 µg/dL [1]. Similarly, in secondary adrenal insufficiency, the increase in cortisol levels after cosyntropin administration is also less than 9 µg/dL, and the maximum value does not exceed 18 µg/dL [5, 6].

Endocrinology: Pathophysiology to Therapy, First Edition. Akuffo Quarde.
© 2024 John Wiley & Sons Ltd. Published 2024 by John Wiley & Sons Ltd.

Historically, the established threshold for post-stimulation cortisol has been 18 mcg/dL, a value determined using older polyclonal antibody-based immunoassays. Recently, newer immunoassays have been developed, such as the Roche Elecsys II assay, which employs monoclonal antibodies and offers a lower detection limit for cortisol. As a result, when using these advanced assays, the acceptable post-stimulation cortisol level at 60 minutes is typically above 15 mcg/dL, rather than the traditional cut-off of 18 mcg/dL [5].

9.1.1.3 Practice Guide

The test involves administering a synthetic form of ACTH (such as cosyntropin) intravenously or intramuscularly to the patient. Venous blood samples are then collected at specified intervals (typically 30 and 60 minutes after administration) to measure cortisol levels [1].

Before undergoing the cortrosyn stimulation test, patients should abstain from glucocorticoids for at least 24 hours, as common exogenous steroids such as hydrocortisone and prednisone can be detected in cortisol assays [7]. Although dexamethasone does not cross-react with the cortisol immunoassay, as such, it will not be spuriously detected as cortisol; it still transiently suppresses the HPA axis and will lead to low cortisol levels at baseline. However, the post-ACTH stimulation levels of cortisol will not be affected in patients exposed to dexamethasone before testing [8]. There are a few essential considerations to keep in mind when performing this test.

The influence of binding proteins on the measurement of total cortisol is crucial. Total cortisol, measured in most immunoassays, is calculated as the sum of free and bound cortisol. Examples of cortisol-binding proteins include corticosteroid-binding globulin (CBG) and albumin. Thus, medical conditions that alter these binding proteins can affect plasma cortisol levels measured in plasma [9]. Estrogen found in combined oral contraceptives increases CBG, which can lead to spuriously elevated total cortisol levels in patients undergoing this test. Furthermore, patients with low serum albumin levels (usually below 2.5 g per dL) will exhibit low total cortisol levels since albumin is a primary binding protein for cortisol [10].

The cortrosyn stimulation test cannot differentiate between primary and secondary adrenal insufficiency. Its primary purpose is to evaluate the adrenal glands' response to exogenous ACTH stimulation. Although the test exhibits high specificity for both primary and secondary adrenal insufficiency, it has low sensitivity for secondary adrenal insufficiency [11]. This is because the adrenal cortex remains responsive to exogenous ACTH stimulation within the first 3 months of the onset of secondary adrenal insufficiency. Consequently, the cortrosyn stimulation test may produce false negative results during the first few months of adrenal insufficiency in patients with secondary adrenal insufficiency [12, 13]. This occurs because, despite the lack of ACTH stimulation of cortisol production, the adrenal cortex can take up to 3 months to develop significant atrophy as such, will continue to maintain an adequate response to exogenous ACTH [14].

Clinical Trial Evidence

This research aimed to assess the diagnostic precision of high-dose (250 mcg) and low-dose (1 mcg) ACTH stimulation tests for the diagnosis of adrenal insufficiency. The authors searched six databases and included 30 studies with 1209 adults and 228 children (with a diagnosis of secondary adrenal insufficiency) and five studies with 100 patients with a diagnosis of primary adrenal insufficiency. The results showed that the high- and low-dose ACTH stimulation tests had similar diagnostic accuracy in adults and children, with low sensitivity and high specificity. The tests were sufficient to confirm, but not exclude, secondary adrenal insufficiency. For primary adrenal insufficiency, data were only available for the sensitivity of the high-dose ACTH stimulation test (92%; 95% confidence interval, 81–97%). The researchers concluded that both tests had comparable diagnostic accuracy, but their confidence in these estimates was low to moderate due to potential bias, heterogeneity, and imprecision [15].

 Clinical Pearl

If you believe a hormone is being overproduced, "suppress it." If you believe it is being underproduced, "stimulate it."

9.1.2 ACTH Stimulation Test (Non-Classic Adrenal Hyperplasia)

9.1.2.1 Physiology

Adrenal steroidogenesis and non-classic congenital adrenal hyperplasia (NCAH) were previously reviewed.

9.1.2.2 Mechanism of Action

NCAH is mainly caused by a partial deficiency of the enzyme 21-hydroxylase, which plays a crucial role in the synthesis of cortisol and aldosterone in the adrenal cortex [16]. This partial enzymatic block results in the shunting of cortisol precursors into the synthesis of androgens. 17-hydroxyprogesterone is a relevant marker of endogenous hyperandrogenemia and is useful in screening patients with NCAH [16–18].

During the ACTH stimulation test, cosyntropin is administered to the patient, usually by intramuscular injection. Cosyntropin stimulates the adrenal glands to produce cortisol and its precursors, including 17-hydroxyprogesterone [19].

In NCAH, the adrenal glands exhibit an exaggerated response to ACTH stimulation, resulting in elevated levels of 17-hydroxyprogesterone. This occurs due to the partial deficiency of 21-hydroxylase, leading to the accumulation of precursor molecules and the overproduction of androgens [20].

9.1.2.3 Practice Guide

When investigating hyperandrogenemia in women, the test should ideally be performed during the early follicular phase of their menstrual cycle. Additionally, oral contraceptive pills should be discontinued at least 8 weeks before the test because the levels of androgens are expected to reach their baseline after approximately 8 weeks of discontinuing combined oral contraceptives [21].

In this test, baseline 17-hydroxyprogesterone and cortisol samples are drawn. 250 mcg of cortrosyn is administered intramuscularly, followed by the collection of 17-hydroxyprogesterone and cortisol samples at the 60-minute mark. If the basal 17-hydroxyprogesterone level is below 200 ng/dL, the diagnosis of NCAH is improbable, and an ACTH stimulation test is unnecessary. However, if the basal 17-hydroxyprogesterone level exceeds 10,000 ng/ml (or 1000 ng/dL), it indicates classic 21-hydroxylase deficiency rather than late-onset congenital adrenal hyperplasia. For patients with basal 17-hydroxyprogesterone levels between 200 ng/ml and 10,000 ng/ml, an ACTH stimulation test is required [22].

Interpretation of the Test

- For patients with non-classic CAH, a value of 17-hydroxyprogesterone at 60 minutes between 1000 and –10,000 ng/dL is diagnostic.
- If the stimulated 17-hydroxyprogesterone at 60 minutes is less than 1000 ng/dL, then the patient is either a heterozygote or is unaffected.
- If the stimulated 17-hydroxyprogesterone at 60 minutes is greater than 10,000 ng/dL, then the patient has classic 21 hydroxylase deficiency [22].

Clinical Trial Evidence
There is a lack of consensus on the optimal cut-off limits for 17-hydroxyprogesterone when distinguishing non-classic CAH from a normal response [23].

9.1.3 Dexamethasone Suppression Test

9.1.3.1 Physiology

The dexamethasone suppression test (DST) is a diagnostic tool used primarily to evaluate cases of suspected endogenous hypercortisolemia. The pathophysiological basis of the DST lies in the ability of dexamethasone, a synthetic glucocorticoid, to exert negative feedback effects on the HPA axis and thus suppress the production of ACTH and cortisol (see Figure 9.1).

In the DST, dexamethasone is administered orally as a low-dose or high-dose test [24]. Low-dose DST is used to screen for Cushing's syndrome, while high-dose DST helps differentiate the etiology of Cushing's syndrome (pituitary vs. ectopic ACTH production) [25]. In a normal HPA axis response, cortisol production should be suppressed after dexamethasone administration. The lack of suppression of cortisol

Circadian rhythm is part of the body's **internal clock**; it follows a 24-hour schedule and regulates the sleep–wake cycle.

During the 24-hour cycle, our hormone levels fluctuate in response to light, particularly **cortisol**.

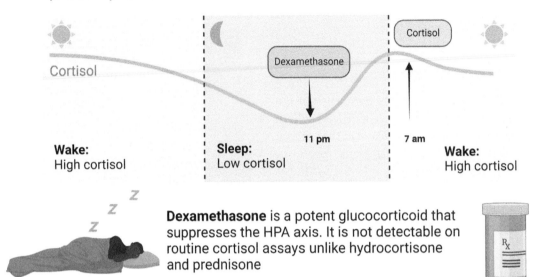

FIGURE 9.1 Circadian rhythm and cortisol regulation.

production may indicate an abnormal HPA axis response, suggesting Cushing's syndrome or another disorder that affects cortisol regulation [26, 27].

9.1.3.2 Mechanism of Action

Dexamethasone, a synthetic glucocorticoid, closely resembles cortisol in structure and function and acts on the same receptors as cortisol. Hence, the administration of dexamethasone suppresses ACTH and cortisol secretion, allowing the evaluation of feedback control of the HPA axis. This helps in potentially identifying cases of Cushing's syndrome or other disorders that affect cortisol regulation [28].

Normal circadian regulation of cortisol curve showing the times of dexamethasone administration and plasma cortisol sampling.

9.1.3.3 Practice Guide

Dexamethasone, an exogenous glucocorticoid, is highly potent (up to 15 times more potent than hydrocortisone) and significantly inhibits the HPA axis [29]. In particular, it does not bind to cortisol-binding globulin, allowing it to cross the blood–brain barrier easily.

A 1 mg dose of dexamethasone is administered between 11 and 12 pm, with serum cortisol sampling occurring between 8 and 9 am (see Figure 9.2). The timing of dexamethasone administration is crucial for suppressing ACTH secretion, which begins at 3 am. and peaks around 7 am. A diagnosis of endogenous hypercortisolemia is suggested when the levels of post-suppression cortisol exceed 1.8 μg/dL (95% sensitivity and 80% specificity) [30]. The HPA axis generally recovers in 24 hours after a single dose of 1 mg of dexamethasone dose [31].

Clinical Trial Evidence

A meta-analysis that included 50 studies with 1531 patients with Cushing's syndrome and 3267 control subjects demonstrated that the 1 mg overnight dexamethasone suppression test (DST), using a cortisol cut-off of 1.8 mcg/dL (50 nmol/L), had the highest sensitivity (98.6%) and specificity (90.6%) compared to other initial diagnostic tests for Cushing's syndrome [32].

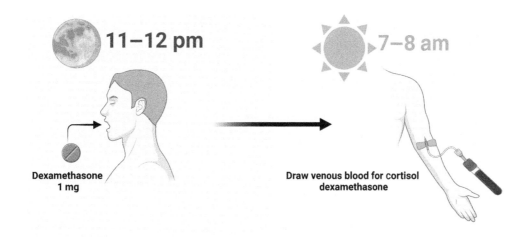

The cutoff for diagnosing endogenous hypercortisolemia is a post suppression cortisol level > 1.8 µg/dL with a sensitivity of 95% and a specificity of 80%.

Dexamethasone level within the expected range after an overnight administration. Dexamethasone level outside the reference range is likely due to rapid or slow metabolism.

FIGURE 9.2   Dexamethasone suppression test. Administration of oral dexamethasone around 11 pm and assessment of venous cortisol around 8 am.

Clinical Pearl

Understanding the clinical application of the Dexamethasone Suppression Test.

The indications and interpretation of various forms of the DST are shown in Table 9.1.

TABLE 9.1   Types of the dexamethasone suppression test.

Type of DST	Indication	Procedure	Interpretation
Two-day low-dose DST	Equivocal results of 24 h UFC, LNSC, or 1 mg ONDST.	Dexamethasone 0.5 mg tablet every 6 h × 48 h.ᵃ Early morning cortisol exactly 6 h after the last dose of dexamethasone.	Serum cortisol >1.8 mcg/dL is suggestive of Cushing's syndrome [33].
1 mg overnight dexamethasone suppression test (low-dose DST)	Evaluation of adrenal incidentaloma and screening for Cushing's syndrome.	Administration of 1 mg of dexamethasone at 11 pm followed by an evaluation of fasting serum cortisol at 8 am	Serum cortisol >1.8 mcg/dL is suggestive of Cushing's syndrome (screening test) [34], or > 3–5 mcg/dL is suggestive of subclinical Cushing's syndrome (adrenal incidentaloma) [30].
8 mg overnight dexamethasone suppression test (high-dose DST)	Differentiating between Cushing's disease and ectopic ACTH production for patients with ACTH-dependent Cushing's syndrome.	Baseline serum cortisol is drawn at 8–9 am, and 8 mg of dexamethasone is administered at 11 pm. Post-suppression cortisol is then drawn around 8–9 am the next morning.	Undetectable cortisol (normal response) [35]. Detectable cortisol but <5 mcg/dL (Cushing's syndrome). Suppression of cortisol >50% is diagnostic of Cushing's disease [36].

(continued)

TABLE 9.1   (Continued)

Type of DST	Indication	Procedure	Interpretation
Dexamethasone-CRH test	Differentiating between Cushing's syndrome and pseudo-Cushing's syndrome.	Dexamethasone 0.5 mg tablet every 6 h × 48 h.[b] Early morning cortisol, exactly 2 h after the last dose of dexamethasone, 100 mcg of ovine CRH (oCRH) is administered as an IV bolus (8 am). Cortisol is then drawn 15 min after oCRH.	Post Dex-CRH cortisol of >1.4 mcg/dL suggests Cushing's syndrome and rules out pseudo-Cushing's syndrome [37].

24 h, UFC 24 hour urinary free cortisol; LNSC, late-night salivary cortisol; 1 mg ONDST, 1 mg overnight dexamethasone suppression test; CRH, corticotropin-releasing hormone.
[a] 8 am, 2 pm, 8 pm, and 2 am
[b] 12 pm, 6 pm, 12 am and 6 am.

9.1.4   Glucagon Stimulation Test

9.1.4.1   Physiology

Glucagon, a peptide hormone secreted by alpha cells of the pancreas, plays a significant role in the regulation of growth hormone (GH) levels. Glucagon stimulates GH release by acting on the hypothalamus and increasing the secretion of growth hormone-releasing hormone (GHRH) [38]. GHRH, in turn, acts on the anterior pituitary gland to stimulate GH synthesis and release. Furthermore, GH is also influenced by other factors such as somatostatin (also known as growth hormone inhibitory hormone, GHIH) and ghrelin, which have inhibitory and stimulatory effects on GH secretion, respectively [39, 40].

The role of glucagon in the regulation of GH levels has been shown in several clinical studies. For example, intravenous glucagon administration leads to a significant increase in plasma GH levels [38]. This effect is believed to be mediated by the stimulation of GHRH secretion, as well as the suppression of somatostatin release, which has an inhibitory effect on GH secretion [39].

In addition to its direct effects on GH release, glucagon indirectly influences GH levels through its role in regulating blood glucose concentrations. For example, an increase in blood glucose levels leads to a decrease in GH secretion [41].

9.1.4.2   Mechanism of Action

Also, see Section 1.2.1 for the effects of glucagon and other GH secretagogues.

9.1.4.3   Practice Guide

The glucagon stimulation test is a diagnostic tool that is used to evaluate GH deficiency in patients suspected of having this condition. The test involves the administration of glucagon, which stimulates the release of GH from the anterior pituitary gland.

- The patient should fast for 8–12 hours before the test to ensure accurate results.
- A baseline blood sample is taken before glucagon administration to measure the patient's initial GH, glucose, and insulin levels.
- Glucagon is administered intramuscularly or subcutaneously, usually at a dose of 1 mg or 1.5 mg (if body weight is greater than 90 kg).
- Blood samples are collected at regular intervals after glucagon administration, typically 30, 60, 90, 120, 150, and 180 minutes. These samples are analyzed to measure GH, glucose, and insulin levels.

The maximum GH level is determined from the collected samples, and the results are interpreted based on the specific laboratory reference range. A maximum GH response less than a certain threshold (e.g. less than 3 ng/mL, though this may vary between laboratories) may indicate GH deficiency [42].

It is important to note that the glucagon stimulation test is not without potential side effects, and some patients may experience nausea, vomiting, or dizziness during the test. Additionally, the test may not be suitable for patients with certain medical conditions, such as pheochromocytoma, due to the risk of fluctuation in blood pressure [43].

Interpretation of the Test

A peak GH level below 3 ng/mL (failure to respond to glucagon) suggests growth hormone deficiency. This diagnostic threshold has sensitivity and specificity of 97% and 88%, respectively, for diagnosing growth hormone deficiency [44].

Clinical Trial Evidence

The study aimed to evaluate the glucagon stimulation test as an alternative to the insulin tolerance test (ITT) in the diagnosis of growth hormone deficiency (GHD). The researchers studied 33 patients with known pituitary disease (age 21–60 years) and a control group of 25 individuals matched in age and sex, selected by ITT if their peak GH response was >5.0 ng/mL. The results showed that the maximum GH after glucagon was significantly lower in the patient group compared to the control group $(0.49 \pm 0.85$ vs. 8.69 ± 5.85 ng/mL, $p = 0.0001)$.

Using receiver operating characteristic (ROC) plot analysis, the area under the curve was 0.982 for the response of the GH peak to glucagon. A 3.0 ng/mL cut-off threshold provided the best sensitivity (97%) and specificity (88%) to define GHD. The study concluded that the glucagon stimulation test demonstrates good performance and high diagnostic accuracy for the diagnosis of GHD, making it a suitable alternative to ITT [44].

9.1.5 Growth Hormone Suppression Test

9.1.5.1 Physiology

The oral glucose tolerance test (OGTT) evaluates the suppression of GH secretion in patients suspected of having acromegaly, a disorder characterized by excessive GH production and its subsequent effects on the body. The pathophysiologic basis of OGTT in evaluating acromegaly is based on the negative feedback regulation of GH secretion by glucose.

In normal individuals, GH secretion is inhibited by increased blood glucose levels, leading to a decrease in GH levels after glucose ingestion [45]. However, this negative feedback mechanism is impaired in patients with acromegaly, thus GH levels remain elevated or inadequately suppressed after glucose intake [46].

9.1.5.2 Mechanism of Action

The exact mechanism of glucose-induced suppression of GH is not fully understood. However, several theories have been proposed to explain the physiological process. Glucose-induced suppression of GH is believed to involve the hypothalamus and anterior pituitary gland, which are essential components of the hypothalamic–pituitary axis responsible for the regulation of GH secretion.

One theory suggests that increased blood glucose levels stimulate the release of somatostatin, also known as GHIH, from the hypothalamus [47]. Somatostatin acts on the anterior pituitary gland to inhibit GH secretion. Increased somatostatin release in response to glucose can result in the suppression of GH levels [48, 49].

Another theory proposes that elevated blood glucose levels may inhibit the secretion of GHRH from the hypothalamus [50]. GHRH is responsible for stimulating the release of GH from the anterior pituitary gland. By inhibiting GHRH release, glucose can suppress GH secretion [51].

Glucose may also have a direct inhibitory effect on the anterior pituitary gland, reducing GH secretion [52]. This mechanism may involve the detection of glucose by pituitary somatotroph cells, which could alter intracellular signaling pathways and decrease GH release.

9.1.5.3 Practice Guide

The GH suppression test is indicated in patients with mild to modest elevations in serum insulin-like growth factor 1 (IGF-1), defined as less than twofold of the upper limit of normal and accompanying equivocal clinical findings of GH excess [53].

To perform the GH suppression test, a modified OGTT is used. The patient must fast overnight before the test. A baseline blood sample is drawn to measure the initial level of GH. The patient ingests a 75 g oral glucose load, and subsequent blood samples are collected at regular intervals, usually every 30 minutes for up to 2 hours (30, 60, 90, and 120 minutes). These samples are analyzed to assess GH levels in response to an oral glucose challenge [54].

In healthy individuals, GH levels must be suppressed to a nadir value below 1 ng/mL after glucose ingestion [54]. In patients with acromegaly, GH levels remain elevated or are inadequately suppressed, suggesting impaired feedback regulation and abnormal GH secretion [55]. This traditionally accepted threshold of <1 ng/mL for the lowest GH level during the OGTT has long been accepted for distinguishing between normal and acromegalic patients. However, with the development of more sensitive GH assays, current guidelines recommend a much lower diagnostic threshold of 0.4 ng/mL. As such, failure to suppress at least one of the timed GH measurements during the OGTT to less than 0.4 ng/dL is suggestive of acromegaly [56].

Clinical Trial Evidence

In this study, the authors aimed to systematically compare sensitive growth hormone (GH), insulin-like growth factor I (IGF-I), and IGF-binding protein-3 (IGFBP-3) assays to define disease status in a large cohort of patients with persistent postoperative acromegaly. The traditional cut-off point for GH suppression, measured by polyclonal radioimmunoassay (RIA), was less than 2.0 μg/L after oral glucose. However, recent advances have suggested a cut-off of less than 1.0 μg/L. The study examined 60 postoperative acromegaly patients and 25 age-matched healthy subjects, assessing nadir GH levels after 100 g oral glucose and baseline IGF-I and IGFBP-3 levels. GH was assayed using polyclonal RIA, a sensitive immunoradiometric assay (IRMA), and a highly sensitive enzyme-linked immunosorbent assay (ELISA).

- GH levels after oral glucose, measured with highly sensitive GH assays, can be much lower in subjects with active disease than previously believed; values less than 1.0 μg/L can be found in up to 50% of patients.
- In 39% of patients in apparent remission with normal levels of IGF-I, GH determined by highly sensitive assays does not usually suppress, raising questions about the risk of recurrence of active disease in these patients.

The study highlights the importance of using modern assays for a more accurate assessment of disease activity in patients with acromegaly [57].

9.1.6 Water Deprivation Test

9.1.6.1 Physiology

The role of AVP in water conservation was reviewed in Chapter 1.

9.1.6.2 Mechanism of Action

The water deprivation test serves as a diagnostic method to differentiate between central diabetes insipidus (CDI) and nephrogenic diabetes insipidus (NDI), both of which cause excessive urination (polyuria) and extreme thirst (polydipsia) [58]. The fundamental principle is to evaluate the ability of a patient to concentrate urine in response to water deprivation and subsequent administration of desmopressin (DDAVP), a synthetic antidiuretic hormone (ADH) [59].

CDI and NDI are characterized by impaired ADH secretion or action, respectively [60]. CDI results from inadequate ADH production or release from the posterior pituitary gland, often due to hypothalamic or pituitary gland dysfunction [61]. On the other hand, NDI arises from the kidney's inability to respond appropriately to ADH action, which can be caused by genetic mutations or specific medications [62].

9.1.6.3 Practice Guide

The Water Deprivation Test (WDT) is a widely used diagnostic tool consisting of two steps: an initial 8-hour period of water deprivation followed by the administration of desmopressin, a synthetic ADH. This test is based on the measurement of urine osmolality to assess renal antidiuretic hormone (AVP) action. Dehydration leads to an increase in plasma sodium concentration, which in turn stimulates AVP release. AVP then acts on the kidneys, causing an increase in urine osmolality. If the stimulus for AVP secretion is sufficient, urine osmolality should increase to more than 700 mOsm/kg, differentiating patients with normal vasopressin secretion and function from those with CDI or NDI, who cannot maximally concentrate urine during dehydration. However, patients with prolonged significant polyuria of any cause may not concentrate their urine maximally due to the effects of chronic polyuria on renal concentrating capacity [58].

The second part of the test, the administration of desmopressin, is designed to differentiate CDI from NDI. In CDI, a physiological increase in urine osmolality should occur after desmopressin administration.

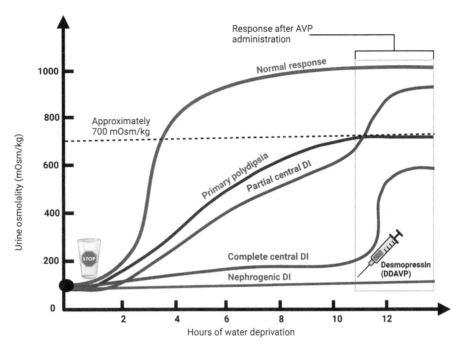

FIGURE 9.3 Results of the water deprivation test. Comparison of urine osmolality and hours of water deprivation. Distinguishing between various cases of polyuria based on the response of urine osmolality to DDVAP administration.

However, different authors have varying opinions on the accepted normal level, ranging from 700 to 800 mOsm/kg (see Figure 9.3). In NDI, urinary concentration remains dilute after desmopressin administration. In the cases of diagnostic uncertainty, a hypertonic saline test with AVP, in addition to measurement of plasma copeptin may be performed [58].

9.1.7 Inferior Petrosal Sinus Sampling

9.1.7.1 Physiology

Inferior Petrosal Sinus Sampling (IPSS) is a specialized diagnostic procedure employed to distinguish the origin of excessive cortisol production in patients with Cushing's syndrome [63]. Cushing's disease, a subtype of Cushing's syndrome, involves increased cortisol production resulting from a pituitary adenoma, which is a nonmalignant tumor in the pituitary gland. The fundamental principles of IPSS are based on the anatomy of the pituitary gland and its associated venous drainage system [64].

The pituitary gland, a small, pea-sized organ, is located at the base of the brain within the sella turcica, a bony structure in the sphenoid bone [65]. This gland is crucial to controlling various hormones in the body, including the ACTH, which stimulates the production of cortisol by the adrenal glands [66].

The inferior petrosal sinuses are paired bilateral venous channels that drain blood from the cavernous sinuses, which receive blood directly from the pituitary gland, and eventually empty into the internal jugular veins [67].

In Cushing's disease, the pituitary gland produces excessive ACTH, leading to increased cortisol production by the adrenal glands. IPSS is performed to verify that the pituitary gland is, in fact, the source of excessive ACTH and not an ectopic source within the body [68].

During the procedure, catheters are inserted into the inferior petrosal sinuses, typically accessed via the femoral veins. Blood samples are collected simultaneously from the inferior petrosal sinuses and a peripheral vein before and after the administration of corticotropin-releasing hormone (CRH) or desmopressin. CRH triggers the pituitary gland to release ACTH, and subsequently, blood samples are analyzed for ACTH levels [69].

In Cushing's disease, ACTH levels in the inferior petrosal sinus blood samples will be markedly higher than those of peripheral blood samples, indicating a pituitary origin of ACTH [70]. Furthermore, the side that exhibits higher ACTH levels may suggest the location of the pituitary adenoma. On the contrary, suppose that the ACTH levels in the inferior petrosal sinus blood samples are not significantly higher than those in peripheral blood. In that case, it implies that excessive cortisol production is not due to an adenoma in the pituitary gland, suggesting ectopic ACTH production or adrenal tumors [69, 71].

9.1.7.2 Mechanism of Action

CRH, a hypothalamic peptide hormone, plays a central role in the regulation of the release of ACTH from the pituitary gland. When CRH binds to its receptors in pituitary corticotroph cells, it stimulates the synthesis and release of ACTH into the bloodstream [72]. The increase in circulating ACTH, in turn, causes the adrenal glands to produce cortisol. In the context of IPSS, the administration of CRH helps confirm whether the excess ACTH is produced by the pituitary gland [73].

Desmopressin, a synthetic analog of vasopressin, can also stimulate the release of ACTH from the pituitary gland. Although vasopressin's primary function is water homeostasis, it also has a secondary function of stimulating ACTH release in certain situations, such as stress [74]. Desmopressin binds to vasopressin V3 receptors on corticotroph cells in the pituitary gland, leading to an increase in intracellular calcium and subsequent release of ACTH [75]. In IPSS, desmopressin can be used instead of CRH when CRH is not available or is contraindicated [69].

9.1.7.3 Practice Guide

IPSS with CRH stimulation is performed after diagnosing ACTH-dependent Cushing's syndrome when an MRI of the pituitary gland is inconclusive (pituitary adenoma measuring less than 6 mm in size) [76]. This test helps to confirm whether the pituitary is the source of ACTH and rules out the production of ACTH by an ectopic tumor [77].

Catheters are placed in the femoral veins and threaded up to the inferior petrosal sinus, with intravenous contrast that ensures the correct placement. Four baseline ACTH measurements are taken before CRH administration, followed by blood sampling from both central and peripheral lines at 2, 5, 10, and 15 minutes [64].

 Interpretation of the Test

Plasma ACTH values are normalized to the prolactin value to account for any catheter location or movement. A central to peripheral ACTH gradient equal to or greater than 2 before CRH administration or equal to or greater than 3 after CRH infusion indicates a pituitary source of ACTH production (Cushing's disease) [64, 78].

Clinical Trial Evidence

The study evaluated the diagnostic accuracy of inferior petrosal sinus sampling (IPSS) compared to pituitary imaging techniques to differentiate between various causes of ACTH-dependent Cushing's syndrome. It involved 97 patients, including 74 with Cushing's disease (CD) and 10 with ectopic ACTH secretion (EAS). The results showed that the diagnostic precision of IPSS, using the basal and post-CRH ACTH inferior petrosal sinus: peripheral (IPS: P) ratios, was significantly higher than magnetic resonance imaging (MRI) and computed tomography (CT). Specifically, diagnostic accuracy was 86% for the basal ratio and 90% for the post-CRH ratio, compared to 50% for MRI and 40% for CT. However, IPSS was less reliable in identifying the site of adenoma found in surgery than MRI or CT. In conclusion, IPSS improves diagnostic performance compared to imaging techniques and can help prevent unnecessary transsphenoidal surgery in patients with EAS patients [78].

9.1.8 TRH Stimulation Test

9.1.8.1 Physiology

The pathophysiological basis for the use of the thyrotropin-releasing hormone (TRH) stimulation test in central hypothyroidism lies in the role TRH plays in regulating the hypothalamic–pituitary–thyroid axis. In central hypothyroidism, hypothalamic or pituitary gland dysfunction leads to decreased thyroid-stimulating hormone (TSH) and, subsequently, low levels of thyroid hormone levels [79]. In normal physiology, TRH, produced by the hypothalamus, stimulates the pituitary gland to release TSH, which, in turn, stimulates the thyroid gland to produce thyroid hormones [80].

The TRH stimulation test is helpful in assessing the pituitary gland's response to TRH, providing information on possible defects in the hypothalamic–pituitary–thyroid axis [79]. By measuring TSH levels before and after TRH administration, we can determine whether the pituitary gland's response is adequate or impaired [80]. An abnormal response may indicate central hypothyroidism and help guide further diagnostic evaluations and treatment strategies.

9.1.8.2 Mechanism of Action

The role of TRH in the HPT axis was reviewed in Chapter 2.

9.1.8.3 Practice Guide

Dynamic testing with TRH does not hold diagnostic significance for secondary hypothyroidism or for forecasting the likelihood of developing TSH deficiency. For these reasons, the TRH stimulation test is rarely used to assess pituitary reserve [81, 82]. Furthermore, intravenous administration of TRH could potentially induce apoplexy in patients with pre-existing pituitary adenomas [83].

Clinical Trial Evidence

The study aimed to evaluate the diagnostic value of the thyrotropin-releasing hormone (TRH) stimulation test for the diagnosis of central hypothyroidism in patients with Sheehan syndrome. The test was performed in 72 patients, and the diagnosis of central hypothyroidism was made based on specific criteria. The results showed that 56 (77.7%) patients had low serum levels of free T4 and free T3 with inappropriately low serum levels of TSH (CH0 group). Ten (13.8%) patients with normal or low normal free thyroid hormone levels did not respond or had a delayed response to the TRH stimulation test (CH1 group). Six (8.3%) patients had normal free T3, free T4, and TSH levels and maximum TSH responses consistent with euthyroidism. In total, 66 (91.6%) of the 72 patients with Sheehan syndrome had central hypothyroidism. The TRH stimulation test proved useful in diagnosing central hypothyroidism, particularly in patients with low normal free T4 or TSH and known hypothalamo-pituitary pathology [84].

9.1.9 GnRH Stimulation Test

9.1.9.1 Physiology

The gonadotrophin-releasing hormone (GnRH) test, also known as the GnRH stimulation test, is a diagnostic tool used in the evaluation of reproductive disorders. Although it has limited diagnostic value in most clinical settings, the test remains relevant for confirming gonadotroph reserve in patients undergoing pulsatile GnRH therapy for infertility [85] and for evaluating precocious puberty [86].

GnRH is a critical component of the hypothalamic–pituitary-gonadal axis (HPG), which controls the reproductive system in males and females [87]. Pulsatile secretion of GnRH stimulates the release of luteinizing hormone (LH) and follicle-stimulating hormone (FSH) from the anterior pituitary, which, in turn, regulate the development and function of the gonads (ovaries and testes) [88].

9.1.9.2 Mechanism of Action

The mechanism of action of GnRH was reviewed in Section 6.1.4.

9.1.9.3 Practice Guide

There is limited use of this dynamic test in clinical practice.

Clinical Trial Evidence

Limited clinical trial data investigating the utility of this test in practice.

9.2 DISORDERS OF THE THYROID GLAND

9.2.1 Levothyroxine Absorption Test

9.2.1.1 Physiology

Levothyroxine absorption occurs mainly in the small intestine, and the majority of the process occurs within the first 3 hours after ingestion. On average, only 60–80% of the dose administered of the drug is absorbed by the body [89]. The physiological process of levothyroxine absorption is influenced by factors such as gastric pH [90], food intake [91], and the presence of certain medications, which can alter the rate and extent of absorption [92]. Furthermore, the bioavailability of levothyroxine can be affected by individual factors such as age, gastrointestinal disorders, and genetic polymorphisms [93]. An in-depth understanding of the various factors that affect levothyroxine absorption is essential to optimize its therapeutic efficacy in patients with thyroid disorders. Indeed, these factors in addition to nonadherence to therapy by patients should be considered as a possible reason for suboptimal response to thyroid hormone replacement therapy.

9.2.1.2 Mechanism of Action

The mechanism of action of thyroid hormone was reviewed in Chapter 2.

9.2.1.3 Practice Guide

The levothyroxine absorption test is recommended for hypothyroid patients who struggle to reach therapeutic thyroid hormone levels despite adhering to the appropriate dose of levothyroxine. This situation is identified by TSH levels that exceed the upper limit of the reference range while taking a daily dose of LT4 dosage of ≥1.9 mcg/kg [94]. The test assesses a patient's ability to absorb levothyroxine by examining serum T4 levels before and after administering a test dose of the drug. The process typically involves the following steps:

- A blood sample is taken to determine the patient's initial serum T4 level.
- The patient receives a test dose of levothyroxine, typically 1000 mcg, which is consumed orally on an empty stomach.
- Another blood sample is drawn 2–4 hours after the test dose to measure the serum T4 level.
- The percentage of levothyroxine absorption is calculated by comparing the pre- and post-dose T4 levels.

Estimation of Levothyroxine Absorption

$$\%\text{absorption} = \left[\text{peak } \Delta\text{T4} \times \text{volume distribution}\left(\text{dL}\right) \right.$$

$$\left. \text{Dose administered of LT4}\left(\text{mcg}\right) \right] \times 100$$

$$\text{Volume distribution}\left(\text{dL}\right)$$
$$= 4.42 \times \text{body mass index}\left(\text{kg/m}^2\right)$$

The normal percentage of levothyroxine absorption is 60–80% [89, 95].

Clinical Trial Evidence

The study aimed to evaluate the levothyroxine absorption test to determine pseudo malabsorption in patients with primary hypothyroidism. The standardization of the test and the criteria for conducting a malabsorption test were unclear. The study involved various groups: euthyroid, newly diagnosed hypothyroid, hypothyroid treated with normalized TSH, hypothyroid with elevated TSH despite an adequate dose of levothyroxine, and subjects with euthyroid with true malabsorption. Participants received levothyroxine (10 µg/kg or a maximum of 600 µg), and their free T4 levels were measured at hourly intervals for 5 hours.

The results showed that free T4 peaked at 3 hours in all groups, with a marginally insignificant decrease at 4 hours. The increases in free T4 in the groups, except for malabsorption, were not statistically different. The mean increment of free T4 in true malabsorption was 0.39 ng/dL, while it was 0.78 ng/dL for other groups combined. A free T4 increase at 3 hours above 0.40 ng/dL had a sensitivity of 97% and a specificity of 80% to exclude true malabsorption (AUC 0.904, $p < 0.001$).

In conclusion, the levothyroxine absorption test can reliably diagnose nonadherence to treatment in subjects with elevated TSH on adequate doses of LT4. An incremental value greater than 0.40 ng/dL (5.14 pmol/L) at 3 hours can help identify individuals whose malabsorption workup is unnecessary [96].

9.2.2 Radioactive Iodine Scans in Thyroid Cancer (Withdrawal)

9.2.2.1 Physiology

The pathophysiological basis of the radioactive iodine (RAI) scan using the withdrawal protocol is based on the preferential uptake of RAI by thyroid cells due to their unique ability to concentrate iodine. This property is used to image the thyroid gland and diagnose various thyroid conditions, such as hyperthyroidism, thyroid cancer, and thyroid nodules [97].

The withdrawal protocol in the context of the management of differentiated thyroid cancer requires discontinuation of thyroid hormone replacement therapy, specifically levothyroxine, for a period of time prior to the scan, typically 4–6 weeks [98]. This protocol aims to increase the levels of TSH in the blood. Elevated TSH levels (typically >30 mIU/mL) stimulate the thyroid gland to absorb more iodine, enhancing the effectiveness of the RAI scan [98].

When the patient undergoes the RAI scan, a small dose of RAI (I-123 or I-131) is administered orally. Thyroid cells absorb RAI, and a gamma camera captures images of the distribution of the radioactive substance in the thyroid gland [99].

9.2.2.2 Mechanism of Action

The role of iodine in thyroid hormone synthesis is reviewed in Chapter 2.

Iodine-131 (I-131) and Iodine-123 (I-123) are RAI isotopes used in nuclear medicine for diagnostic and therapeutic purposes, particularly to assess thyroid function [100].

I-131 is a beta and gamma-emitting isotope with an 8-day half-life, used primarily to diagnose and treat hyperthyroidism and thyroid cancer [101]. It is absorbed by the thyroid gland similarly to non-RAI, allowing evaluation of thyroid function and visualization of the structure of the gland. Due to the longer half-life and increased radiation exposure, I-131 has limitations for some diagnostic applications [102].

I-123, a gamma-emitting isotope with a 13-hour half-life, is more suitable for certain diagnostic purposes than I-131 due to its lower radiation exposure [103]. I-123 is not used for therapeutic purposes, as it lacks beta particle emissions necessary to destroy thyroid cells [104].

9.2.2.3 Practice Guide

A practical guide to interpreting radioactive iodine scans during the evaluation of differentiated thyroid cancers is shown in Table 9.2.

Clinical Trial Evidence

This study investigated the use of recombinant human thyrotropin (rhTSH) as an alternative to the withdrawal of thyroid hormone for radioiodine detection in patients with differentiated thyroid cancer. The research included 127 patients who underwent whole-body radioiodine scanning using both methods. The results showed that the rhTSH-stimulated scans were equivalent to thyroid hormone withdrawal scans in 66% of the patients with positive scans, superior in 5%, and inferior in 29%. When considering all patients, both methods were equivalent in 83% of cases. Patients experienced fewer symptoms of hypothyroidism and mood disturbances with rhTSH administration. Although rhTSH scanning has lower sensitivity, it offers a viable alternative to the withdrawal of thyroid hormone with reduced side effects [106].

9.2.3 Radioactive Iodine Scans in Thyroid Cancer (Thyrogen)

9.2.3.1 Physiology

RAI scans are used to assess patients with thyroid cancer, particularly differentiated thyroid cancer, to detect residual or recurrent disease after thyroidectomy. Thyrogen, also known as rhTSH, is a synthetic form of TSH [107].

The hypothalamic–pituitary–thyroid axis was reviewed in Chapter 2.

TABLE 9.2 Interpretation of radioactive iodine scans.

Imaging findings	Management plan
Absent radioiodine uptake in the thyroid bed	Suboptimal TSH stimulation Poor adherence to a low-iodine diet
Increased focus of uptake in the thyroid bed	Possible excess remnant tissue or persistent thyroid cancer. The patient may require repeat surgery or fine needle biopsy
Focus of uptake outside the thyroid bed	Additional testing is required. Evaluate metastatic disease and consider dosimetrically guided instead of empiric I-131 activities for treatment

Source: Adapted from Ref. [105].

9.2.3.2   Mechanism of Action

In patients who have undergone thyroidectomy, the administration of recombinant human TSH (thyrogen) stimulates any remaining thyroid tissue or metastatic thyroid cancer cells to increase iodine uptake. This is because TSH acts on thyroid cells to increase sodium-iodide symporter (NIS) activity, which is responsible for the transport of iodine into the cells [108].

9.2.3.3   Practice Guide

Recombinant human TSH (rhTSH) was created to stimulate TSH without the withdrawal of thyroid hormone and the associated risks of clinical hypothyroidism. Administered by two consecutive daily injections, rhTSH leads to short-term elevation of TSH, which could potentially reduce the risks of tumor stimulation risks [109].

Clinical Trial Evidence

This study investigated the use of human thyroid stimulating hormone (rhTSH) recombinant as an alternative to thyroid hormone withdrawal (THW) to enhance iodine-131 uptake in patients with differentiated thyroid cancer (DTC) after thyroidectomy. Although rhTSH has potential benefits, its efficacy for residual or metastatic DTC has not been prospectively assessed.

This study analyzed four trials with 223 patients with DTC, finding no significant differences between rhTSH and THW in ablation rate. However, rhTSH treatment showed benefits in reduced radiation exposure to the blood and bone marrow and some improvement in health-related quality of life scores. No serious adverse effects or deaths were reported in either group. However, the study lacks sufficient data on metastatic DTC and long-term outcomes.

The authors concluded that rhTSH is as effective as THW for ablation of thyroid remnants with iodine-131. More randomized controlled trials are needed to evaluate the effectiveness of lower doses of iodine-131 and guide treatment selection for metastatic DTC [110].

9.3   DISORDERS OF THE ADRENAL GLANDS

9.3.1   Oral Sodium Loading Test

9.3.1.1   Physiology

The pathophysiologic basis of this test is based on the fact that aldosterone is responsible for sodium reabsorption in the kidneys. In primary hyperaldosteronism, there is an excess of aldosterone, leading to increased sodium reabsorption, which in turn leads to volume expansion and hypertension. By challenging the system with high sodium intake, the test aims to differentiate between normal physiology (in which aldosterone secretion should be suppressed) and primary hyperaldosteronism (in which aldosterone secretion remains inappropriately high) [111].

9.3.1.2   Mechanism of Action

See Chapter 3 for the role of aldosterone in the conservation of sodium and water.

9.3.1.3   Practice Guide

The patient is asked to consume a high-sodium diet for several days (typically 3 days). This high sodium intake suppresses the renin–angiotensin–aldosterone system (RAAS) in healthy individuals, leading to a decrease in aldosterone levels. Urinary sodium and aldosterone levels are measured after a high-sodium diet. In healthy individuals, increased sodium intake results in the suppression of aldosterone, while in patients with primary hyperaldosteronism, aldosterone secretion remains inappropriately high despite sodium loading [112].

If the urinary aldosterone level remains elevated (> 12 µg/24 hours) and the urinary sodium level is high (>200 mEq/24 hours) after sodium loading, it suggests that the patient has primary hyperaldosteronism [113]. This is because aldosterone levels should have been suppressed by high sodium intake if the RAAS were functioning normally [114].

Clinical Trial Evidence

This prospective study aimed to compare the captopril suppression test with the salt loading approach in confirming primary aldosteronism. A total of 49 patients with a suspected diagnosis of primary aldosteronism were included. Of the 49 patients, 44 had non-suppressible aldosterone concentrations, 22 had a unique adenoma, and 22 had presumed bilateral hyperplasia. A significant correlation was found between plasma aldosterone values in salt-loaded patients and values 2 hours after captopril administration ($r = 0.8$, $P < 0.01$). The study concluded that the captopril suppression test is as effective as sodium loading in confirming the diagnosis of primary aldosteronism diagnosis [115].

9.3.2 Intravenous Saline Suppression Test

9.3.2.1 Physiology

The pathophysiological basis of the saline suppression test is similar to what was described for the oral salt loading test in Section 9.3.1.

9.3.2.2 Mechanism of Action

See Chapter 3 for the role of aldosterone in the conservation of sodium and water.

9.3.2.3 Practice Guide

The Saline Infusion Test (SIT) involves administering 2 l of 0.9% saline intravenously over 4 hours to patients in the sitting position. Blood samples for aldosterone, renin, and cortisol are then collected before and after the infusion. Medications that could interfere with aldosterone and renin measurements are generally replaced by alpha-adrenoceptor blockers (e.g. doxazosin, prazosin), vasodilators (e.g. hydralazine), or non-dihydropyridine calcium channel blockers (e.g. verapamil) [116, 117].

Clinical Trial Evidence

This study aimed to prospectively investigate the precision of the saline infusion test (SIT) in diagnosing primary aldosteronism (PA). Of the 1115 patients screened in the PAPY study, 317 underwent plasma aldosterone, cortisol, and renin activity measurements after an intravenous infusion of 2 L of isotonic saline for 4 hours. The study found that 120 patients (37.9%) had PA, 46 (38.3%) had aldosterone-producing adenoma (APA), and 74 (61.7%) had idiopathic hyperaldosteronism (IHA). The SIT was safe and had no adverse effects. The area under the receiver–operator characteristic curves (AUC) was significantly higher than under the diagonal, indicating that the test was accurate in diagnosing PA, APA, and IHA. However, the study found that the test had moderate sensitivity and specificity due to overlapping values between patients with and without the disease and could not discriminate between APA and IHA. In conclusion, SIT was safe and specific in excluding PA, but was not effective in differentiating between APA and IHA [118].

9.3.3 Clonidine Suppression Test

9.3.3.1 Physiology

The clonidine suppression test (CST) is used to diagnose pheochromocytoma, a rare tumor of the adrenal gland that produces excessive amounts of catecholamines, such as epinephrine and norepinephrine. The pathophysiological basis of the CST lies in the effect of clonidine on the central nervous system and its ability to suppress catecholamine release [119].

Clonidine is an alpha-2 adrenergic agonist that acts on the central nervous system. It stimulates alpha-2 adrenergic receptors in the brain, which in turn inhibits the release of norepinephrine from nerve endings [120]. In a healthy individual, this leads to a decrease in circulating catecholamines (epinephrine and norepinephrine) and, therefore, to a reduction in blood pressure.

In the case of pheochromocytoma, tumor cells produce and secrete catecholamines independently of the control of the central nervous system. Consequently, when clonidine is administered during the suppression test, it will not significantly suppress the release of catecholamines from the tumor, as does in a healthy individual [121].

9.3.3.2 Mechanism of Action

Clonidine can reduce norepinephrine levels in the blood of healthy individuals by activating central alpha-adrenergic receptors. As the natural increase in catecholamines relies on the activation of the sympathetic nervous system, while the tumor-related release is thought to occur independently, clonidine can help differentiate between a healthy state and a true pheochromocytoma. This is because it inhibits catecholamine release that is triggered by the nervous system but not autonomous secretion caused by pheochromocytomas [122].

9.3.3.3   Practice Guide

The CST is performed in patients between 8:00 am and 9:00 am. Patients are instructed to avoid certain medications, smoking, and food for 12 hours prior to the test. During the test, the patients remained supine, with their blood pressure and heart rate monitored every 30 minutes. Blood samples are then collected after 30 minutes of supine rest and 3 hours after ingestion of clonidine, with the dose adjusted according to body weight. A CST result is considered normal if catecholamine levels are below age-adjusted upper reference limits (URL) or decrease by at least 40% compared to baseline after clonidine administration [123].

Clinical Trial Evidence

In a single-center prospective study involving 60 patients with suspected pheochromocytoma/paraganglioma (PPGL), the clonidine suppression test (CST) was evaluated for its role in the diagnosis of PPGL in patients with adrenal tumors and/or arterial hypertension. Of the 46 patients who entered the final analysis, CST demonstrated 100% specificity in excluding false positive normetanephrine (NMN) results. The sensitivity of CST increased from 85% to 94% when tumors with an increase in isolated metanephrine (MN) were not considered. CST accurately identified all patients without PPGL who had elevated baseline NMN. The study concluded that CST is a useful diagnostic tool for evaluating elevated plasma-free NMN in patients with suspected PPGL, correctly identifying all false positive NMN screening results [123].

9.3.4   Insulin Tolerance Test

9.3.4.1   Physiology

The pathophysiological basis for using insulin tolerance testing (ITT) in the evaluation of adrenal insufficiency lies in the body's response to induced hypoglycemia. ITT involves the administration of insulin, leading to a rapid decrease in blood glucose levels. This drop in blood glucose serves as a powerful physiological stressor, causing the hypothalamus to release CRH [124].

CRH stimulates the anterior pituitary gland to secrete ACTH, which, in turn, triggers the adrenal cortex to produce cortisol. Cortisol is a crucial hormone that promotes gluconeogenesis and restores plasma glucose levels.

In individuals with normal adrenal function, cortisol levels will increase in response to ITT-induced hypoglycemia. However, in patients with adrenal insufficiency, the cortisol response will be inadequate or absent due to impaired adrenal gland function, ACTH deficiency, or issues with the hypothalamic–pituitary–adrenal (HPA) axis.

Therefore, the insulin tolerance test serves as a valuable tool for assessing the integrity of the HPA axis and identifying adrenal insufficiency by evaluating the cortisol response to hypoglycemic stress.

9.3.4.2   Mechanism of Action

Insulin-mediated hypoglycemia triggers a stress response that involves the release of CRH, ACTH, and eventually cortisol.

9.3.4.3   Practice Guide

ITT is associated with an increased risk of complications and requires close medical supervision. Therefore, it is no longer routinely used in the evaluation of adrenal insufficiency or GH deficiency anymore [125].

Clinical Trial Evidence

See the practice guide.

9.3.5   Adrenal Venous Sampling

9.3.5.1   Physiology

Adrenal vein sampling (AVS) is a diagnostic procedure used to evaluate the cause of hyperaldosteronism, a condition characterized by excessive production of aldosterone, a hormone that regulates blood pressure and electrolyte balance [126]. Hyperaldosteronism can be due to primary aldosteronism (PA) or secondary aldosteronism [127].

AVS is used in the evaluation of hyperaldosteronism due to its diagnostic utility in differentiating between unilateral and bilateral adrenal diseases [128]. Unilateral adrenal disease, typically caused by an aldosterone-producing adenoma (APA) or unilateral adrenal hyperplasia (UAH), can be treated surgically, while bilateral adrenal hyperplasia (BAH) is treated medically [129].

9.3.5.2   Mechanism of Action

ACTH plays a crucial role in AVS, as it helps minimize the variability caused by the pulsatile secretion of aldosterone and the stress reaction during the procedure [130]. Pulsatile aldosterone secretion can create artifactual gradients between the right and left adrenal glands when blood sampling is performed sequentially, particularly if the interventionist is not proficient and fast enough [131]. The stress reaction that occurs when starting AVS can also exacerbate these problems and affect the assessment of lateralization [132].

To overcome these issues, some centers use ACTH infusion during the AVS procedure, known as ACTH-stimulated AVS [133]. ACTH is a hormone that stimulates the adrenal cortex to produce and release cortisol and aldosterone. When a continuous infusion of synthetic ACTH is administered, the adrenal glands are stimulated, reducing variability in aldosterone secretion and helping to obtain more consistent and accurate aldosterone-to-cortisol ratios (ACR) [134]. This, in turn, improves the interpretation of the lateralization index, a crucial determinant for differentiating unilateral and bilateral adrenal hyperaldosteronism [135].

9.3.5.3   Practice Guide

During AVS, both adrenal veins are sequentially accessed through a percutaneous bilateral femoral approach using fluoroscopic guidance. A 5 or 6 French vascular catheter is inserted into the femoral vein, allowing placement of 4 and 5 French catheters in each adrenal vein [136]. The accurate positioning of the catheter tip is verified by contrast enhancement. To minimize the time gap between the samples, the right adrenal vein (the most challenging) is sampled first, followed by the left adrenal vein, and finally, the external iliac vein. Blood samples are collected from each site to measure aldosterone and cortisol levels.

A continuous infusion of cosyntropin (at a rate of 50 mcg per hour) is initiated at least 30 minutes before adrenal gland sampling and continues throughout the procedure [137]. This helps counteract stress-induced increases in aldosterone production. Furthermore, cosyntropin enhances the cortisol gradient (comparing the adrenal gland to the inferior vena cava) and maximizes aldosterone secretion from the source of hyperaldosteronism, whether it is an APA or adrenal hyperplasia [138].

The interpretation of AVS is discussed in Chapter 4.

Clinical Trial Evidence

This study aimed to assess the impact of lateralization cut-off points from adrenal venous sampling (AVS) on surgical outcomes in 377 primary aldosteronism (PA). Clinical benefit and complete biochemical success were measured using the aldosterone lateralization index (LI). Clinical benefit was observed in 29 of 47 patients (LI 2–4), 66 of 101 patients (LI 4–10), and 158 of 203 patients (LI > 10). Complete biochemical success was achieved in 27 of 42 patients (LI 2–4), 60 of 76 patients (LI 4–10), and 127 of 155 patients (LI > 10). The study concluded that the use of a strict diagnostic threshold led to a relatively small difference in clinical outcomes, while an LI > 4 was sufficient to achieve a biochemical cure and appropriate to identify unilateral disease in PA patients [135].

9.4   DISORDERS OF THE PANCREAS

9.4.1   Oral Glucose Tolerance Test

9.4.1.1   Physiology

See Chapter 4 for the role of insulin in glucose homeostasis.

9.4.1.2   Mechanism of Action

Under normal physiological conditions, carbohydrate ingestion leads to the breakdown of complex sugars into glucose, which subsequently enters the bloodstream. The resulting elevation in blood glucose levels stimulates pancreatic insulin secretion, a hormone that facilitates cellular glucose uptake and maintains glucose homeostasis [139, 140].

Individuals with insulin resistance, as observed in prediabetes (impaired glucose tolerance) or type 2 diabetes mellitus, experience persistent hyperglycemia after oral glucose challenge due to the diminished capacity of insulin to promote glucose uptake by cells [141].

9.4.1.3   Practice Guide

The OGTT is a diagnostic procedure used to assess an individual's ability to metabolize glucose and is particularly helpful in diagnosing diabetes.

The patient must fast for at least 8 hours prior to the test to ensure accurate results. Patients should be instructed to not consume any food or caloric beverages during this period. A blood sample is taken from the patient before the glucose load is administered. This fasting blood glucose measurement serves as a baseline for comparison with subsequent samples. The patient receives a glucose-containing solution to drink, which typically contains 75 g of glucose for adults or a weight-adjusted dose for children [142]. Blood samples are collected at specific intervals after the patient has consumed the glucose solution. These intervals usually include 1 and 2 hours after ingestion, although additional time points can be included depending on the specific protocol followed [143].

Blood samples are analyzed to determine glucose levels at each time point. These measurements are then compared to the baseline fasting blood glucose level and established diagnostic criteria. Based on blood glucose levels obtained during the OGTT, a diagnosis of normal glucose tolerance, impaired glucose tolerance (prediabetes), or diabetes can be made. In general, higher blood glucose levels and slower return to baseline levels indicate a reduced ability to metabolize glucose, suggesting the presence of diabetes or prediabetes.

For adults, the standard diagnostic criteria for an OGTT are as follows.

Blood glucose 2 hours after consuming the glucose solution.

Normal: less than 140 mg/dL (7.8 mmol/L)

Impaired glucose tolerance (prediabetes): 140–199 mg/dL (7.8–11.0 mmol/L)

Diabetes: 200 mg/dL (11.1 mmol/L) or higher [144].

Clinical Trial Evidence

This study aimed to determine to what extent insulin sensitivity and release could be predicted from an oral glucose tolerance test (OGTT). The researchers evaluated insulin sensitivity using the euglycemic-hyperinsulinemic clamp and insulin release using the hyperglycemic clamp in 104 non-diabetic volunteers who also underwent an OGTT. Demographic parameters, plasma glucose, and insulin values were used in multiple linear regression models to predict glucose metabolic clearance rate (MCR), insulin sensitivity index (ISI), and insulin release in the first phase (first PH) and second phase (second PH) insulin release.

The resulting equations for MCR and ISI, which included BMI, insulin (120 min) and glucose (90 minutes), demonstrated strong correlations with measured MCR ($r = 0.80$, $P < 0.00005$) and ISI ($r = 0.79$, $P < 0.00005$). Similarly, the equations for the first and second PH, which included insulin (0 and 30 minutes) and glucose (30 minutes), showed strong correlations with the first PH ($r = 0.78$, $P < 0.00005$) and the second PH ($r = 0.79$, $P < 0.00005$). The study concluded that insulin sensitivity and release could be predicted with reasonable precision using demographic parameters and values obtained during an OGTT. The derived equations could be useful in clinical settings where clamping is used, or the minimal model would be impractical [145].

9.4.2   The 72-Hour Fast

9.4.2.1   Physiology

When hypoglycemia occurs, there is a marked decrease in insulin production by pancreatic beta cells. Subsequently, this is followed by an increase in glucagon secretion from alpha cells of the pancreas. If hypoglycemia continues, additional counterregulatory hormones are released. The release of epinephrine leads to the characteristic hyperadrenergic symptoms associated with hypoglycemia. Finally, GH and cortisol are secreted as the final stress responses to hypoglycemia [146].

Symptoms that trigger behavioral defense of food consumption typically develop at an average plasma glucose concentration of approximately 55 mg/dL

(3.0 mmol/L). At this concentration and lower, insulin secretion is almost completely suppressed; plasma insulin levels fall below 3 U/mL (18 pmol/L), C-peptide levels drop below 0.6 ng/mL (0.2 nmol/L), and proinsulin levels are below 5.0 pmol/L [147].

9.4.2.2 Mechanism of Action

See Section 4.3.5.

9.4.2.3 Practice Guide

See Section 4.3.5.

Clinical Trial Evidence

The aim of this study is to evaluate the need for a full 72-hour fast for the diagnosis of insulinoma.

Patients with suspected hypoglycemia and documented glucose levels below 45 mg/dL were admitted to the NIH. Data from a supervised fast of patients with pathologically confirmed insulinoma over a 30-year period were reviewed. A total of 127 patients with insulinoma were identified, with an average age of 42.7 ± 15.9 years and a predominance of women (62%). Among them, 107 had benign tumors, 20 had malignant insulinomas, and 15 had multiple endocrine neoplasia type 1.

The fast was stopped due to hypoglycemia in 44 patients (42.5%) in 12 hours, 85 patients (66.9%) by 24 hours, and 120 (94.5%) by 48 hours. Seven patients fasted for 48 hours despite subtle neuroglycopenic symptoms and glucose and insulin levels indicative of insulinoma. Immunoreactive proinsulin was elevated at the beginning of the fast in 90% of 42 patients. Proinsulin levels in noninsulinoma patients, in contrast to insulinoma patients, are usually suppressible, so samples taken in the suppressed state provide the greatest diagnostic value.

The study concludes that with current insulin and proinsulin assays, the diagnosis of insulinoma can be made within 48 hours of a supervised fast [148].

9.4.3 The Secretin Stimulation Test

9.4.3.1 Physiology

Secretin, a peptide hormone consisting of 27 amino acids, was initially discovered by Starling and is synthesized in various human tissues such as the small intestine, hypothalamus, and neocortex [149]. By binding to its specific receptors found in pancreatic ductal and acinar cells, secretin plays a crucial role in stimulating the secretion of a bicarbonate-rich fluid [150]. This fluid is essential for neutralizing gastric acid present in the small intestine, thus maintaining an optimal environment for the digestion and absorption of nutrients [151].

9.4.3.2 Mechanism of Action

Secretin stimulates the release of pancreatic juices while inhibiting gastric acid secretion and intestinal motility at the same time [152]. In normal physiology, secretin stimulates the release of pancreatic fluid (containing bicarbonate), which, upon reaching the duodenum plays a pivotal role in neutralizing gastric acid and raising the duodenal pH. In so doing, this exerts a negative feedback inhibition that regulates secretin release.

In patients with gastrin-secreting tumors, secretin causes a paradoxical increase in gastrin release rather than its inhibition, as occurs in normal physiology. This forms the basis for the secretin stimulation test performed to diagnose hypergastrinemia [153].

9.4.3.3 Practice Guide

Secretin Stimulation Test Procedure

- Ensure that the patient has not consumed any food for a minimum of 12 hours prior to the test.
- Insert an intravenous cannula (heplock) to maintain easy access to the patient's veins during the test.
- Collect a venous blood sample at the beginning of the test to establish the patient's basal fasting serum gastrin levels. Obtain at least two baseline samples.
- Administer an intravenous bolus of secretin in 30 seconds, using a dose of 0.4 mcg per kg of body weight of synthetic human secretin.
- Measure gastrin levels after secretin injection in the following time intervals: 2, 5, 10, 15, and 20 minutes (using a gold top tube).
- Remove intravenous access and label the collected samples.
- Keep in mind that different authors suggest various diagnostic thresholds, leading to a range of sensitivities and specificities. Consider an

increase in gastrin levels after secretin administration (relative to baseline) of 200 pg/mL, 120 pg/mL, or 110 pg/mL [154].

Clinical Trial Evidence

Evaluating fasting serum gastrin (FSG) is crucial to diagnosing and managing Zollinger–Ellison syndrome (ZES). However, existing studies on FSG levels in patients with gastrinoma have limitations due to small sample sizes, varied methodologies, and the absence of correlations with clinical, laboratory, or tumor characteristics in patients with ZES. To address this, a prospective National Institutes of Health (NIH) study was conducted of 309 patients with ZES, and its results were compared to those of 2229 patients with ZES patients in 513 smaller studies and case reports in the literature.

The findings revealed that normal FSG values were rare (0.3–3%) among patients with ZES, as well as very high FSG levels >100-fold normal (4.9–9%). Two-thirds of gastrinoma patients had FSG values <10-fold normal, which overlapped with levels seen in more prevalent conditions such as *Helicobacter pylori* infection or antral G-cell hyperplasia/hyperfunction. In these cases, FSG levels alone were not diagnostic for ZES, necessitating provocative gastrin tests for a definitive diagnosis.

Most clinical variables did not correlate with FSG levels, but a strong correlation was found between FSG values and certain clinical characteristics, such as prior gastric surgery, diarrhea, and the time from onset to diagnosis. Furthermore, increasing basal acid production (but not maximal acid production) was closely correlated with increasing FSG. Several tumor characteristics, including location, primary size, and extent, were also found to correlate with FSG levels [154].

9.5 DISORDERS OF THE REPRODUCTIVE ORGANS

9.5.1 Progestin Challenge Test

9.5.1.1 Physiology

Normal menstrual cycles are regulated by a complex interplay of hormones involving the hypothalamic-pituitary-ovarian (HPO) axis. The pulsatile release of GnRH from the hypothalamus stimulates the anterior pituitary gland to secrete FSH and LH. FSH and LH act on the ovaries, promoting follicular growth and the production of estrogen. During the midcycle, a spike in LH levels triggers ovulation and the formation of the corpus luteum, which secretes progesterone [155].

Estrogen plays a vital role in the proliferation of the endometrial lining during the follicular phase, while progesterone, secreted during the luteal phase, stabilizes and prepares the endometrium for potential implantation. If fertilization does not occur, the corpus luteum regresses, leading to a decrease in progesterone levels and shedding of the endometrial lining, presenting as a normal menstruation. See Figure 6.5.

9.5.1.2 Mechanism of Action

The mechanism of action is reviewed in Chapter 7.

9.5.1.3 Practice Guide

The Progestin Challenge Test assesses the presence of adequate estrogen levels and the endometrial response to progesterone. Synthetic progestin (e.g. medroxyprogesterone acetate) is administered for a short period, typically 5–10 days, to mimic progesterone's effect on the endometrium during the luteal phase [156]. If there is adequate estrogen, the endometrium will proliferate and respond to progestin.

Withdrawal bleeding after stopping progestin administration indicates a normal estrogen level and an intact HPO axis, suggesting that amenorrhea is probably due to anovulation or hypothalamic–pituitary dysfunction. In such cases, further evaluation is required to identify the cause of anovulation or hormonal imbalance.

In contrast, the absence of withdrawal bleeding after the progestin challenge implies insufficient estrogen levels, an unresponsive endometrium, or an obstruction of the outflow tract. Low estrogen levels could be due to ovarian failure, hypothalamic amenorrhea, or pituitary dysfunction. Additional diagnostic tests, such as measuring serum estrogen levels, FSH, and LH, or performing a hysteroscopy, may be warranted to elucidate the cause of amenorrhea.

Clinical Trial Evidence

In this clinical study, 41 amenorrheic patients were divided into two groups according to whether they experienced withdrawal uterine bleeding after intramuscular administration of progesterone. The study aimed to investigate the correlation between withdrawal bleeding and ovarian volume, morphology (specifically, the presence or absence of follicles and their stage of development), and steroidogenic function in these patients.

Most of the patients who experienced progesterone-induced uterine bleeding had relatively large ovaries with highly developed follicles (tertiary-Graafian follicle) and demonstrated an increase in urinary excretion of total estrogens at 24 hours in response to exogenously administered human menopausal gonadotropin (HMG) and human chorionic gonadotropin (HCG). On the contrary, most patients without progesterone-induced uterine bleeding had smaller ovaries with no follicles or those in a lower developmental stage (primordial-secondary follicle) and did not respond to exogenous HMG and HCG.

The study findings suggest that the presence or absence of progesterone-induced uterine bleeding in amenorrheic patients is strongly associated with ovarian volume, morphology, and steroidogenic function. This correlation allows the classification of pathological amenorrhea into two distinct groups using the progesterone challenge test. This clinical categorization could prove valuable in the diagnosis and treatment of patients with amenorrhea [157].

PRACTICE-BASED QUESTIONS

1. A 46-year-old woman presents with generalized fatigue, weight loss, and hyper-pigmentation, especially in skin folds and mucous membranes. She has a history of hypothyroidism, which is well controlled on medication. The laboratory workup shows low serum cortisol and ACTH levels. An ACTH stimulation test is ordered for further evaluation.

   Which of the following results of the ACTH stimulation test would be consistent with the diagnosis of secondary adrenal insufficiency?

   a. A peak cortisol level of 20 mcg/dL
   b. A peak cortisol level of 17 mcg/dL
   c. A peak cortisol level of 16 mcg/dL
   d. A peak cortisol level of 14 mcg/dL

2. A 28-year-old woman presents with irregular periods, hirsutism, and obesity. Her fasting blood glucose and insulin levels are within normal limits. The physician suspects non-classic adrenal hyperplasia (NCAH) and decides to perform an ACTH stimulation test.

   Which result of the ACTH stimulation test is consistent with a diagnosis of NCAH?

   a. Baseline 17-hydroxyprogesterone level of 500 ng/dL and a stimulated level of 800 ng/dL
   b. Baseline 17-hydroxyprogesterone level of 1500 ng/dL and a stimulated level of 2500 ng/dL
   c. Baseline 17-hydroxyprogesterone level of 180 ng/dL and a stimulated level of 600 ng/dL
   d. Baseline 17-hydroxyprogesterone level of 3000 ng/dL and a stimulated level of 5000 ng/dL

   Answer: B) Baseline 17-hydroxyprogesterone level of 1500 ng/dL and a stimulated level of 2500 ng/dL. **Explanation:** Non-classic adrenal hyperplasia (NCAH) is often characterized by an exaggerated response to ACTH stimulation with increased 17-hydroxyprogesterone levels. In NCAH, a value of 17-hydroxyprogesterone at the 60-minute sample between 1000 and 10,000 ng/dL is diagnostic. Therefore, a baseline 17-hydroxyprogesterone level of 1500 ng/dL and a stimulated level of 2500 ng/dL is consistent with NCAH.

3. A 35-year-old male patient with a history of being significantly taller than his peers presents with coarse facial features, enlarged hands and feet, and joint pain. A glucagon stimulation test was performed with the maximum GH level determined as 2.7 ng/mL. What does this result suggest?

   a. The patient has acromegaly.
   b. The patient has a growth hormone deficiency.
   c. The patient has pheochromocytoma.
   d. The patient has no endocrine abnormalities.

   Answer: b. **Explanation:** This patient presents with features suggestive of acromegaly, a condition characterized by excessive GH secretion. However, the glucagon stimulation test shows a maximum GH level of 2.7 ng/mL, which falls below the typical threshold of 3 ng/mL, suggesting a growth hormone deficiency. This indicates a possibility of diagnostic discordance, necessitating further diagnostic workup.

4. A 50-year-old female with a history of hypertension presents with mild hypoglycemic episodes, unexplained weight loss, and an adrenal incidentaloma identified on imaging. Given the clinical presentation and her medical history, which of the following would be the most appropriate reason for not performing a glucagon stimulation test in this patient?

   a. The patient's age
   b. The presence of an adrenal incidentaloma
   c. The patient's weight loss
   d. The patient's hypoglycemic episodes

   Answer: b. **Explanation:** The glucagon stimulation test may not be suitable for patients with pheochromocytoma, a tumor that originates from the adrenal medulla and is associated with fluctuating blood pressure. In this case, the patient's adrenal incidentaloma could potentially be a pheochromocytoma, increasing the risk of blood pressure fluctuations during the test.

5. A 40-year-old male patient with a suspected diagnosis of acromegaly underwent an oral glucose tolerance test. Which of the following GH levels after glucose ingestion would most likely confirm the diagnosis?

   a. GH level decreases to 0.2 ng/mL
   b. GH level remains constant at 2 ng/mL
   c. GH level increases to 4 ng/mL
   d. GH level decreases to 1 ng/mL

   Answer: b. **Explanation:** In healthy individuals, GH levels are suppressed to below 0.4 ng/mL after glucose ingestion. In patients with acromegaly, GH levels remain elevated or are inadequately suppressed, suggesting impaired feedback regulation and abnormal GH secretion. Therefore, a GH level remaining constant at 2 ng/mL after glucose ingestion would most likely confirm the diagnosis of acromegaly.

6. Which of the following is the correct sequence of events in the normal regulation of growth hormone (GH) release?

   a. Increased glucose -> increased somatostatin -> decreased GH release
   b. Increased glucose -> decreased GHRH -> decreased GH release

   c. Increased glucagon -> increased GHRH -> increased GH release
   d. All of the above

   Answer: d. **Explanation:** All of the provided sequences are correct. Increased blood glucose levels stimulate the release of somatostatin, which inhibits GH secretion (a), and may also inhibit the secretion of GHRH, which stimulates GH release (b). Glucagon stimulates the release of GHRH, leading to an increase in GH release (c).

7. A 43-year-old female presents with a history of polyuria and polydipsia. A water deprivation test is conducted, and her urine osmolality is found to be significantly less than 700 mOsm/kg after the 8-hour period of water deprivation. Subsequent administration of desmopressin does not increase her urine osmolality. What is the most likely diagnosis?

   a. Normal vasopressin secretion and function
   b. Central diabetes insipidus (CDI)
   c. Nephrogenic diabetes insipidus (NDI)
   d. Psychogenic polydipsia

   Answer: c. Nephrogenic diabetes insipidus (NDI). **Explanation:** In the water deprivation test, the failure to concentrate urine (urine osmolality <700 mOsm/kg) after an 8-hour period of water deprivation indicates either CDI or NDI. However, in NDI, despite the administration of desmopressin, urine osmolality does not increase, differentiating NDI from CDI.

8. A 58-year-old male has been diagnosed with Cushing's syndrome. During Inferior Petrosal Sinus Sampling (IPSS), ACTH levels in the inferior petrosal sinus blood samples are not significantly higher than those in peripheral blood. What does this finding suggest?

   a. Cushing's disease
   b. An ectopic ACTH source
   c. Addison's disease
   d. Hyperaldosteronism

   Answer: b. An ectopic ACTH source. **Explanation:** In Cushing's disease, the pituitary gland produces excessive ACTH, leading to increased cortisol production. If ACTH levels in the inferior petrosal sinus blood samples are not significantly higher than those in peripheral blood, it suggests that the excessive ACTH is not coming from the pituitary gland, suggesting an ectopic ACTH source or adrenal tumors.

9. A 36-year-old woman with Sheehan syndrome presents with symptoms suggestive of hypothyroidism. A TRH stimulation test shows a delayed response. What is the most likely diagnosis?

 a. Primary hypothyroidism
 b. Central hypothyroidism
 c. Graves' disease
 d. Hashimoto's thyroiditis

Answer: b. Central hypothyroidism. **Explanation:** The TRH stimulation test assesses the pituitary gland's response to TRH. A delayed or nonresponse may indicate central hypothyroidism, where the dysfunction lies at the level of the hypothalamus or pituitary gland.

10. A 55-year-old female who has been recently diagnosed with differentiated thyroid cancer has just undergone thyroidectomy. She is now on levothyroxine replacement therapy. A radioactive iodine scan using a withdrawal protocol is planned.

 Why is it necessary to discontinue her levothyroxine replacement therapy before the scan?

 a. To suppress TSH levels
 b. To increase TSH levels
 c. To decrease iodine uptake by thyroid cells
 d. To enhance iodine excretion from the body

Answer: b) To increase TSH levels. **Explanation:** The withdrawal protocol for a radioactive iodine scan requires discontinuation of thyroid hormone replacement therapy (levothyroxine), typically 4–6 weeks before the scan. This is done to increase the levels of thyroid-stimulating hormone (TSH) in the blood. Elevated TSH levels stimulate thyroid cells to absorb more iodine, which enhances the effectiveness of the radioactive iodine scan.

11. A 45-year-old man with differentiated thyroid cancer undergoes a radioactive iodine scan after the administration of thyrogen

 Why is thyrogen administered before the radioactive iodine scan?

 a. To decrease iodine uptake by thyroid cells
 b. To increase iodine uptake by thyroid cells
 c. To suppress TSH levels
 d. To enhance iodine excretion from the body

Answer: b) To increase iodine uptake by thyroid cells. **Explanation:** Thyrogen, or recombinant human thyrotropin (rhTSH), is a synthetic form of thyroid-stimulating hormone (TSH). In patients who have undergone thyroidectomy, the administration of rhTSH stimulates any remaining thyroid tissue or metastatic thyroid cancer cells to increase iodine uptake, thereby enhancing the effectiveness of the radioactive iodine scan.

12. A 62-year-old woman, known to have hypertension, shows evidence of high aldosterone levels. A physician decides to proceed with an oral sodium loading test.

 Why is an oral sodium loading test performed?

 a. To stimulate the renin–angiotensin–aldosterone system
 b. To suppress the renin–angiotensin–aldosterone system
 c. To increase aldosterone secretion
 d. To enhance sodium excretion

Answer: b) To suppress the renin–angiotensin–aldosterone system. **Explanation:** An oral sodium loading test is done by consuming a high-sodium diet for several days. This high sodium intake suppresses the renin–angiotensin–aldosterone system (RAAS) in healthy individuals, decreasing aldosterone levels. If aldosterone secretion remains inappropriately high despite sodium loading, it suggests that the patient has primary hyperaldosteronism.

REFERENCES

1. Bornstein, S.R., Allolio, B., Arlt, W. et al. (2016). Diagnosis and treatment of primary adrenal insufficiency: an endocrine society clinical practice guideline. *J. Clin. Endocrinol. Metab.* 101: 364–389.

2. Charmandari, E., Tsigos, C., and Chrousos, G. (2005). Endocrinology of the stress response. *Annu. Rev. Physiol.* 67: 259–284.

3. Smith, S.M. and Vale, W.W. (2006). The role of the hypothalamic-pituitary-adrenal axis in neuroendocrine responses to stress. *Dialogues Clin. Neurosci.* 8: 383–395.

4. Herman, J.P. and Tasker, J.G. (2016). Paraventricular hypothalamic mechanisms of chronic stress adaptation. *Front Endocrinol. (Lausanne)* 7: 137.

5. Javorsky, B.R., Raff, H., Carroll, T.B. et al. (2021). New cutoffs for the biochemical diagnosis of adrenal insufficiency after ACTH stimulation using specific cortisol assays. *J. Endocrine Soc.* 5: bvab022.

6. Ortiz-Flores, A.E., Santacruz, E., Jiménez-Mendiguchia, L. et al. (2018). Role of sampling times and serum cortisol cut-off concentrations on the routine assessment of adrenal function using the standard cosyntropin test in an academic hospital from Spain: a retrospective chart review. *BMJ Open* 8: e019273.

7. Krasowski, M.D., Drees, D., Morris, C.S. et al. (2014). Cross-reactivity of steroid hormone immunoassays: clinical significance and two-dimensional molecular similarity prediction. *BMC Clin. Pathol.* 14: 33.

8. Bower, A.N. and Oyen, L.J. (2005). Interaction between dexamethasone treatment and the corticotropin stimulation test in septic shock. *Ann. Pharmacother.* 39: 335–338.

9. Cizza, G. and Rother, K.I. (2012). Cortisol binding globulin: more than just a carrier? *J. Clin. Endocrinol. Metab.* 97: 77–80.

10. Dubey, A. and Boujoukos, A.J. (2005). Measurements of serum free cortisol in critically ill patients. *Crit. Care* 9: E2.

11. Suliman, A.M., Smith, T.P., Labib, M. et al. (2002). The low-dose ACTH test does not provide a useful assessment of the hypothalamic-pituitary-adrenal axis in secondary adrenal insufficiency. *Clin. Endocrinol.* 56: 533–539.

12. Birtolo, M.F., Antonini, S., Saladino, A. et al. (2023). ACTH stimulation test for the diagnosis of secondary adrenal insufficiency: light and shadow. *Biomedicine* 11: 904.

13. Fleseriu, M., Gassner, M., Yedinak, C. et al. (2010). Normal hypothalamic-pituitary-adrenal axis by high-dose cosyntropin testing in patients with abnormal response to low-dose cosyntropin stimulation: a retrospective review. *Endocr. Pract.* 16: 64–70.

14. Alexandraki, K.I. and Grossman, A. (2000-2023). Diagnosis and management of adrenal insufficiency. In: *Endotext [Internet]* (ed. K.R. Feingold, B. Anawalt, M.R. Blackman, et al.). South Dartmouth (MA): MDText.com, Inc. https://www.ncbi.nlm.nih.gov/books/NBK279122/.

15. Ospina, N.S., Al Nofal, A., Bancos, I. et al. (2016). ACTH stimulation tests for the diagnosis of adrenal insufficiency: systematic review and meta-analysis. *J. Clin. Endocrinol. Metab.* 101: 427–434.

16. Chesover, A.D., Millar, H., Sepiashvili, L. et al. (2020). Screening for nonclassic congenital adrenal hyperplasia in the era of liquid chromatography-tandem mass spectrometry. *J. Endocrine Soc.* 4: bvz030.

17. Tsai, W.-H., Wong, C.-H., Dai, S.-H. et al. (2020). Adrenal tumor mimicking non-classic congenital adrenal hyperplasia. *Front. Endocrinol.* 11.

18. Nordenström, A. and Falhammar, H. (2019). Management of endocrine disease: diagnosis and management of the patient with non-classic cah due to 21-hydroxylase deficiency. *Eur. J. Endocrinol.* 180: R127–R145.

19. Dessinioti, C. and Katsambas, A. (2009). Congenital adrenal hyperplasia. *Dermatoendocrinol* 1: 87–91.

20. Carmina, E., Dewailly, D., Escobar-Morreale, H.F. et al. (2017). Non-classic congenital adrenal hyperplasia due to 21-hydroxylase deficiency revisited: an update with a special focus on adolescent and adult women. *Hum. Reprod. Update* 23: 580–599.

21. Sánchez, L.A., Pérez, M., Centeno, I. et al. (2007). Determining the time androgens and sex hormone-binding globulin take to return to baseline after discontinuation of oral contraceptives in women with polycystic ovary syndrome: a prospective study. *Fertil. Steril.* 87: 712–714.

22. Speiser, P.W., Arlt, W., Auchus, R.J. et al. (2018). Congenital adrenal hyperplasia due to steroid 21-hydroxylase deficiency: an endocrine society clinical practice guideline. *J. Clin. Endocrinol. Metab.* 103: 4043–4088.

23. Domagala, B., Trofimiuk-Muldner, M., Krawczyk, A. et al. (2021). What cut-off value of 17-hydroxyprogesterone should be an indication to perform a 250 µg cosyntropin stimulation test when NCCAH is suspected? - a retrospective study. *J. Endocr. Soc.* 5: A102.

24. Katabami, T., Obi, R., Shirai, N. et al. (2005). Discrepancies in results of low-and high-dose dexamethasone suppression tests for diagnosing preclinical Cushing's syndrome. *Endocr. J.* 52: 463–469.

25. Wagner-Bartak, N.A., Baiomy, A., Habra, M.A. et al. (2017). Cushing syndrome: diagnostic workup and imaging features, with clinical and pathologic correlation. *AJR Am. J. Roentgenol.* 209: 19–32.

26. Esfahanian, F. and Kazemi, R. (2010). Overnight dexamethasone suppression test in the diagnosis of Cushing's disease. *Acta Med. Iran.* 48: 222–225.

27. Ceccato, F. and Boscaro, M. (2016). Cushing's syndrome: screening and diagnosis. *High Blood Press Cardiovasc. Prev.* 23: 209–215.

28. Tuck, M.L., Sowers, J.R., Asp, N.D. et al. (1981). Mineralocorticoid response to low dose adrenocorticotropin infusion. *J. Clin. Endocrinol. Metab.* 52: 440–446.

29. Lacroix, A., Feelders, R.A., Stratakis, C.A., and Nieman, L.K. (2015). Cushing's syndrome. *Lancet* 386: 913–927.

30. Martin, N.M., Dhillo, W.S., and Meeran, K. (2007). The dexamethasone-suppressed corticotropin-releasing hormone stimulation test and the desmopressin test to distinguish Cushing's syndrome from pseudo-Cushing's states. *Clin. Endocrinol.* 67: 476.

31. Buliman, A., Tataranu, L., Paun, D. et al. (2016). Cushing's disease: a multidisciplinary overview of the clinical features, diagnosis, and treatment. *J. Med. Life* 9: 12–18.

32. Galm, B.P., Qiao, N., Klibanski, A. et al. (2020). Accuracy of laboratory tests for the diagnosis of cushing syndrome. *J. Clin. Endocrinol. Metab.* 105: dgaa105.

33. Kennedy, L., Atkinson, A.B., Johnston, H. et al. (1984). Serum cortisol concentrations during low dose dexamethasone suppression test to screen for Cushing's syndrome. *Br. Med. J. (Clin. Res. Ed.)* 289: 1188–1191.

34. Wood, P.J., Barth, J.H., Freedman, D.B. et al. (1997). Evidence for the low dose dexamethasone suppression test to screen for Cushing's syndrome – recommendations for a protocol for biochemistry laboratories. *Ann. Clin. Biochem.* 34 (Pt 3): 222–229.

35. Liddle, G.W. (1960). Tests of pituitary-adrenal suppressibility in the diagnosis of Cushing's syndrome. *J. Clin. Endocrinol. Metab.* 20: 1539–1560.

36. Bruno, O.D., Rossi, M.A., Contreras, L.N. et al. (1985). Nocturnal high-dose dexamethasone suppression test in the aetiological diagnosis of Cushing's syndrome. *Acta Endocrinol.* 109: 158–162.

37. Yanovski, J.A., Cutler, G.B., Chrousos, G.P., and Nieman, L.K. (1993). Corticotropin-releasing hormone stimulation following low-dose dexamethasone administration. A new test to distinguish Cushing's syndrome from pseudo-Cushing's states. *JAMA* 269: 2232–2238.

38. Müller, E.E., Locatelli, V., and Cocchi, D. (1999). Neuroendocrine control of growth hormone secretion. *Physiol. Rev.* 79: 511–607.

39. Giustina, A. and Veldhuis, J.D. (1998). Pathophysiology of the neuroregulation of growth hormone secretion in experimental animals and the human. *Endocr. Rev.* 19: 717–797.

40. Kojima, M., Hosoda, H., Date, Y. et al. (1999). Ghrelin is a growth-hormone-releasing acylated peptide from stomach. *Nature* 402: 656–660.

41. Rizza, R.A., Cryer, P.E., and Gerich, J.E. (1979). Role of glucagon, catecholamines, and growth hormone in human glucose counterregulation. Effects of somatostatin and combined alpha- and beta-adrenergic blockade on plasma glucose recovery and glucose flux rates after insulin-induced hypoglycemia. *J. Clin. Invest.* 64: 62–71.

42. Dichtel, L.E., Yuen, K.C.J., Bredella, M.A. et al. (2014). Overweight/Obese adults with pituitary disorders require lower peak growth hormone cutoff values on glucagon stimulation testing to avoid overdiagnosis of growth hormone deficiency. *J. Clin. Endocrinol. Metab.* 99: 4712–4719.

43. Hosseinnezhad, A., Black, R.M., Aeddula, N.R. et al. (2011). Glucagon-induced pheochromocytoma crisis. *Endocr. Pract.* 17: e51–e54.

44. Conceição, F.L., da Costa e Silva, A., Leal Costa, A.J., and Vaisman, M. (2003). Glucagon stimulation test for the diagnosis of GH deficiency in adults. *J. Endocrinol. Investig.* 26: 1065–1070.

45. Rabinowitz, D., Klassen, G.A., and Zierler, K.L. (1965). Effect of human growth hormone on muscle and adipose tissue metabolism in the forearm of man. *J. Clin. Invest.* 44: 51–61.

46. Freda, P.U., Bruce, J.N., Reyes-Vidal, C. et al. (2021). Prognostic value of nadir GH levels for long-term biochemical remission or recurrence in surgically treated acromegaly. *Pituitary* 24: 170–183.

47. Tannenbaum, G.S. and Martin, J.B. (1976). Evidence for an endogenous ultradian rhythm governing growth hormone secretion in the rat. *Endocrinology* 98: 562–570.

48. Thorner, M.O., Vance, M.L., Hartman, M.L. et al. (1990). Physiological role of somatostatin on growth hormone regulation in humans. *Metabolism* 39: 40–42.

49. Córdoba-Chacón, J., Gahete, M.D., Culler, M.D. et al. (2012). Somatostatin dramatically stimulates growth hormone release from primate somatotrophs acting at low doses via somatostatin receptor 5 and cyclic AMP. *J. Neuroendocrinol.* 24: 453–463.

50. Ho, K.Y., Veldhuis, J.D., Johnson, M.L. et al. (1988). Fasting enhances growth hormone secretion and

amplifies the complex rhythms of growth hormone secretion in man. *J. Clin. Invest.* 81: 968–975.

51. Hage, M., Kamenický, P., and Chanson, P. (2019). Growth hormone response to oral glucose load: from normal to pathological conditions. *Neuroendocrinology* 108: 244–255.

52. Møller, N., Jørgensen, J.O., Schmitz, O. et al. (1990). Effects of a growth hormone pulse on total and forearm substrate fluxes in humans. *Am. J. Phys.* 258: E86–E91.

53. Subbarayan, S.K., Fleseriu, M., Gordon, M.B. et al. (2012). Serum IGF-1 in the diagnosis of acromegaly and the profile of patients with elevated IGF-1 but normal glucose-suppressed growth hormone. *Endocr. Pract.* 18: 817–825.

54. Giustina, A., Chanson, P., Bronstein, M.D. et al. (2010). A consensus on criteria for cure of acromegaly. *J. Clin. Endocrinol. Metab.* 95: 3141–3148.

55. Feelders, R.A., Bidlingmaier, M., Strasburger, C.J. et al. (2005). postoperative evaluation of patients with acromegaly: clinical significance and timing of oral glucose tolerance testing and measurement of (free) insulin-like growth factor I, acid-labile subunit, and growth hormone-binding protein levels. *J. Clin. Endocrinol. Metabol.* 90: 6480–6489.

56. Katznelson, L., Atkinson, J.L.D., Cook, D.M. et al. (2011). American association of clinical endocrinologists medical guidelines for clinical practice for the diagnosis and treatment of acromegaly-2011 update. *Endocr. Pract.* 17: 1–44.

57. Freda, P.U., Post, K.D., Powell, J.S., and Wardlaw, S.L. (1998). Evaluation of disease status with sensitive measures of growth hormone secretion in 60 postoperative patients with acromegaly. *J. Clin. Endocrinol. Metab.* 83: 3808–3816.

58. Tomkins, M., Lawless, S., Martin-Grace, J. et al. (2022). Diagnosis and management of central diabetes insipidus in adults. *J. Clin. Endocrinol. Metabol.* 107: 2701–2715.

59. Robertson, G.L. (1995). Diabetes insipidus. *Endocrinol. Metab. Clin. N. Am.* 24: 549–572.

60. Christ-Crain, M., Bichet, D.G., Fenske, W.K. et al. (2019). Diabetes insipidus. *Nat. Rev. Dis. Primers.* 5: 54.

61. Verbalis, J.G. (2003). Diabetes insipidus. *Rev. Endocr. Metab. Disord.* 4: 177–185.

62. Kavanagh, C. and Uy, N.S. (2019). Nephrogenic diabetes insipidus. *Pediatr. Clin. N. Am.* 66: 227–234.

63. Raff, H. and Carroll, T. (2015). Cushing's syndrome: from physiological principles to diagnosis and clinical care. *J. Physiol.* 593: 493–506.

64. Manni, A., Latshaw, R.F., Page, R., and Santen, R.J. (1983). Simultaneous bilateral venous sampling for adrenocorticotropin in pituitary-dependent cushing's disease: evidence for lateralization of pituitary venous drainage. *J. Clin. Endocrinol. Metab.* 57: 1070–1073.

65. Wiggam, M.I., Heaney, A.P., McIlrath, E.M. et al. (2000). Bilateral inferior petrosal sinus sampling in the differential diagnosis of adrenocorticotropin-dependent Cushing's syndrome: a comparison with other diagnostic tests. *J. Clin. Endocrinol. Metab.* 85: 1525–1532.

66. Findling, J.W., Kehoe, M.E., Shaker, J.L., and Raff, H. (1991). Routine inferior petrosal sinus sampling in the differential diagnosis of adrenocorticotropin (ACTH)-dependent Cushing's syndrome: early recognition of the occult ectopic ACTH syndrome. *J. Clin. Endocrinol. Metab.* 73: 408–413.

67. Akobo, S., Bernard, S., Granger, A., and Tubbs, R.S. (2020). Chapter 11 - The inferior petrosal sinus. In: *Anatomy, Imaging and Surgery of the Intracranial Dural Venous Sinuses* (ed. R.S. Tubbs), 109–116. Philadelphia: Elsevier.

68. Perlman, J.E., Johnston, P.C., Hui, F. et al. (2021). Pitfalls in performing and interpreting inferior petrosal sinus sampling: personal experience and literature review. *J. Clin. Endocrinol. Metab.* 106: e1953–e1967.

69. Feng, M., Liu, Z., Liu, X. et al. (2018). Tumour lateralization in Cushing's disease by inferior petrosal sinus sampling with desmopressin. *Clin. Endocrinol.* 88: 251–257.

70. Pereira, C.A., Ferreira, L., Amaral, C. et al. (2021). Diagnostic accuracy of bilateral inferior petrosal sinus sampling: the experience of a tertiary centre. *Exp. Clin. Endocrinol. Diabetes* 129: 126–130.

71. Vassiliadi, D.A., Mourelatos, P., Kratimenos, T., and Tsagarakis, S. (2021). Inferior petrosal sinus sampling in Cushing's syndrome: usefulness and pitfalls. *Endocrine* 73: 530–539.

72. Vale, W., Spiess, J., Rivier, C., and Rivier, J. (1981). Characterization of a 41-residue ovine hypothalamic peptide that stimulates secretion of corticotropin and beta-endorphin. *Science* 213: 1394–1397.

73. Zampetti, B., Grossrubatscher, E., Dalino Ciaramella, P. et al. (2016). Bilateral inferior petrosal sinus sampling. *Endocr. Connect.* 5: R12–R25.

74. Engelmann, M., Landgraf, R., and Wotjak, C.T. (2004). The hypothalamic-neurohypophysial system regulates the hypothalamic-pituitary-adrenal axis under stress: an old concept revisited. *Front. Neuroendocrinol.* 25: 132–149.

75. de Keyzer, Y., Lenne, F., Auzan, C. et al. (1996). The pituitary V3 vasopressin receptor and the corticotroph phenotype in ectopic ACTH syndrome. *J. Clin. Invest.* 97: 1311–1318.

76. Yogi-Morren, D., Habra, M.A., Faiman, C. et al. (2015). Pituitary MRI findings in patients with pituitary and ectopic ACTH-dependent cushing syndrome: does a 6-mm pituitary tumor size cut-off value exclude ectopic acth syndrome? *Endocr. Pract.* 21: 1098–1103.

77. Pecori Giraldi, F., Cavallo, L.M., Tortora, F. et al. (2015). The role of inferior petrosal sinus sampling in ACTH-dependent Cushing's syndrome: review and joint opinion statement by members of the Italian Society for Endocrinology, Italian Society for Neurosurgery, and Italian Society for Neuroradiology. *Neurosurg. Focus.* 38: E5.

78. Colao, A., Faggiano, A., Pivonello, R. et al. (2001). Inferior petrosal sinus sampling in the differential diagnosis of Cushing's syndrome: results of an Italian multicenter study. *Eur. J. Endocrinol.* 144: 499–507.

79. Persani, L., Brabant, G., Dattani, M. et al. (2018). 2018 European Thyroid Association (ETA) guidelines on the diagnosis and management of central hypothyroidism. *Eur. Thyroid J.* 7: 225–237.

80. Beck-Peccoz, P., Rodari, G., Giavoli, C., and Lania, A. (2017). Central hypothyroidism – a neglected thyroid disorder. *Nat. Rev. Endocrinol.* 13: 588–598.

81. Judd, S.J. and Lazarus, L. (1976). A combined test of anterior pituitary reserve. *Aust. NZ J. Med.* 6: 30–36.

82. Gual, C., Wilber, J.F., Tello, C., and Ríos, E. (1972). Administration of synthetic thyrotropin releasing hormone (TRH) as a clinical test for pituitary thyrotropin reserve. *Rev. Investig. Clin.* 24: 35–55.

83. Yamamoto, T., Yano, S., Kuroda, J. et al. (2012). Pituitary apoplexy associated with endocrine stimulation test: endocrine stimulation test, treatment, and outcome. *Case Rep. Endocrinol.* 2012: 826901.

84. Atmaca H, Tanriverdi F, Gokce C, Unluhizarci K, Kelestimur F (2007) Do we still need the TRH stimulation test? *Thyroid* https://doi.org/10.1089/thy.2006.0311

85. Chen, M., Luo, L., Wang, Q. et al. (2020). Impact of gonadotropin-releasing hormone agonist pre-treatment on the cumulative live birth rate in infertile women with adenomyosis treated with IVF/ICSI: a retrospective cohort study. *Front. Endocrinol.* 11.

86. Ab Rahim, S.N., Omar, J., and Tuan Ismail, T.S. (2020). Gonadotropin-releasing hormone stimulation test and diagnostic cutoff in precocious puberty: a mini review. *Ann. Pediatr. Endocrinol. Metab.* 25: 152–155.

87. Acevedo-Rodriguez, A., Kauffman, A.S., Cherrington, B.D. et al. (2018). Emerging insights into Hypothalamic-pituitary-gonadal (HPG) axis regulation and interaction with stress signaling. *J. Neuroendocrinol.* 30: e12590.

88. Marques, P., Skorupskaite, K., Rozario, K.S. et al. (2000-2023). Physiology of GnRH and gonadotropin secretion. In: *Endotext [Internet]* (ed. K.R. Feingold, B. Anawalt, M.R. Blackman, et al.). South Dartmouth (MA): MDText.com, Inc. https://www.ncbi.nlm.nih.gov/books/NBK279070/.

89. Colucci, P., Yue, C.S., Ducharme, M., and Benvenga, S. (2013). A review of the pharmacokinetics of levothyroxine for the treatment of hypothyroidism. *Eur. Endocrinol.* 9: 40–47.

90. Virili, C., Bruno, G., Santaguida, M.G. et al. (2022). Levothyroxine treatment and gastric juice pH in humans: the proof of concept. *Endocrine* 77: 102–111.

91. Wiesner, A., Gajewska, D., and Paśko, P. (2021). Levothyroxine interactions with food and dietary supplements–a systematic review. *Pharmaceuticals (Basel)* 14: 206.

92. Irving, S.A., Vadiveloo, T., and Leese, G.P. (2015). Drugs that interact with levothyroxine: an observational study from the thyroid epidemiology, audit and research study (TEARS). *Clin. Endocrinol.* 82: 136–141.

93. Caron, P., Grunenwald, S., Persani, L. et al. (2022). Factors influencing the levothyroxine dose in the hormone replacement therapy of primary hypothyroidism in adults. *Rev. Endocr. Metab. Disord.* 23: 463–483.

94. Gonzales, K.M., Stan, M.N., Morris, J.C. et al. (2019). The levothyroxine absorption test: a four-year experience (2015–2018) at The Mayo Clinic. *Thyroid* 29: 1734–1742.

95. Yildirim Simsir, I., Soyaltin, U.E., and Ozgen, A.G. (2019). Levothyroxine absorption test results in patients with TSH elevation resistant to treatment. *Endocrine* 64: 118–121.

96. Ghosh, S., Pramanik, S., Biswas, K. et al. (2020). Levothyroxine absorption test to differentiate

pseudomalabsorption from true malabsorption. *Eur. Thyroid J.* 9: 19–24.

97. Iqbal, A. and Rehman, A. (2023). *Thyroid Uptake and Scan*. StatPearls.

98. Haugen, B.R., Alexander, E.K., Bible, K.C. et al. (2016). 2015 American Thyroid Association Management guidelines for adult patients with thyroid nodules and differentiated thyroid cancer: the American Thyroid Association Guidelines Task Force on thyroid nodules and differentiated thyroid cancer. *Thyroid* 26: 1–133.

99. Hänscheid, H., Lassmann, M., Luster, M. et al. (2006). Iodine biokinetics and dosimetry in radioiodine therapy of thyroid cancer: procedures and results of a prospective international controlled study of ablation after rhTSH or hormone withdrawal. *J. Nucl. Med.* 47: 648–654.

100. Silberstein, E.B. (2012). Radioiodine: the classic theranostic agent. *Semin. Nucl. Med.* 42: 164–170.

101. Galasko, G.T. (2017). 29 - Pituitary, thyroid, and parathyroid pharmacology. In: *Pharmacology and Therapeutics for Dentistry*, 7e (ed. F.J. Dowd, B.S. Johnson, and A.J. Mariotti), 417–428. Mosby.

102. Wyszomirska, A. (2012). Iodine-131 for therapy of thyroid diseases. Physical and biological basis. *Nucl. Med. Rev. Cent. East. Eur.* 15: 120–123.

103. Kim, P.D. and Tran, H.D. (2023). *I-123 Uptake*. StatPearls.

104. Mettler FA, Guiberteau MJ (2012) 4 - Thyroid, parathyroid, and salivary glands. In: Mettler FA, Guiberteau MJ (eds) *Essentials of Nuclear Medicine Imaging* (6). W.B. Saunders, Philadelphia, pp. 99–130

105. Van Nostrand, D. (2019). Radioiodine imaging for differentiated thyroid cancer: not all radioiodine images are performed equally. *Thyroid* 29: 901–909.

106. Ladenson, P.W., Braverman, L.E., Mazzaferri, E.L. et al. (1997). Comparison of administration of recombinant human thyrotropin with withdrawal of thyroid hormone for radioactive iodine scanning in patients with thyroid carcinoma. *N. Engl. J. Med.* 337: 888–896.

107. Dueren, C., Dietlein, M., Luster, M. et al. (2010). The use of thyrogen in the treatment of differentiated thyroid carcinoma: an intraindividual comparison of clinical effects and implications of daily life. *Exp. Clin. Endocrinol. Diabetes* 118: 513–519.

108. Kogai, T., Taki, K., and Brent, G.A. (2006). Enhancement of sodium/iodide symporter expression in thyroid and breast cancer. *Endocr. Relat. Cancer* 13: 797–826.

109. Zagar, I., Schwarzbartl-Pevec, A.A., Vidergar-Kralj, B. et al. (2012). Recombinant human thyrotropin-aided radioiodine therapy in patients with metastatic differentiated thyroid carcinoma. *J. Thyroid. Res.* 2012: 670180.

110. Ma, C., Xie, J., Liu, W. et al. (2010). Recombinant human thyrotropin (rhTSH) aided radioiodine treatment for residual or metastatic differentiated thyroid cancer. *Cochrane Database Syst. Rev.* 2010: CD008302.

111. Ahmed, A.H., Cowley, D., Wolley, M. et al. (2014). Seated saline suppression testing for the diagnosis of primary aldosteronism: a preliminary study. *J. Clin. Endocrinol. Metab.* 99: 2745–2753.

112. Clarkson, M.R., Magee, C.N., and Brenner, B.M. (ed.) (2011). Chapter 22 - Hypertension. In: *Pocket Companion to Brenner and Rector's The Kidney*, 8e, 439–467. Philadelphia: W.B. Saunders.

113. Morera, J. and Reznik, Y. (2019). Management of endocrine disease: the role of confirmatory tests in the diagnosis of primary aldosteronism. *Eur. J. Endocrinol.* 180: R45–R58.

114. Thakkar, R.B. and Oparil, S. (2007). Primary aldosteronism: a practical approach to diagnosis and treatment. *J. Clin. Hypertens. (Greenwich)* 3: 189–195.

115. Agharazii, M., Douville, P., Grose, J.H., and Lebel, M. (2001). Captopril suppression versus salt loading in confirming primary aldosteronism. *Hypertension* 37: 1440–1443.

116. Eisenhofer, G., Kurlbaum, M., Peitzsch, M. et al. (2022). The saline infusion test for primary aldosteronism: implications of immunoassay inaccuracy. *J. Clin. Endocrinol. Metabol.* 107: e2027–e2036.

117. Fuss, C.T., Brohm, K., Kurlbaum, M. et al. (2021). Confirmatory testing of primary aldosteronism with saline infusion test and LC-MS/MS. *Eur. J. Endocrinol.* 184: 167–178.

118. Rossi, G.P., Belfiore, A., Bernini, G. et al. (2007). Prospective evaluation of the saline infusion test for excluding primary aldosteronism due to aldosterone-producing adenoma. *J. Hypertens.* 25: 1433–1442.

119. Remde, H., Pamporaki, C., Quinkler, M. et al. (2022). Improved diagnostic accuracy of clonidine suppression testing using an age-related cutoff for plasma normetanephrine. *Hypertension* 79: 1257–1264.

120. Giovannitti, J.A., Thoms, S.M., and Crawford, J.J. (2015). Alpha-2 adrenergic receptor agonists: a review of current clinical applications. *Anesth. Prog.* 62: 31–38.

121. Bravo, E.L. and Tagle, R. (2003). Pheochromocytoma: state-of-the-art and future prospects. *Endocr. Rev.* 24: 539–553.

122. Bravo, E.L., Tarazi, R.C., Fouad, F.M. et al. (1981). Clonidine-suppression test. *N. Engl. J. Med.* 305: 623–626.

123. Tsiomidou, S., Pamporaki, C., Geroula, A. et al. (2022). Clonidine suppression test for a reliable diagnosis of pheochromocytoma: when to use. *Clin. Endocrinol.* 97: 541–550.

124. Drummond, J.B., Soares, B.S., Pedrosa, W., and Ribeiro-Oliveira, A. (2021). Revisiting peak serum cortisol response to insulin-induced hypoglycemia in children. *J. Endocrinol. Investig.* 44: 1291–1299.

125. Maghnie, M., Uga, E., Temporini, F. et al. (2005). Evaluation of adrenal function in patients with growth hormone deficiency and hypothalamic-pituitary disorders: comparison between insulin-induced hypoglycemia, low-dose ACTH, standard ACTH and CRH stimulation tests. *Eur. J. Endocrinol.* 152: 735–741.

126. Daunt, N. (2005). Adrenal vein sampling: how to make it quick, easy, and successful. *Radiographics* 25 (Suppl 1): S143–S158.

127. Dominguez, A., Muppidi, V., and Gupta, S. (2023). *Hyperaldosteronism.* StatPearls.

128. So, C.B., Leung, A.A., Chin, A., and Kline, G.A. (2022). Adrenal venous sampling in primary aldosteronism: lessons from over 600 single-operator procedures. *Clin. Radiol.* 77: e170–e179.

129. Betz, M.J. and Zech, C.J. (2022). Adrenal venous sampling in the diagnostic workup of primary aldosteronism. *Br. J. Radiol.* 95: 20210311.

130. Rossi, G.P., Auchus, R.J., Brown, M. et al. (2014). An expert consensus statement on use of adrenal vein sampling for the subtyping of primary aldosteronism. *Hypertension* 63: 151–160.

131. Seccia, T.M., Miotto, D., De Toni, R. et al. (2009). Adrenocorticotropic hormone stimulation during adrenal vein sampling for identifying surgically curable subtypes of primary aldosteronism: comparison of 3 different protocols. *Hypertension* 53: 761–766.

132. Seccia, T.M., Miotto, D., Battistel, M. et al. (2012). A stress reaction affects assessment of selectivity of adrenal venous sampling and of lateralization of aldosterone excess in primary aldosteronism. *Eur. J. Endocrinol.* 166: 869–875.

133. Laurent, I., Astère, M., Zheng, F. et al. (2019). Adrenal venous sampling with or without adrenocorticotropic hormone stimulation: a meta-analysis. *J. Clin. Endocrinol. Metabol.* 104: 1060–1068.

134. Lee, S.-E., Park, S.W., Choi, M.S. et al. (2021). Primary aldosteronism subtyping in the setting of partially successful adrenal vein sampling. *Ther. Adv. Endocrinol. Metab.* 12: 2042018821989239.

135. Umakoshi, H., Tsuiki, M., Yokomoto-Umakoshi, M. et al. (2018). Correlation between lateralization index of adrenal venous sampling and standardized outcome in primary aldosteronism. *J. Endocr. Soc.* 2: 893–902.

136. Deipolyi, A.R. and Oklu, R. (2015). Adrenal vein sampling in the diagnosis of aldosteronism. *JVD* 3: 17–23.

137. Young, W.F., Stanson, A.W., Thompson, G.B. et al. (2004). Role for adrenal venous sampling in primary aldosteronism. *Surgery* 136: 1227–1235.

138. Wannachalee, T., Zhao, L., Nanba, K. et al. (2019). Three discrete patterns of primary aldosteronism lateralization in response to cosyntropin during adrenal vein sampling. *J. Clin. Endocrinol. Metab.* 104: 5867–5876.

139. Norton, L., Shannon, C., Gastaldelli, A., and DeFronzo, R.A. (2022). Insulin: the master regulator of glucose metabolism. *Metabolism* 129: 155142.

140. Giugliano, D., Ceriello, A., and Esposito, K. (2008). Glucose metabolism and hyperglycemia. *Am. J. Clin. Nutr.* 87: 217S–222S.

141. Kuo, F.Y., Cheng, K.-C., Li, Y., and Cheng, J.-T. (2021). Oral glucose tolerance test in diabetes, the old method revisited. *World J. Diabetes* 12: 786–793.

142. Jagannathan, R., Neves, J.S., Dorcely, B. et al. (2020). The oral glucose tolerance test: 100 years later. *Diabetes Metab. Syndr. Obes.* 13: 3787–3805.

143. Eyth, E., Basit, H., and Swift, C.J. (2023). *Glucose Tolerance Test.* StatPearls.

144. American Diabetes Association (2020). 2. Classification and diagnosis of diabetes: standards of medical care in diabetes-2020. *Diabetes Care* 43: S14–S31.

145. Stumvoll, M., Mitrakou, A., Pimenta, W. et al. (2000). Use of the oral glucose tolerance test to assess insulin release and insulin sensitivity. *Diabetes Care* 23: 295–301.

146. Sprague, J.E. and Arbeláez, A.M. (2011). Glucose counterregulatory responses to hypoglycemia. *Pediatr. Endocrinol. Rev.* 9: 463–475.

147. Cryer, P.E., Axelrod, L., Grossman, A.B. et al. (2009). Evaluation and management of adult hypoglycemic disorders: an Endocrine Society Clinical Practice Guideline. *J. Clin. Endocrinol. Metab.* 94: 709–728.

148. Hirshberg, B., Livi, A., Bartlett, D.L. et al. (2000). Forty-eight-hour fast: the diagnostic test for insulinoma. *J. Clin. Endocrinol. Metab.* 85: 3222–3226.

149. Afroze, S., Meng, F., Jensen, K. et al. (2013). The physiological roles of secretin and its receptor. *Ann. Translational Med.* 1: 29–29.

150. Mollapour, E. and Shetzline, M.A. (2004). Secretin. In: *Encyclopedia of Gastroenterology* (ed. L.R. Johnson), 335–339. New York: Elsevier.

151. Chey, W.Y. and Chang, T.-M. (2003). Secretin, 100 years later. *J. Gastroenterol.* 38: 1025–1035.

152. Giusti, F., Cioppi, F., Fossi, C. et al. (2022). Secretin stimulation test and early diagnosis of gastrinoma in MEN1 syndrome: survey on the MEN1 florentine database. *J. Clin. Endocrinol. Metabol.* 107: e2110–e2123.

153. Deveney, C.W., Deveney, K.S., Jaffe, B.M. et al. (1977). Use of calcium and secretin in the diagnosis of gastrinoma (Zollinger-Ellison syndrome). *Ann. Intern. Med.* 87: 680–686.

154. Berna, M.J., Hoffmann, K.M., Serrano, J. et al. (2006). Serum gastrin in Zollinger-Ellison syndrome: I. Prospective study of fasting serum gastrin in 309 patients from the National Institutes of Health and comparison with 2229 cases from the literature. *Medicine (Baltimore)* 85: 295–330.

155. Mikhael, S., Punjala-Patel, A., and Gavrilova-Jordan, L. (2019). Hypothalamic-pituitary-ovarian axis disorders impacting female fertility. *Biomedicine* 7: 5.

156. Schlaff, W.D. and Coddington, C.C. (2020). Use of the progestin challenge test in diagnosing amenorrhea: the time has come to say goodbye. *Fertil. Steril.* 113: 51–52.

157. Nakano, R., Hashiba, N., Washio, M., and Tojo, S. (1979). Diagnostic evaluation of progesterone: challenge test in amenorrheic patients. *Acta Obstet. Gynecol. Scand.* 58: 59–64.

Appendix A

A.1 CARDIOVASCULAR OUTCOME TRIALS IN DIABETES CARE

TABLE A.1 Selected trials of GLP-1 agonists.

Clinical trial	Drug
LEADER	Liraglutide
SUSTAIN-6	Semaglutide
ELIXA	Lixisenatide
PIONEER	Oral semaglutide
HARMONY	Albiglutide
REWIND	Dulaglutide
FREEDOM-CVO	Canagliflozin

TABLE A.2 Selected trials of SGLT-2 inhibitors.

Clinical trial	Drug
EMPA-REG OUTCOME	Empagliflozin
CANVAS	Canagliflozin
DAPA-HF	Dapagliflozin
VERTIS CV	Ertugliflozin
DECLARE-TIMI 58	Dapagliflozin
CREDENCE	Canagliflozin
EMPEROR-Preserved	Empagliflozin
EMPEROR Reduced	Empagliflozin

TABLE A.3 Selected trials of DPP-4 inhibitors.

Clinical trial	Drug
EXAMINE	Alogliptin
SAVOR-TIMI 53	Saxagliptin
TECOS	Sitagliptin
CARMELINA	Linagliptin
CAROLINA	Linagliptin vs glimepiride

TABLE A.4 Other selected clinical trials.

Clinical trial	Drug
DEVOTE	Insulin degludec vs. insulin glargine
IRIS	Pioglitazone
ACE	Acarbose

TABLE A.5 Landmark diabetes trials.

Clinical trial	Drug
DCCT	Intensive vs. conventional insulin therapy
EDIC	Early intensive insulin therapy
UKPDS	Intensive blood-glucose control
ACCORD	Intensive vs. standard glycemic control
ADVANCE	Intensive blood glucose control
VADT	Intensive vs. standard glycemic control

Endocrinology: Pathophysiology to Therapy, First Edition. Akuffo Quarde.
© 2024 John Wiley & Sons Ltd. Published 2024 by John Wiley & Sons Ltd.

Zoledronic Acid Recurrent Fracture Trial :
Zoledronic Acid in Reducing Clinical Fracture and Mortality after Hip Fracture.
A randomized, double-blind, placebo-controlled trial

Rationale : Mortality is increased after a hip fracture, and strategies that improve outcomes are needed. Patients received IV zoledronic acid within 90 days after surgical repair of a hip fracture.

N = 2127

IV Zoledronic Acid 5mg yearly
(Median follow-up of 1.9 years)

New Clinical Fracture
(Hip, vertebral OR nonvertebral)

☑ Men and Women 50 years of age or older.

☑ Within 90 days after surgical repair of a hip fragility fracture.

☑ Being ambulatory before the hip fracture.

8.6%
Zoledronic Acid

13.9%
Placebo

Primary Outcome

Hazard ratio, 0.65 ; 95% CI, 0.50 to 0.84; P value of 0.001

Practice Changing Pearls

An annual infusion of zoledronic acid within 90 days after repair of a low-trauma hip fracture was associated with a reduction in the rate of new clinical fractures and improved survival.

Journal: N Engl J Med 2007; 357:1799-1809   MyEndoConsult.com

Sample infographic of an important clinical trial in endocrinology. Review other infographics of landmark trials at https://myendoconsult.com/learn/clinical-trials/.

A.2 COMMON SIDE EFFECTS OF ENDOCRINE TREATMENTS (BOARD REVIEW)

A.2.1   Pituitary Therapies

Pasireotide: Hyperglycemia.

Retinoic Acid: Dry skin and increased sensitivity to sunlight.

Dopaminergic agonists: Nausea, dizziness, and orthostatic hypotension.

Steroidogenesis inhibitors: Adrenal insufficiency, gastrointestinal upset, and rash.

Mifepristone: Abdominal pain, nausea, and fatigue.

Somatostatin analogs: Gastrointestinal upset, gallstones, and injection site reactions.

Growth hormone receptor antagonists: Injection site reactions, elevated liver enzymes.

Growth hormone: Joint pain and slipped capital femoral epiphysis.

Desmopressin: Hyponatreamia.

Natriuretic agents: Dizziness, headache, and electrolyte imbalance.

Clofibrate, Chlorpropamide, and Carbamazepine: Gastrointestinal upset, dizziness, and skin rash.

Vaptans: Hyponatremia.

A.2.2   Thyroid Therapies

Thionamides: Skin rash, joint pain, and liver problems.

Lugol's iodine: Metallic taste.

Glucocorticoids: Weight gain, insomnia, and mood changes.

Beta-blockers: Fatigue.

Lithium: Increased thirst, hand tremors, and weight gain.

Teprotumumab: Muscle cramps, nausea, and hair loss.

Rituximab: Infusion reactions, infections, and fatigue.

Tyrosine kinase inhibitors: Diarrhea, rash, and fatigue.

Radioactive iodine ablation: Dry mouth, taste changes, and neck tenderness.

mTOR inhibitors: Mouth sores, diarrhea, and elevated blood sugar levels.

A.2.3   Adrenal Therapies

Glucocorticoids: Increased appetite and weight gain.

Mineralocorticoids: Fluid retention.

Androgens: Acne and oily skin and male pattern baldness in women.

Mineralocorticoid antagonists: Hypotensive symptoms.

Alpha-blockers: Hypotensive symptoms, dizziness, and fainting, nasal congestion.

Calcium channel blockers: Leg edema and dizziness.

A.2.4   Pancreas-Related Therapies

Insulin: Hypoglycemia and weight gain.

Biguanides: Diarrhea, metformin-associated lactic acidosis.

Meglitinides: Hypoglycemia, weight gain, and joint pain.

Sulfonylureas: Hypoglycemia and weight gain,

PPAR-gamma agonists: Fluid retention, bone fractures, and bladder cancer (rare).

GLP-1 agonists: Nausea, vomiting, diarrhea, and pancreatitis (rare but serious).

SGLT-2 inhibitors: Increased urination, yeast infections, and low blood pressure.

DPP-4 inhibitors: Nasopharyngitis (common cold), headache, and joint pain.

Alpha-glucosidase inhibitors: Bloating and diarrhea.

Amylin agonists: Nausea, vomiting, and hypoglycemia.

Somatostatin analogs: Diarrhea, nausea, abdominal pain, and gallstones.

Diazoxide and diuretics: Fluid retention, low blood pressure, and hyperglycemia.

Phenytoin: Gum overgrowth.

A.2.5   Parathyroid-Related Therapies

Calcimimetics: Nausea, decreased appetite, and muscle aches.

Bisphosphonates: Bone pain (acute phase reaction).

Thiazide diuretics: Hypokalemia.

Calcium: Constipation, polyuria, and urolithiasis.

Calcitonin: Flushing.

RANK-L inhibitors: Hypocalcemia and increased risk of infections.

Anti-sclerostin inhibitors: Cardiovascular risk.

Hormone Replacement Therapy (Estrogen): Breast tenderness, bloating, nausea, and increased risk of blood clots (rare).

A.2.6   Obesity and Lipid-Related Therapies

Ezetimibe: Diarrhea and abdominal pain.

Statins: Muscle pain and weakness, liver damage (rare), increased risk of diabetes (in some people).

PCSK9-inhibitors: Injection site reactions and flu-like symptoms.

Omega-3 Fatty Acids: Fishy aftertaste.

Fibrates: Upset stomach.

Phentermine-Topiramate: Dry mouth and tachycardia.

Bupropion-Naltrexone: Suicidal ideation.

Intestinal lipase inhibitor: Gas, oily spotting, and increased risk of liver damage (rare).

A.3   BRAND NAMES OF COMMON MEDICATIONS IN ENDOCRINOLOGY

A.3.1   Diabetes Therapies

Metformin: Glucophage, Glucophage XR, Glumetza, Riomet, Fortamet

Glimepiride: Amaryl

Glipizide: Glucotrol, Glucotrol XL

Glyburide: Diabeta, Glynase, Micronase

Pioglitazone: Actos

Rosiglitazone: Avandia

Sitagliptin: Januvia

Saxagliptin: Onglyza

Linagliptin: Tradjenta

Alogliptin: Nesina

Canagliflozin: Invokana

Dapagliflozin: Farxiga

Empagliflozin: Jardiance

Ertugliflozin: Steglatro

Liraglutide: Victoza, Saxenda

Exenatide: Byetta, Bydureon

Dulaglutide: Trulicity

Semaglutide: Ozempic, Rybelsus

Albiglutide: Tanzeum

Lixisenatide: Adlyxin

Acarbose: Precose

Miglitol: Glyset

Repaglinide: Prandin

Nateglinide: Starlix

Insulin Glargine: Lantus, Basaglar, Toujeo

Insulin Detemir: Levemir

Insulin Aspart: NovoLog, Fiasp

Insulin Lispro: Humalog, Admelog

Insulin Glulisine: Apidra

Insulin Degludec: Tresiba

Regular insulin: Humulin R, Novolin R

NPH insulin: Humulin N, Novolin N

70/30 insulin: Humulin 70/30, Novolin 70/30

A.3.2   Pituitary-Related Therapies

Pasireotide: Signifor, Signifor LAR

Mifepristone: Korlym

Ketoconazole: Nizoral (off-label use for Cushing's disease)

Osilodrostat: Isturisa

Octreotide: Sandostatin, Sandostatin LAR Depot

Lanreotide: Somatuline Depot

Pegvisomant: Somavert

Pasireotide: Signifor, Signifor LAR

Cabergoline: Dostinex

Bromocriptine: Parlodel

Desmopressin: DDAVP, Minirin, Stimate, Noqdirna, Nocdurna

Somatropin: Genotropin, Humatrope, Norditropin, Nutropin, Omnitrope, Saizen, Zomacton

Aminoglutethimide: Cytadren (off-label use for Cushing's disease)

Bromocriptine: Parlodel (less common for treating acromegaly)

Quinagolide: Norprolac (not available in the United States)

Vasopressin: Vasostrict, Pitressin (less common than desmopressin for treating central diabetes insipidus)

Sermorelin: Geref (less common for treating growth hormone deficiency)

Corticosteroids: Hydrocortisone (Cortef), prednisone (Deltasone), dexamethasone (Decadron)

Testosterone: AndroGel, Testim, Androderm, Axiron

Estradiol: Estrace, Climara, Vivelle-Dot

Medroxyprogesterone: Provera, Depo-Provera

A.3.3   Thyroid Hormone Therapies

Levothyroxine: Synthroid, Levoxyl, Tirosint, Unithroid, Euthyrox

Liothyronine: Cytomel, Triostat

Natural desiccated thyroid (NDT): Armour Thyroid, Nature-Throid, WP Thyroid, NP Thyroid

Methimazole: Tapazole, Thiamazole

Sorafenib: Nexavar

Lenvatinib: Lenvima

Vandetanib: Caprelsa

Cabozantinib: Cometriq

Teprotumumab: Tepezza

A.3.4 Reproductive Endocrinology Therapies

Clomiphene: Clomid, Serophene

Letrozole: Femara

Spironolactone: Aldactone, CaroSpir

Letrozole: Femara

Gonadotropins: Follistim AQ, Gonal-F, Menopur, Bravelle, Pergoveris

Human Chorionic Gonadotropin (hCG): Pregnyl, Novarel, Ovidrel

Progesterone: Prometrium, Endometrin, Crinone

Leuprolide: Lupron, Lupron Depot, Eligard

Goserelin: Zoladex

Nafarelin: Synarel

Ganirelix: Antagon

Cetrorelix: Cetrotide

Estradiol: Estrace, Climara, Vivelle-Dot, Alora, Divigel, Estring, Estradot, EstroGel

Conjugated Estrogens: Premarin

Estropipate: Ogen

Ethinyl Estradiol + Norethindrone: Loestrin, Microgestin, Junel, Femhrt

Ethinyl Estradiol + Levonorgestrel: Alesse, Aviane, Lessina, Levora, Lutera, Sronyx

Ethinyl Estradiol + Drospirenone: Yasmin, Yaz, Nikki, Loryna

Norethindrone: Camila, Errin, Heather, Jencycla, Ortho Micronor, Nor-QD

Medroxyprogesterone: Depo-Provera, Depo-subQ Provera 104

Etonogestrel: Nexplanon

Levonorgestrel-releasing IUD: Mirena, Skyla, Liletta, Kyleena

Copper IUD: Paragard

Testosterone Gel: AndroGel, Testim, Fortesta, Vogelxo

Testosterone Patch: Androderm

Testosterone Cream: Axiron (applied to underarms)

Testosterone Injections: Depo-Testosterone, Xyosted, Aveed, Testopel (pellets)

Testosterone Buccal System: Striant

Testosterone Nasal Gel: Natesto

Clomiphene: Clomid, Serophene

Anastrozole: Arimidex

Letrozole: Femara

Choriogonadotropin alfa: Ovidrel

Chorionic Gonadotropin: Novarel, Pregnyl

Gonadorelin: Factrel, Lutrepulse

Leuprolide: Lupron, Lupron Depot, Eligard

A.3.5 Obesity and Lipid-Lowering Therapies

Phentermine: Adipex-P, Lomaira

Phendimetrazine: Bontril PDM, Bontril Slow Release

Diethylpropion: Tenuate, Tenuate Dospan

Lorcaserin: Belviq (withdrawn from the market due to safety concerns)

Orlistat: Xenical (prescription strength), Alli (over-the-counter strength)

Phentermine and Topiramate: Qsymia

Bupropion and Naltrexone: Contrave

Liraglutide: Saxenda

Semglutide: Wegovy

Tirzepatide: Mounjaro

Atorvastatin: Lipitor

Simvastatin: Zocor

Lovastatin: Mevacor, Altoprev

Pravastatin: Pravachol

Rosuvastatin: Crestor

Fluvastatin: Lescol, Lescol XL

Pitavastatin: Livalo, Zypitamag

Fenofibrate: Tricor, Antara, Fenoglide, Lipofen, Lofibra, Triglide

Gemfibrozil: Lopid

Cholestyramine: Questran, Questran Light, Prevalite

Colestipol: Colestid

Colesevelam: Welchol

Ezetimibe: Zetia

Icosapent ethyl: Vascepa

Omega-3-acid ethyl esters: Lovaza, Omtryg

Omega-3-carboxylic acids: Epanova

Evolocumab: Repatha

Alirocumab: Praluent

Inclisiran: Leqvio

Index

Note: Page numbers followed by *f* refer to figures and *t* refer to tables.

Endocrinology: Pathophysiology to Therapy, First Edition. Akuffo Quarde.
© 2024 John Wiley & Sons Ltd. Published 2024 by John Wiley & Sons Ltd.